Women's Health in Primary Care

AN INTEGRATED APPROACH

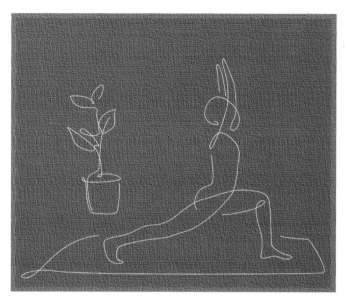

Women's Health in Primary Care

AN INTEGRATED APPROACH

LISA L. FERGUSON, DNP, APRN, WHNP-BC, CNE

*Women's Health Nurse Practitioner, Ocala, Florida; Formerly, Assistant Clinical Professor,
College of Nursing, University of Florida, Gainesville, Florida*

SUSAN M. KENDIG, JD, MSN, RN, WHNP-BC, FAANP

*Attorney/Health Policy Consultant and Principal, Health Policy Advantage, LLC, Ballwin, Missouri;
Teaching Professor, College of Nursing, University of Missouri-St. Louis, St. Louis, Missouri*

SARAH B. FREEMAN, PHD, ARNP, FAANP

Professor Emeritus, Emory University, Atlanta, Georgia

KELLY ELLINGTON, DNP, WHNP-BC, RNC-OB

*Assistant Professor, University of North Carolina Wilmington, Wilmington, North Carolina; Women's
Health Nurse Practitioner, Kamm McKenzie OB/GYN
Raleigh, North Carolina*

ELSEVIER

Elsevier
3251 Riverport Lane
St. Louis, Missouri 63043

Notice

Practitioners and researchers must always rely on their own experience and knowledge in evaluating and using any information, methods, compounds or experiments described herein. Because of rapid advances in the medical sciences, in particular, independent verification of diagnoses and drug dosages should be made. To the fullest extent of the law, no responsibility is assumed by Elsevier, authors, editors or contributors for any injury and/or damage to persons or property as a matter of products liability, negligence or otherwise, or from any use or operation of any methods, products, instructions, or ideas contained in the material herein.

Executive Content Strategist: Lee Henderson
Content Development Manager: Danielle Frazier
Publishing Services Manager: Julie Eddy
Project Manager: Becky Langdon
Design Direction: Brian Salisbury

Printed in India

Last digit is the print number: 9 8 7 6 5 4 3 2 1

Working together to grow libraries in developing countries

www.elsevier.com • www.bookaid.org

Meredith Annon, MSN, CNM, WHNP-BC
Certified Nurse Midwife
Obstetrics & Gynecology
Jefferson Health
Washington Township, New Jersey

Kala K. Blakely, DNP, CRNP, NP-C, CNE, FAANP
Assistant Professor
School of Nursing
University of Alabama at Birmingham
Birmingham, Alabama

Lorraine Byrnes, PhD, APRN, FNP-BC, PMHNP-BC, FAANP
Associate Professor (ret.)
Nursing
Hunter College
New York, New York

Ginny Cassidy-Brinn, MSN, AP
Nurse Practitioner
Reproductive Health
Ravenna Women's Health
Seattle, Washington

Carolyn K. Clevenger, DNP, RN, GNP-BC, AGPCNP-BC, FAANP, FGSA
Associate Dean for Transformative Clinical Practice
Nell Hodgson Woodruff School of Nursing
Emory University
Atlanta, Georgia

Kelly Convery, BSN, RN, IBCLC
Clinical Quality Manager
Keriton LLC
Narberth, Pennsylvania

Diana Drake, DNP, APRN, WHNP-BC, FNAP, FAAN
Clinical Professor ad Honorem
School of Nursing
University of Minnesota;
Adjunct Professor
Earl E. Bakken Center for Spirituality and Healing
University of Minnesota
Minneapolis, Minnesota

Simon Adriane Ellis, MSN, CNM, ARNP, FACNM
Certified Nurse Midwife
Quilted Health
Renton, Washington

Lisa L. Ferguson, DNP, APRN, WHNP-BC, CNE
Women's Health Nurse Practitioner
Ocala, Florida;
Formerly, Assistant Clinical Professor
College of Nursing
University of Florida
Gainesville, Florida

Rachel Fidino, MSN, ARNP, WHNP-BC, AGN-BC, DNP
CEO
Gynecology
New U Women's Clinic & Aesthetics
Kennewick, Washington

Sarah B. Freeman, PhD, ARNP, FAANP
Professor Emeritus
School of Nursing
Emory University
Atlanta, Georgia

Kimberly Gray, MSN, APRN-BC
Nurse Practitioner
Washington University School of Medicine
St. Louis, Missouri

Ayanna Gray-Bolden, CRNP
Nurse Practitioner
Philadelphia, Pennsylvania

Dana Renee Cummings, MSN, BSN, FNP-BC
Nurse Practitioner, Penn Medicine
University of Pennsylvania Health System
Philadelphia, Pennsylvania

Alison Hathaway, MSN, WHNP-BC, ANP-C
Women's Health & Adult Nurse Practitioner
Patient Care
Planned Parenthood
Oakland, California

Ashley L. Hodges, PhD, CRNP, PMHNP-BC, WHNP-BC, FAANP, FAAN
Clinic Director and Nurse Practitioner
UAB School of Nursing Clinic at the WellHouse
Birmingham, Alabama

Susan E. Hoffstetter, PhD, WHNP, FAANP
Professor
Department of Obstetrics, Gynecology, and Women's Health
Saint Louis University School of Medicine
St. Louis, Missouri

Aimee Chism Holland, DNP, WHNP-BC, FNP-C, FAANP, FAAN
Professor
Nursing
University of Alabama at Birmingham
Birmingham, Alabama

Shavondra Huggins, DNP, CNS, WHNP-BC, FNP-C, APRN, CNE
Clinical Assistant Professor
University of Florida
College of Nursing
Gainesville, Florida

Debra Ilchak, DNP, RN, FNP-BC, CNE
Clinical Associate Professor
Edison College of Nursing and Health Innovation
Arizona State University
Phoenix, Arizona

Cori Cunningham Johnson, DNP, CRNP, AGNP-C
Assistant Professor
Acute, Chronic, and Continuing Care
University of Alabama at Birmingham School of Nursing
Birmingham, Alabama

Beth M. Kelsey, EdD, APRN, WHNP-BC, FAANP
Editor in Chief
Women's Healthcare: A Clinical Journal for NPs
National Association of Nurse Practitioners in Women's Health
Washington, DC

Mariya Kovaleva, RN, PhD, MS, AGPCNP-BC
Assistant Professor
College of Nursing
University of Nebraska Medical Center
Omaha, Nebraska

Michele J. LaMarr-Suggs, CNM
Certified Nurse Midwife
Obstetrics and Gynecology
Penn OBGYN and Midwifery Care, Pennsylvania Hospital
Philadelphia, Pennsylvania

Randee Masciola, DNP, APRN-CNP, WHNP-BC, FAANP
Associate Clinical Professor
College of Nursing
The Ohio State University
Columbus, Ohio

Jamille Nagtalon-Ramos, EdD, MSN, WHNP-BC, IBCLC, FAANP
Assistant Professor
School of Nursing
Rutgers University
Camden, New Jersey

Stacy Selbert, APRN, WHNP-BC, MSN
Women's Health Nurse Practitioner
Department of Obstetrics & Gynecology
Washington University School of Medicine
St. Louis, Missouri

Natasha Seth-McCoy, DNP, MSN, FNP, WHNP-BC
Nurse Practitioner
Penn Medicine, University of Pennsylvania Health System
Philadelphia, Pennsylvania

Annelle Taylor, RN, MSN, NP-C, WHNP-BC
Nurse Practitioner
Women's Health and Adult Primary Care Nurse Practitioner
The Bronx Health Collective at Montefiore Medical Center
Bronx, New York

Laura Thiem, DNP, RN, FNP-BC, PMHCNS-BC, PMHNP-BC, CNE
Interim Associate Dean of Academics, Clinical Associate Professor
School of Nursing and Health Studies
University of Missouri–Kansas City
Kansas City, Missouri

Holly B. Buckley, DNP, APRN, WHNP-BC, ANP-BC, NCMP
Nurse Practitioner
Primary Care Consultant
Rebel Health & Wellness, PLLC, Telemedicine
Owner, Provider
Bradford, New Hampshire

Tamika Dowling, DNP, FNP-c
Assistant Professor
United States University
San Diego, California

Kathleen S. Jordan, DNP, RN, FNP-BC, ENP-C, SANE-P, FAEN, FAANP
Clinical Associate Professor
School of Nursing
The University of North Carolina at Charlotte;
Nurse Practitioner
Emergency Department
Mid-Atlantic Emergency Medicine Associates
Charlotte, North Carolina

Yvette Lowery, DNP, MSN/Ed, FNP-c, CCRN, CEN, PCCN
Emergency Nurse Practitioner
North Florida Regional Medical Center
Gainesville, Florida

PREFACE

INTRODUCTION

Primary care clinicians are expected to know a breadth of information to care for their population, whether that population is the family, adults, or children. Having a broad base of knowledge forces the clinician to be more familiar with patient response to more commonly seen disease processes and does not allow for expertise in more specialized care. This completely new textbook for nurse practitioners (NPs), physician assistants (PAs), and other practitioners responsible for primary health care of women provides a strong, evidence-based clinical foundation for primary care of women.

ORGANIZATION

This text is the only primary care women's health book organized by the latest AWHONN/NPWH and national well-woman guidelines. Divided into three sections, the material provides a basis for understanding the uniqueness of female patients beginning with Foundational Concepts in Women's Health. Section II provides guidance on Well-Woman Care Throughout the Life Span, concentrating on care that is distinctive to being female. Section III concludes with Common Conditions Affecting Women. Chapters in Sections II and III are organized to give an overview of the information to follow, discuss a focused history and physical examination, explore differential diagnoses, and provide interventions. Interventions encompass pharmacological, nonpharmacological, patient education, counseling, and interprofessional collaboration/referral.

FEATURES

Women's Health in Primary Care: An Integrated Approach has several unique features not found in other women's health textbooks. This book provides a holistic, woman-centered foundation in women's health for primary care with a full breadth of foundational women's health content. Included in the content are foundational concepts, well-woman care throughout the life span and primary care management of common conditions affecting women.

Quick-reference features for busy clinicians include "Not to Be Missed" boxes that call attention to such "red flags" as signs of human trafficking, breast lumps, low back pain in pregnancy, and the need for HIV counseling/testing. "Patient-Centered Care" boxes demonstrate how to tailor care to patients in special populations or situations, such as LGBTQ patients, those with disabilities, older women, military veterans, racial/ethnic variations, religious/cultural variations, and more. "Safety Alerts" call attention to special precautions to protect patients and ensure their safety.

In this text, we provide a strong emphasis on patient diversity, including LGBTQ issues, global health, and underserved populations. Because primary care of women increasingly requires interprofessional collaboration, interprofessional collaborative practice is a key thread throughout the book. Also featured is a strong emphasis on the emerging trend of clinical integration, encouraging providers to collaborate with other services to coordinate timely and effective patient-focused care. There is a great need to address the various disparities seen in the current healthcare system.

Arming today's providers with the unique features found in this text will help improve clinical efficiency, provide perspective and language to effectively communicate with varied population groups, increase patient safety, and improve health outcomes for the patients we serve.

* * *

We hope that this completely new text meets the needs of a wide range of providers who are responsible for the primary care of women. We welcome your feedback for future editions as you use this book!

ACKNOWLEDGMENTS

First, I'd like to acknowledge Sue Kendig and Sarah Freeman, without whose vision this text would have never come into being. This work was their concept, and as the result of a multitude of challenges, I was asked to bring it to fruition. It is such an honor to be trusted by such accomplished women's health experts to continue their work! Thank you Sue and Sarah for your vote of confidence!

Second, I would like to thank Beck Rist, former Senior Content Development Specialist at Elsevier, who was my hand-holder, cheerleader, and confidant; without her constant support I would not have been able to complete this project. To Lee Henderson, Executive Content Strategist, Nursing Content at Elsevier, your flexibility, support, and encouragement was also instrumental in helping me get this text across the finish line.

To Kelly Ellington, whose guidance in chapter editing was so helpful to get me started on this adventure. Although we only worked together for a short time, you taught me a few invaluable lessons.

To Melanie Cole, without whose expertise in locating appropriate drawings, figures, tables, and other graphic material I would have been so lost. Thank you.

To Peggy Mancuso, PhD, CNM, thank you for my first opportunity to write a textbook chapter with you. None of this would have happened if you hadn't offered me that opportunity. You always believed in me and my abilities, much more than I did.

Finally, to my family who always believes in me, no matter what crazy situation I get myself into. To my husband, Glen, your patience and support mean the world to me. Thank you for encouraging me to fly into new adventures! To Mom, my sounding board, thank you for listening to me complain about things you didn't understand and for just listening. To my sister Diane, thank you for your invaluable advice when I was stuck, when I had writer's block, or when I just needed a kick in the pants! To my sisters and brother, Sharon, Nancy, and Reed, thank you for your unconditional love and support always. You were constantly there to cheer me on in my accomplishments and I love you all. Dad in heaven, thank you for encouraging me to read when I was young and to continue my education. You always believed I could accomplish anything.

Lisa L. Ferguson

This textbook is dedicated to all the nurses and nurse practitioners who sacrifice so much, every day, to ensure that quality, compassionate patient care is delivered to those in need.

CONTENTS

1

A Clinically Integrated Approach to Women's Health Care

Sarah B. Freeman

OBJECTIVES

- Analyze the effect of gender on the health care of women with chronic disease.
- Evaluate the impact of adequate health care for women on the woman, family, and society in general.
- Compare the interaction of biological and sociological factors as they relate to the development and progression of chronic disease in women.

- Integrate knowledge of the effects of reproduction on health into the assessment, evaluation, and treatment of women throughout the life span.
- Evaluate the influence of social determinants of health on the health care of women.

INTRODUCTION

The effect of gender on health care and health care outcomes is multifactorial. When discussing gender and health, it is important to note that it is both psychosocial as well as biological in origin. There is a uniqueness to being female that greatly affects health care. Both the social determinants of health as well as any biological factors must be considered to get a clear picture of gender and health.

NOT TO BE MISSED

Some of the major risk factors for chronic diseases, including physical inactivity, inadequate diet, weight, alcohol use, and smoking, also relate in complex ways to sex, gender, income, and education.

DETERMINANTS OF HEALTH

There is evidence that chronic disease affects women and men differently. Consequently, until recent years, there was an intrinsic gender bias in research. Not only were women not included in some research, but the analysis of the data did not consider sex and gender to be a relevant factor when studying chronic disease. With the use of sex- and gender-based analysis (SGBA), both constructs are now providing valuable insights into the prevention and management of chronic diseases.[1] We are now better able to provide a plan that includes the multiple determinants of health (Fig. 1.1; Box 1.1). Diseases are now being examined in relation to not only sex and gender but also to ethnicity, education, income, and the multiple psychosocial factors that affect health (Table 1.1).[2] Combined with the study of

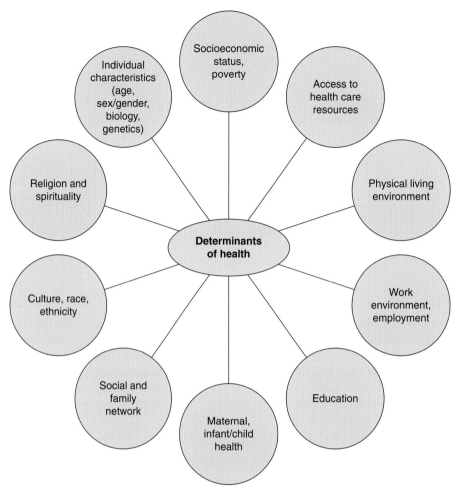

Fig. 1.1 Social determinants of health. (Modified from Johnson C, Green BN. Public health, wellness, prevention, and health promotion: considering the role of chiropractic and determinants of health. *J Manipulative Physiol Ther.* 2009;32[6]:405–412.)

BOX 1.1   Social Determinants of Health Care[2]

Women and men tend to manage their chronic disease differently because of their gender. Chronic disease can affect people differently related to the following:
- Cultural background
- Geographic location
- Economic condition
- Education

---

the biological differences in both the presentation and outcome of a disease, the clinician should be able to better develop a course of treatment appropriate to the individual patient.

There are many differences between men and women across the spectrum of disease. The importance of biology is paramount, but other psychosocial differences are also important. When discussing gender and sex differences in health, one must always consider sex- and gender-specific diseases. Specific diseases of the reproductive tract are gender-specific and can help account for the differences seen in visits to the provider's office. Women seem to seek health care at a greater rate than men. Women also carry the burden of prevention of pregnancy, and the most effective method requires regular visits to a health care provider. The same is true of pregnancy and childbirth. Women have a greater number of health care visits during a lifetime because of their role in the reproductive process.

TABLE 1.1 The Leading Causes of Death in Women and Men (2017)			
Women	%	Men	%
1. Heart disease	21.8	1. Heart disease	24.2
2. Cancer	20.7	2. Cancer	21.9
3. Chronic lower respiratory disease	6.2	3. Unintentional injuries	7.6
4. Stroke	6.2	4. Chronic lower respiratory disease	5.2
5. Alzheimer disease	6.1	5. Stroke	4.3
6. Unintentional injuries	4.4	6. Diabetes	3.2
7. Diabetes	2.7	7. Suicide	2.6
8. Influenza and pneumonia	2.1	8. Alzheimer disease	2.6
9. Kidney disease	1.8	9. Influenza and pneumonia	1.8
10. Septicemia	1.6	10. Chronic liver disease	1.8

This fact makes comparison of the number of office visits difficult and misleading.

Women have lower mortality rates than men and a longer life expectancy. Although they live longer, women tend to be sicker and experience greater morbidity and thus may be overrepresented in health statistics.[3] In addition to overall mortality and morbidity, there is a disparity associated with certain diseases and their occurrence by gender. For example, gender-based diseases that are more common in women include dementia, depression, and rheumatic diseases.[4]

The biomedical interpretation would argue that the variations in health and life span between men and women can be accounted for strictly by their biological differences. This is an oversimplification of a very complex issue. The use of a wider approach that also includes the psychosocial dimensions gives us a more complete look at the effects of gender on health.

PATIENT-CENTERED CARE: An examination of the social determinants of health that negatively affect each woman is key to providing patient-centered care.

One needs to look at gender roles in society as well as gender behavior and the economic conditions of women to give us a complete picture of the relationship of sex and gender to health and well-being. By remembering that biological differences between women and men are just one part of the total picture, we can begin to look more holistically at patients. Only with this holistic approach can we begin to look at programs that will help promote health and improve the outcomes of management for our patients. With a holistic approach, we can gain a much deeper understanding of chronic disease.

BOX 1.2   Needs of Women in the Health Care System

- Related to sexual and reproductive function
- Related to a reproductive system that is vulnerable to dysfunction or disease
- Diseases of other body systems that can affect women. These disease patterns often differ from those of men because of the following:
  - Genetic differences
  - Hormonal differences
  - Gender-related lifestyle behavior
- Social problems that affect physical, mental, or social health
  - Female genital mutilation
  - Sexual abuse and domestic violence

NOT TO BE MISSED

Provision of women's health should be a priority for all providers. Women have unique health care needs and issues that require special attention. Because women are the primary caregivers in many societies, helping women achieve and maintain health will affect the health of the family.

EFFECT OF REPRODUCTION ON WOMEN'S HEALTH

Being a woman has implications for health care. Women experience differences in both receipt of services and health outcomes. Health needs of women are broadly classified under four categories (Box 1.2).[5] Diseases of other body systems as well as their treatments may interact with conditions and functions of the reproductive system.

Before we discuss the outcome of diseases on women, it is important to look at the effect of reproduction on the overall health of women. Both the function and dysfunction of the reproductive system is crucial to the health of women. Women need sexual and reproductive health services from adolescence through menopause.

Many of the causes of both mortality and morbidity are related to reproduction in women 15 to 45 years of age.[5] Although both contraception and pregnancy can be safe, women need health care services to help ensure their safety and a successful outcome. Looking at reproductive health care worldwide, there has been a decrease in both maternal and infant mortality.[6] The greatest disparities are among women who have appropriate access to health care versus those who do not.

There is still a worldwide difference related to the ability to obtain adequate prenatal care. According to the Guttmacher Institute, of the approximately 127 million women who give birth each year in low- to middle-income countries, fewer than 50 million make the minimum[4] of antenatal visits recommended by the World Health Organization (WHO); 31 million are not delivered in a safe health care facility; 16 million do not receive needed care for major obstetric complications; 13 million have newborns that do not receive needed care for health complications; and 1.4 million are living with HIV, with approximately 19% not receiving needed antiretroviral care.[7]

Each year, 100 million women have a pregnancy that ends in miscarriage, stillbirth, or abortion. Of these women, many are not receiving the medical care they need: 2 million do not receive needed care after a miscarriage; 35 million receive abortions in unsafe conditions; and 9 million with complications from unsafe abortions do not receive postabortion care.[7]

Although contraception is both safe and effective, it is not universally available worldwide. In the United States, the most effective methods of contraception are too costly for many women to afford, essentially making them unavailable. An estimated 218 million women worldwide who want to avoid pregnancy are not using the most effective contraceptive method because of issues with access. Because increases in the use of highly effective contraceptive methods have barely kept up with growing populations, this number has essentially not changed since the report was issued in 2008.[7]

If all women attempting to avoid pregnancy used highly effective methods of contraception and all pregnant women and their newborns received care at the standards recommended by the WHO, the safety of both pregnancy and contraception would be greatly improved. Compared with what we see today, we would expect to see the following:

- The burden of disability related to pregnancy and delivery experienced by women and newborns would decrease by two-thirds.
- Unintended pregnancies would decrease by 68% (111 million to 35 million per year).
- Maternal deaths would decrease by 62% (299,000 to 113,000 per year).
- Newborn deaths would decrease by 69% (2.5 million to 755,000 per year)[7]

In keeping with the internationally recognized right to good health, investing in sexual and reproductive health can save lives and reduce health-related problems among women and their children. The immediate health benefits alone are well worth the cost; however, the benefits are even greater when considering the long-term benefits for women, their partners and families, and societies.

It is estimated that fully meeting the need for modern contraceptive services would cost $12.6 billion. When you compare this to the cost of maternal and newborn care, it is clear how cost-effective contraception can be. The estimated cost is as follows:

- $24.9 billion to provide the recommended levels of maternal and newborn health care for women who have a live birth
- $2 billion to provide the recommended care for women whose pregnancies end in miscarriage, stillbirth, or abortion[7]

When the reproductive needs of a woman are met by society, the woman and, by extension, the family is healthier. These types of services affect both the individual and the family and are a large part of the provision of services provided in a women's health care setting (see Box 1.2).

CHRONIC DISEASES

Women develop the same chronic diseases that men do; however, there may be a difference in both presentation and outcome for women based on their determinants of health. The leading causes of death are similar in men and women, with heart disease as the leading cause of

TABLE 1.2	Modifiable Risk Factors for Cardiovascular Disease in Women	
Risk Factor	How It Differs from Men	Modification to Make
Smoking	In women, smoking is a greater risk factor for heart disease than it is in men.[1]	Quit smoking
Overweight and obesity	More women are obese than men (40.4% vs. 35%), and about 9.9% of women are considered to have extreme or morbid obesity.[18]	Lose weight, and try to reach and maintain a normal BMI. Eat a healthy diet that includes whole grains, a variety of fruits and vegetables, low-fat or fat-free dairy products, and lean meats.
Physical activity	Women may be more inactive than men according to some research.	Exercise at least 3 times a week for at least 30 minutes, and try to increase up to 4–6 times per week for 45 minutes or more.
Alcohol	Women absorb and metabolize alcohol differently than men and have higher concentrations of blood alcohol. They become more impaired than men after drinking equivalent amounts of alcohol.[16]	No amount of alcohol is recommended in the Dietary Guidelines for Americans because the potential risks and harms outweigh any benefit.
Stress	Women and men are at risk for different types of stress-related disorders, with women at greater risk for depression and anxiety and men at greater risk for alcohol-use disorders.[19] Both can be related to heart disease.	Develop a program of stress management.
Diabetes	Diabetes increases the risk of heart disease in women more than it does in men.[1]	Maintain good control of diabetes with an A1C of 6.5 or less.
Hypertension	There is a higher prevalence of hypertension in women than in men.[1]	Maintain good control of blood pressure at below 140/90 mm Hg.
Cholesterol/ triglycerides	Men and premenopausal women have important differences in cholesterol. Young women tend to have lower LDL levels than young men, and from puberty on, women tend to have higher HDL levels than men, thus decreasing the risk of heart disease. When estrogen production declines after menopause, HDL levels decrease greatly. After 55 years of age, women tend to have higher LDL and VLDL levels than men. Both changes increase a woman's chances of heart disease after menopause.	Maintain cholesterol and triglycerides at a normal level.

BMI, Body mass index; *LDL,* low-density lipoprotein; *VLDL,* very-low-density lipoprotein.

death in both (Table 1.2).[8,9] Although men and women have similar causes of death, the morbidity is higher in women. Because of the increased morbidly and differences in presentation, it is important to look at some of the most common chronic diseases and how they differ in presentation between men and women.

Heart Disease

Heart disease is the leading killer of both of men and women; 1 in 3 women in the United States dies from heart disease.[10] The WHO definition of cardiovascular disease (CVD) is found in Box 1.3.[9] The older a woman gets, the more at risk she is for developing heart disease; however, women of all ages should know the signs and symptoms and be informed about heart disease. Because women have more morbidity associated with heart disease, it is a major course of disability for the aging woman.

General facts about heart disease in women point to the increased need for the clinician to be aware of the difference in both presentation and outcome. When looking at stroke along with heart disease, the death rate for

BOX 1.3 World Health Organization Definition of Cardiovascular Disease

- Disease of the vessels of the heart: coronary heart disease
- Disease of the vessels supplying the brain: cerebrovascular disease
- Disease of the vessels of the extremities: peripheral arterial disease
- Damage to the heart muscle and valves from streptococcal bacteria: rheumatic heart disease
- Malformation of the heart from birth: congenital heart disease
- Blood clots in the legs: deep vein thrombosis
- Blood clots that dislodge and block the lung: pulmonary embolism

BOX 1.4 Nonmodifiable Risk Factors for Cardiovascular Disease

- Gender
- Age
- Family history (genetics)
- Race

NOT TO BE MISSED

Heart disease affects women of all ages. For younger women, the combination of birth control pills and smoking boosts the risk of heart disease by 20%. Risks increase with age. Obesity and lack of exercise are two of the biggest and modifiable risk factors for women.

All women are at risk for heart disease, though many are unaware of the risk and the signs and symptoms. To provide good care for women across the life span, it is important that the educational deficit related to heart disease be corrected. The modifiable risk for heart disease in women (Box 1.4)[11-14] should be a part of the education of women starting in early adulthood. Because their risk reduction can lead to prevention, it is important that this becomes part of the routine care that women receive. There are also some risks that are nonmodifiable (see Box 1.4). Becoming aware of risks and their uniqueness to women can help protect you.

women is 1 in 3 each year, killing approximately 1 woman every 80 seconds.[10] Other statistics are as follows:

- An estimated 44 million women are affected by CVDs.
- Hispanic women are likely to develop heart disease 10 years earlier than Caucasian women.
- 90% of women have one or more risk factors for heart disease or stroke.
- Women have a higher lifetime risk of stroke than men.
- 80% of heart disease and stroke may be prevented by lifestyle changes and education.
- Fewer women than men survive their first heart attack.[10]

There are also many ethnic differences seen in women with heart disease. Although the leading cause of death for African American women is also heart disease, killing over 50,000 annually, only 36% of them are aware of the risk. African American women also develop heart disease at an earlier age. Of women 20 years of age and older, 49% have some degree of disease present, yet only 58% of African American women are aware of the symptoms of a myocardial infarction.

The leading cause of death for Hispanic women is also heart disease, with nearly 301,000 deaths annually.[11] They are also likely to develop heart disease as much as 10 years earlier than Caucasian women. As with African American women, only a small percentage (34%) are aware of the risk and symptoms. In the United States, Hispanic women are least likely to have a usual source of health/medical care. Only 1 in 3 Hispanic women know that heart disease is their number-one killer.[10]

NOT TO BE MISSED

Important gender differences exist in the symptoms and pathology of heart disease and must be taken into consideration to prevent, diagnose, and treat heart disease in women.

The symptoms of heart attack can be different in women versus men. Although women can experience the same symptoms, research has shown that the presenting symptoms are usually different. Men tend to experience chest pain or discomfort as the primary sign of a heart attack, while the primary symptom for women is shortness of breath. Although chest pain and discomfort are found in a large percent of women (87%), it is usually a combination of not only chest discomfort but also back, neck, and jaw pain or tightness as well as a burning sensation in the chest similar to heartburn.[15]

Women are also more likely to experience prodromal symptoms up to 1 month before a cardiac event.

TABLE 1.3 **Symptoms of a Cardiac Event in Women**[15]			
Prodromal (>1 Month Prior)	**%**	**Acute Symptoms**	**%**
Unusual fatigue	70.7	Shortness of breath	57.9
Sleep disturbance	47.8	Weakness	54.8
Shortness of breath	42	Unusual fatigue	42.9
Indigestion	39.4	Cold sweats	39
Anxiety	36	Nausea	36
Heart racing	27	Arms weak/heavy	35
Arms weak/heavy	25		

In a 2003 survey, 95% of women reported one or more symptoms for at least 1 month before the heart attack. Of the symptoms reported (Table 1.3), fatigue and sleep pattern alteration were rated as severe.[15] The presence of prodromal symptoms creates an opportunity to intervene early and possibly prevent a heart attack. Clinicians must be aware of these symptoms and use them to provide screening and referral when indicated.

Recognizing that women are at risk for heart disease and that the risk factors may affect women differently from men is paramount to providing care. The only clinician that many reproductive age women see is their women's health care practitioner. If we are to provide preventive services, then we must be aware of the risks and their effects on women. CVD may be one of the most preventable diseases that affect women, but it is still the leading cause of death. Women must be made aware of the problem, and routine care should include preventive strategies that help modify risks. It is important to remember the following:

- CVD, including heart attack and stroke, is the leading cause of death in women.
- CVD presents differently in men and women.
- Women develop CVD at a greater rate after menopause, but it can develop earlier.
- Women have several risk factors for CVD, and they affect each woman differently.
- Diabetic women have a greater risk of CVD than diabetic men.
- Smoking presents a greater risk in women than in men.
- Smoking and the use of combined hormonal contraception increases the risk at an earlier age.

> **PATIENT-CENTERED CARE:** Providing information to every woman during each visit with a provider about chronic illness risk factors that are tailored to the patients' ethnicity is paramount to providing patient-centered preventive care.

Diabetes

Diabetes is a major health concern for people all over the world. It is the seventh leading cause of death in the United States and is associated with an increase in CVD, stroke, and dementia. As with other chronic diseases, diabetes has some unique components as related to women (Table 1.4). In the same way as other chronic diseases, the burden in women is greater than in men. Overall diabetes and prediabetes are considered a major health problem as a result of the following factors:

- **Prevalence:** In 2018, 34.2 million people (10.5% of the population) had diabetes, and approximately 32.6 million had type 2 diabetes.
- **Undiagnosed:** Of the 34.2 million adults with diabetes, only 26.8 million were diagnosed, making underdiagnosis a major problem.
- **Prevalence in older adults:** The percentage of people older than 64 years of age is high, at 26.8%, or 14.3 million (diagnosed and undiagnosed).
- **New cases:** 1.5 million new cases are diagnosed every year.
- **Prediabetes:** In 2015, 88 million people older than 18 years of age had prediabetes.
- **Deaths:** Diabetes is the seventh leading cause of death in the United States. In 2017, 83,564 death certificates listed diabetes as the underlying cause of

TABLE 1.4	Diabetes and Women: The Biological Difference[18]	
Condition	Effect	Plan of Care
Cancer	Associated with increased risk of colorectal, liver, and pancreatic cancer. Women are 30% more likely to be diagnosed with breast cancer.	Careful screening is important.
Cardiovascular disease	Diabetes is the greatest risk factor for heart disease in women. Women are at greater risk for developing heart attack and stroke, especially if disease is poorly controlled. In diabetic women, there is a greater risk of heart disease at a younger age compared with nondiabetic women.	Screening and management of risk factors for cardiovascular disease is important.
Depression	Twice as high as in men with diabetes	Screen and treat.
Osteoporosis	Type 1: reduced bone mass and fragility Type 2: also more at risk for low trauma fracture, especially hip	Screen at an earlier age, and evaluate fall risk.

death, and 270,702 death certificates listed diabetes as an underlying or contributing cause of death.[16]

The cost of care for persons with diabetes is also a problem. The average medical cost among people with diagnosed diabetes was 2.3 times higher than for those without diabetes. In the United States in 2017, the total cost of diagnosed diabetes was $327 billion, with $237 billion for direct medical costs and $90 billion in decreased productivity at work.[16]

When looking at the gender differences between men and women, one of the first things noted is the difference in mortality. Between 1971 and 2000, the death rate for men decreased, but the rate for women did not change. The effects of type 1 diabetes on mortality in women were reported to be 37% greater in than in men, and the effects of type 2 diabetes were 13% higher in women, making both the mortality and morbidity burden greater in women.[17] This is thought to be due to the increased rate of heart disease that is seen with women with diabetes. Whereas the risk of heart disease in men with diabetes is increased two- to threefold, the risk for women is increased sixfold.

NOT TO BE MISSED

Data has shown that women with diabetes are more likely than men with the disease to have the following:
- Poor blood glucose control
- Obesity
- High blood pressure
- Abnormal cholesterol levels
- Kidney disease

These differences can be related to both biology and gender disparity. The effect on cholesterol levels appears to be even more problematic. HDL cholesterol, which is normally higher in women than in men, may be a part of the biological disparity. When women develop diabetes, the high triglycerides drive down HDL levels. The combination of high triglycerides and low HDL leads to a greater risk of heart disease.

Another biological condition that affects women and leads to an increased risk for diabetes is polycystic ovarian syndrome (PCOS). The hormonal condition of anovulation and increased androgen production is associated with insulin resistance and type 2 diabetes. Women with PCOS should be identified and managed to help prevent the development of diabetes.

Sociologically, there is evidence that women with diabetes may receive less effective health care. One problem perhaps is perception. Again, this relates to the relationship of diabetes to CVD. Because CVD is less prevalent in premenopausal women, the clinician may not be concerned about the disease in the reproductive middle-age woman. However, women with diabetes are not less likely to have CVD, and clinicians must be aware of this fact and realize that the diabetic woman needs aggressive screening and aggressive management of any risk factors identified.[17] Other sociological factors may also contribute to the increased risk experienced by women with diabetes. Complicating factors for diabetes in women relate to the following:
- Women experience poverty. By 65 years of age, women are twice as likely as men to fall below the poverty level.

- Women receive lower pay, receive fewer benefits, and face significant challenges to balance job and family responsibilities.
- Women are uninsured and/or lack access to health care. Approximately 1 in 7 women lack health insurance. There is also a lack of access to adequate health care for women in rural areas, notably women of childbearing age and older adults.[18,16]

Because it can affect both the course and outcome of pregnancy, diabetes provides some unique challenges for clinicians working with women. Gestational diabetes is associated with both immediate and long-term implications for women. Diabetes is also associated with fetal problems. Spontaneous abortion and birth defects are higher in pregnancies affected by diabetes. Women with gestational diabetes have a recurrence rate of 25% to 45% for subsequent pregnancies. They are also at risk for development of nongestational diabetes. The rate of development is from 17% to 63% during the 5 to 16 years following the pregnancy. Gestational diabetes occurs in 16.6% of all pregnancies that result in a live birth.[19]

The relationship between diabetes and gender is complex. Many of the risk factors for diabetes such as weight gain and lack of physical activity along with gender bias in the health care system have made diabetes a women's issue. Diabetes is a disease in which the interaction of the biological, behavioral, and social factors affect the progression of the disease in women. To promote the health of women, all of these factors must be considered when managing the woman with diabetes.

Arthritis and Rheumatic Arthritis

Arthritis is defined as inflammation of one or more joints. Arthritis also affects the surrounding tissues and other connective tissues. Although the term *arthritis* includes more than 100 different diseases, the two most common forms of arthritis are osteoarthritis (OA), a degenerative joint disease, and rheumatoid arthritis (RA), a systemic autoimmune disease. OA affects more than 27 million people, and RA affects over 1.5 million people. Although OA and RA are distinctly different, they share several things in common, with both occurring more frequently in women than in men; 25.9% of women have arthritis compared with only 18.3% of men.

Arthritis is the leading cause of disability in the United States.[20] Arthritis affects about 1 in 4 adults. In the United States, 54.4 million adults (22.7% of all adults) had clinician-diagnosed arthritis, and 23.7 million (9.8%) had

TABLE 1.5   Prevalence of Arthritis and Rheumatic Disorders by Gender

Disease	Ratio (Female-to Male)
Sjögren syndrome	9:1
Systemic lupus erythematosus	10:1
Rheumatoid arthritis	3:1
Systemic sclerosis	3:1
Scleroderma	3:1
Osteoarthritis	2:1

arthritis-attributable activity limitation. About 43.5% of people with arthritis had activity limitations.[21]

Rheumatic diseases, arthritis, and other diseases of the muscles, joints, and bones are common and affect the health and well-being of nearly 50 million people in the United States. The most severe of these inflammatory diseases can cause joint and organ destruction, leading to severe pain and disability. They affect quality of life and can be a life-changing event. Rheumatic diseases may be caused by an immune system problem as demonstrated by RA. Although rheumatic diseases can affect anyone, women are more likely to be affected than men. These disorders affect 5% of men and 8.4% of women, thus making them a problem for the clinician working in women's health.[22]

NOT TO BE MISSED

Facts About Rheumatic Disorders in Women

- Of the 1.3 million people living with RA, 75% are female.
- Women are two to three times more likely to develop RA and 10 times more likely to develop lupus than men.
- RA often strikes between 35 and 50 years of age, while lupus often develops between 15 and 44 years of age.

Table 1.5 compares the most common rheumatic diseases as well as OA by gender and shows that the rate for women is generally higher than the rate for men.[23]

The increased risk of these diseases seems to be related to both hormones and bony structure in the woman. Women have less muscle mass to support the bony structure, which can lead to increased stress on joint structure. Studies have shown an increased rate of cartilage destruction compared with men, especially in OA of the knee.[24]

Hormones may also play a part in the disparity of disease in women. Estrogen and prolactin are both pro-inflammatory hormones that may, in part, explain the high female-to-male ratio when looking at rheumatic disorders.[25] The longer the lifetime period of menstruation, the greater the lifetime exposure to estrogen. An early age of menarche has been associated with doubling the risk of systemic lupus erythematosus (SLE). This increase has also been found for the risk of RA. Very irregular menses associated with anovulatory cycles and increased estrogen levels were also found to be associated with an increased risk of RA.[25]

As with other chronic diseases, both OA and rheumatic disorders are more frequent and can be more problematic in women. Clinicians must be aware of gender differences to provide adequate care for women. Preventing disease-related disability and helping women maintain a good quality of life depends on helping them cope with these diseases. The simple treatment goals are to control pain and improve joint function. This can be done by helping women achieve a healthy lifestyle.

▌KEY POINTS

- Gender and health care is a complex issue that must be addressed daily when providing care for women.
- The burden of chronic disease is different in men than in women. Clinicians must be aware of these differences and approach patient care with these in mind.
- It is important to remember that the disparity we see in the health care of women is related to the interaction of biology, sociology, and the environment in which we live.
- It is important to consider all aspects of a woman's life to provide an environment that helps her maximize her health regardless of the diagnosis.
- Childbearing increases morbidity and mortality for women and increases the risk of chronic health problems.
- When society meets the reproductive needs of a woman, the woman and by extension the family is healthier.

REFERENCES

1. Gender Imbalance in Health Research Policy Brief #5, The ENGENDER Project. October 2011. https://euro-health.ie/wp-content/uploads/2012/02/PB5-Draft.pdf.
2. Matthews D. Sociology in nursing 3: how gender influences health inequalities. *Nursing Times*. 2015;111(43):21–23.
3. Broom D. Gender and health. In: Germov J, ed. *Second Opinion: An Introduction to Health Sociology*. Melbourne: Oxford University Press.
4. Annandale E. *The Sociology of Health and Medicine: A Critical Introduction*. Cambridge: Polity Press 2012; 2014.
5. Fathalla MF. Issues in reproductive health. http://www.un.org/womenwatch/daw/csw/issues.htm.
6. United Nations, Department of Economic and Social Affairs, Population Division. *World Mortality*; 2019. *Highlights*. https://www.un.org/en/development/desa/population/publications/pdf/mortality/WMR2019/WMR2019_Highlights.pdf.
7. Sully, E, et al. Adding It Up: Investing in Sexual and Reproductive Health 2019. https://www.guttmacher.org/report/adding-it-up-investing-in-sexual-reproductive-health-2019.
8. Centers for Disease Control and Prevention. (n.d.). Health, United States, 2019—Data finder, Table 6. Leading causes of death and numbers of deaths, by sex, race, and Hispanic origin: United States, 1980 and 2018. https://www.cdc.gov/nchs/data/hus/2019/006-508.pdf.
9. Women and cardiovascular disease. *Policy Brief*. European Institute of Women's Health. https://eurohealth.ie/women-and-cardiovascular-disease/.
10. American Heart Association. *Go Red for Women. About women and heart disease*. https://www.goredforwomen.org/en/about-heart-disease-in-women.
11. Lichtman JH, et al. Sex differences in the presentation and perception of symptoms among young patients with myocardial infarction. *Circulation*. 2018;137:781–790.
12. U.S. Department of Health and Human National Institute of Diabetes and Digestive and Kidney Disease. https://www.niddk.nih.gov/health-information/health-statistics/overweight-obesity#prevalence.
13. National Institute on Alcohol Abuse and Alcoholism. *National Institute on Alcohol Abuse and Alcoholism: Women and alcohol*. 2021. https://www.niaaa.nih.gov/publications/brochures-and-fact-sheets/women-and-alcohol.
14. Chaplin TM, et al. Gender difference in response to emotional stress: An assessment across subjective, behavioral, and physiological domains related to alcohol craving. *Alcohol Clin Exp Res*. 2008;32(7):1242–1250.
15. McSweeney JC, et al. Women's early warning symptoms of acute myocardial infarction. *Circulation*. 2003;108(21):2619–2623.
16. The American Diabetes Association. Statistics about Diabetes. http://www.diabetes.org/diabetes-basics/statistics/.
17. Xu G, You D, Wong L, et al. Risk of all-cause and CHD mortality in women versus men with type 2 diabetes: A

systematic review and meta-analysis. *Eur J Endocrinol.* 2019;180(4):243–255.

18. Sex and Gender in Diabetes. Policy Brief. European Gender Medicine; 2015.

19. International Diabetes Federation. (n.d.). Gestational diabetes. https://www.idf.org/our-activities/care-prevention/gdm.

20. Hardin J, Crow MK, Diamond B. Get the facts: Women and arthritis. Arthritis Foundation. http://www.arthritis.org/New-York/-Files/Documents/Spotlight-on-Research/Get-the-Facts-Women-and-Arthritis.pdf.

21. Arthritis Foundation. *Arthritis By the Numbers/Book of Trusted Facts & Figures*; 2019:v3.

22. Marder W, Vinet É, Somers EC. Rheumatic autoimmune diseases in women and midlife health. *Women's Midlife Health.* 2015;1:11.

23. van Vollenhoven RF. Sex differences in rheumatoid arthritis: more than meets the eye. *BMC Med.* 2009;7:12.

24. Price MD, Herndon JH. Gender differences in osteoarthritis. *Menopause.* 2009;16(4):624–625.

25. Oliver JE, Silman JA. Why are women predisposed to autoimmune rheumatic diseases? *Arthritis Res Ther.* 2009;11(5):252.

2

Female Reproductive Anatomy and Physiology

Beth M. Kelsey

OBJECTIVES

- Differentiate normal and abnormal assessment findings related to female reproductive anatomy.
- Apply knowledge of female reproductive physiology in diagnostic reasoning and management decisions.

- Educate adolescent and adult females about normal changes that occur from puberty through menopause.
- Educate adolescent and adult females about their own anatomy and physiology to empower their reproductive and health care decisions through the life span.

INTRODUCTION

This chapter provides a review of the female reproductive anatomy and physiology from puberty through menopause. The focus is on normal anatomy and physiology. It is recognized that not all individuals who were born with female reproductive anatomy and that experience the reproductive physiological events described in this chapter identify as female. Information is inclusive of all individuals who have these anatomical and physiological characteristics. Use of the terms *female, girl,* and *woman* in this chapter is not intended to exclude people with these characteristics who do not identify as female.

The nurse practitioner providing care for adolescent girls and adult women must be knowledgeable about the female reproductive anatomy to discern normal findings, variations of normal, and abnormal findings during a physical examination. Additionally, the nurse practitioner should be able to provide adolescent girls and adult women with information about their bodies to include parts of their anatomy not often discussed. This anatomy should not be a mystery to females as they move from puberty to reproductive age to menopause and beyond. It is an important part of practice to educate patients regarding their body and its function.

Just as it is important for the nurse practitioner providing health care for adolescent girls and adult women to be knowledgeable about female reproductive anatomy, it is also crucial to have a solid understanding of the basics of the female reproductive physiology. During routine well visits, this knowledge allows the nurse practitioner to educate and support patients as they go through the normal changes that occur from puberty through menopause. Reproductive health care includes attention to contraception and conception mediated by female hormones. The health care of patients with conditions related to alterations in female hormone production such as menstrual disorders, infertility, hyperandrogenic disorders, some breast conditions, and some sexual dysfunction requires the ability to apply diagnostic reasoning and make management decisions based on knowledge of female reproductive physiology.

FEMALE REPRODUCTIVE ANATOMY

The female reproductive anatomy includes the internal genitalia (the uterus, fallopian tubes, ovaries, and vagina) and the external genitalia (the mons pubis, labia majora, labia minora, clitoris, vaginal orifice and hymen, and the openings of the paraurethral (Skene) glands and greater vestibular (Bartholin) glands. This section focuses on a description of the genitalia and also includes the breast as it is usually considered part of the female reproductive anatomy. Knowledge of female reproductive anatomy should go beyond the internal and external genitalia. The nurse practitioner should understand the structure of the pelvic bones and joints and the location and function of the ligaments and muscles that support the genitalia. Therefore this review of female reproductive anatomy also provides a discussion of the supporting structures including bones, muscles, and joints. Ligaments are described as associated with specific organs and structures making up the internal genitalia.

Pelvic Bones and Joints

The skeletal component of the pelvis includes two innominate or hip bones, the sacrum, and the coccyx, which form a pelvic girdle surrounding the pelvic cavity. This cavity contains the reproductive organs and the rectum. The hip bones consist of the ilium, ischium, and pubis that fuse after puberty. The ilium is the uppermost and largest portion of the hip bone. The edge of the ilium forms the iliac crest and the body of each of the ilium joints with the sacrum at the sacroiliac joint. The ischium forms the lower portion of the

hip bone below the ilium and behind the pubis. The ischium has three parts: the body, superior ramus, and posterior ramus. The body of each ischium contains an ischial spine with a notch above it (greater sciatic notch) and below it (lesser sciatic notch). The ischial spines are of clinical importance, as they provide landmarks for assessing fetal descent during childbirth as well as for administration of a pudendal nerve block for analgesia of the vaginal introitus and perineum. The superior ramus projects downward and backward from the body of the ischium. Its posterior end forms the ischial tuberosity. Its anterior end joins with the inferior ramus. The inferior ramus is the thin, flat part of the ischium that joins with the pubic bone. The pubis or pubic bone is the most anterior portion of the hip bone. The pubic bones join at the symphysis pubis. The pubic arch is formed by the convergence of the ischium and pubis below and on either side of the symphysis pubis.[1,2]

The sacrum is a large, triangular bone formed by fusing of five sacral vertebrae in early adulthood. The upper part of the sacrum connects with the last lumbar vertebra, and the lower part connects with the coccyx. The broadest, uppermost part of the sacrum tilts forward as the sacral promontory, forming the posterior margin of the pelvic inlet. The coccyx is formed by fusion of three to four rudimentary vertebrae (Fig. 2.1).[1,2]

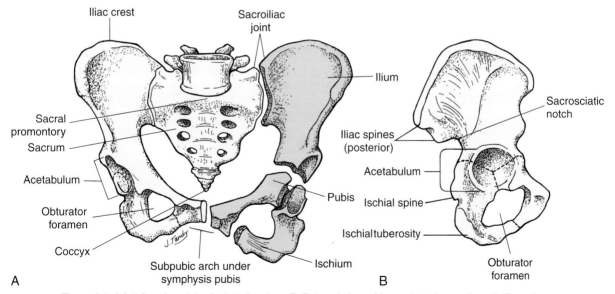

Figure 2.1 Adult female pelvis. **A,** Anterior view. **B,** External view of innominate bones (fused). (From Lowdermilk DL, Perry SE, Cashion K, Alden KR, Olshansky EF. *Maternity & Women's Health Care.* 12th ed. St. Louis: Elsevier; 2020: Figure 4.4.)

The pelvis is described as being divided into what are called a *false (greater) pelvis* and a *true (lesser) pelvis*. The false pelvis is the upper portion above the iliac spines with its boundaries consisting of the iliac fossa on each side, the lumbar vertebrae posteriorly, and the abdominal wall anteriorly. The true pelvis contains the pelvic organs and is the curved bony passageway through which the fetus passes during vaginal birth. The boundaries of the true pelvis are the ischium on either side, the sacrum and coccyx posteriorly, and the pubis anteriorly (Fig. 2.2).[1-3] During pregnancy, the relative dimensions of the true pelvis are estimated with examination techniques referred to as *clinical pelvimetry.*

The four pelvic joints include two sacroiliac joints, the sacrococcygeal joint, and the symphysis pubis. These joints usually have very little mobility. During pregnancy, under the influence of increased levels of the hormones relaxin and progesterone, these joints soften and become more elastic, allowing for enlargement of pelvic dimensions to facilitate labor and birth. The relaxation and increased mobility varies and may result in some discomfort with walking and contribute to the "waddle" of pregnancy.[1-3]

Pelvic Muscles

The muscles supporting the contents of the pelvis include those that make up the pelvic diaphragm and two triangular groups of muscles referred to as the *perineal body.* The pelvic diaphragm consists of the levator ani and the coccygeus muscles. The paired levator ani muscles originate from the pubic bones, extend and fuse together posteriorly at the coccyx, and span the opening within the bony pelvis. The three components of the levator ani muscles, the pubococcygeus muscle, puborectalis muscle, and iliococcygeus muscle, form the greater part of the pelvic diaphragm. The pubococcygeus muscle forms the bulky medial section encompassing a narrow hiatus through which the terminal portions of the urethra, vagina, and rectum pass.[2,4,5]

The pubococcygeus muscle in its normal resting tone squeezes the urethra, vagina, and rectum closed by compressing them against the pubic bone. The puborectalis muscle originates on each side of the pubococcygeus muscle forming a sling behind the rectum. The iliococcygeus muscle arises from the lateral pelvic walls forming a shelf for the pelvic organs. The coccygeus muscle is located posterior to the levator ani extending from the ischial spines and attaching to the lateral margins of the sacrum and coccyx.[2,4,5]

The bladder, urethra, vagina, uterus, and rectum are all supported within the pelvis by the levator ani muscles. Impairment of the levator ani muscles contributes to pelvic organ prolapse as well as urinary and fecal incontinence.[6,7] An assessment of levator ani muscle tone or more specifically pubococcygeus muscle tone can be conducted during a digital vaginal examination. Pelvic floor muscle therapy that includes exercises to squeeze and hold the levator ani muscles in a state of contraction may be a component of treatment for pelvic organ prolapse and stress urinary incontinence.[7]

Below the pelvic diaphragm is the perineal body made up of an anterior urogenital triangle, also called the *urogenital diaphragm,* spanning the pelvic outlet and a posterior anal triangle. The anterior urogenital triangle includes the ischiocavernosus muscles running along either side of the pelvic outlet and bulbocavernosus muscles extending from the glans of the clitoris under the labia minora and connecting at the perineum. The urogenital muscles support the pelvic contents, allow for voluntary contraction and relaxation of the vagina, and contribute to bladder control. The deep transverse

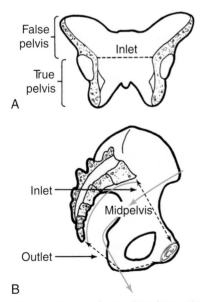

Figure 2.2 Female pelvis. A, Cavity of the false pelvis. B, Cavity of the true pelvis. (From Lowdermilk DL, Perry SE, Cashion K, Alden KR, Olshansky EF. *Maternity & Women's Health Care.* 12th ed. St. Louis: Elsevier; 2020: Figure 4.5.)

perineal muscle forms the base and separates the urogenital and anal triangles. The anal triangle is the posterior part of the perineal body and contains the external anal sphincter muscle (Fig. 2.3).[2,4-6]

Internal Genitalia

The internal female genitalia include the uterus, ovaries and fallopian tubes (adnexa), and the vagina. These structures are evaluated during a pelvic examination, thus it is important for the nurse practitioner to know the normal parameters and normal variations. As well, knowledge of internal female genitalia anatomy provides a basis for understanding the function of these structures. Figures 2.4 and 2.5 provide illustrations of the internal female genitalia.

Uterus

The uterus is a pear-shaped, muscular organ divided anatomically into the corpus and the cervix. The corpus extends upward from the cervix behind the symphysis pubis between the bladder and the rectum. It consists of a convex upper segment referred to as the *fundus* that extends above the points of insertion of the fallopian tubes, a main portion or body, and a lower segment or narrowed isthmus that is adjacent to the cervix. In a person who has never been pregnant, the corpus is approximately 8 cm long, 5 cm wide, and 2.5 cm thick.[6] The corpus contains a cavity or potential space that can accommodate a pregnancy. After childbirth, the corpus may remain slightly larger by about 1 to 1.5 cm in each of the dimensions.[6]

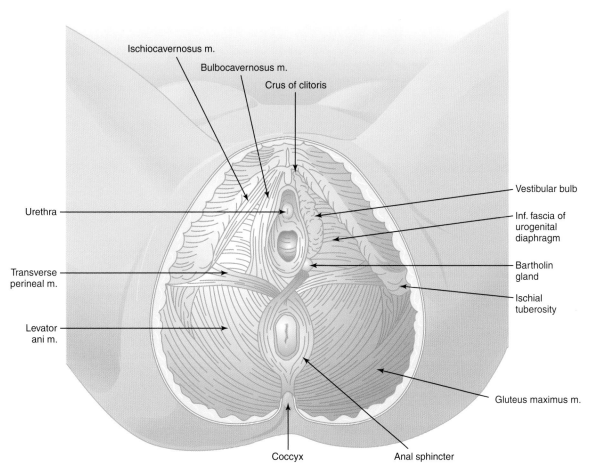

Figure 2.3 The perineum, showing superficial structures *(left)* and deeper structures *(right)*. (From Lowdermilk DL, Perry SE, Cashion K, Alden KR, Olshansky EF. *Maternity & Women's Health Care*. 12th ed. St. Louis: Elsevier; 2020: Figure 3.2.)

The external portion of the corpus is the myometrium, which is composed of thick, smooth muscles. The internal portion is the endometrium or uterine lining. It is a highly vascular mucous membrane composed of columnar epithelium. The endometrium has three layers. The superficial compact layer and spongy middle layer are functional layers responsive to ovarian hormones.[6] Between puberty and menopause, these functional layers proliferate and slough with each menstrual cycle. The basal layer of the endometrium is attached to the myometrium. This layer regenerates the functional layers after each slough (menstruation).

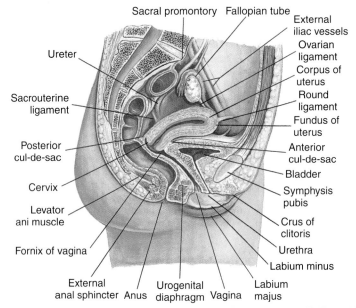

Figure 2.4 Midsagittal view of the female pelvic organs. (From Ball JW, Dains JE, Flynn JA, Solomon BS, Stewart RW. *Seidel's Guide to Physical Examination: An Interprofessional Approach*. St. Louis: Elsevier; 2019: Figure 19.3.)

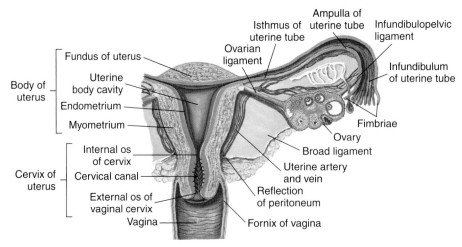

Figure 2.5 Cross-sectional view of internal female genitalia and pelvic contents. (From Ball JW, Dains JE, Flynn JA, Solomon BS, Stewart RW. *Seidel's Guide to Physical Examination: An Interprofessional Approach*. 9th ed. St. Louis: Elsevier; 2019: Figure 19.4.)

The parietal peritoneum is an outer serous membrane that covers most of the uterus, except for the cervix and a portion of the anterior corpus. The parietal peritoneum extends downward behind the uterus into a cul-de-sac called the *rectouterine pouch* (Pouch of Douglas) that separates the uterus from the large intestines.[6] You can just reach this area on rectovaginal examination. In a patient who has endometriosis, you may palpate nodularity in the rectouterine pouch.

The cervix, composed mostly of fibrous connective tissue, is a round, firm terminus to the uterus that extends from the uterine isthmus and protrudes into the vagina. The normal consistency of the cervix in a nonpregnant individual is sometimes described as feeling like the tip of the nose. The diameter of the cervix varies from about 2 to 3 cm depending on parity. The length of the cervix is approximately 2 to 3 cm.[6] Shiny, pink, squamous epithelium covers the cervical body or *ectocervix*. This surface of the cervix is generally smooth, although single or multiple translucent nodules called *nabothian cysts* may be present and are of no pathologic significance. The external os visible at the center of the ectocervix is small and round or oval in a nulliparous individual. It is larger in the parous individual and may appear slitlike or stellate after vaginal births.[3,8]

The endocervix is the canal between the external os of the cervix proximal to the vagina and the internal os proximal to the uterine cavity. The endocervix is lined with plushy, red columnar epithelium. The secretory cells of the endocervix produce mucus that varies in amount and consistency in response to ovarian hormones during the menstrual cycle.

The squamocolumnar (SC) junction is the area of the cervix where the squamous epithelium and the columnar epithelium meet. Before puberty, the SC junction is located on the outer surface of the cervix. During puberty, the SC junction may be visible as a broad band of columnar epithelium encircling the external os called the *ectropion*. After puberty, under the influence of estrogen, the SC junction begins to recede back toward the external os.[3,8]

The transformation zone is the area around the SC junction where squamous metaplasia occurs. Squamous metaplasia is the process whereby columnar cells of the endocervix are replaced by mature squamous epithelium. The SC junction is the most frequent site of changes associated with the development of cervical dysplasia.[3,8]

NOT TO BE MISSED

Cells from both the SC junction and the ectocervix should be obtained for a Pap test to screen for cervical cancer.

The uterus is supported by several ligaments that allow for its mobility within the pelvis and accommodate its increase in size during pregnancy. The cardinal ligaments connected to the lateral margins of the uterus are a portion of the broad ligament and contain uterine blood vessels and ureters. The round ligaments originate on either side of the uterine fundus and pass through the inguinal canals to attach to the labia majora.[2] During pregnancy, the round ligaments stretch as the uterus grows. It is speculated that sudden movements pulling on an already stretched round ligament cause the occasional sharp pain in the groin area experienced by pregnant individuals.[1] The anterior ligament extends from the anterior cervix to the bladder. The posterior ligament extends from the posterior cervix to the rectum. Uterosacral ligaments extend from the lateral portions of the cervix over the rectum to the sacral vertebrae holding the cervix in place.[2]

The position of the uterus within the pelvis is described in terms of the direction in which the corpus is inclined or tilted and the flexion between the corpus and cervix (Fig. 2.6). The most common position is anteverted in which the corpus is tilted toward the bladder. The term *anteflexed* is used when the anterior surface of the anteverted corpus bends toward the cervix. Other normal variations include *retroverted* with the corpus tilted toward the rectum, *retroflexed* when the posterior surface of the retroverted corpus bends toward the cervix, and *midposition*. Although these are all normal variations, there is some clinical significance. A retroverted or retroflexed uterus that is fixed in position may be an examination finding when there are pelvic adhesions caused by endometriosis or chronic pelvic inflammation. Unrecognized anteflexion or retroflexion can increase the risk for uterine perforation during intrauterine contraception placement.[6]

! SAFETY ALERT

Reduce the risk for uterine perforation by carefully determining the position of the uterus before intrauterine contraception placement.

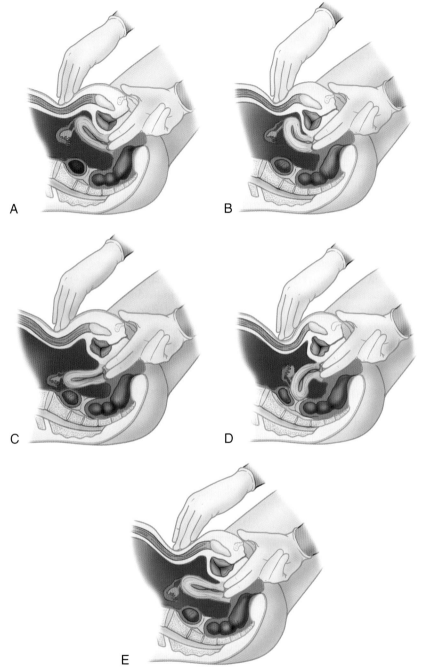

Figure 2.6 Varying positions of uteri. **A,** Anteverted. **B,** Anteflexed. **C,** Retroverted. **D,** Retroflexed. **E,** Midpo-sition of the uterus. (From Ball JW, Dains JE, Flynn JA, Solomon BS, Stewart RW. *Seidel's Guide to Physical Examination: An Interprofessional Approach.* St. Louis: Elsevier; 2019: Figure 19.27.)

Adnexa

The term *adnexa* refers to the fallopian tubes, ovaries, and supporting ligaments. The fallopian tubes, also referred to as *oviducts,* attach to the uterine fundus and curve around each ovary, providing a passage for the ovum into the uterus. The length of these tubes ranges from 10 to 14 cm, and the diameter is less than 1 cm, except at the fimbriated ends, which flare out like a funnel.[6] The interstitial portion of the fallopian tube is the narrowest part passing through the myometrium and opening into the uterine cavity. The isthmus is the main body, and the ampulla is the portion adjacent to the ovary. Ova are usually fertilized by sperm in the ampulla portion of the tubes. The infundibulum is the most distal portion. It is funnel shaped and covered with fimbriae that guide the ovum into the ampulla of the tube by creating a wavelike motion. Cilia that line the tubes continue the wavelike motion and along with peristaltic activity of the muscles of the tubes transport the ovum through the tubes to the uterus. The fallopian tubes are not normally palpable on bimanual pelvic examination.

The ovaries are endocrine organs with the major functions of production of ova and secretion of steroid hormones, estrogen, progesterone, and androgens. They are located below and behind the fimbriated ends of the fallopian tubes. The ovaries are smooth, almond shaped, and approximately 3 cm by 2 cm by 2 cm in the reproductive-age person.[6] They may or may not be palpable on a bimanual pelvic examination depending on the amount of abdominal adipose tissue and the degree to which the patient is able to relax the abdominal muscles.

NOT TO BE MISSED

The ovaries atrophy after menopause and should not be palpable.

The external surface of each ovary is covered with a thin epithelium. Underneath the epithelium is the ovarian stroma, a connective tissue framework. The stroma is divided into a central part called the *medulla* and an outer part called the *cortex*. The medulla contains blood vessels, lymphatic vessels, and nerves that enter at the hilum. The *hilum* is the point of ovarian attachment to the mesovarium, a peritoneal fold on the posterior surface of the broad ligament.[5]

The cortex of the ovary is a dynamic structure containing the follicles and ova at various stages of development. At birth, the cortex of each ovary contains approximately 1 to 2 million potential ova within immature ovarian follicles.[5,6] By puberty, the number is reduced significantly through the process of atresia, and only about 300,000 potential ova remain.[6] Ovarian

follicles grow and undergo atresia continuously throughout the reproductive years.

Vagina

The vagina is an elastic, fibromuscular canal that connects the external genitalia to the uterus. It lies between the urethra and part of the bladder and rectum. The length of the vagina is approximately 6 to 9 cm anteriorly and 8 to 12 cm posteriorly.[5] The upper part of the vagina surrounds the cervix, creating recessed spaces called *fornices* (anterior, posterior, and lateral). The posterior fornix is usually deeper than the anterior fornix because of the angle of the cervix which is most often about 90 degrees. The rectouterine pouch separates the posterior fornix and the rectum. The fornices are of clinical importance because the internal pelvic organs can be palpated through their thin walls. To examine the adnexal area and ovaries, the nurse practitioner inserts internal examining fingers into the lateral fornix, pressing inward and upward, and presses the corresponding external examining fingers deeply inward on the abdomen to meet the internal examining fingers with a sweeping movement toward the symphysis pubis.

The vagina has three layers. The innermost layer consists of a reddish, pink mucous membrane composed of nonkeratinized squamous epithelial cells that is continuous with the epithelial membrane of the ectocervix. This epithelial layer thickens under the influence of estrogen, forming transverse folds called *rugae* that allow for distention during coitus and childbirth. After menopause, the epithelium becomes thinner, and the mucous membrane has a pale and smooth appearance.

Underlying the mucous membrane of this inner vaginal layer is connective tissue called the *lamina propria*. The lamina propria contains elastic fibers and capillaries that provide a rich vascular bed and allow for transudation of fluid across the mucous membrane. During sexual arousal, the lamina propria becomes engorged with blood, pushing more fluid to the surface of the mucous membrane and providing vaginal lubrication.[6] The mucous membrane does not itself contain any mucus-secreting glands. However, secretions from the endocervical glands do drain into the vagina. A constant natural sloughing of dead epithelial cells along with the secretions within the vagina cause the normal thin, clear or white vaginal discharge.

Smooth muscle with both circular and longitudinal fibers forms the middle layer of the vagina. The outer layer of the vagina, called the *adventitia,* is composed of dense connective tissue that blends with looser connective tissue containing blood and lymphatic vessels as well as nerve fibers.

> **CLINICAL SURVIVAL TIP:** To examine the adnexal area and ovaries, the nurse practitioner inserts internal examining fingers into the lateral fornix, pressing inward and upward, and presses the corresponding external examining fingers deeply inward on the abdomen to meet the internal examining fingers with a sweeping movement toward the symphysis pubis.

External Genitalia

Structures comprising the external genitalia include the mons pubis, labia majora, labia minora, clitoris, vaginal orifice and hymen, and the openings of the paraurethral (Skene) glands and greater vestibular (Bartholin) glands. Typically, the urethral orifice is also included in descriptions of the external genitalia. Collectively, these structures are referred to as the *vulva.* The vulva is bordered by the symphysis pubis anteriorly, the buttocks posteriorly, and the thighs laterally (Fig. 2.7). The mons pubis is the rounded pad of subcutaneous fatty tissue that overlies the symphysis pubis. In adult females, it

is covered by course pubic hair in an inverted triangle pattern. The labia majora are the two longitudinal folds of adipose and connective tissue that extend from the mons pubis downward to the perineum enclosing the other external genital structures. The pigmented skin of the labia majora is partially covered with pubic hair and contains both sweat and sebaceous glands. The labia minora are thin folds of squamous epithelial tissue that lie inside and parallel to the labia majora. The color, size, and shape of the labia minora is variable. The skin of the labia minora contains sebaceous glands and a rich blood and nerve supply but is without hair follicles or sweat glands. The folds of the labia minora form a vestibule with the prepuce at the anterior border and the fourchette at the posterior border above the perineum. Within the vestibule are the clitoris, vaginal orifice and hymen, the openings of the Skene glands and Bartholin glands, and the urethral orifice.

The clitoris lies at the anterior junction of the labia minora under the prepuce, which provides a hoodlike covering, protecting the clitoris anteriorly. It is located just above the urethral orifice. It consists of the glans, the body, and the crura. The glans, partially covered by the prepuce, has an abundant supply of sensory nerve endings. Only the glans is visible, with an average length of 1.5 to 2 cm and a diameter of less than 1 cm.[5] The body of the clitoris contains a pair of corpora cavernosa,

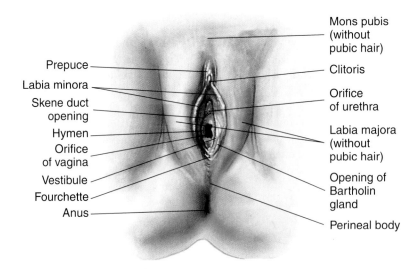

Figure 2.7 External female genitalia. (From Lowdermilk DL, Perry SE, Cashion K, Alden KR, Olshansky EF. *Maternity & Women's Health Care.* 12th ed. St. Louis: Elsevier; 2020: Figure 4.1.)

spongy cylinders of tissue that fill with blood and cause the clitoris to become erect during sexual arousal. These spongy cylinders are covered by the bulbocavernosus muscles. The body of the clitoris extends superiorly and divides into two crura that together provide a *V*-shaped attachment to the undersurface of the symphysis pubis. Two elongated vestibular bulbs formed of erectile tissue also extend from the glans of the clitoris along the sides of the vaginal orifice and beneath the labia majora. The vestibular bulbs become engorged and expand during sexual arousal.[5,6]

The opening of the vagina is referred to as the *introitus*. It may be partially covered by a membrane of connective tissue known as the *hymen*. Characteristics of the hymen are variable. The presence or absence of a hymen can neither confirm nor rule out sexual experience.

The urethral orifice lies anterior to the vaginal introitus and below the clitoris within the vestibule. Just posterior to and on each side of the urethral orifice are the openings of the Skene glands, which may or may not be visible. The Skene glands are similar in morphology to the male prostate gland. They may secrete a small amount of fluid during female sexual orgasm. The pea-sized Bartholin glands are located slightly posterior and on both sides of the vaginal introitus and are usually not palpable. The Bartholin gland openings or ducts, usually not visible, are at the 4 o'clock and 8 o'clock positions. These glands, similar in morphology to the male bulbourethral glands, secrete a small amount of mucus during sexual arousal, providing some vaginal lubrication. The fourchette is a band of mucous membrane at the point where the labia majora and labia minora merge at the posterior border. The perineum is the area located between the fourchette anteriorly and the anus posteriorly.

Blood Supply, Lymphatics, and Innervation

Blood is supplied to the pelvis primarily from arteries branching from the internal iliac arteries. Major pelvic arteries include the uterine, vaginal, pudendal, and perineal arteries. Ovarian arteries branch directly from the aorta.[2,5,6]

Lymph from the internal genitalia, including the upper vagina, flows into pelvic and abdominal lymph nodes, which are not palpable. Lymph from the lower vagina and external genitalia drains into the inguinal nodes.[2,6]

The internal genitalia are innervated primarily by the sacral and coccygeal spinal nerves and the pelvic portion of the autonomic nervous system. The pudendal nerve arising from the sacral plexus supplies motor and sensory innervation for most of the external genitalia and the perineum.[2,5]

Breasts

The female breasts are mammary glands responsible for lactation. They also serve as a stimulus for sexual arousal. The breasts are located within the superficial fascia of the anterior chest wall over the pectoral muscles with the inferior margins over the serratus anterior muscles. Breast tissue extends from the clavicle and second rib down to sixth rib and from the sternum across the midaxillary line. A triangle of breast tissue referred to as the tail of Spence extends laterally across the anterior axillary fold. The breasts are attached to the skin and the underlying muscle by fibrous connective tissue. Suspensory ligaments referred to as Cooper's ligaments support the glandular structures of the breasts allowing for their mobility on the chest wall. Adipose tissue surrounds the superficial and peripheral areas of the breasts. With aging, the proportion of adipose tissue in the female breast increases and the glandular component decreases. In some individuals, a firm transverse ridge of compressed breast tissue may be present along the lower edge of the breast called the inframammary ridge.[1,3]

Each breast is made of lobes that are divided into lobules. The lobes, 15 to 20 for each breast, are composed of glandular tissue surrounded by fatty and connective tissue radiating around the nipple. Lobules are small branching glands within each lobe containing tiny, hollow sacs called alveoli. The alveoli are the functional unit of the breasts containing the milk-secreting acini cells. Each lobe empties into a single lactiferous duct that opens out through the nipple. Lactiferous ducts enlarge behind the nipple to form small reservoirs called *lactiferous sinuses*[1,3] (Fig. 2.8).

The nipples form the terminus into which the lactiferous sinuses secrete milk. Each nipple is composed of epithelial tissue containing smooth muscle fibers that contract in response to tactile, sensory, or autonomic stimuli and has multiple duct openings.

A circular pigmented area, the areola, surrounds the nipple. The color of the areola may be pink, brown, or black depending on race or ethnicity, and it may darken

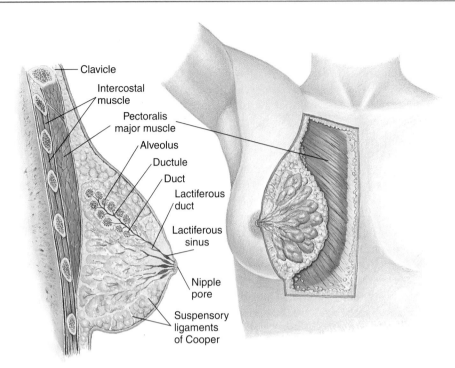

Figure 2.8 Anatomy of the breast showing position and major structures. (From Ball JW, Dains JE, Flynn JA, Solomon BS, Stewart RW. *Seidel's Guide to Physical Examination: An Interprofessional Approach.* St. Louis: Elsevier; 2019: Figure 17.1.)

during pregnancy and lactation. On the surface of the areola are sebaceous glands referred to as *Montgomery glands.* A few hair follicles may be present around the periphery of the areola.[1,3]

Usually the nipples are everted, protruding out from the surface of the breast. Occasionally they may be inverted or depressed below the areolar surface. Long-standing inversion is usually a normal variant and does not generally affect the ability to breastfeed. However, a recent or fixed flattening or depression of the nipple constitutes retraction and may be caused by an underlying cancer.[3,8]

NOT TO BE MISSED

Although long-standing inversion of nipples is usually a normal variant, recent or fixed flattening or depression of the nipple constitutes retraction and may be caused by an underlying cancer.

Supernumerary nipples with a small amount of breast tissue are occasionally found along an embryonic ridge of mammary tissue, sometimes referred to as a *milk line,* extending from the axilla, over the breasts, and down toward the groin. These extra nipples are commonly mistaken for a mole and have no pathological significance.[3,8]

Each breast contains a network of superficial lymphatics that drain the skin and deep lymphatics that drain the mammary lobules. Lymphatics from most of the breast drain toward the axilla. The central (midaxillary) nodes are located high in the axilla between the anterior and posterior axillary folds. These are the nodes that are most likely to be palpable. The anterior (pectoral), posterior (subscapular), and lateral axillary nodes along the upper humerus drain into the central nodes. The central nodes drain into the infraclavicular and supraclavicular nodes. An internal mammary chain also drains into the infraclavicular nodes[3,8] (Fig. 2.9).

FEMALE REPRODUCTIVE PHYSIOLOGY

Female reproductive physiology entails a complex series of endocrine and hormonal actions that change over

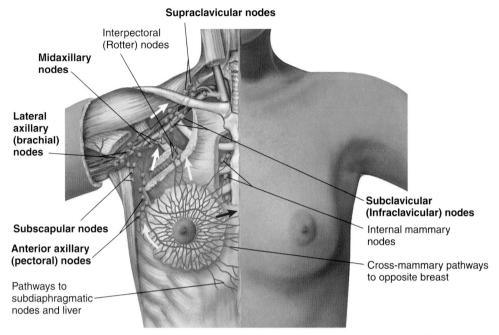

Figure 2.9 Lymphatic drainage of the breast. (From Ball JW, Dains JE, Flynn JA, Solomon BS, Stewart RW. *Seidel's Guide to Physical Examination: An Interprofessional Approach.* St. Louis: Elsevier; 2019: Figure 17.3.)

time from puberty through the reproductive years and to menopause. Additionally, these endocrine and hormonal actions fluctuate in a cyclic manner during the reproductive years. To understand the basics of female reproductive physiology, one must first understand the hypothalamic-pituitary-ovarian axis.

Hypothalamic-Pituitary-Ovarian Axis

Three endocrine organs, the hypothalamus, pituitary gland, and ovaries work together in an intricate and coordinated manner responding to positive and negative feedback loops to regulate female steroid hormone production. Thus we refer to the *hypothalamic-pituitary-ovarian* (HPO) axis in the discussion of female reproductive physiology. The hypothalamus is located at the base of the brain and is connected to the pituitary gland by a stalklike passageway called the *infundibulum.* The pituitary gland sits below the hypothalamus within a concave surface in the sphenoid bone called the *sella turcica.* The pituitary gland has an anterior and posterior component. The hypothalamus communicates with the posterior pituitary gland through neurosecretory neurons. The anterior pituitary gland and hypothalamus communicate through a unique hypophyseal portal system in which blood flows from one capillary bed to another without going through the general circulation. Gonadotropin-releasing hormone (GnRH) produced in the hypothalamus passes through this portal system directly to the anterior pituitary gland, where it stimulates the synthesis and release of the two female gonadotropins: follicle stimulating hormone (FSH) and luteinizing hormone (LH).[9-11]

FSH and LH enter the general circulation and travel to their target site, the ovaries. In response to FSH and LH, the ovaries produce the steroid hormones estrogen, progesterone, and androgens. In turn, negative and positive feedback systems related to estrogen and progesterone levels control FSH and LH secretion. That is, when estrogen or progesterone reach levels above a set point, the hypothalamus decreases GnRH secretion with a resultant decrease in FSH or LH secretion. When estrogen or progesterone levels fall below the set point, the hypothalamus increases GnRH secretion. These two responses to estrogen and progesterone levels are considered negative feedback loops. Additionally, there is one positive feedback loop. Just before ovulation when estrogen levels reach a peak, the hypothalamus increases GnRH secretion, causing a surge of FSH and LH secretion (primarily LH) and subsequent release of a mature ovum from the ovary.[10,11]

Although the target site for FSH and LH is the ovaries, the ovarian steroid hormones act both within the ovaries as well as circulate to target tissues and organs throughout the body exerting specific effects.

Ovarian Steroid Hormones

Three major classes of steroid hormones are produced by the ovarian follicles during their development and by the corpus luteum formed from the ruptured dominant follicle after ovulation: estrogens, progesterone, and androgens. These hormones are all derived from cholesterol through a process called *steroidogenesis*. Steroidogenesis of the ovarian steroid hormones is a complex process, however a description of pathways helps one to see the flow and various conversions that occur along the way.

Within the cells of developing follicles, cholesterol is converted through an enzymatic process to a precursor steroid, pregnenolone. Further conversion of pregnenolone follows one of two pathways. In one pathway, pregnenolone goes through a series of conversions within the follicles from 17-hydroxypregnenolone to the androgen dehydroepiandrosterone (DHEA) and then to the androgen androstenedione. In the other pathway, predominant in the corpus luteum after ovulation, pregnenolone is converted to progesterone. Progesterone either enters the general circulation to act on target tissues or undergoes conversion to 17-hydroprogesterone

and then to androstenedione.[10,11] Estrogens are produced from further conversion of androstenedione to testosterone and then to estradiol, the most potent and abundant of the estrogens during the reproductive years, through an enzymatic process called *aromatization*. The other two estrogens, estriol and estrone, are also synthesized in smaller amounts through these pathways (Fig. 2.10).

Once released into the blood, the ovarian steroid hormone molecules attach to serum-binding proteins, mainly sex hormone–binding globulin (SHBG). The hormone molecules while protein-bound are able to move through the general circulation to target tissues throughout the body. These target tissues are those that have receptors specific for the particular hormone. Thus, although all body tissues may be exposed to the ovarian steroid hormones, only target tissues are responsive to a given hormone.

Additionally, SHBG releases only a certain number of hormone molecules at a time to maintain an equilibrium between unbound and bound molecules. Only unbound molecules are able to leave the circulation and attach to receptors to exert an effect on these tissues. SHBG levels are influenced by several factors. For example, hyperthyroidism, pregnancy, and the administration of exogenous forms of estrogen such as oral contraceptives increase SHBG levels. Obesity, hyperinsulinemia, and androgens decrease SHBG levels.[9-11]

Thus the biological activity of these hormones in particular tissues is dependent on the presence of specific receptors, the number of available receptors, and the local concentration of unbound hormone.

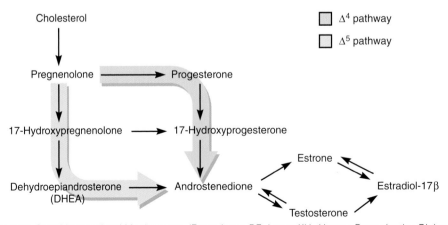

Figure 2.10 Steroidogenesis within the ovary. (From Jones RE, Lopez KH. *Human Reproductive Biology*. 4th ed. San Diego: Elsevier Academic Press; 2014: Figure 2.5)

Estrogens

Estrogens are a group of hormones primarily responsible for the growth and development of female sexual characteristics and reproductive function. There are three types of estrogen produced by women. Estradiol, the primary estrogen produced by the ovaries, is the predominant estrogen during the reproductive years in terms of estrogenic activity. After menopause, estrone becomes the predominant estrogen. Estrone is derived mostly from metabolism of estradiol and from the aromatization of androstenedione in adipose tissue and muscle. A small amount of estrone comes from the ovaries and adrenal glands. During pregnancy, estriol, produced by the placenta, predominates.[10,11]

Estrogen initiates the development of the breasts, causes growth of the bony pelvis, and contributes to increased deposits of subcutaneous fat. Growth and development of the external genitalia and the vagina, fallopian tubes, and uterus occur under the influence of estrogen.[11] Cyclic fluctuations in estrogen levels result in proliferation of the endometrium, ovulation, and menstruation. During pregnancy, estrogen influences some of the physiological adaptations that occur, such as uterine enlargement, hypertrophy of smooth muscles of the vagina, relaxation of pelvic joints and ligaments, and growth of mammary glands with proliferation of lactiferous ducts and lobule tissue.[1]

Estrogen receptors are found throughout the body including but not limited to the uterus, vagina, bladder, urethra, breasts, liver, bones, colon, vascular epithelium, cardiovascular tissues, brain, and skin. To some degree, estrogen affects physiology beyond the reproductive organs wherever there are estrogen receptors. These effects may become more apparent when estrogen levels dramatically change during puberty, pregnancy, menopause, and with some hormonally mediated diseases. Knowledge about the role of estrogen receptors and estrogen action in various parts of the body has provided a better understanding about strategies for both prevention and treatment of such diseases as breast cancer and osteoporosis. As this knowledge evolves, more clinical implications will likely become apparent.

Progesterone

Progesterone is produced by the ovaries, with the largest amounts secreted from the corpus luteum in the luteal phase of the menstrual cycle. Small amounts of progesterone are also secreted by the adrenal glands.

Progesterone receptors are found in the uterus, ovaries, and breasts. Increased levels of progesterone just before and after ovulation cause activation of blood vessels and glands within the endometrium. This in turn causes an accumulation of glycogen and enzymes in preparation for possible implantation of a fertilized ovum.[1,11,12] Progesterone contributes to breast development. During pregnancy, progesterone is first produced by the corpus luteum and then by the placenta. The role of progesterone during pregnancy is to maintain the endometrium, decrease contractility of the uterus, and stimulate development of breast alveoli.[1]

Androgens

Androgens are produced by the ovaries, the adrenal glands, and through peripheral conversion of circulating androstenedione and DHEA to testosterone. Androgens are responsible for the growth of pubic and axillary hair, contribute to the skeletal growth spurt, and activate sebaceous glands. Additionally, androgens have a role in sex drive. As noted earlier, androgens are the primary precursor for the synthesis of estrogens.[11]

Nonsteroidal Hormones and Ovarian Function

Several nonsteroidal hormones and growth factors also contribute to ovarian function, further demonstrating the complex, yet well-coordinated nature of the female reproductive physiology. Among the nonsteroidal hormones are activin, inhibin-A, inhibin-B, and follistatin. Each of these polypeptide hormones exerts a direct effect on ovulatory function by fine-tuning pituitary FSH secretion and ovarian response. Activin, synthesized in both the ovaries and pituitary gland, stimulates FSH secretion and augments its action by increasing FSH receptors in the ovaries. Both forms of inhibin act directly on pituitary cells to inhibit FSH secretion. Follistatin is produced in the pituitary gland but found primarily in the follicles, where it binds to activin, resulting in inhibition of FSH synthesis and secretion.[11,13]

Anti-Müllerian hormone (AMH) is produced exclusively by primordial or undeveloped follicles. AMH inhibits FSH-dependent follicular growth of these primordial follicles and thus may play a role in the selective recruitment of follicles that will continue to grow and develop. Because serum AMH levels are positively correlated with the number of small, primordial follicles within the ovaries, it is sometimes measured as a marker of ovarian reserve.[9,13] AMH levels usually begin to decrease as early as the late twenties and thirties, and it is undetectable about 5 years before menopause.[14]

Although they are not hormones, insulin-like growth factors (IGFs) are polypeptides produced in the liver and ovaries that contribute to steroidogenesis. In the ovaries, IGFs stimulate an increase in size and number of FSH and LH receptors. IGFs also contribute to growth and differentiation throughout the body in response to growth hormone.[10,13] Table 2.1 provides a summary of the source and function of the major female reproductive hormones.

Puberty

Puberty is the transition period between childhood and becoming a sexually mature adult capable of reproduction. During puberty, a complex series of interrelated endocrine and physiological changes occur, primarily as a result of sex steroid hormone production. An increase in sex steroid hormone production is regulated by a maturing HPO axis.

Timing of Puberty

The age of onset of puberty in the United States gradually declined from the early 1900s until 1970 and has remained stable since then.[15] This decline in age has been seen in most developed countries and likely reflects improvements in nutritional status and healthier living conditions.[10,13,15] In the United States at the time of this writing, the first visible changes of puberty in girls are generally noted between about 8 and 10 years of age.[10,11,15]

It is likely that multiple factors interact to trigger the onset of puberty. A genetic influence is recognized as one of the most important factors. There is a positive correlation between the ages at which a mother and daughter as well as sisters go through puberty. Other factors that may influence the timing of puberty include nutritional status, exposure to daylight, altitude, and body weight. Girls who live near the equator or at lower altitudes and those who are mildly obese tend to begin puberty earlier than those who live at more northern latitudes or higher altitudes and those who are normal weight.[10,11]

It is also hypothesized that a critical body weight and fat composition may be crucial in regulating the onset of puberty. This hypothesis is supported by the relationship between an increase in leptin levels and the beginning of puberty. Leptin is a peptide hormone secreted from adipose tissue that circulates in the blood. It acts on the central nervous system to regulate eating behavior and energy balance. Leptin levels increase by 50% just before the onset of puberty and then return to baseline as pubertal changes progress. A critical amount of adipose tissue is necessary for leptin to reach its threshold level. Overweight children have higher leptin levels than normal weight children and tend to enter puberty at an earlier age. Girls with anorexia nervosa and/or low body fat have low levels of leptin and often have delayed puberty. Consequently, leptin is believed to have some role in the initiation of puberty by acting as a messenger between body fat and the central nervous system.[10,13,15]

Mechanism of Puberty

Before puberty, the hypothalamus is highly sensitive to low levels of estrogen, thus GnRH secretion is not stimulated. LH and FSH are suppressed to very low levels. As puberty approaches, the hypothalamus loses this sensitivity, and low levels of circulating estrogen begin to stimulate a pulsatile secretion of GnRH. Initially this GnRH secretion is only nocturnal. In response to GnRH, the anterior pituitary gland secretes FSH and LH in pulses. Nocturnal pulses of LH and to a lesser extent FSH exhibit greatly increased amplitude and increased frequency. As puberty progresses, FSH and LH levels approach the adult pattern of pulsatile secretion without a significant day and night variation.[10,15]

FSH and LH stimulate increased production of the steroid hormones estrogen and progesterone by the ovaries. Even with the initial increase in levels of these steroid hormones, the decreased sensitivity of the hypothalamus to estrogen results in continued GnRH secretion, leading to continued increased FSH and LH secretion by the anterior pituitary gland. The resultant increased levels of estrogen and progesterone are responsible for the development of secondary sexual characteristics and eventually menstruation and ovulation.

Sequence of Pubertal Events

The physical changes that occur during puberty are largely under the influence of increasing estrogen levels along with an increase in adrenal and ovarian androgen production. Although there is individual variation, these changes usually follow a predictable pattern. The beginning of the growth spurt and widening of the pelvis are early changes. Skeletal growth in the pubertal female is

TABLE 2.1   Female Reproductive Hormones

Hormone	Source	Function/Definition
Activin	Ovarian follicular fluid and anterior pituitary gland	Polypeptide that stimulates FSH secretion
Androgens	Ovaries and adrenal cortex	Contribute to long bone growth and growth of pubic and axillary hair
Androstenedione	Ovaries and adrenal cortex	Weak androgen that serves as a precursor for estrogen synthesis
Anti-Müllerian hormone (AMH)	Small, undeveloped, or primordial follicles	Inhibits FSH-dependent follicular growth of primordial follicles and has a role in selective recruitment of follicles that will continue to grow and develop
Estradiol	Ovarian follicle and corpus luteum; small amounts from adrenal cortex	Most potent and plentiful estrogen in reproductive years; see *estrogen* for function
Estriol	Placenta and small amounts in ovaries as a metabolite of estradiol and estrone	Major source of estrogen during pregnancy; see *estrogen* for function
Estrogen	Ovaries, adrenal cortex, peripheral conversion of androgens in adipose tissue, placenta	Needed for maturation of reproductive organs, development of secondary sex characteristics, closure of long bones, regulation of the menstrual cycle, and maternal physiological adaptations in pregnancy; has metabolic effects on several other organs
Estrone	Ovaries, adrenal cortex, conversion of androgens in peripheral adipose tissue	Major source of estrogen after menopause; see *estrogen* for function
Follicle-stimulating hormone (FSH)	Anterior pituitary gland	Stimulates ovarian follicle growth and estrogen production
Follistatin	Produced by anterior pituitary gland and found in ovarian follicular fluid	Inhibits FSH secretion by binding to activin
Gonadotropin-releasing hormone (GnRH)	Hypothalamus	Neurohormone that stimulates LH and FSH secretion from the anterior pituitary gland
Inhibin	Ovarian follicular fluid	Inhibits FSH secretion
Insulin-like growth factors	Liver and ovaries are major sources; multiple sites throughout the body	Involved in growth and differentiation in response to growth hormone; promote steroidogenesis by stimulating an increase in size and number of FSH and LH receptors
Luteinizing hormone (LH)	Anterior pituitary gland	Stimulates secretion of progesterone from the corpus luteum
Sex hormone–binding globulin (SHBG)	Liver	Serum protein that binds to estrogens and androgens in the blood
Progesterone	Ovaries, corpus luteum, small amount from adrenal cortex	Contributes to mammary gland development, regulation of the menstrual cycle, and maternal physiological adaptations in pregnancy
Testosterone	Ovaries, adrenal cortex, peripheral conversion of other androgens in adipose tissue	Androgen that serves as a precursor in estradiol synthesis; see *androgens* for other functions

dependent on the interaction of growth hormone, IGF-1, estrogen, and androgens. A growth spurt typically begins around 9 years of age along with a beginning shift to higher body fat levels and less lean body mass.[10,15]

However, the first easily recognizable change around this same time is breast budding. The growth of pubic and axillary hair usually begins after breast budding. In about one of three girls, pubic hair growth may be noted before breast budding. On average, girls reach their peak height velocity about 2 years after breast budding and 1 year before menarche.[10,15] As estrogen levels increase, long bone growth slows and epiphyseal closure occurs. Bone growth usually is complete by about 15 years of age, although some females may continue to have some increase in height over another several years. During puberty, females experience a significant increase in body fat and decrease in lean body mass.[11,15]

Breast Development. Thelarche or breast development occurs over several years and generally follows a predictable pattern that allows for correlation with other puberty events. Although the average age for beginning breast development is typically between about 9 to 11 years of age, it is not abnormal to have breast budding as early as 6 to 7 years of age.[10,13] In about 1 of 10 girls, breasts develop at slightly different rates, so there is some noticeable asymmetry.[15] This usually resolves

with the completion of breast development. There are five defined stages of breast development called *Tanner sex maturity rating* (SMR) stages (Fig. 2.11). The Tanner SMR stages for breast development are as follows:[11,15,16]

- Stage 1: preadolescent with elevation of nipple only
- Stage 2: breast bud stage with elevation of breast and nipple into a small mound and enlargement of the diameter of the areola
- Stage 3: further enlargement of the breast and areola with no separation of their contours
- Stage 4: further elevation of the areola and nipple to form a secondary mound above the level of the breast
- Stage 5: mature stage with projection of the nipple only; the areola recedes to the general contour of the breast; in some individuals, the areola continues to form a secondary mound

Breast growth and differentiation occur under the influence of a variety of hormones, primarily estrogen and progesterone. Other hormones necessary for the full differentiation of breasts include prolactin, growth hormone, thyroid and parathyroid hormones, insulin, and cortisol. Estrogen promotes the development of mammary and lactiferous ducts, increased glandular tissue, and increased vascularity. Progesterone stimulates the development of epithelial cells lining the alveoli. Growth of the milk-producing system of the mammary glands

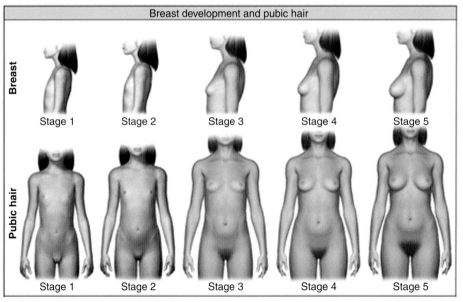

Figure 2.11 Pubertal rating according to Tanner stage. (From Herring JA. Tachdjian's Pediatric Orthopedics: From the Texas Scottish Rite Hospital for Children. 5th ed. Philadelphia: Elsevier; 2014.)

occurs in two sequences. The initial development occurs during puberty. The final differentiation of the alveolar epithelial cells into mature milk-secreting cells occurs with the increase in estrogen and progesterone levels during pregnancy. Secretory activity occurs with the presence of prolactin as pregnancy progresses. Nulliparous individuals will not reach this final stage of mammary gland development.[11]

Pubic Hair Growth. Adrenarche or the growth of pubic hair also follows a predictable pattern that allows for correlation with other puberty events. Increased secretion of the major adrenal androgens— androstenedione, DHEA, and dehydroepiandrosterone sulfate (DHEA-S)—accelerates in late childhood and continues through puberty in both girls and boys. Once puberty begins, there is a rapid increase in androstenedione levels as it is then produced by both the adrenal glands and ovaries. These androgens are responsible for the growth of axillary and pubic hair, slight lowering of the voice, development of sebaceous glands, growth of the long bones, and increased sex drive in the pubescent female.[11]

Although the growth of pubic hair usually starts after breast budding, it may normally occur as early as 7 years of age. Early development of pubic hair without other signs of maturation may occur as a normal variant in some children. Other pubertal events usually occur at the expected time as in other children.[10]

There are Tanner sex maturity rating (SMR) stages for pubic hair growth (see Fig. 2.11). The Tanner SMR stages for pubic hair development are as follows:[8,11,15,16]
- Stage 1: preadolescent with no pubic hair
- Stage 2: sparse growth of long, slightly pigmented, downy hair that is straight or slightly curled along the labia
- Stage 3: darker, coarser, curlier hair that spreads sparsely over the symphysis pubis
- Stage 4: coarse and curly hair as in adults, with a covered area greater than in stage 3 but not yet including the thighs
- Stage 5: adult female inverted triangle hair distribution with spread to the medial surfaces of the thighs

The use of Tanner SMR staging is helpful in assessing growth and development of older children and adolescents. Using pictures of SMR staging can also be helpful in explaining these changes to adolescents. The SMR is calculated by averaging the stage of breast development and pubic hair growth. This rating is used to relate secondary sexual characteristic development with other

physiological changes during puberty. Most children complete physical maturation within 2 to 3 years of reaching SMR stage 2. Menarche generally occurs in SMR stage 4 or breast stages 3 or 4.[8] Although there is significant variation in the age of onset and completion of puberty, the stages normally occur in a predictable fashion.

Delayed onset of puberty in which secondary sexual characteristics begin development later than the average age is usually a normal variant. These children will have a later growth spurt. Often parents will have had a similar development pattern. Once pubertal changes begin, these adolescents follow the same sequence of development, often in a shorter time span. Ultimate height is usually not affected. Medically speaking, delayed puberty is defined as no breast growth by 14 years of age or no skeletal growth spurt by 15 years of age.[11] *Precocious puberty* refers to breast or pubic hair development before 7 years of age in White girls or 6 years of age in Black girls.[11] Although precocious puberty is idiopathic in 75% of cases, an evaluation is needed to rule out congenital causes such as congenital adrenal hyperplasia or neoplastic causes such as virilizing ovarian or adrenal tumors.[15]

NOT TO BE MISSED

Precocious puberty is usually idiopathic. However, evaluation is needed to rule out congenital abnormalities or neoplastic processes as potential causes.

CLINICAL SURVIVAL TIP: Failure of adolescents to develop breasts by 13 years of age or begin menstruation by 16 years of age may be a sign of delayed or absent sexual development caused by chromosomal abnormalities, autoimmune disorders, or other disorders such as diabetes, inflammatory bowel disease, anemia, or cystic fibrosis. Delayed puberty should be evaluated to rule out these causes.

Menarche. Late in the pubertal sequence, the HPO axis reaches maturation. At this time, increasing levels of estrogen exert a positive feedback mechanism on the anterior pituitary gland. There is increased secretion of FSH and LH. Initially, this increase in gonadotropin secretion is not enough to result in ovulation, but it does cause enough fluctuation in ovarian estrogen production so menstruation occurs. The average age of first menses or menarche in the United States is 12 to 13 years of age.[10,11,15] In the first 12 to 18 months after menarche, anovulation is common while the HPO axis continues to mature. Menses may be irregular with heavy bleeding in these anovulatory cycles. The pubertal process lasts on average 4.5 years with a range of 1.5 to 6 years considered within normal limits; the process is considered complete when the individual begins to have ovulatory menstrual cycles.[15] Of note, however, as many as 25% to 50% of adolescents may still have anovulatory cycles up to 4 years after menarche.[10]

Internal and External Genitalia Growth and Development. Although the most apparent pubertal changes involve height, body fat distribution, breast development, pubic hair growth, and menarche, there are significant changes in external and internal genitalia during this time. The labia minora become more vascular, and the clitoris becomes more vascular and erectile. The labia majora become more prominent, with an increase in fatty tissue, growth of pubic hair on the lateral surfaces, and development of sebaceous glands on the hairless medial surfaces. The mons pubis develops its moundlike shape with increased fat deposits under the skin and becomes covered with pubic hair. Sebaceous and sweat gland activity increases in this area. The vaginal walls thicken and become more vascular and elastic. The uterus, fallopian tubes, and ovaries mature and reach adult size.

Menstrual Cycle

The normal menstrual cycle consists of three successive phases: follicular/proliferative, peri-ovulatory, and luteal/secretory. As discussed previously, hormonal control of these three phases depends on the complex interactions among the hypothalamus, anterior pituitary gland, and ovaries.

Each menstrual cycle normally lasts 28 days (+/− 7 days). Variations in cycle length generally reflect differences in the length of the follicular phase. The length of the luteal phase remains constant at 14 years of age (+/− 1 day) once regular ovulatory cycles are established[1,9] (Fig. 2.12).

Follicular/Proliferative Phase

Because menstruation is an observable event, it is standard to consider the first day of menses as the first day of the menstrual cycle. During menstruation, the functional layer of the endometrium degenerates and is discharged through the vagina. The first day of menses coincides with the beginning of the follicular phase.

At the beginning of the follicular phase, estradiol levels are low, which leads to increased GnRH secretion followed by increased FSH secretion. A cohort of primary follicles is recruited in response to increasing FSH levels. As estradiol levels increase, the number of FSH receptors on the largest of the recruited follicles increase so it will in turn produce greater amounts of estradiol. The increasing estradiol level along with the action of inhibin provides negative feedback to the anterior pituitary gland so FSH secretion begins to decrease. The follicle that has the most FSH receptors and produces the most estradiol becomes the dominant follicle. As the FSH level decreases, the dominant follicle survives and the other recruited follicles undergo atresia. The dominant follicle continues to mature and produce high levels of estradiol in the latter half of the follicular phase. Generally, it takes the dominant ovarian follicle 10 to 17 days to fully mature.[9,11]

Estradiol also causes the cells of the endometrium to proliferate during the ovarian follicular phase, thus there is a corresponding endometrial proliferative phase. During this proliferative phase, the endometrium thickens as a result of an increasing number and size of endometrial cells and extension of spiral vessels. There is an increase of blood flow to the endometrium. Estradiol also stimulates the formation of progesterone receptors on endometrial cells during this phase. Proliferation of the endometrium peaks at about days 8 to 10 of the menstrual cycle when circulating estradiol levels peak. By the end of the follicular phase and at the time of ovulation, the endometrium thickens to 12 mm compared with an average thickness of 1 to 2 mm immediately after menstruation.[9]

Peri-Ovulatory Phase

When estradiol reaches a critical blood level, it exerts positive feedback on the anterior pituitary gland, which causes a surge of LH and FSH. Estradiol reaches its peak level about 24 hours before ovulation. Increasing LH also causes increased progesterone production. Progesterone, proteolytic enzymes, and prostaglandins cause thinning and digestion of the follicular wall and contraction of smooth muscle cells of the follicle. Ovulation occurs when the follicle ruptures and the mature oocyte and follicular fluid exude from the ovary. This

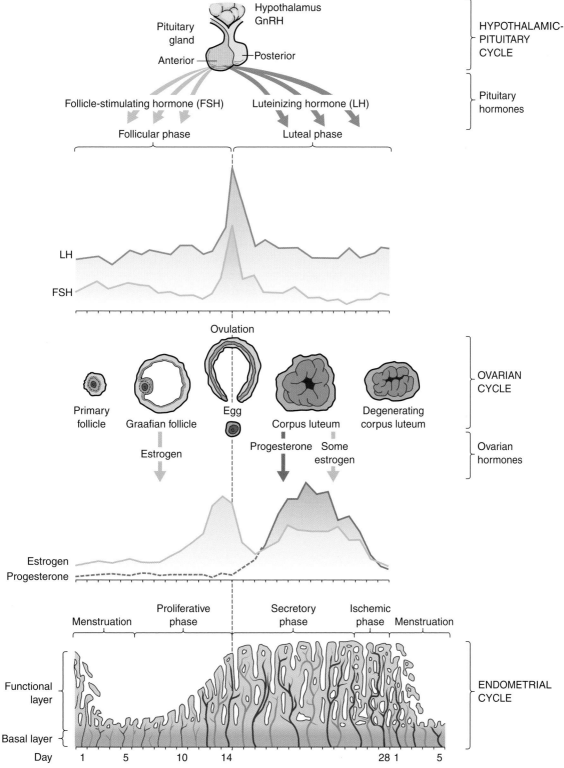

Figure 2.12 Menstrual cycle: hypothalamic-pituitary, ovarian, and endometrial. (From Lowdermilk DL, Perry SE, Cashion K, Alden KR, Olshansky EF. *Maternity & Women's Health Care*. 12th ed. St. Louis: Elsevier; 2020: Figure 4.7.)

occurs about 32 hours after onset of the LH surge and about 16 hours after the LH peak.[9] The LH surge is a reliable indicator of impending ovulation. Ovulation predictor kits are designed to detect this LH surge. Some individuals experience *mittelschmerz* or localized lower abdominal pain related to the rupture of the ovarian follicle and leaking of follicular fluid into the abdominal cavity.[1]

Luteal/Secretory Phase

The luteal phase begins after ovulation. The LH surge transforms the cells of the ruptured follicle into the corpus luteum. There is a shift from estrogen dominance to progesterone dominance in the luteal phase. Progesterone suppresses new follicular growth and causes secretory changes in the endometrium that correspond with the ovarian luteal phase. During this secretory phase, the endometrium does not grow in thickness but takes on a cushiony characteristic as the glands become torturous, the stroma becomes edematous, and the spiral vessels become coiled. This endometrium secretes nutritive proteins necessary for implantation if fertilization occurs.

There is a peak in progesterone production about 7 days after the LH surge that corresponds with the time of implantation if fertilization occurs.[1] Progesterone also causes an increase in basal body temperature (BBT). Daily measurement of BBT can be used to determine if ovulation has or has not occurred. Because the BBT rise does not occur until after ovulation, it cannot be used to predict when ovulation is going to occur. The length of the luteal phase is more constant than the follicular phase, lasting approximately 14 days (+/− 1 day).[1,9]

If implantation and pregnancy occur, the corpus luteum is maintained by human chorionic gonadotropin (hCG) produced initially by the implanted blastocyst and later by the placenta. If pregnancy does not occur, the corpus luteum begins to degenerate rapidly about 9 to 11 days after ovulation.[1,9] Estrogen and progesterone levels decrease. The endometrium begins to degenerate with withdrawal of hormonal influence. Proteolytic enzymes begin to digest endometrial cells. Prostaglandins initiate contractions of the uterine smooth muscle and sloughing of the degraded endometrial tissue. About 14 days after ovulation, menstruation occurs with the discharge through the vagina of the degraded endometrial tissue, red blood cells, inflammatory exudates, and proteolytic enzymes. The enzymes also destroy some of the clotting factors found in the menstrual blood, so clots do not generally form with a normal amount of bleeding. Menstrual flow usually lasts 3 to 5 days, but anywhere from 2 to 7 days is considered within normal limits.[15] The normal amount of blood lost during menses ranges from 10 to 80 mL, with an average of 35 mL.[9]

The decline in estrogen and progesterone levels at the end of the luteal phase and beginning of the follicular phase cause an increase in GnRH secretion; FSH and LH levels begin to increase, starting another cycle.

Summary of Events of the Menstrual Cycle

A summary of the events that take place during the menstrual cycle are as follows (see Figure 2.12).

- Menstruation with low levels of estradiol and progesterone
- Increase in GnRH secretion → increase in FSH and LH, predominantly FSH
- Cohort of follicles recruited and begins to grow, producing estradiol
- Dominant follicle develops more FSH receptors and produces more estradiol
- Other recruited follicles undergo atresia
- Dominant follicle continues to mature, producing high levels of estradiol
- Endometrium undergoes proliferative growth during the follicular phase
- Estradiol reaches a critical level causing a surge in LH and FSH, predominantly LH
- LH surge promotes final maturation of the dominant follicle and the beginning increase in progesterone production
- Mature follicle ruptures and releases an oocyte
- Ruptured follicle becomes the corpus luteum, producing increasing amounts of progesterone
- Progesterone level peaks 7 to 8 days after the LH surge
- Endometrium undergoes secretory changes during the luteal phase
- Corpus luteum begins to degenerate 9 to 11 days after ovulation → decrease in estradiol and progesterone levels
- Endometrium begins to degenerate with withdrawal of estradiol and progesterone
- Menstruation occurs with the low levels of estradiol and progesterone

Cyclic Changes in Reproductive Organs

All of the reproductive organs and the breasts respond to the cyclic changes in estradiol and progesterone levels during the reproductive years. Some of these changes are subtle, while others are detectable by the individual.

Under the influence of estradiol in the follicular phase, the superficial epithelial cells of the vaginal lining grow, and a layering of these cells occurs. In the luteal phase, there is a thinning of the squamous epithelium making up the vaginal mucosal membrane. Near the end of the luteal phase, leukocytes invade the vaginal epithelium, removing the outer layer in a process called *decornification*.[10]

The cervix and cervical mucous respond to the cyclic changes in estradiol and progesterone. Under the influence of estradiol in the follicular phase, cervical vascularity increases, causing softening and swelling of the cervix. There is some eversion of the external cervical os. Cervical mucous becomes clear, copious, and elastic, a condition termed *spinnbarkeit* (Fig. 2.13). These changes become more apparent as ovulation approaches, facilitating sperm penetration from the vagina into the fallopian tubes. After ovulation, under the influence of progesterone, the cervix becomes firmer, and the external cervical os inverts. Cervical mucous becomes turbid, scant, and thick. These changes prevent microorganisms and sperm from entering the uterine cavity.[1] Individuals can learn to assess these changes in their own bodies to determine when they are most likely to be fertile or infertile.

Estrogen and progesterone also affect the fallopian tubes. Estrogen increases the number of cilia in the tubes. Progesterone increases ciliary movement and egg transport.[11] This movement facilitates transport of the ovum through the tube.

As discussed earlier, estrogen and progesterone are responsible for maturation of the female breasts during puberty. Cyclic changes in the breasts also occur with the menstrual cycle. During the follicular phase, high estradiol levels increase breast tissue vascularity, and proliferation of ductal cells occurs. These changes are sustained under the influence of progesterone. During the luteal phase, progesterone is responsible for dilation of the ducts and differentiation of alveolar cells into secretory cells. The cyclic glandular and nonglandular changes in the breasts are prominent enough so most individuals notice some degree of breast fullness, tenderness, and/or nodularity before each menses. Because

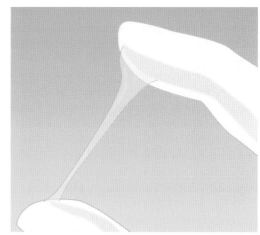

Figure 2.13 Spinnbarkeit. (From Hacker NF, Gambone JC, Hobel CJ. *Hacker & Moore's Essentials of Obstetrics and Gynecology.* 6th ed. Philadelphia: Elsevier; 2016: Figure 34.3.)

these changes do not entirely regress by the start of a new cycle, breast growth may continue at a slow rate until approximately 35 years of age.[10]

Menopause

Menopause, by definition, is the final menstrual period (FMP) resulting from a permanent decline in female steroid hormone levels. Menopause is confirmed by 12 months of amenorrhea in individuals with a uterus. In individuals without a uterus, menopause is confirmed by a history of bilateral oophorectomy, typical symptoms, and/or serial measurement of hormonal markers.[14] The age of menopause is mostly affected by genetics. Individuals with less body fat tend to reach menopause at a slightly younger age. Those who smoke have a mean age of menopause that is 1 to 2 years sooner than in nonsmokers.[17] Age of menopause does not seem to be influenced by age of menarche, number of pregnancies, breastfeeding, or hormonal contraceptive use. In the United States, the average age of menopause is around 51 to 52 years of age, with most individuals reaching menopause between 50 and 55 years of age.[14,18] Although there has been an increase in life expectancy over the years, the age of menopause has not changed. What has changed is that most women now spend at least one-third of their lives in the postmenopause stage.[14]

Hormonal Changes of Menopause

The time span beginning when hormonal changes start to occur and ending with the FMP is referred to as the *menopause transition. Perimenopause* extends from the beginning of the menopause transition until 12 months after the FMP. *Postmenopause* refers to the years following menopause.[14]

The STRAW (Stages of Reproductive Aging Workshop) reproductive-aging continuum provides a standardized definition of reproductive aging based on specific clinical criteria, endocrine parameters, and characteristic markers. Menstrual cycle changes are considered the principle clinical criteria, and characteristic markers include vasomotor symptoms and symptoms of urogenital atrophy. Endocrine parameters including FSH, AMH, and inhibin B are considered supportive criteria not typically measured for the purposes of staging reproductive aging or menopause.[14]

Ovarian aging is the predominant event leading to menopause. At birth, females have 1 to 2 million follicles. As one ages, the number of follicles falls at a constantly increasing rate through the process of follicular atresia. Decreasing AMH levels coincide with follicular atresia, reaching an undetectable range up to 5 years before menopause.[14,17] As the number of responsive follicles decreases, so does the production of estradiol. This decrease in estradiol induces a negative feedback to the hypothalamus and anterior pituitary gland, resulting in an increase in FSH. There is also a decrease in the production of ovarian inhibin B, removing this previous inhibitory effect on FSH secretion. During the menopause transition, there is variability in hormone secretion and inconsistent ovulation. There may be extreme fluctuations in FSH levels shifting between postmenopausal levels and those consistent with reproductive capability. Estradiol levels likewise will fluctuate.

NOT TO BE MISSED

Measuring FSH and/or estradiol levels is not a reliable method to determine menopause.

In the early menopause transition with fluctuating hormone levels, menstrual cycle length becomes variable. As the transition progresses, there are typically intervals of amenorrhea (≥60 days). Individuals may have different patterns. Heavy, prolonged bleeding may occur during anovulatory cycles. The hallmark for the end of the menopause transition and initiation of the postmenopause is the FMP.

During the first 1 to 2 years postmenopause, there is a 10- to 15-fold increase in FSH and LH, with a greater increase in FSH. There is then a gradual and slight decrease and stabilization in both FSH and LH levels.[14] Estrogen production by the ovaries ceases with menopause. Postmenopause circulating estradiol levels are approximately 10 to 20 pg/mL compared with 40 to 400 pg/mL in the reproductive age years.[14] Most of this estradiol comes from peripheral conversion of estrone, which is primarily derived from peripheral conversion of androstenedione. The ovaries and adrenal glands continue to secrete androstenedione and testosterone, with levels gradually decreasing over time. However, as estrogen levels decrease at menopause, SHBG levels, which bind testosterone in the circulation, also decrease. Increased levels of free testosterone are thought to contribute at least in part to increased sexual desire in some women during the perimenopause stage.

About 75% to 85% of individuals experience some degree of vasomotor symptoms (VMS), commonly referred to as *hot flashes,* during the perimenopause and extending into the early postmenopause years.[14,18] VMS, by definition, are recurrent, transient episodes of flushing accompanied by a sensation of warmth to intense heat involving the upper body and face. Profuse sweating and palpitations may occur. The specific mechanism causing VMS is not known. There seems to be a gonadotropin-related effect on the central thermoregulatory function of the hypothalamus. An increase in core body temperature leads to an increase in body surface temperature, resulting in peripheral vasodilation, followed by a decrease in the core body temperature. Hot flashes typically begin in the late perimenopause stage, reach the greatest frequency and intensity within the first 2 years after the FMP, and then decrease over time. Some individuals continue to have VMS for 10 or more years after the FMP.[14,17]

Menopausal Changes in Reproductive Organs and Genitalia

The labia major and minora, clitoris, urethra, vagina, and trigone area of the bladder all have high concentrations of estrogen receptors and are affected by decreased levels of circulating estrogen. The labia majora and minora become thinner and less prominent with loss of subcutaneous tissue. There is a decrease of blood flow to the clitoris and atrophy of the clitoral prepuce. The urethral meatus may become more prominent as the labia minora thins. The vagina shortens and narrows with decreased elasticity. The vaginal epithelium thins, and rugae disappear. A decrease in cervical secretions and vaginal blood flow results in reduced vaginal lubrication. The number of lactobacilli is reduced, and the pH of the vagina becomes alkaline with a pH usually greater than 5.[17] The uterine body and cervix decrease in size. The cervical os may appear flush with the vaginal walls and may become stenotic. The ovaries also decrease in size and are not normally palpable within a few years after menopause.

Up to 50% of individuals experience significant symptoms related to the anatomical and physiological changes related to menopause. The term *genital syndrome of menopause* (GSM) is used to describe the collection of symptoms and physical findings in these urogenital areas of the body associated with decreased estrogen and other sex steroid hormones.[14] Symptoms include varying levels of genital dryness, burning, and irritation. Dyspareunia and impaired sexual response may occur. Urinary symptoms may include frequency, nocturia, urgency, dysuria, and recurrent urinary tract infections.

> **PATIENT-CENTERED CARE:** It is important to determine how menopausal changes affect the quality of life of each patient and advise them on ways to mitigate the impact on their lives.

Other Hormone-Related Menopausal Changes

There is a beginning decrease in glandular breast tissue as women reach their mid-thirties to mid-forties. After menopause, glandular tissue is further reduced, and there is an increase in adipose tissue. This typically results in some reduction in breast size and firmness.[19]

Like the genitourinary tract, the skin also has significant numbers of estrogen receptors. In the postmenopause stage, there is a decrease in skin collagen and skin thickness. Exposure to sunlight and tobacco smoke over the years are also important factors in skin aging. Because there is a significant change in the androgen-to-estrogen ratio, some menopausal women experience mild acne and facial hair growth.[14,18]

Weight gain is likely more related to aging and lifestyle than to the hormonal changes of menopause. Lean body mass decreases with age. As women age, they may become less physically active, resulting in an increase in body fat and weight. There has been a demonstrated association between menopause and a shift of body fat to the abdominal region.[14]

Decreased estrogen and testosterone may contribute to changes in sexual function for menopausal women. This effect is variable as general health, interpersonal factors, and psychological factors also influence one's sexual functioning. As previously discussed, vaginal changes may cause discomfort with sexual intercourse. Extra lubrication and time may be necessary for a satisfactory sexual experience. Sexual desire may decrease in both men and women as testosterone levels decline. Women who are 70 years of age and older have testosterone levels that are one-half of what they were in their early twenties.[14]

KEY POINTS

- Knowledge about female reproductive anatomy and physiology from puberty through the reproductive years to menopause and beyond is critical when providing health care for women.
- The SC junction is the most frequent site of changes associated with the development of cervical dysplasia. Cells from both the SC junction and the ectocervix should be obtained for a Pap test to screen for cervical cancer.
- Unrecognized anteflexion or retroflexion can increase the risk for uterine perforation during intrauterine contraception placement.

- The ovaries may or may not be palpable on a bimanual pelvic examination in the reproductive age individual. The ovaries atrophy after menopause and should not be palpable.
- Long-standing inversion of the nipple is usually a normal variant. However, a recent or fixed flattening or depression of the nipple constitutes retraction and may be caused by an underlying cancer.
- Three endocrine organs (the hypothalamus, pituitary gland, and ovaries) work together in an intricate and coordinated manner responding to positive and negative feedback loops to regulate female steroid hormone production.

- Delayed onset of puberty in which secondary sexual characteristics begin development later than the average age is usually a normal variant. These children will have a later growth spurt.
- *Precocious puberty* refers to female breast or pubic hair development before 7 years of age in White girls or 6 years of age in Black girls. In 75% of cases, precocious puberty is idiopathic, but evaluation is important to rule out congenital or neoplastic causes.

- In the first 12 to 18 months after menarche, anovulation is common while the HPO axis continues to mature. Menses may be irregular with heavy bleeding in these anovulatory cycles.
- During the menopause transition, there is variability in hormone secretion and inconsistent ovulation. There may be extreme fluctuations in FSH and estradiol levels. Thus measuring FSH and/or estradiol levels is not a reliable method to determine menopause.

REFERENCES

1. Lowdermilk DL, Perry SE, Cashion K, Alden KR. *Maternity and Women's Health Care*. 11th ed. St. Louis: Elsevier Mosby; 2016.
2. O'Rahilly R. *Basic Human Anatomy: A Regional Study of Human Structure*. Hanover, NH: Dartmouth Medical School; 2008. http://www.dartmouth.edu/~humananatomy.
3. Ball JW, Dains JE, Flynn JA, Solomon BS, Stewart RW. *Seidel's Guide to Physical Examination*. 8th ed. St. Louis: Elsevier Mosby; 2015.
4. Herschorn S. Female pelvic floor anatomy, the pelvic floor, supporting structures, and pelvic organs. *Rev Urol*. 2004;6(suppl 5):S2–S10.
5. Valea FA. Reproductive anatomy. In: Lobo RA, Gershenson DA, Lentz GM, Valea FA, eds. *Comprehensive Gynecology*. 7th ed. Philadelphia: Elsevier; 2017:48–76.
6. Gambone JC. Female reproductive anatomy and embryology. In: Hacker NF, Gambone JC, Hobel CJ, eds. *Hacker and Moore's Essentials of Obstetrics & Gynecology*. 6th ed. Philadelphia: Elsevier; 2016:23–36.
7. Rosenman AE. Pelvic floor disorders. In: Hacker NF, Gambone JC, Hobel CJ, eds. *Hacker and Moore's Essentials of Obstetrics & Gynecology*. 6th ed. Philadelphia: Elsevier; 2016:291–303.
8. Bickley LS. *Bates' Guide to Physical Examination and History Taking*. 12th ed. Philadelphia: Lippincott Williams & Wilkins; 2016.
9. Douglas NC, Lobo RA. Reproductive endocrinology. In: Lobo RA, Gershenson DA, Lentz GM, Valea FA, eds. *Comprehensive Gynecology*. 7th ed. Philadelphia: Elsevier; 2017:77–107.
10. Fritz MA, Speroff L. *Clinical Gynecologic Endocrinology and Infertility*. Philadelphia: Lippincott Williams & Wilkins; 2011.
11. Jones RE, Lopez KH. *Human Reproductive Biology*. 4th ed. San Diego: Elsevier Academic Press; 2014.
12. Gambone JC. Female reproductive physiology. In: Hacker NF, Gambone JC, Hobel CJ, eds. *Hacker and Moore's Essentials of Obstetrics & Gynecology*. 6th ed. Philadelphia: Elsevier; 2016:37–49.
13. Jameson JL, deKrester D, Marshall JC. *Reproductive Endocrinology: Adult and Pediatric*. 6th ed. Philadelphia: Elsevier Saunders; 2010.
14. North American Menopause Society. *Menopause Practice: A Clinician's Guide*. 5th ed. Mayfield Heights, OH: North American Menopause Society; 2014.
15. Churchill S, Alexander CJ. Puberty and disorders of pubertal development. In: Hacker NF, Gambone JC, Hobel CJ, eds. *Hacker and Moore's Essentials of Obstetrics & Gynecology*. 6th ed. Philadelphia: Elsevier; 2016:370–379.
16. Lobo RA. Primary and secondary amenorrhea and precocious puberty: Etiology, diagnostic evaluation, management. In: Lobo RA, Gershenson DA, Lentz GM, Valea FA, eds. *Comprehensive Gynecology*. 7th ed. Philadelphia: Elsevier; 2017:829–852.
17. Lobo RA. Menopause and care of the mature woman. In: Lobo RA, Gershenson DA, Lentz GM, Valea FA, eds. *Comprehensive Gynecology*. 7th ed. Philadelphia: Elsevier; 2017:258–293.
18. Gambone JC. Menopause and perimenopause. In: Hacker NF, Gambone JC, Hobel CJ, eds. *Hacker and Moore's Essentials of Obstetrics & Gynecology*. 6th ed. Philadelphia: Elsevier; 2016:406–413.
19. Sandadi S, Rock DT, Orr JW, Valea FA. Breast disorders. In: Lobo RA, Gershenson DA, Lentz GM, Valea FA, eds. *Comprehensive Gynecology*. 7th ed. Philadelphia: Elsevier; 2017:294–328.

3

Adolescent Women's Health

Dana Renee Cummings

OBJECTIVES

- Define and identify the stages of female adolescence.
- Discuss reproductive and wellness assessments and evaluation, screening tools, and the vaccination schedule for adolescent females.
- Identify key risk behaviors and causes of mortality and morbidity among adolescent females.
- Examine the mental health concerns of adolescent females.

INTRODUCTION

According to the World Health Organization (WHO) report on mortality, morbidity, and disability in adolescence, the mortality rate for adolescents continues to be lower in comparison with other age groups. In general, the rates among 10- to 14-year-old adolescents have declined in the past decade. However, even with a decline in rates, there is still a significant level of mortality among adolescents. The WHO reported in 2020 an estimated 1.1 million adolescents died, down from 1.5 million in 2019. Globally, the leading causes of death among adolescents in 2019 were road traffic injuries, suicide, and interpersonal violence. The WHO surveyed for adolescent morbidity issues to identify important health problems that affect the adolescent population. Issues identified were mental health problems, followed by health-compromising behaviors (e.g., tobacco and alcohol use) and health-compromising conditions (e.g., obesity). Other issues identified were noncommunicable diseases (e.g., asthma, diabetes) followed by acute conditions (e.g., fevers, headaches, common cold).

Adolescence marks the period from 11 to 21 years of age.[1] Adolescence is a dynamic period of development, with rapid changes in body size, shape, and composition. Along with physical changes, cognitive, psychological, and social development occur, making this a very important period in a person's life. *Puberty* is described as the transitional period between childhood and the reproductive maturity of adulthood. However, adolescence is a biopsychosocial process, and cognitive changes may start before the appearance of secondary sexual characteristics and may go well beyond attainment of reproductive maturity and cessation of physical growth. For females, the development of secondary sexual characteristics is based on pubic hair and breast development. As clinicians, it is important to remember that there are vast individual variations, not only in the time of initiation of puberty but also in the time between the different stages of breast and pubic hair development.[2]

REPRODUCTIVE ASSESSMENT AND EVALUATION

The initial screening for reproductive preventive health care services and guidance should occur between 13 and 15 years of age.[3] Growth in any one developmental area including cognitive, psychosocial, or physical development, may or may not correspond with the chronological age of the female. The scope of the initial visit is tailored to the patient's individual needs, including medical history as well as physical and emotional development. The level of care received from other health care providers may not include reproductive health. Patients seeing a range of clinicians for other services (e.g., mental health or physical therapy) may not have addressed reproductive health, making it important to assess for comprehensive care including reproductive care.[3]

The office environment for the initial visit should be one that is less intimidating to adolescents. Rooms designated for adolescent females with culturally inclusive reading materials for youth, including the use of diagrams, charts, and models, allow younger patients to feel comfortable and openly communicate with the provider. The use of culturally sensitive materials is helpful, providing the opportunity to teach about the anatomy and physiology of the reproductive tract. Appointments scheduled before and after school are more favorable and convenient for adolescents.[3]

> **PATIENT-CENTERED CARE:** The office environment for the initial visit should be one that is less intimidating to adolescents. Rooms designated for adolescent females with culturally inclusive reading materials for youth, including diagrams, charts, and models, allow younger patients to feel comfortable and openly communicate with the provider.

Confidentiality is vital to adolescent care and should be discussed with both the adolescent and parent before the examination. When appropriate, the patient's request for privacy from the parent should be accommodated. If the caregiver desires time alone with the provider to address questions and concerns, this should also be discussed with the adolescent, and the discussion should occur before the evaluation. Both parents and adolescents must be made aware of state and local statutes regarding clinical practice as well as legal restrictions that prohibit the provider from maintaining confidentiality. Laws and regulations addressing provision of care to adolescents and confidentiality requirements may vary from state to state. Examples of such requirements include disclosure of evidence of a major medical problem, risk of bodily harm to herself or others, and mandatory reporting of physical and/or sexual abuse of minors. Clinicians should familiarize themselves with their state and local statutes regarding the rights of minors to consent to health care services and the federal and state laws that affect confidentiality.[4]

Assessment

History assessment should include but not be limited to the patient's general medical history, family medical

> **NOT TO BE MISSED**
>
> Laws and regulations addressing provision of care to adolescents and confidentiality requirements may vary from state to state.

history, and immunization status. The family medical history should include questions regarding cardiovascular disease, diabetes, hypertension, venous thromboembolism, mental illness, substance abuse, and delayed puberty. An assessment of breast, ovarian, colon, and uterine cancers should be performed along with assessment of familial gynecological conditions such as leiomyomas and endometriosis.

Menarche and subsequent menses are physiologically and emotionally important milestones for female adolescents. Detailed questions about the patient's menstrual cycle should be addressed at office visits. Special populations including adolescents with disabilities and developmental delays may especially benefit from an initial reproductive health-based visit.

Adolescents with physical or developmental disabilities have needs similar to their peers in regard to menstruation, fertility, hygiene, and contraception, and they should receive care and education that is developmentally appropriate.[5] Female adolescents who identify themselves as gay or lesbian should also have their first reproductive health care visit between 13 and 15 years of age. Transgender teenagers who have female reproductive organs or who are taking female hormones are also in need of female reproductive health care.

A discussion regarding pregnancy prevention/contraception and sexually transmitted infections (STIs) is crucial, as some adolescents may have engaged in sexual activity or are contemplating having sex (including noncoital sexual activity), which commonly occur with coital behavior.[6]

Forty percent of adolescents 15 to 19 years of age have engaged in intercourse, and the incidence of sexual activity increases with age. The Guttmacher Institute reported that 20% of 15-year-old individuals and nearly 66% of 18-year-old individuals admit to sexual activity. Noncoital sexual activity rates among adolescents are similar to coital sexual activity, with oral sex reported at 45% and anal sex described much lower at 9%.[7] Many adolescents are unlikely to use barrier protection when engaging in oral and anal sex. Adolescents perceive increased safety with vaginal sex.

Adolescents and young adults may engage in sexual play or noncoital sex falsely believing there is a reduced risk of pregnancy and STIs. Clinicians have the opportunity to improve outcomes by providing education regarding high-risk sexual practices. Adolescents are at risk of STIs as transmission may be spread through oral/anal sex as well as coital sex. Adolescents require education of risks about possible infection exposure and transmission including human immunodeficiency virus (HIV), human papillomavirus (HPV), herpes simplex virus (HSV), hepatitis virus (types A, B, and C), syphilis, gonorrhea, and chlamydial infections.[6]

Sending sexual messages and/or pictures (sexting) has been associated with early initiation of sexual behaviors and intercourse. The use of electronic mobile communication between adolescents is high, suggesting that clinicians should discuss healthy screen time as well as provisions for monitoring safety with patients and caregivers.[8]

The initial reproductive visit is also an appropriate time to screen for high-risk behaviors including substance abuse, tobacco use, and alcohol use. Other issues to consider addressing include eating disorders, anxiety/depression, and physical, sexual, and emotional abuse.[6] The dual systems model, which examines cognitive control in adolescence, suggests that decision making occurs under conditions that excite or activate the socioemotional system (Fig. 3.1). Adolescents are more prone than other age groups to pursue exciting, novel, and risky behaviors. Risky behaviors with poor decision making are often under the influence of peer pressure. Emotionally arousing circumstances can influence adolescents to react based on immediate reward.[9]

A useful screening tool when interviewing adolescents and young adults is the Home, Education, Activity, Drugs, Sex/Stress (HEADSS) model (Table 3.1). This assessment includes questions regarding home, education and employment, activities, drugs, sexuality, suicide, and depression. These principles are universally relevant to youth and can be integrated within preventive, chronic, and acute care encounters. The use of HEADSS creates awareness of issues; facilitates conversations among providers, patients, and caregivers; and helps avoid and/or solve relevant problems. It also creates dialogue around health and health care within the important domains of adolescent development.[10]

> **PATIENT-CENTERED CARE:** HEADSS is a useful screening tool when interviewing adolescents and young adults. The assessment includes questions regarding home, education and employment, activities, drugs, sexuality, suicide, and depression.

Examination

The adolescent initial examination does not require an internal pelvic examination unless indicated by a pelvic complaint such as abnormal discharge, abnormal bleeding, or pelvic pain.[3] The pelvic examination or speculum examination should be thoroughly explained before performing it. Clinicians have the opportunity to discuss the differences between a pelvic examination (external and internal) and a Pap smear test (screening for cervical cancer). Adolescents and parents are uncertain and unaware of the differences and indications for a pelvic examination and/or pap smear. Patients who have engaged in sexual activity should be screened for chlamydia and gonorrhea at the initial visit and annually. STI serum screening should also be considered including HIV testing, especially if the patient has had unprotected sexual activity.

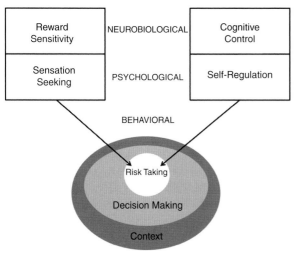

Figure 3.1 Dual systems model. Constructs implicated in the dual systems model of adolescent risk-taking arranged by level of analysis. (Modified from Shulman EP, Smith AR, Silva K, et al. The dual systems model: Review, reappraisal, and reaffirmation. *Dev Cogn Neurosci.* 2016;17:103–117.)

> **CLINICAL SURVIVAL TIP** Patients that have engaged in sexual activity should be screened for chlamydia and gonorrhea at the initial visit and annually. It is also recommended that testing for HIV be performed at least once.

TABLE 3.1	**HEADSSS Assessment Tool for Adolescent Patients***	
H	Home	• Who lives with you? • Do you share a room with anyone? • Do you get along with everyone in your home? • Who can you talk to at home when you are upset?
E	Education and employment	• Do you still go to school or college? • Do you have a job? How many hours do you work? • What are your goals in the future? • Do you have any specific careers in mind? • Do you have friends at school or work?
A	Activities	• What do you like to do in your spare time? • How easy do you find it to relax? • Do you like doing any exercise? • Do you like doing these activities by yourself or with friends?
D	Drugs, smoking, and alcohol	• Have you ever tried drugs, smoking, or alcohol? • Do you feel pressured to try drugs, smoking, or alcohol? • Where do you get the money to do these things? • Are you interested in stopping or cutting down?
S	Sex and relationships	• Are you in a relationship with anyone at the moment? • Is it with a male, female, or both? • Have you ever had sex? • Do you ever feel pressured into sexual relations? • Do you know anything about contraception?
S	Self harm, depression, and self-image	• How is your mood at the moment? • What makes you feel sad or stressed? • Do you ever have any thoughts about hurting yourself? • Have you ever told anyone about these thoughts? • How do you feel about yourself?
S	Safety and Abuse	• Do you feel safe at home? • Is there anyone in your life who makes you feel unsafe? • Are you ever made to do things that you do not want to?

*HEADSSS is an international tool that can be used to structure a rapid psychological assessment for adolescent patients, either in the emergency department or the ward setting.
Courtesy Dr. Zoë Johnson, MbChB.

The U.S. Preventive Services Task Force (USPSTF)[11] recommends against screening for cervical cancer in females younger than age 21 years. Chlamydia and gonorrhea screening should be done using nucleic acid amplification techniques. The use of urine or vaginal swab by speculum examination may be determined by both the patient and health care provider. A vaginal swab is more sensitive than a urine test; however, both have been found to be acceptable to young patients.[3] Annual chlamydia and gonorrhea screening for all sexually active females younger than 25 years of age is recommended.[12]

The Centers for Disease Control and Prevention (CDC) STD and HIV screening recommendations state that all adults and adolescents from 13 to 64 years of age should be tested at least once for HIV. The U.S. Preventive Services Task Force[13] recommends that clinicians screen adolescents and adults 15 to 65 years of age for HIV infection. Younger adults who are at increased risk should be screened. The risk factors identified include unprotected vaginal or anal intercourse, HIV-infected sexual partners, bisexual or injection drug users, and the exchanging of sex for drugs or money. Other identified behaviors include men who have sex with men (MSM) or those that have acquired or request testing for other sexually transmitted infections.[13]

NOT TO BE MISSED

The CDC STI Provider Pocket Guides is a helpful resource for treatment recommendations and can be found at https://www.cdc.gov/std/products/provider-pocket-guides.htm.

The Pederson or Huffman speculum is typically used for a pelvic examination (Fig. 3.2). The patient's pubertal development, hymenal opening, and sexual experience may guide the choice of speculum.[3] The Graves speculum should be avoided because the wider width may cause unnecessary discomfort. Plastic disposable specula are available in variety of appropriate sizes. Specula with self-contained lighting can make visualization easier.[14] Water-based lubricants provide lubrication for the speculum and have not been shown to interfere with either Pap or STI testing. Chaperones are strongly recommended regardless of whether or not the provider and patient are the same gender. Use of a chaperone may help avoid any false accusations to the clinician. Chaperones can assist clinicians during the examination, improving efficiency in collecting specimens. The examination may include inspection of the external genitalia, internal examination with a speculum, and a bimanual examination.

CLINICAL SURVIVAL TIP Chaperones are strongly recommended regardless of whether or not the provider and patient are the same gender. Use of a chaperone may help avoid any false accusations to the clinician.

Young females with physical disabilities may require modification of the physical examination because of a limb, pelvic, or spine deformity or immobility. Patients with behavioral or developmental disability may require examination under anesthesia. Clinicians should advise patients that the examination may be uncomfortable but should not be painful in the absence of a pelvic abnormality. It is important to encourage patients to offer feedback during the examination if they are not comfortable physically or emotionally.[14]

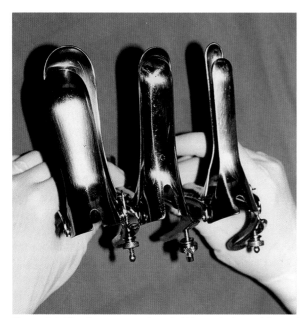

Figure 3.2 The Graves speculum *(left)* is 1.5 inches wide, and the Pederson speculum *(center)* is 1 inch wide. The narrow Pederson speculum *(right)* is 0.75 inches wide and is ideal for placement in a young adolescent to view the vagina and cervix. (Courtesy of Diane F. Merritt, MD, Saint Louis, Missouri.)

PATIENT-CENTERED CARE: Water-based lubricants provide lubrication for the speculum and have not been shown to interfere with either Pap or STI testing.

Physical findings, diagnosis, and treatment, if required, should be addressed with the patient at the conclusion of the examination. Any areas of concern for the patient should be discussed, and education regarding vaccination for human papilloma virus (HPV) and contraception (including emergency and long-acting reversible contraception) should be offered. A conversation between the patient and provider regarding normal pubertal development and menstruation is vital. Instruction on menstrual flow, hygiene, symptoms, duration, and frequency of bleeding should be given. Patients should be encouraged to include caregivers in their planning and decision making.[3]

OTHER REPRODUCTIVE HEALTH CONCERNS TO CONSIDER

Menstruation

The median age at menarche worldwide and within the U.S. population continues to be between 12 and 13 years of age across well-nourished populations in developed countries. According to the U.S. National Health and Nutrition Examination survey, there has been no significant change in the median age of menarche occurring over the past 30 years. One exception was found among non-Hispanic blacks demonstrating a 5.5 month earlier median age of menarche. Higher body mass index during childhood is attributed to earlier onset of puberty. Environmental considerations including socioeconomic conditions, nutrition, and access to preventive health care may influence the timing and progression of puberty.[15] The patient's menstrual cycle should be included as an additional vital sign during primary and reproductive health screenings. Reproductive health visits provide opportunities to educate adolescent females and caregivers on what to expect with the onset of menarche. The range of normal cycle length with subsequent menses should be reviewed.

Menarche on average occurs within 2 to 3 years after thelarche (breast budding) at Tanner stage 4 breast development and rarely before Tanner stage 3 development (see Fig. 2.11 for Tanner stage development). Evaluation for primary amenorrhea should be considered for any adolescent who does not reach menarche by 15 years of age or within 3 years of thelarche. Lack of breast development by 13 years of age should be evaluated.

Irregular menstrual cycles often occur during adolescence, especially during the interval from the first cycle to the second cycle. On average, most females bleed 2 to 7 days during their first menses; 90% of cycles are in the range of 21 to 45 days, though short cycles of less than 20 days and long cycles of more than 45 days may occur. Nearly 80% of menstrual cycles are 21 to 34 days by year 3, typical of an adult pattern.[15]

Adolescent girls may seek medical attention for cycle variations. These variations may fall within normal range or may be attributable to other medical issues. Identification of abnormal menstrual patterns in adolescence may improve early recognition of potential health concerns for adulthood.[15] Dysmenorrhea (painful menses) in adolescent females is associated with absenteeism from school or work and limitation of other daily activities. Medical treatment for dysmenorrhea includes nonsteroidal antiinflammatory drugs (NSAIDs), oral contraceptive pills (OCPs), or surgical intervention. Unresponsiveness to medical treatment for dysmenorrhea may be indicative of underlying pelvic disease and requires further evaluation.[16]

Various medical conditions can cause abnormal uterine bleeding characterized by unpredictable timing and variable amount of flow. Menstrual flow requiring a change of feminine products every 1 to 2 hours is considered excessive and should be evaluated. Adolescents who have amenorrhea (absence of menses) for more than 3 months or 90 days should also be evaluated. Pregnancy, sexual trauma, and STIs should be ruled out in cases of menstrual irregularity or abnormal uterine bleeding.[15]

> **⚠ SAFETY ALERT**
>
> Menstrual flow requiring a change of feminine products every 1 to 2 hours is considered excessive and should be evaluated.

Clinicians should always ask the patient's first day of her last menstrual period and the pattern of menses at every visit. Education on charting of menses may be beneficial if a patient's menstrual history is too vague or considered to be inaccurate. The use of smart phone applications may assist patients with remembering.[15]

Teen Pregnancy

In 2019, teen birth rates in the United States declined to record lows for nearly all age, race, and Hispanic-origin groups. As a result of these declines, particularly with large long-term declines for the groups with higher rates, differences in rates across race and Hispanic-origin groups have narrowed for teenagers 15 to 19 years of age, and for both younger teenagers (15 to 17 years of age) and older teenagers (18 to 19 years of age). Birth rates declined to 11.4% for non-Hispanic White, 29.2% for American Indian or Alaskan Native, 25.8% for non-Hispanic Black, and 25.3% for Hispanic female teenagers 15 to 19 years of age. Levels for Asian or Pacific Islander teenagers remained unchanged. Despite the large declines in teen childbearing outlined in this report, the U.S. birth rate remains higher than in other industrialized countries, and disparities in proportions of teen childbearing by race and Hispanic origin persist (CDC, n.d.a.).

This reinforces the importance of counseling and pregnancy prevention planning as well as the need to have an open dialogue with adolescents at each visit regardless of why the patient is being evaluated.

Contraception

In the United States, 42% of adolescents 15 to 19 years of age have had sexual intercourse. With many reporting some use of contraception during their lifetime, generally the methods selected are least effective. Adolescents commonly use contraceptive methods with higher failure rates including condoms, withdrawal, or OCPs. Failure rates are reflected in the high percentages of unintended adolescent pregnancies in the United States secondary to nonuse and inconsistent use of contraception. In 2011, 75% of adolescent pregnancies were unplanned; this accounts for one-sixth of all unintended pregnancies in the United States, indicating the unmet need for acceptable, reliable, and effective contraceptive methods for female adolescents.[17]

The use of long-acting reversible contraception (LARC) methods including intrauterine devices (IUDs) and the contraceptive implant are safe and appropriate contraceptive methods for adolescents and should be discussed. Providers should encourage adolescent females to consider IUDs and implants because they are the best reversible methods for preventing unintended pregnancy, rapid repeat pregnancy, and abortion in young females.[17]

Short-acting contraceptive methods including condoms, OCPs, the vaginal ring, contraceptive patch, and depot medroxyprogesterone acetate (DMPA) injections continue to be prime choices for adolescent females. Short-acting methods have lower continuation rates and higher pregnancy rates than LARC methods. LARC methods are increasing in popularity, with use increasing from 2.4% of all U.S. females using contraception in 2002 to 8.5% in 2009 to 11.6% in 2012.[18] Approximately 5.8% of females 15 to 19 years of age are currently using a LARC, with the most common choice an IUD. The etonogestrel single-rod contraceptive implant that was approved by the U.S. Food and Drug Administration in 2006 is used by 1.3% of U.S. females using contraception and 2.8% of those 15 to 19 years of age.[17]

Clinicians discussing contraception with patients at the reproductive health visit or primary care visit should include LARCs as first-line safe and reliable forms of contraception and be knowledgeable about concerns adolescents may have. Those concerns may include pain or difficulty with insertion/placement, infertility, expulsion, and side effects including changes in bleeding pattern.[16]

Clinicians should consider barriers to LARCs including cost, which can be a deterrent for use. Adolescents with insurance coverage through their parents may not want to use the benefit secondary to confidentiality concerns. Knowledge of or referral to publicly funded facilities offering LARCs may be necessary, as some adolescents may be uninsured or have insurance that excludes coverage for LARC methods.[17] Health care providers should continue to advise the use of barrier methods (condoms) to decrease the risk of STIs including HIV.

The first reproductive health visit is important for numerous female adolescents. For many, it may serve as an introduction into the health care system. It is vital for adolescents to learn how to navigate and advocate for themselves regarding their specific reproductive health care needs. The initiation of reproductive care affords providers with the opportunity to build patient-centered relationships that can encourage lifelong healthy behaviors.

WELLNESS AND PREVENTIVE HEALTH

Vaccinations

HPV is a very common virus that can lead to cancer. Nearly 42 million people are currently infected with HPV in the United States. Approximately 13 million people, to include teenagers, become infected with HPV annually. About 36,000 people in the United States each year are affected by an HPV-related cancer. Although there is screening available for cervical cancer for females, there is no screening for the other cancers caused by HPV infection like cancers of the mouth/throat, anus/rectum, penis, vagina, or vulva. HPV vaccination provides safe, effective, and lasting protection against the HPV infections that most commonly cause cancer (CDC, n.d.b.).

NOT TO BE MISSED

- HPV vaccine is recommended for routine vaccination at 11 or 12 years of age (vaccination can be started at 9 years of age).
- Vaccination is also recommended for boys and girls 13 to 26 years of age.
- Adolescents should be vaccinated before they are exposed to HPV. However, those who have already been infected with one or more HPV types can still receive protection from other HPV types with the vaccine.[19]

NOT TO BE MISSED

Dosing Schedules for Human Papillomavirus Vaccination

- Two doses of HPV vaccine are recommended for all persons starting the series before their 15th birthday.
- The second dose of HPV vaccine should be given 6 to 12 months after the first dose.
- Adolescents who receive two doses less than 5 months apart will require a third dose of HPV vaccine.
- Three doses of HPV vaccine are recommended for teenagers and young adults who start the series at 15 to 26 years of age and for immunocompromised persons. The recommended three-dose schedule is 0 months, 1 to 2 months, and 6 months. Three doses are recommended for immunocompromised persons (including those with HIV infection) 9 to 26 years of age.[20]

! SAFETY ALERT

Contraindications and Precautions With Human Papillomavirus Vaccination

A severe allergic reaction (e.g., anaphylaxis) to a vaccine component or following a prior dose of HPV vaccine is a contraindication to receive the HPV vaccine.

- 9-valent HPV vaccine is produced in *Saccharomyces cerevisiae* (baker's yeast) and is contraindicated for persons with a history of immediate hypersensitivity to yeast.
- A moderate or severe acute illness is a precaution to vaccination, and vaccination should be deferred until symptoms of the acute illness improve.
- A minor acute illness (e.g., diarrhea or mild upper respiratory tract infection, with or without fever) is not a reason to defer vaccination.
- HPV vaccination is not recommended for use during pregnancy (CDC, n.d.b.).

Other vaccines to consider include the following:

- Influenza vaccine is recommended yearly for adolescents and young adults 11 to 21 years of age.
- All 11- to 12-year-olds should receive a single shot of a quadrivalent meningococcal conjugate vaccine (MenACWY). A booster shot is recommended at 16 years of age.
- Teenagers 16 to 18 years of age may be vaccinated with a meningococcal vaccine.
- Adolescents 11 to 12 years of age should receive one dose of tetanus, diphtheria, and acellular pertussis

(Tdap) vaccine. Females should get a Tdap vaccine during every pregnancy, preferably during gestational weeks 27 to 36. A tetanus and diphtheria (Td) booster is recommended every 10 years.[21]

Primary Care

Bright Futures outlines the screening and physical assessment needed for adolescents 11 to 21 years of age in addition to reproductive health. The following sections outline both universal and select screening.[22] Hearing screening with audiometry should be conducted once between 11 and 14 years of age, once between 15 and 17 years of age, and once between 18 and 21 years of age. Oral health care should include identification of a dental provider at the well visit. Dyslipidemia screening should occur once between 9 and 11 years of age and once between 17 and 21 years of age.

ISSUES AFFECTING FEMALE ADOLESCENTS

Alcohol, Tobacco, and Substance Abuse

The use of alcohol, tobacco, and other drugs is a leading cause of injury and death for adolescents. In comparison with nonsmoking females, females who smoke tobacco have a greater risk for reproductive health problems, gynecological and other cancer types, coronary/vascular disease, chronic obstructive lung disease, and osteoporosis.[23] Misuse of prescription drugs is highest among adults 18 to 25 years of age, with 2.2% of youth 12 to 17 years of age reporting nonmedical use of prescription drugs. Perception of risk versus benefit, social approval versus disapproval, and the availability of drugs within communities are key factors influencing adolescent substance use. The influence of alcohol or other drugs places adolescents at increased risk for unprotected sexual activity and interpersonal violence.[1]

Screening and Intervention

Clinicians should obtain information from adolescents during their visit regarding whether they or their friends have ever tried/used tobacco, alcohol, or other drugs. The USPSTF recommends that clinicians screen adults 18 years of age and older for alcohol misuse and provide those engaged in risky or hazardous drinking with brief behavioral counseling interventions to reduce alcohol misuse.[24] The USPSTF recommends that clinicians provide interventions, including education or brief counseling, to prevent initiation of tobacco use in school-age children and adolescents.

> **PATIENT-CENTERED CARE:** The USPSTF recommends that clinicians screen adults 18 years of age and older for alcohol misuse and provide those engaged in risky or hazardous drinking with brief behavioral counseling interventions to reduce alcohol misuse.

Peer Relationships and Interpersonal Violence

Bullying is often associated with poor school adjustment and academic success. There are multiple forms of bullying. These include verbal, physical, relational, extortion, and cyberbullying. Bullying rarely occurs in private settings, therefore health care professionals who suspect that a patient is being bullied or witness bullying should encourage disclosure.[1]

Providers should counsel adolescents about healthy relationships and discuss coercive and abusive relationships with intimate partners. Adolescents with disabilities are more likely to be sexually abused because of dependence on others for intimate care and increased exposure to various caregivers and settings.[1]

> **! SAFETY ALERT**
>
> Adolescents with disabilities are more likely to be sexually abused because of dependence on others for intimate care and increased exposure to various caregivers and settings.

The USPSTF recommends that clinicians screen females of childbearing age for intimate partner violence, such as domestic violence, and provide or refer females who screen positive to intervention services. This recommendation applies to females who do not have signs or symptoms of abuse.[25]

Mental Health

Bright Futures informs that 1 in 5 teenagers experiences significant symptoms of emotional distress, and 1 in 10 is emotionally impaired with a common mental health disorder including depression, attention-deficit/hyperactivity disorder (ADHD), anxiety, and substance use disorder. One-half of all lifetime cases of mental health disorder begin by 14 years of age, with three-fourths

manifesting by 24 years of age.[1] Suicide is the third leading cause of death for adolescents. The CDC Youth Risk Behavior Surveillance System (YRBSS) from 2013 showed that 17% of high school students reported seriously considering attempting suicide; 13.6% had a plan made, and 8.0% had made a suicide attempt with attempts being almost twice as high among girls in comparison with boys.[1] The burden is highest in low- and middle-income countries. Depression is associated with substantial present and future morbidity. The strongest risk factors for depression in adolescents are a family history of depression and exposure to psychosocial stress.[26]

Screening and Referral

One useful screening tool for adolescents is *The Patient Health Questionnaire-2* (PHQ-2), which is used to screen adolescents for depression (Table 3.2). A study that was conducted on 499 individuals 13 to 17 years of age who were enrolled in an integrated health care system and participated in a full assessment using the PHQ-2, the PHQ-9 (Patient Health Questionnaire 9-item depression screen), and a structured mental health interview (Diagnostic Interview Schedule for Children) revealed that participants with a PHQ-2 score ≥3 had a sensitivity of 74% and specificity of 75% for detecting youth who met criteria for major depression in the *Diagnostic and Statistical Manual of Mental Disorders,* fourth edition.[27] The PHQ-2 has good sensitivity and specificity for detecting major depression. These properties, coupled with the brief nature of the instrument, make this tool promising as a first step for screening for adolescent depression in primary care.[27] Screening is not diagnostic, and clinicians must be able to communicate openly with patients. Mental wellness should be assessed at each visit.

> **CLINICAL SURVIVAL TIP** Clinicians must be able to communicate openly with patients, and mental wellness should be assessed at each visit.

Providers referring for mental health services based on screening results should initiate the process early and address the concerns of the patient and family, including stigmas often associated with receiving services. Discussion of cultural views regarding mental health and wellness may affect acceptance and should be acknowledged to enhance the success of the referral process.[1]

TABLE 3.2   The Patient Health Questionnaire-2 (PHQ-2)*

Over the past *2 weeks,* how often have you been bothered by any of the following problems?	Not At All	Several Days	More Than Half the Days	Nearly Every Day
1. Little interest or pleasure in doing things	0	1	2	3
2. Feeling down, depressed, or hopeless	0	1	2	3

Proposed Treatment Actions: The PHQ-2 consists of the first two questions of the PHQ-9. Scores range from 0 to 6. The recommended cut point is a score of 3 or greater. Recommended actions for persons scoring 3 or higher are *one* of the following:
• Administer the full PHQ-9.
• Conduct a clinical interview to assess for major depressive disorder.

For office coding: _____ 0_____ +_____ +_____ +_____ = Total Score _____
Modified from Kroenke K, Spitzer RL, Williams JB. The Patient Health Questionnaire-2: Validity of a Two-Item Depression Screener. *Med Care.* 2003;41(11):1284–1292; Kroenke K, Spitzer RL, Williams JB, Lowe B. The Patient Health Questionnaire Somatic, Anxiety, and Depressive Symptom Scales: a systematic review. *Gen Hosp Psychiatry.* 2010;32(4):345–359; The Patient Health Questionnaire (PHQ) Screeners. https://www.phqscreeners.com/ (see website for additional information and translations).

KEY POINTS

• Adolescence marks the period from 11 to 21 years of age.
• Adolescence is a dynamic period of development, with rapid changes in body size, shape, and composition.
• The leading causes of death among adolescents in 2019 were road injury, suicide, and interpersonal violence.
• The initial screening for reproductive preventive health care services and guidance should occur between 13 and 15 years of age.
• Confidentiality is vital to adolescent care and should be discussed with both the adolescent and caregiver before examination.
• Menarche and subsequent menses are physiologically and emotionally important milestones for female adolescents.
• A discussion regarding pregnancy prevention/contraception and STIs is crucial.
• Confidentiality is vital to adolescent care and should be discussed with both the adolescent and caregiver before examination.
• The initial reproductive visit is also an appropriate time to screen for high-risk behaviors including substance abuse, tobacco use, and alcohol use.

• The use of LARC methods including IUDs and the contraceptive implant are safe and appropriate contraceptive methods for adolescents and should be discussed.
• HPV is a very common virus that can lead to cancer.
• Routine HPV vaccination is recommended at 11 or 12 years of age (vaccination can be started at 9 years of age).
• 1 in 5 teenagers experience significant symptoms of emotional distress, and 1 in 10 is emotionally impaired with a common mental health disorder including depression, ADHD, anxiety, and substance use disorder.

REFERENCES

1. Hagan J, Shaw J, Duncan P. *Bright Futures: Guidelines for Health Supervision of Infants, Children and Adolescents.* Elk Grove Village, IL: American Academy of Pediatrics; 2017.
2. Strasburger Victor C, et al. *Adolescent Medicine: A Handbook for Primary Care.* Wolters Kluwer Health; 2017.
3. American College of Obstetricians and Gynecologists (ACOG). *Committee Opinion Number 811: Committee on Adolescent Health Care. The Initial Reproductive Health Visit;* 2020. https://www.acog.org/clinical/clinical-guidance/committee-opinion/articles/2020/10/the-initial-reproductive-health-visit.

4. American College of Obstetricians and Gynecologists (ACOG). *Committee Opinion Number 803: Committee on Adolescent Health Care. Confidentiality in Adolescent Health Care*; 2020. https://www.acog.org/clinical/clinical-guidance/committee-opinion/articles/2020/04/confidentiality-in-adolescent-health-care.

5. Birdsall R. *Contraception & Menstrual Management*; 2020. https://www.medicalhomeportal.org/clinical-practice/common-issues-for-cyshcn/contraception-and-menstrual-management.

6. American College of Obstetricians and Gynecologists (ACOG). *Committee Opinion Number 582: Committee on Adolescent Health Care and Committee on Gynecologic Practice. Addressing Health Risks of Noncoital Sexual Activity.* (December 2013, Reaffirmed 2020). https://www.acog.org/clinical/clinical-guidance/committee-opinion/articles/2013/12/addressing-health-risks-of-noncoital-sexual-activity.

7. Guttmacher Institute. *Adolescent Sexual and Reproductive Health in the United States.* (September 2019). https://www.guttmacher.org/fact-sheet/american-teens-sexual-and-reproductive-health?gclid=Cj0KCQiA-eeMBhCpARIsAAZfxZBHwMdsrR9q1RYj5QpkIY4gtLG7AKUsdvs32wsVmpjIBxQDGh1XmzIaAp6CEALw_wcB#.

8. Houck CD, Barker D, Rizzo C, Hancock E, Norton A, Brown LK. Sexting and sexual behavior in at-risk adolescents. *Pediatrics.* 2014;133(2):e276–e282.

9. Shulman EP, Smith AR, Silva K, et al. The dual systems model: Review, reappraisal, and reaffirmation. *Dev Cogn Neurosci.* 2016;17:103–117.

10. Scal P. Improving health care transition services: just grow up, will you please. *JAMA Pediatr.* 2016;170(3):197–199.

11. U.S. Preventive Services Task Force (USPSTF). *Cervical Cancer: Screening.* 2018a. https://www.uspreventiveservicestaskforce.org/uspstf/recommendation/cervical-cancer-screening.

12. Centers for Disease Control and Prevention (CDC). *Table 1. Recommended Child and Adolescent Immunization Schedule for Ages 18 Years or Younger, United States, 2021.* 2021. https://www.cdc.gov/vaccines/schedules/hcp/imz/child-adolescent.html#.

13. U.S. Preventive Services Task Force (USPSTF). *Human immunodeficiency virus (HIV) Infection: Screening*; 2019. https://www.uspreventiveservicestaskforce.org/uspstf/recommendation/human-immunodeficiency-virus-hiv-infection-screening#bootstrap-panel--6.

14. Braverman PK, Breech L, Committee on Adolescence. American Academy of Pediatrics. Clinical report—gynecologic examination for adolescents in the pediatric office setting. *Pediatrics.* 2010;126(3):583–590.

15. American College of Obstetricians and Gynecologists (ACOG). *Committee Opinion Number 651: Committee on Adolescent Health Care. Menstruation in Girls and Adolescents: Using the Menstrual Cycle as a Vital Sign.* (December 2015, Reaffirmed 2020). https://www.acog.org/clinical/clinical-guidance/committee-opinion/articles/2015/12/menstruation-in-girls-and-adolescents-using-the-menstrual-cycle-as-a-vital-sign.

16. Vincenzo De Sanctis MD, Soliman A, Bernasconi S, et al. Primary dysmenorrhea in adolescents: prevalence, impact and recent knowledge. *Pediatr Endocrinol Rev (PER).* 2015;13(2):512–520.

17. American College of Obstetricians and Gynecologists (ACOG). *Committee Opinion Number 735: Adolescents and Long-Acting Reversible Contraception: Implants and Intrauterine Devices.* (May 2018, Reaffirmed 2021). https://www.acog.org/clinical/clinical-guidance/committee-opinion/articles/2018/05/adolescents-and-long-acting-reversible-contraception-implants-and-intrauterine-devices.

18. American College of Obstetricians and Gynecologists (ACOG). *Committee Opinion Number 186: Committee on Practice Bulletins-Gynecology. Long-Acting Reversible Contraception: Implants and Intrauterine Devices.* (November 2017, Reaffirmed 2021). https://www.acog.org/clinical/clinical-guidance/practice-bulletin/articles/2017/11/long-acting-reversible-contraception-implants-and-intrauterine-devices.

19. Centers for Disease Control and Prevention (CDC). (n.d.b.). *Human Papillomavirus (HPV) Vaccination & Cancer Prevention.* https://www.cdc.gov/vaccines/vpd/hpv/.

20. Meites E, Kempe A, Markowitz LE. Use of a 2–dose schedule for human papillomavirus vaccination—updated recommendations of the Advisory Committee on Immunization Practices. *Am J Transplant.* 2017;17(3):834–837.

21. Centers for Disease Control and Prevention (CDC). *Sexually Transmitted Infections Treatment Guidelines, 2021*;2021. https://www.cdc.gov/std/treatment-guidelines/screening-recommendations.htm.

22. *Bright Futures/American Academy of Pediatrics.* Periodicity Schedule; 2021. https://downloads.aap.org/AAP/PDF/periodicity_schedule.pdf.

23. American College of Obstetricians and Gynecologists (ACOG). *Committee Opinion Number 503: Committee on Health Care for Underserved Women. Tobacco Use and Women's Health.* (September 2011, Reaffirmed 2017). https://www.acog.org/clinical/clinical-guidance/committee-opinion/articles/2011/09/tobacco-use-and-womens-health.

24. U.S. Preventive Services Task Force (USPSTF). *Unhealthy Alcohol Use in Adolescents and Adults: Screening and Behavioral Counseling Interventions*; 2018b. https://www.uspreventiveservicestaskforce.org/uspstf/recommendation/unhealthy-alcohol-use-in-adolescents-and-adults-screening-and-behavioral-counseling-interventions.

25. U.S. Preventive Services Task Force (USPSTF). *Intimate Partner Violence, Elder Abuse, and Abuse of Vulnerable Adults: Screening*; 2018c. https://www.uspreventiveservicestaskforce.org/uspstf/recommendation/intimate-partner-violence-and-abuse-of-elderly-and-vulnerable-adults-screening.

26. Thapar A, Collishaw S, Pine DS, Thapar AK. Depression inadolescence. *Lancet.* 2012;379(9820):1056–1067.

27. Richardson LP, Rockhill C, Russo JE, et al. Evaluation of the PHQ-2 as a brief screen for detecting major depression among adolescents. *Pediatrics.* 2010;125(5):e1097–e1103.

28. Merritt DF. Genital trauma in the pediatric and adolescent female. *Obstet Gynecol Clin North Am.* 2009;36(1):85–98.

4

Older Women's Health

Carolyn Clevenger and Mariya Kovaleva

OBJECTIVES

- Describe the aging population as it relates to women.
- Examine interventions to maintain a woman's mobility, independence in activities of daily living (ADLs) and instrumental activities of daily living (IADLs), and safety.
- Develop a plan of care for the assessment of the geriatric woman that includes frailty, cognitive impairment, and polypharmacy.

- Design a plan of care for the caregiver that includes assessment and intervention to assist with the caregiver role.
- Explore women as caregivers of the aging population.

INTRODUCTION

By 2040, the cluster of the U.S. population 65 years of age and older will increase to up to 80.8 million, accounting for over 20% of the population. By 2060, the population of Americans 65 years of age and older will be 94.7 million, just short of double the population of 52.4 million of the same age cluster in 2018. Older females outnumber older males at 29.1 to 23.3 million. It is imperative to consider the unique health care needs of this population, including those of older females. The population estimates of older adults project females as the majority sex with a gap that increases with age groups, so females comprise 55.3% of the oldest old (85 years of age and older).[1]

Increases in the aging population yield opportunities and challenges. Studies find that older adults have greater emotional stability, reporting fewer negative emotions and lability than younger counterparts.[2] They get along with more people. They often bring experience to complex tasks and thus demonstrate superior problem-solving abilities.[2] On the other hand, rates of chronic disease and disability increase with age, challenging clinicians to meet the health care needs of the aging population.

As of 2018, among Medicare fee-for-service beneficiaries, the percentage of females living with at least two chronic conditions exceeds that of males (Fig. 4.1). Common chronic conditions include diabetes, cardiovascular disease, chronic obstructive pulmonary disease, asthma, cancer, and arthritis.[3] Additionally, despite the neurotrophic and neuroprotective role of estrogen in brain function, the incidence of Alzheimer's disease is higher in females than in males.[4]

NOT TO BE MISSED

The risk for most chronic conditions increases with age, and the conditions are not mutually exclusive.

DEMOGRAPHICS AND POPULATION HEALTH TRENDS

Compared with males, older females are more likely to be single, live alone, and live in poverty.[1] In addition to differences in these social determinants of health, there is a significant contrast in the overall burden and susceptibility to certain chronic diseases. Although testosterone-induced immunosuppression[5] confers higher immune

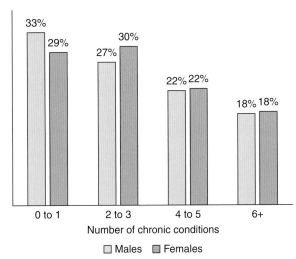

Figure 4.1 Distribution of American males and females according to the number of chronic conditions that they have. (Data from Centers for Medicare and Medicaid Services. *Chartbook and Charts.* https://www.cms.gov/Research-Statistics-Data-and-Systems/Statistics-Trends-and-Reports/Chronic-Conditions/Chartbook_Charts.)

functioning to females than males, it makes females more susceptible to autoimmune disease. Additionally, males are more susceptible to illnesses that may be immediately fatal rather than illnesses that follow a long-term trajectory.[6] For instance, the incidence of myocardial infarction or fatal coronary heart disease is greater among males after 45 years of age.[7] Females, however, are more vulnerable to the morbidity of chronic conditions and to the insidious syndrome of frailty.[8] Females have a higher prevalence of asthma[9] and arthritis;[10] males have a higher prevalence of heart disease,[7] cancer,[11] and diabetes.[12] Finally, life expectancy at 65 years of age remains highest for females. Females who are 65 years of age can expect to live another 20.5 years (2.5 years longer than males). At 85 years of age, females can expect to live another 7 years (1.1 years longer than males).[13]

> **PATIENT-CENTERED CARE:** Males are more susceptible to immediately fatal illnesses, and females are more likely to suffer from chronic conditions. Females tend to live longer than males.

The greater frailty risk for females may stem from their likelihood of suffering from mental illness: their lifetime risk of developing depression and/or anxiety is higher than that for males. Importantly, in middle and late adulthood, depressive symptoms are associated with poor functioning, well-being, and health perception. Depressive symptoms typically contribute more toward dysfunction and poor health perception than chronic conditions, cognitive impairment, and visual and hearing problems.[14] Anxiety and/or depression often lead to prescription of benzodiazepines, which may contribute to falls and injuries,[6] leading to frailty. Depressive symptoms and antidepressant use are also associated with frailty among females 65 to 79 years of age.[15] However, a comparison of mental health in males and females calls for the notion of reporting bias. In western society, males are socialized to emphasize instrumental abilities, self-efficacy, efficiency, assertiveness, and goal orientation (which may cause their underreporting of depression or anxiety).[16]

COMPREHENSIVE GERIATRIC ASSESSMENT

The value of the comprehensive assessment extends beyond an accurate depiction of the older adult's status and prognosis. Care planned for older adults should center on their ability to care for themselves and interact with their world independently. Both longevity and quality of life depend on these factors. In the care of older adults, the clinician walks a fine line between overly aggressive interventions and clinical inertia. Each end of the spectrum is dangerous and represents poor clinical care.

The typical physical examination, social history, and psychosocial background together may not yield a complete—or helpful—assessment of the aging patient's well-being. Assessment of function and engagement allow the clinician to offer meaningful and helpful interventions that improve the quality of care and provide care in line with the patient's values and goals.

A review of valid measures for function, mobility, cognition, and mood is included in this chapter. Many measures inform the care plan by defining the prognosis and the relevance and appropriateness of interventions. Although advance care planning is part of primary care for all patients (not only older adults), planning becomes more specific when informed by data gleaned from these assessments (Box 4.1).

Mobility

Measures of physical mobility take little time, can be obtained by office staff during the rooming process, and

BOX 4.1   **Components of the Comprehensive Geriatric Assessment**

A comprehensive geriatric assessment includes the following measures:
- Mobility
- Function
- Cognition
- Mood

! **SAFETY ALERT**

The longevity and quality of life for an older female patient depends on a care plan that centers on her ability to care for self and interact with the world independently.

BOX 4.2   **Gait Speed Assessment**

- If possible, use a computerized gait mat to assess several gait parameters (speed, variability, balance, and acceleration)
- Use a stopwatch
- Instruct the person to walk at a usual pace from the starting point to the point of 3 m (10 feet). After this instruction is provided, do not give additional instructions or encouragement[17]
- Conduct three attempts
- The average of three attempts represents the final result of gait speed
- Use of assistive devices is acceptable
- Consult publications/free applications for age and sex norms for gait speed

require little or no special equipment. A powerful measure of vitality is gait speed. Gait speed represents the overall function of the cardiopulmonary, musculoskeletal, and neurological systems. Any of these areas are targets for intervention, and evidence suggests that improvements in gait speed increase the likelihood of 5-year survival. Compared with lengthier measures to evaluate overall well-being and vitality of older adults, use of just three factors—age, sex, and gait speed—is nearly equivalent to more complex tools used to predict survival.[17]

A simple stopwatch and marked path provides the information on overall mortality risk. Instructions are provided to walk at usual pace from the starting point to the point of 3 m (10 feet). A final score is calculated based the average of three attempts. Use of assistive devices is acceptable (Box 4.2). Age and sex norms are readily available in publications and in many free applications. A more comprehensive measure of mobility includes metrics of speed, variability, balance, and acceleration, which requires a computerized gait mat. The results of such assessment provide detailed information to inform intervention by physiotherapists.

Falls are the leading cause of accidental death among older adults.[18] To assess balance and fall risk, the clinician may conduct the Timed Up and Go Test.[19] This screening tool evaluates fall risk with enough detail to allow for a meaningful intervention by the clinician. The measure is completed with use of a chair and marked line at 3 m (10 feet). A standard scoring sheet and stopwatch are required for completion. The patient is instructed to rise from the chair, walk at usual pace to

the designated line, turn, walk back to the chair at usual pace, and sit down.

The scoring sheet is shown in Table 4.1. The clinician should carefully review the scoring sheet for specific assessments and potential interventions. Differences in performance on each component of the test may be relevant and provide guidance on the appropriate interventions. Potential interventions for slow walking speed can be found earlier in the chapter in the discussion of gait speed. Loss of balance during turning may indicate further evaluation of vestibular function, and the patient may respond to Tai Chi, which has demonstrated improvements in balance.[20] The inability to rise from a chair without support indicates an opportunity for improving joint flexibility or muscle strength, and referral for physical therapy may be indicated. A time over 12 seconds indicates an increased fall risk.[19]

Information on these and other fall risk measures and guidance on interventions to reduce fall risk can be found in the Centers for Disease Control and Prevention (CDC) STEADI toolkit.[21] Measures of mobility and strength have implications for the concept of frailty, discussed later in this chapter.

CLINICAL SURVIVAL TIP Gait speed, balance, and fall risks may be assessed in clinical settings with minimal equipment and using scoring sheets provided at the end of this chapter or on the CDC website: https://www.cdc.gov/steadi/pdf/steadi_tool_kit_materials_handout-a.pdf.

TABLE 4.1	Scoring Sheet for the Test of Walking Speed and the Timed Up and Go Test	
Direction	**Result**	**Result**
Gait Speed Assessment		
1. Follow directions in Table 1	Record gait speed: m/s	Faster than 1.2 m/s suggests exceptional life expectancy Faster than 1.0 m/s suggests more favorable outcomes Slower than 0.6 m/s suggests higher probability of impaired health and function
The Timed Up and Go Test 1. Use a stopwatch Patients must wear their regular shoes and may use a walking aid if needed.		
2. The test begins with the patient sitting back in a standard chair.		
3. Identify a point that is 3 m (10 feet) away from the chair.		

4. Give the following instructions to the patient: When I say "go," please:
  a. Stand up
  b. At your normal pace, walk to the line on the floor
  c. Then turn
  d. At your normal pace, walk back to the chair
  e. Sit down		

5. Timing starts when you say "Go."		
6. After the patient sits back down, stop the stopwatch and record the time in seconds.	Record time: seconds	12 seconds or longer suggests the patient is at high risk for falling
7. While the patient is completing the task, observe sway, stride length, gait, and postural stability.		
8. Check all that apply:	a. Slow hesitant pace b. Balance loss c. Short strides d. Little to no arm swing e. Uses walls to steady self f. Shuffling gait g. Turning with the entire body at once h. Unable to use walking aids properly	
9. Summarize all findings to make a conclusion about the patient's fall risk. Counsel the patient and family accordingly.		

Modified from Centers for Disease Control and Prevention. The Timed Up and Go (TUG) Test. https://www.cdc.gov/steadi/pdf/TUG_Test-print.pdf; Cesari M, Kritchevsky SB, Penninx BW, et al. Prognostic value of usual gait speed in well-functioning older people—results from the Health, Aging and Body Composition Study. *J Am Geriatr Soc.* 2005;53(10):1675–1680; Studenski S, Perera S, Wallace D, et al. Physical performance measures in the clinical setting. *J Am Geriatr Soc.* 2003;51(3):314–322.

Function

Measures of function include one's ability to perform basic activities of daily living (ADLs) and instrumental activities of daily living (IADLs) and interact with their environment. IADLs (light and heavy housework, preparing meals, using the telephone, driving) are measured on an eight-point scale, with higher scores indicating higher independence. ADLs (bathing, transferring, toileting oneself) are measures on a six-point scale, with higher scores indicating higher independence. Standardized tools include the Katz[22] (Table 4.2) and Lawton-Brody[23-29] (Table 4.3) scales, which list activities and degrees of dependence.

Given the nature of functional assessment—one's daily interactions with their environment—the measures are typically self- or informant-reported and based on typical behavior patterns. Scoring of these tools is especially helpful with repeated measurement to observe for overall progression. Often ADL/IADL behaviors reported by the individual represent an overestimation of independence. Likewise, the ADL/IADL behaviors reported by an informant often represent an underestimation of independence. The clinician may include follow-up or clarifying questions to add value to the instrument's raw score. Again, the value of this score lies in comparison with previous performance in the same individual.

The Life Space Assessment (LSA) is a global measure of an individual's interaction with their environment including the immediate home as well as community.[30] Although less commonly administered in primary care, this measure has several compelling features to support its use. The measure is self-reported, requiring no office staff time or space to administer. It is not afflicted with the ceiling effect that occurs with ADL/IADL measures, especially among community-dwelling older adults. The measure is sensitive enough to account for the use of an assistive device or another person. The LSA overall score and change in score predicts mortality as short as 6 months. In addition to mortality and prognostication, the results demonstrate the influence of social factors on the older adult's mobility. It also measures the impact and burden of the individual's morbidity and symptom severity beyond the presence or absence of chronic conditions.

TABLE 4.2	**Activities of Daily Living**	
Circle the response option that corresponds to the patient's ability.		
Activity	**Independent**	**Dependent**
	Does not require supervision, personal assistance, or direction	Requires supervision, personal assistance, direction, or total care
Bathing	(1 point) Bathes self completely or needs help in bathing only in a single part of the body such as the back, genital area, or disabled extremity	(0 points) Needs help with bathing more than one part of the body, getting in or out of the tub or shower. Requires total bathing
Dressing	(1 point) Gets clothes from closets and drawers and puts on clothes and outer garments complete with fasteners	(0 points) Needs help with dressing self or needs to be completely dressed
Toileting	(1 point) Goes to toilet, gets on and off, arranges clothes, cleanses genital area without help	(0 points) Needs help transferring to the toilet, and cleansing self, or uses bedpan or commode
Transferring	(1 point) Moves in and out of bed or chair unassisted. Mechanical transferring aids are acceptable	(0 points) Needs help in moving from bed to chair or requires a complete transfer
Continence	(1 point) Exercises complete self-control over urination and defecation	(0 points) Is partially or totally incontinent of bowel and bladder
Feeding	(1 point) Gets food from plate into mouth without help. Preparation of food may be done by another person	(0 points) Needs partial or total help with feeding or requires parenteral feeding
Calculate total points	_____ points	6—Patient is independent 0—Patient is very dependent

Modified from Katz S, Down TD, Cash HR, Grotz RC. Progress in the development of the index of ADL. *Gerontologist.* 1970;10(1):20-30; Shelkey M, Wallace M. Katz Index of Independence in Activities of Daily Living. *J Gerontol Nurs.* 1999;25(3):8–9.

TABLE 4.3 Instrumental Activities of Daily Living[23-29]

Circle the response option that corresponds to the patient's ability.

Ability to Use Telephone

1. Operates telephone on own initiative (e.g., looks up and dials numbers).	1
2. Dials a few well-known numbers.	1
3. Answers telephone, but does not dial.	1
4. Does not use telephone at all.	0

Shopping

1. Takes care of all shopping needs independently.	1
2. Shops independently for small purchases.	0
3. Must be accompanied on any shopping trip.	0
4. Completely unable to shop.	0

Food Preparation

1. Plans, prepares, and serves adequate meals independently.	1
2. Prepares adequate meals if supplied with ingredients.	0
3. Heats and serves prepared meals, or prepares meals but does not maintain adequate diet.	0
4. Needs to have meals prepared and served.	0

Housekeeping

1. Maintains the house alone or with occasional assistance (e.g., "heavy-work domestic help").	1
2. Performs light daily tasks such as dishwashing and bed making.	1
3. Performs light daily tasks, but cannot maintain acceptable level of cleanliness.	1
4. Needs help with all home maintenance tasks.	1
5. Does not participate in any housekeeping tasks.	0

Laundry

1. Does personal laundry completely.	1
2. Launders small items (e.g., rinses socks, stockings)	1
3. All laundry must be done by others.	0

Mode of Transportation

1. Travels independently on public transportation or drives own car.	1
2. Arranges own travel via taxi, but does not otherwise use public transportation.	1
3. Travels on public transportation when assisted or accompanied by another.	1
4. Travel limited to taxi or automobile with assistance of another.	0
5. Does not travel.	0

Responsibility for Own Medications

1. Is responsible for taking medication in correct dosages at correct time.	1
2. Takes responsibility if medication is prepared in advance in separate dosages.	0
3. Is not capable of dispensing own medication.	0

Ability to Handle Finances

1. Manages financial matters independently (budgets, writes checks, pays rent and bills), collects and keeps track of income.	1
2. Manages day-to-day purchases, but needs help with banking, major purchases, and so on.	0
3. Incapable of handling money.	0

Calculate total score by adding scores in the sub-scales:
Higher score corresponds to the greater level of independence

The LSA is based on an individual's mobility through their home and community over a 4-week period preceding the assessment. The questionnaire asks about the distance an individual travels from their "home base," conceptualized as the bed or bedroom, the frequency with which one makes the travel, and the level of assistance required to do so (Fig. 4.2). The composite score ranges from 0 to 120 with higher scores indicating higher mobility. The scores can be normalized for age, as age-related decline can be seen in population reports. The clinical value for the individual patient lies in changes over time, with a 10-point change representing a clinically meaningful decline. The LSA can be performed as often as every 6 months or annually, possibly as part of an annual wellness visit (Table 4.4). These assessments can be considered in hierarchy—with dependence in basic ADLs as being most disabled. Given the hierarchical nature of the measures, the tool choice may be made based on appropriateness. All community-dwelling older adults are appropriate candidates for LSA, whereas ADL/IADL assessments provide little value in patients whose only affiliation with "geriatrics" is their chronological age.

Frailty

The term *frailty* lacks a single accepted definition. Broadly, it represents "a multidimensional syndrome of loss of reserves (energy, physical ability, cognition, health) that gives rise to vulnerability."[31] Frailty is associated with advancing age[32] and risks for morbidity, disability, falls, hospitalization, institutionalization, and mortality.[33] Frailty is separate from disability as "a biologic syndrome of decreased reserve and resistance to stressors, resulting from cumulative declines across multiple physiologic systems, and causing vulnerability to adverse outcomes."[34] Frailty markers include low activity and a decline in strength, endurance, walking performance, balance, and lean body mass (Box 4.3). Several parameters must be present simultaneously for an individual to be considered frail.[35]

> **CLINICAL SURVIVAL TIP** The patient's performance in ADLs and IADLs should be measured with the standardized tools. The score may be supplemented by commentary from the patient and/or caregiver. The patient's function should be assessed objectively and not derived from the clinician's "intuition" or caregiver's report alone.

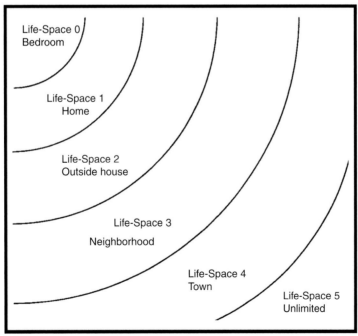

Life-Space 0
Bedroom

Life-Space 1
Home

Life-Space 2
Outside house

Life-Space 3
Neighborhood

Life-Space 4
Town

Life-Space 5
Unlimited

Figure 4.2 Conceptual model of life-space levels. (From Peel C, Sawyer Baker P, Roth DL, Brown CJ, Brodner EV, Allman RM. Assessing mobility in older adults: the UAB Study of Aging Life-Space Assessment. *Phys Ther.* 2005;85[10]:1008–1119)

TABLE 4.4   Life-Space Assessment Worksheet

Life-Space Level	Frequency			Independence		Score
During the past four weeks have you been to	How often did you get there?			Did you use aids or equipment? Did you need help from another person?		Level X Frequency X Independence
Life-Space Level 1 . . . Other rooms of your home besides the room where you sleep?	Yes 1 / No 0	Less than 1/ week	1–3 times/ week	4–6 times/ week	Daily	1 = Personal assistance 1.5 = Equipment only 2 = No equipment or personal assistance
Score						Level 1 Score
Life-Space Level 2 . . . An area outside your home such as your porch, desk or patio, hallway (of an apartment building) or garage, in your own yard or driveway?	Yes 1 / No 0	Less than 1/ week	1–3 times/ week	4–6 times/ week	Daily	1 = Personal assistance 1.5 = Equipment only 2 = No equipment or personal assistance
Score						Level 2 Score
Life-Space Level 3 . . . Places in your neighborhood, other than your own yard or apartment building?	Yes 1 / No 0	Less than 1/ week	1–3 times/ week	4–6 times/ week	Daily	1 = Personal assistance 1.5 = Equipment only 2 = No equipment or personal assistance
Score						Level 3 Score
Life-Space Level 4 . . . Places outside your neighborhood, but within your town?	Yes 1 / No 0	Less than 1/ week	1–3 times/ week	4–6 times/ week	Daily	1 = Personal assistance 1.5 = Equipment only 2 = No equipment or personal assistance
Score						Level 4 Score
Life-Space Level 5 . . . Places outside your town?	Yes 1 / No 0	Less than 1/ week	1–3 times/ week	4–6 times/ week	Daily	1 = Personal assistance 1.5 = Equipment only 2 = No equipment or personal assistance
Score						Level 5 Score
Total Score	Add subscores for the five levels					Total Score

Modified from Peel C, Sawyer Baker P, Roth DL, Brown CJ, Bodner EV, Allman RM. Assessing mobility in older adults: the UAB Study of Aging Life-Space Assessment. *Phys Ther.* 2005;85(10):1008–1119.

In a landmark study, frailty was defined as a clinical syndrome in which at least three of the following five criteria were met: self-reported exhaustion, unintentional weight loss (10 lbs. in the past year), weakness as measured by grip strength, low physical activity, and slow walking speed. Criteria were differentiated for males and females for the last three parameters. Frailty was associated with Black race ethnicity, being female, being older, having less education and lower income, and having more comorbidities and disability. Frail individuals had significantly higher rates of pulmonary and cardiovascular diseases, diabetes, arthritis, and depressive symptomatology as well as lower cognition.[34]

Frailty affects health and well-being. The phenotype independently predicts risk of hospitalization, falls, worsening disability in ADLs and mobility, and death.[34] This set of characteristics (self-reported exhaustion, weakness, slow walking speed, unintentional weight loss, and low physical activity) has received the term the *Fried phenotype*. The Fried phenotype is currently the most frequently used operational definition of frailty in research studies.[36]

Frailty is more common in females than in males,[37] no matter how *frailty* is defined. Although females live longer than males, they are more likely to have poor health. It is difficult to identify factors that cause a higher prevalence of frailty among females, but proposed risks include their higher rates of autoimmune disorders, mental health concerns with subsequent exposure to treatments,[38] and rates of abdominal obesity leading to increased inflammation.[39]

NOT TO BE MISSED

The frequency of frailty and the opportunity for meaningful intervention make it an important concept for the clinician to recognize, treat, and/or minimize its repercussions. Frailty is not inevitable.

Standardized Tool to Measure Frailty

Similar to the importance of using instruments to screen for functional status, it is critical to rely on evidence to determine one's frailty status, rather than attribute frailty merely to the patient's appearance. In case of frailty, the Fried frailty phenotype[34] serves as a screening tool (Table 4.5). According to the Fried phenotype, individuals are grouped into three categories: *robust* (without frailty characteristics); *intermediate frailty*, or *prefrail* (one or two characteristics out of the five in the phenotype); and *frail* (at least three characteristics in the phenotype). Although those who are frail are at the highest risk for the adverse outcomes stated earlier, those who are prefrail are at intermediate risk for these outcomes. Furthermore, prefrail individuals have an over two times

---

BOX 4.3   Frailty Markers*

- Weakness
- Slow gait
- Fatigue
- Weight loss
- Low physical activity
- Declines in endurance, walking performance, lean body mass, and balance
- Cognitive impairment
- Depressive symptoms
- Excessive vulnerability to stressors
- Lack of physiological reserve
- Incontinence
- Dependence in instrumental and noninstrumental activities of daily living
- At an increased risk of health concerns, including episodes of delirium, falls, fractures, disability, hospitalizations, and death

* These characteristics are not a set of a defined phenotype (e.g., Fried phenotype), but rather a compilation of features attributed to frailty in various studies. Nor does it mean that individuals who have one or several of these characteristics at any point in time are frail (e.g., fatigued and depressed). Rockwood et al. (2005) present a list with 70 signs and symptoms that are used to characterize frailty.[31]

TABLE 4.5   Fried Frailty Phenotype

Characteristics	Interpretation
Weakness	Robust • No characteristics
Slow gait	Prefrail • 1–2 characteristics
Fatigue	Frail • 3 or more characteristics
Weight loss	
Low physical activity	

From Fried LP, Tangen CM, Walston J, et al. Frailty in older adults: evidence for a phenotype. *J Gerontol A Biol Sci Med Sci.* 2001;56(3):M146–156.

greater risk of becoming frail in the period between 3 and 4 years compared with those who are robust.[34] This underscores the importance for clinicians to screen for frailty and intervene.

Interventions for Frailty

Frailty does not equate irreversible deterioration. Interventions are feasible and include exercise, multicomponent programs, and nutritional interventions.[40] Many exercise programs are beneficial in terms of frailty outcomes. A progressive course of high-intensity resistance exercise increases muscle strength among very elderly frail adults. This exercise increases gait velocity, stair-climbing power, and level of spontaneous physical activity. Individuals who are the weakest at baseline (but without significant muscle atrophy) benefit from the training the most. Importantly, multinutrient supplementation without an accompanying training program neither improves muscle strength nor adds to exercise-associated gains.[41] Additionally, gradual increase in intensity of exercise improves skeletal muscle strength, balance, and perceived health status for frail individuals. Intervention staging from less intense (focused on flexibility, balance, coordination) to more intense (resistance and endurance training) over the course of 9 months is intended to condition individuals and prevent injury.[42] The benefits of resistance training cannot be overestimated because frailty is associated with an increased risk of recurrent falls, non-spine fractures, hip fractures, and death. This risk is pertinent to females over the spectra of age (from 69 to older than 80 years of age) and body mass index (BMI), including those with a BMI $\geq$30 kg/m². Likewise, Tai Chi reduces the risk of multiple falls by 47.5% and is associated with less pronounced loss of grip strength, lowered systolic blood pressure after a 12-minute walk, and less fear of falling, making it an effective intervention for frail persons.[20]

Overweight and obese females are at risk for frailty and should be screened for it routinely. Additionally, the high prevalence of frailty among those who are overweight or obese underscores the importance of screening all older female patients for frailty because females who are overweight and obese as a result of body type may not "appear" frail to clinicians.[43] Contrary to appearance, overweight and obese frail persons have relative sarcopenia as a result of low muscle mass relative to body weight, a phenomenon

of sarcopenic obesity.[44] Obesity accelerates age-related physical function decline and is linked to impairment in mobility and ADLs and worsened physical performance, leading to frailty.[45] The use of the Fried phenotype allows for the identification of frail females among those with a BMI $\geq$18.5 kg/m². Likewise, in females who are overweight and frail at the same time (according to the Fried phenotype), clinicians should educate patients and families that even though the patient may be overweight or obese, she fits the definition of frailty, and interventions aimed to increase muscle strength, level of energy, and walking speed are recommended.

In light of the contribution of obesity to frailty, a multicomponent intervention with a combination of exercise and moderate weight loss improves physical function and mitigates frailty. This intervention leads to objective improvements in endurance, strength, balance, gait, and health-related quality of life (a subjective measure).[44] Furthermore, a combination of weight loss through dietary modification and exercise leads to greater physical function improvement than either intervention alone. A multicomponent exercise program is recommended and should include aerobic exercise, resistance training, flexibility, and balance training. The combination of exercise and weight loss via diet reduces the relative sarcopenia caused by the decrease of fat mass relative to lean body mass.[46]

NOT TO BE MISSED

Overweight and obese females are at risk for frailty and should be screened for it routinely.

Barriers to engagement in resistance training include weight-bearing pain caused by arthritis, fear of falling, difficulty transferring, cognitive impairment, illness, deconditioning and significant frailty, as well as safety issues in an unsupervised environment. Clinicians should address modifiable obstacles to promote exercise participation for frail individuals. Understanding the reasons why frail patients may not exercise highlights the importance of a thorough comprehensive approach and an inquiry about the environment where they may exercise, financial means required to exercise, or availability of a group or caregiver to assist with exercise. It is essential to inquire about and control arthritic pain and reinforce the principle that although pain accompanies exercise for persons affected by arthritis, lack of exercise will make pain and stiffness worse. Difficulty transferring may require that a caregiver, trainer, or a physical therapist assists the woman with exercise. Facilitation of exercise may require teamwork with other health care professionals, such as social workers, to find suitable outlets and means for females to exercise. Similarly, it is important to counter a potential untrue perception (that could be raised by the patient or family) that a person is too frail to exercise. Although severe deconditioning and extreme frailty would indeed make exercise impossible, those who are frail could engage in some exercise and would benefit from it. Strength training and resistance training can be done in both the sitting and reclining position, so most individuals are able to do them.

Prehabilitation, functional decline prevention among frail persons who have not yet sustained acute illness or injury, is another example of a multicomponent intervention for frail patients. It involves balance training and conditioning exercises for upper and lower extremities. It also incorporates instructions for transferring, indoor gait and outdoor mobility, use of assistive devices, and environmental modifications to enhance safety.[47]

> **! SAFETY ALERT**
>
> Frail individuals are capable of appropriately tailored exercise, and exercise may prevent further deterioration. Only the most frail individuals may not be able to exercise as this would jeopardize their safety.

Good nutritional status and diet supplementation with macronutrients and micronutrients reduce risk of frailty onset.[48] Malnutrition leads to frailty because weight loss is accompanied by slower walking speed, reduced physical activity, weakness, and exhaustion. Malnourished older adults are usually frail, making nutritional screening (nutritional and medical history, blood tests, and anthropometry) a priority among frail persons. A consultation with a dietician may be warranted to develop a diet plan for frail females, both for those who suffer from unintentional weight loss and those who have relative sarcopenia and are overweight. A detailed overview of frailty interventions is shown in Table 4.6.

> **! SAFETY ALERT**
>
> Judiciously consider the necessity of diagnostic and invasive procedures: Will they jeopardize a frail patient's status? Would undergoing them cause more harm than benefit or vice versa? Assess the impact of such procedures, and make your recommendation according to the patient's prognosis, without failing to treat.

Frailty Implications

Frailty is often a predictor of adverse outcomes, including death. Clinicians should judiciously prescribe diagnostic and invasive procedures with attention to their necessity and likelihood of improvement of quality of life in case a frail patient does undergo them. Such procedures include mammography, colonoscopy, and Pap smear. For instance, a patient or family members may inquire about a procedure that the female patient has been having routinely (e.g., mammography, Pap smear). There are two major considerations in this scenario: direct (dehydration during colonoscopy) and indirect (falls resulting from dehydration or lingering anesthetic medication effects). These considerations may determine that the risk of a given procedure is greater than its potential benefit.

Additionally, frailty should be considered in the preoperative assessment. In this setting, frailty has been calculated as a composite of several measures: mobility, function, cognition, comorbidity, and other physiological measures (Table 4.7). Frail patients have longer hospital stays and higher 30-day readmission rates.[49] Frailty likewise independently predicts discharge to a skilled nursing facility or assisted living facility following surgery.[50] A preoperative frailty assessment may be conducted in the primary care setting as a screening tool for a patient who may consider a surgery, such that recommendations may be made with respect to surgery outcomes.

Frailty is an important clinical syndrome that should be screened for among all older female patients to determine the course of treatment, suitability of diagnostic procedures and surgeries, and interventions that may be implemented to prevent prefrailty or frailty or ameliorate frailty and the risk of associated adverse outcomes. Aging does not equate to frailty. It is critical to implement strategies, including exercise and adequate nutrition, to ensure quality of life for older females. Table 4.8

TABLE 4.6   Frailty Interventions

Intervention Type	Description	Benefits
Resistance exercise	• Progressive course of high-intensity resistance training of the hip and knee extensors 3 days a week (45 minutes daily, with 1 day of rest between exercises) for 10 weeks.[41]	• Increase in muscle strength, gait velocity, stair-climbing power, and level of spontaneous physical activity. • Individuals who are the weakest at baseline benefit from this training the most. • Gradual increase in intensity improves skeletal muscle strength, balance, and perceived health status. • Conditioning and injury prevention: staging from less intense (flexibility, balance, coordination) to more intense (resistance and endurance training) over 9 months.[42] • Strength and resistance training can be accomplished in sitting or reclining positions, thus it can be completed by most individuals
Tai Chi	• Exercises derived from martial arts, aimed to improve balance and body awareness.[20]	• Reduces the risk of multiple falls, decreases the rate of grip strength loss, lowers systolic blood pressure after a 12-minute walk, reduces fear of falling.[20]
Multicomponent interventions: exercise and weight loss	• Combination of exercise and moderate weight loss for frail females who are overweight or obese. Includes aerobic, resistance, balance, and flexibility training.[46]	• Improves strength, endurance, balance, gait, and health-related quality of life.[44] • Reduces relative sarcopenia (decrease of fat mass in relation to lean body mass).[46] • Exercise combined with weight loss via diet leads to better physical function improvement than either intervention alone.[46]
Multicomponent interventions: prehabilitation	• Prevention of functional deterioration among persons who have not yet had an acute illness or injury. • Exercises for balance; upper and lower extremities' conditioning; instructions for transferring, indoor and outdoor gait mobility, use of assistive equipment, and environmental adjustments to increase safety. • Program implemented by a physical therapist. Guided by principles: identification and amelioration of deficits relevant for mobility and activities of daily living; engaging in interventions that are most relevant for individuals; tailoring interventions to individuals' preferences, comorbid conditions, and contraindications; use of equipment that is appropriate for home setting.[47]	• Feasible home-based program. For many frail individuals, a home-based program is preferred to any activity that would involve leaving the house.[47] • However, a home-based program may provide less incentive to engage in training compared with programs conducted outside the house.[47] • Cost-effective, could be incorporated into the list of services rendered by home health agencies.[47] • A potential challenge to this program is that many older adults may not wish to adjust their home settings, despite recommendations.[47]
Nutrition	• Maintenance of a good nutritional status.[48] • Diet supplementation with macronutrients and micronutrients.[48,156] • Increased intake of protein and amino acids.[156]	• Reduction of the risk of frailty onset.[48,156]

TABLE 4.7 Preoperative Frailty Measures

Measure	Positive (Abnormal) Finding
The Timed Up and Go Test[49]	≥15 seconds
Activities of daily living[22,155]	Dependence in one or more activities of daily living
Mini-Cog[157]	Score ≤3
Charlson Comorbidity Index[158]	Score ≥3
Anemia	Hematocrit <35%
Poor nutrition	Serum albumin <3.4 g/dL
Fall history	At least one fall in the 6 months before surgery

TABLE 4.8 Frailty Considerations

Category	Activity
Screening	• Apply the Fried phenotype[34]

Pre-frailty or frailty confirmed	• Develop a plan of interventions:
	  • Exercise
	  • Nutrition
	  • Multicomponent interventions

Diagnostic procedures and treatments	• Judiciously consider juxtaposition of the person's frailty status with the benefits that the proposed diagnostic procedure/treatment may afford.
Surgery	• Estimate frailty for preoperative assessment;[49] recommend for or against surgery based on frailty status
Patient and family education	• Educate about the role of frailty in life expectancy, quality of life, and measures taken to improve pre-frailty and frailty status • Reinforce that individuals may not "appear frail" yet meet other criteria for frailty • Emphasize that frailty or pre-frailty do not equate to terminal conditions: interventions can help improve the person's health and functional status

summarizes activities that a clinician performs to screen for frailty and implement interventions.

> **CLINICAL SURVIVAL TIP** Screen for frailty using the Fried phenotype: assess for weakness, weight loss, self-reported fatigue/exhaustion, low physical activity, and slow gait.

PHARMACOTHERAPY IN THE OLDER ADULT PATIENT

Pharmacotherapeutic Considerations

Scope of Prescriptive Medication Use in Older Adults

Older adults represent 16% of the total U.S. population and 33% of the consumers of prescription drugs.[1,51] Beyond age- and disease-related changes, prescribing for older adults should be done cautiously because of drug-drug interactions. Although medications are meant to be beneficial, they come with risk. In all decisions on prescribing, continuing, or de-prescribing, the goal is to balance the benefits against the risks.

Harmful prescribing, including use of inappropriate medications, underuse of appropriate medications, and polypharmacy, is one of the most common iatrogenic illnesses among older adults. Although generally considered a negative outcome of clinical care, harmful prescribing is a quality measure that is challenging to quantify or evaluate for its degree of severity. Adults older than 65 years of age are a heterogeneous group of individuals whose well-being is influenced by multiple components: biological, environmental, and psychosocial. Thus, it is difficult to make sweeping generalizations regarding appropriate prescribing based on age alone. Other factors, such as frailty syndrome, may be considered. But geriatric syndromes such as frailty are rarely included in standard medical records. On the other hand, the topic warrants attention as safe prescribing is imperative among older adults, a group highly vulnerable to medication-related harm.

Falls are the leading cause of accidental death among older adults. Many adverse effects of medications follow an indirect path to falls. Other effects include arrhythmias, sedation, central nervous system depression, and lightheadedness. These adverse effects increase the risk of falls and dehydration, which is an ambulatory care–sensitive condition. Adverse events such as life-threatening hypoglycemia or hemorrhage may result in emergency hospitalization.[52]

> **⚠ SAFETY ALERT**
>
> Prescribe, de-prescribe, and adjust medications for older adults with extra caution, paying attention to dosages, drug-drug interactions, and geriatric considerations for each drug. Consult the most up-to-date guidelines on geriatric pharmacotherapy. Adverse effects may be exacerbated in older adults, leading to arrhythmias, sedation, lightheadedness, dehydration, falls, hypoglycemia, or hemorrhage.

Polypharmacy

With the frequency of co-occurring chronic conditions and clinical guidelines recommending multiple therapies, it is no surprise that older adults can easily take 10 or more prescription drugs. *Polypharmacy* is a frequently used term in health care literature. *Polypharmacy* has been used in reference to taking anywhere from two to seven drugs. Although taking four or more medications is associated with a greater frailty incidence,[53] taking five or more medications is the most frequently used cutoff point for polypharmacy.[54] Nonetheless, particularly when applying this term to patient subgroups (e.g., older adults with cancer), no cutoff point is useful for predicting adverse events.[55] *Hyperpolypharmacy* indicates taking 10 or more medications.[56]

Pharmacokinetics in Older Adults

Pharmacokinetic processes in older adults differ from those in younger adults either as a result of normal age-related changes or disease-related changes. Prescription drugs commonly used in younger individuals are either no longer appropriate or must be used with greater caution because of the older adults' vulnerability to adverse effects. For example, a medication that causes loss of appetite and subsequently unintentional weight loss may lead to frailty, which is an independent predictor of mortality. The differences in absorption, distribution, metabolism, and excretion of medications must be considered. An overview of these functions and their considerations is shown in Table 4.9.

Although absorption is not directly influenced by age-related changes, there are important comorbidity considerations. Many chronic conditions alter the gastrointestinal tract from the oral mucosa to the intestines. Decreased hydrochloric acid production (achlorhydria), tube feedings, and concurrent medications may influence absorption; however, overall, age is less likely to influence absorption compared with drug-drug and drug-food interactions.

Distribution of drugs is subject to age and disease effect. Age leads to an increase in the fat-to-water ratio of drugs, such that lipid-soluble drugs have a larger volume of distribution. Age is also associated with a decrease in plasma albumin. This means that medications that are highly protein-bound achieve higher free concentration. Conditions such as heart failure and ascites increase body water content.

> **CLINICAL SURVIVAL TIP** Lipid-soluble drugs achieve a higher volume of distribution because older adults have an increased fat-to-water ratio. Medications that are highly protein-bound achieve a higher free concentration in serum because older adults have decreased plasma albumin (plasma protein level).

Drug metabolism is directly affected by age. Liver mass and liver blood flow decrease with age, reducing drug clearance. Enzyme CYP2C19 may undergo age-related changes, whereas enzymes CYP3A4 and 2D6 are not affected. Because of age-related effects on drug metabolism, lower dosages may be recommended. Nonetheless, modifiable risk factors (smoking, other drugs, alcohol, and caffeine) and nonmodifiable risk factors (genotype) bear a greater influence on metabolism than aging.

Elimination is likewise affected by age, specifically renal elimination, as a result of an age-related

TABLE 4.9 Changes in Pharmacokinetics and Pharmacodynamics Caused by Age

Pharmacokinetic Step	Age Effect	Disease Factor Effect	Prescribing Implications
Absorption	Rate and extent are usually unaffected	Achlorhydria, concurrent medications, tube feedings	Drug-drug and drug-food interactions are more likely to alter absorption
Distribution	Increase in fat:water ratio; decreased plasma protein, particularly albumin	Heart failure, ascites, and other conditions increase body water	Fat-soluble drugs have a larger volume of distribution; highly protein-bound drugs have a greater (active) free concentration
Metabolism	Decrease in liver mass and liver blood flow decrease drug clearance; may be age-related changes in CYP2C19, while CYP3A4 and 2D6 are not affected	Smoking, genotype, other medications, alcohol, and caffeine have more effect than aging on metabolism	Lower dosages may be therapeutic
Elimination	Primarily renal; age-related decrease in glomerular filtration rate	Acute and/or chronic kidney impairment; decreased muscle mass can result in misleadingly low serum creatinine (Cr) levels	Serum Cr may not be a reliable measure of kidney function; best to estimate Cr clearance using formula
Pharmacodynamics	Less predictable and often altered drug response at usual or lower concentrations	Drug-drug and drug-disease interactions may alter responses	Prolonged pain relief with opioids at lower dosages; more sedation and postural instability from benzodiazepines; altered sensitivity to β-blockers

From American Geriatrics Society. Geriatrics Evaluation & Management Tools. *Appropriate Prescribing.* 2021.

reduction in glomerular filtration rate. Importantly, serum creatinine is a nonreliable measure of kidney function among older adults as opposed to younger adults. The reason for this is that acute and/or chronic kidney disease and lower muscle mass can disguise serum creatinine as low. Thus instead of measuring serum creatinine directly, it must be estimated with a formula.

> **CLINICAL SURVIVAL TIP** Use a formula to calculate serum creatinine in older adults.

Pharmacodynamics in Older Adults

Drug response becomes less predictable at usual or lower doses. Drug-disease and drug-drug interactions may change the effect of any given drug. Examples of age-related pharmacodynamic changes include increased risk of anticholinergic side effects caused by antihistamines and anticholinergics (confusion, xerostomia, constipation); risk of orthostatic hypotension caused by peripheral alpha-1 blockers and central alpha blockers; and increased risk of gastrointestinal bleeding from nonsteroidal antiinflammatory drugs (NSAIDs).[57]

Potentially Inappropriate Medications

Medications are described as *potentially inappropriate medications* (PIMs) because of their interaction with normal age-related changes or common geriatric syndromes or conditions. PIMs necessitate careful prescribing (lower doses increased gradually), close monitoring of medication response and adverse effects, and using safer alternatives whenever possible.

Because adverse drug events causing injuries or disabilities requiring interventions are rare, it is difficult to build an evidence base to guide prescribers in drugs to use or not use. Similar to polypharmacy, health services research in this area is logistically challenging. Illness presentation to the provider's office is typically coded for the presenting symptom rather than an "adverse drug event." The same is usually true in emergency departments and hospital admissions. In this area, the concept of PIMs is more helpful than simply placing medications in a category of "never-use" or "always-use."

Clinical Guidelines and Resources

Evidence-based guidelines for medications to avoid, use with caution, or replace can be found in two published guidelines: the Beers Criteria[57] and the STOPP/START.[58] The Beers Criteria were originally developed by Mark Beers, a geriatric pharmacist, for use in nursing homes. The list focused on frail older adults but excluded those under palliative care or hospice services. In 2011, the American Geriatrics Society adopted responsibility for updating and maintaining the list, which is one of the most frequently consulted guides for safe prescribing in older adults. Updates are expected every 3 years, and a published guide often accompanies the clinical guideline available for order from the organization.

> **CLINICAL SURVIVAL TIP** Familiarize yourself with the Beers Criteria, and have the reference available while in clinical practice.

Failure to Prescribe

The omission of appropriate medications for older adults also represents poor prescribing practices. Providers may not prescribe clinically indicated therapies because of ignorance of evidence or bias. For example, appropriate aggressive, guideline-driven diabetes care is lacking for all patient groups. Older adults are even less likely to be prescribed antidiabetic therapies, based on cognitive and functional abilities, than younger counterparts. In the initial study of medication errors *of omission,* the majority of older adults who were admitted to the hospital were missing at least one medication considered safe and appropriate. The likelihood of an omission error was higher for the 85 years and older age group and among females compared with males.[59]

> **CLINICAL SURVIVAL TIP** Do not assume that older adults by default need less medications and lower dosages. This will lead to medication errors of omission and will harm patients.

Strategies for Reducing Polypharmacy

There is no agreed-upon, validated number of prescriptions an older adult "should" have. The general consensus is that having fewer prescriptions is better. Older adults who take five or more prescription medications have a 6.2% increased drug expenditure;[60] an 88% increased risk of adverse drug reactions;[61] are four times more likely to be hospitalized with an adverse drug reaction;[62] have an increased risk of hepatic enzyme–mediated drug-drug interactions;[63] and have an increased risk of IADL deficits.[64] Patients taking more than five medications have an increased risk of cognitive impairment.[65] The American Society of Consultant Pharmacists, a professional organization of pharmacists who are board-certified in geriatrics, provides general guidance for choosing medications to discontinue as an ongoing resource.[66]

Some medications are inappropriate for subgroups of older adults – but not universally – so they do not make the "cut" for the PIM list. In these cases, the clinician must consider the comorbidities, the extent that age-related changes would be expected to alter pharmacokinetics (robust versus frail individuals), and social determinants, including medication assistance and social support (Box 4.4).

> ### BOX 4.4   Medication Review Considerations
>
> During a detailed medication review, consider the following:
> - Does this medication treat a specific diagnosis? Is the diagnosis still relevant?
> - Is this medication intended to treat the side effect of another medication?
> - Is there a medication that could address multiple issues?
> - Is there a valid nonpharmacological option that could be used instead?
> - Is it time for a medication holiday to determine continued efficacy?

COGNITIVE IMPAIRMENT

Overview

Major neurocognitive disorders, commonly referred to as *dementias*, are a major source of disability for older females. For a female in her 60s, the likelihood of developing dementia in her lifetime is twice as high as that of developing cancer.[67] In 2021, an estimated 6.2 million Americans lived with Alzheimer's disease—the most common dementia type (60% to 80% of all dementia cases). Other dementia types include frontotemporal, vascular, Lewy body, and mixed dementia. All dementias are progressive and currently incurable neurodegenerative diseases. The incidence of dementia is growing in the United States; the number of cases of Alzheimer's disease is expected to reach 13.8 million by 2060 unless there is a medical breakthrough in the prevention, slowing, or cure of this disease.[68]

Age is the greatest risk factor for developing dementia for all individuals. However, females who are older than 85 years of age are more likely to have dementia than males in the same age group.[13] Notably, having more years of formal education is associated with lower Alzheimer's disease risk,[69] thus higher education levels in males may protect against the disease. Physical activity may reduce Alzheimer's disease risk,[70] and greater engagement in physical activity in males may also explain the higher Alzheimer's disease incidence among females.

High-quality dementia care starts in the primary care practice with recognition of impaired memory or another cognitive domain (e.g., perceptual-motor function, language, social cognition, attention, or executive function).[71] Dementia is not screened for routinely; thus the prevalence of missed and delayed dementia diagnoses is high.[72] Both the Alzheimer's Association and the American Academy of Neurology have endorsed a list of 10 warning signs.[73,74] The Department of Veterans Affairs, likewise, endorses a similar list.[75] Each list of warning signs captures recent, observable changes in memory, language, and self-care ability (Table 4.10). Although the *Warning Signs* are not diagnostic, comprehensive primary care for older female patients includes

TABLE 4.10	Dementia Warning Signs	
Ten Warning Signs of Dementia (Alzheimer's Association)[73]	**Dementia Warning Signs (Department of Veterans Affairs)[75]**
Memory loss that impairs daily life	*Clinician Observed:*
Difficulties in planning or problem-solving	Inattentive to personal appearance
Difficulty performing familiar activities (home, work, or leisure settings)	Forgetful, "poor historian"
Losing track of time, getting lost in familiar surroundings	Does not keep appointments, appears for appointments on the wrong day or time
Trouble understanding visual images (e.g., difficulty reading) and spatial relationships (determining distance between objects)	Has unexplained weight loss or other vague complaints (weak, dizzy)
Difficulties with speaking and writing (e.g., problems finding words, repeating oneself)	Repeatedly and apparently unwilling or unable to follow instructions (take medications)
Misplacing objects in unusual places, unable to go back to find them	Defers to caregiver or family to answer questions
Difficulties with judgment or decision making (e.g., giving out large amounts of money to telemarketers)	*Patient or Caregiver Reported:*
Withdrawal from work, social, and leisure activities	Asking the same questions over and over
Personality or mood changes (e.g., increased suspiciousness, anxiety, fear, depression)	Gets lost in familiar settings
	Unable to follow directions
	Confusion with respect to time, places, and people
	Difficulties with self-care, including bathing, eating, and safety

TABLE 4.11	Diagnostic Workup for Dementia[22,23,78,79,81,82,84,87-91]
Area of Testing	**Recommended Tests**
Cognition	Montreal Cognitive Assessment (MoCA)[78]
	St. Louis University Mental Status (SLUMS)[79]
Function	Lawton Instrumental Activities of Daily Living[23]
	Katz Activities of Daily Living[22]
	Functional Assessment Questionnaire[81]
Related symptoms	Geriatric Depression Scale (15-item)[82,83]
	Patient Health Questionnaire-9 (PHQ-9)[84]
	Revised Memory and Behavior Problem Checklist[91]
	Neuropsychiatric Inventory[87-90]
Laboratory tests	Complete blood count
	Comprehensive metabolic panel
	Thyroid panel
	Vitamin B_{12} level
	Folate level
Imaging	Computer tomography
	Magnetic resonance imaging

an intentional process to observe for these symptoms along with protocols for further evaluation. The diagnostic workup includes a standardized assessment of cognition and related symptoms, a thorough history of present illness, and radiological imaging along with measures to rule out reversible causes.[76] The diagnostic workup for dementia is shown in Table 4.11.

> **CLINICAL SURVIVAL TIP** Familiarize yourself with the warning signs of dementia. Remember that these signs are not diagnostic, and a comprehensive workup is required to diagnose dementia.

Cognitive Measures and Related Assessments

Standardized measures of cognition are helpful in the diagnosis of dementia.[77] In the primary care setting, appropriate tests capture multiple cognitive domains including memory, attention, language, visuospatial abilities, and executive function. Two such validated instruments are the Montreal Cognitive Assessment (MoCA)[78] and the Saint Louis University Mental Status

(SLUMS) examination.[79] Support staff, trained in the specific tool, typically administers the tests. The interpretation is the clinician's responsibility. For individuals who perform below their expected level (based on norms for age, sex, and education), a referral for neuropsychological testing may be warranted. Keep in mind that additional testing may not be appropriate for those with scores indicating late-stage disease (MoCA or SLUMS score less than 7).

A diagnosis of dementia requires measurable impairment in at least two cognitive domains as well as functional impairment.[80] Functional assessment is integral to dementia staging. A basic functional assessment is best completed by the affected individual as well as by someone who observes the individual regularly (e.g., a family member or close friend). Generally, affected individuals will overestimate their functional abilities and level of independence, and the observer will underestimate the functional abilities; the truth is likely somewhere between the two. Commonly used tools include the Katz[22] and Lawton-Brody[23] scales for ADLs and IADLs and the Functional Assessment Questionnaire (FAQ).[81] Beyond the current state, the clinician should ascertain the degree to which functional status represents a change from baseline (6 months to 1 year prior).

> **NOT TO BE MISSED**
>
> Use standardized tools to evaluate the patient's function. These scores will enable the clinician to see a trajectory of change in the patient's function.

The coexistence of depression and neuropsychiatric symptoms with dementia is high, and clinical guidelines support the assessment of each at the time of cognitive testing. There are a number of reliable and valid instruments to screen for depression in older adults. For most individuals undergoing an initial evaluation for dementia, these tools remain acceptable. Commonly used measures include the Geriatric Depression Scale (GDS), 15-item version,[82,83] and the Patient Health Questionnaire, 9-item version (PHQ-9).[84] For patients with significant cognitive impairment, the Cornell Scale for Depression in Dementia (CSDD) is most appropriate.[85] The GDS and PHQ-9 may be administered by technical staff. The CSDD is a clinician-administered instrument that takes approximately 20 minutes. Evidence supports each of these tools, so the ultimate choice is often based on logistical aspects, including the tool's availability in the electronic medical record and the overall care plan. The PHQ-9 is the best tool at determining response to therapy as it is designed to detect change over time. The CSDD is the most specific to those living with dementia.

The measurement and aggressive management of neuropsychiatric symptoms in dementia is one of the most meaningful contributions the clinician can make to the quality of life for the patient and caregiver(s). Additionally, the timing of the appearance of the symptoms provides important clues to the probable dementia type. Behavioral and psychological symptoms of dementia are categorized into mood disorders (e.g., apathy, depression); psychotic symptoms (e.g., delusions, hallucinations); sleep disturbances (e.g., insomnia, hypersomnia, sleep-wake cycle reversal); and agitation (e.g., pacing, wandering, verbal and physical aggression, sexual disinhibition).[86] Standardized measures for neuropsychiatric symptoms include the Neuropsychiatric Inventory-Questionnaire (NPI-Q)[87-90] and the Revised Memory and Problem Behavior Checklist (RMBPC).[91] The determination to use one over the other may be based on workflow, practically speaking. The NPI-Q is often administered by staff through an interview, whereas the RMBPC may be self-administered (by a caregiver) with reliability.

During the full assessment, the clinician should rule out other possible causes of or contributors to impaired cognition including vitamin B_{12} deficiency, hypothyroidism, depression, anemia, infection, or electrolyte disturbances.[92] It is important to consider that abnormal values on these tests represent opportunities to intervene and correct the cognitive changes. The presence of an abnormality does not exclude a coexisting dementia. It is entirely possible to have Alzheimer's type dementia and hypothyroidism, for example. Treatment of the thyroid condition will optimize cognitive function but not return the affected individual to his or her premorbid cognitive abilities.

CLINICAL SURVIVAL TIP Rule out other causes of impaired cognition by assessing the following:
- Comprehensive metabolic panel
- Complete blood count
- Vitamin B_{12} level
- Thyroid hormones
- Electrolytes
- Depressive symptoms
- Infection

NOT TO BE MISSED

The presence of an abnormality does not exclude a co-existing dementia.

Structural neuroimaging is commonly ordered during the diagnostic workup in the form of magnetic resonance imaging (MRI) of the brain without contrast. If MRI is contraindicated, head computer tomography (CT) without contrast is acceptable. Information gleaned from imaging includes identification of atrophy areas, evidence of cerebrovascular disease, and identification of potentially reversible issues such as normal pressure hydrocephalus. Similar to neuropsychological testing, the decision to order imaging involves the balance of what the patient can reasonably tolerate. A patient with advanced dementia whose symptoms follow the known trajectory of Alzheimer's type may require sedating medication to complete radiological testing. Sedating medication is associated with risks for older adults in general. Furthermore, people with dementia are typically more susceptible to these reactions. In this scenario, a probable diagnosis may be made in the absence of neuroimaging. Once a diagnosis is suspected, referral to a specialist might be indicated.

Stages and Stage-Based Care

Assigning the stage of dementia is helpful for both the family and clinician to plan for care, to consider appropriate interventions, and in the prognostication process. Disease staging is based primarily on functional ability. The most commonly used scale is the Functional Assessment for STaging dementia (FAST) scale.[93-97] The commonly used stages are: mild cognitive impairment (MCI); early stage; early-middle stage; late-middle stage, and late stage. More specific staging frameworks exist such as The GEMS: Brain Change Model[98] for lay audiences. Although it is not clinically used, it may be very helpful in caregiver education and coaching.

MCI is staged when a patient has measurable cognitive impairment on neuropsychological testing in only one cognitive domain or with no impairment in functional abilities. For example, a patient may have significantly impaired memory, but language, executive function, and visuospatial skills remain intact. These individuals typically remain independent in IADLs and ADLs. Formerly referred to as *pre-dementia*, it is now known that individuals with MCI may or may not progress to a dementia diagnosis in the future. MCI is categorized in two ways: (1) amnestic and non-amnestic (according to the presence or absence of memory loss) and (2) single-domain and multi-domain (according to the number of cognitive domains that are impaired). Individuals diagnosed with amnestic or multi-domain MCI have higher likelihood of progression to dementia than those in the other categories.

> **CLINICAL SURVIVAL TIP** MCI can be amnestic or non-amnestic (based on presence or absence of memory loss). It can also be single-domain or multi-domain (based on the number of cognitive domains that are impaired).

Early-stage dementia exists when the affected person has met the criteria for a major neurocognitive disorder (impairment in two or more cognitive domains).[80] This stage represents an initial need for complementary services to offset new declines in IADLs. Daily skills such as medication management and household finances may require additional support and/or delegation to another responsible party. The exact type of assistance recommended should match the cognitive domains that are declining. For those with prominent memory loss, appropriate interventions would focus on reminders and cues that may derive from the built environment. For those with impaired visuospatial abilities, driving becomes a concern early in the disease process. Universally recommended interventions at this stage include a structured routine and schedule and attention to a healthy lifestyle. Generally, the clinician should consider people with early-stage dementia at a lower threshold for stress, emotional distress, and physical symptoms. Although all adults benefit from a full night of restful sleep, increased fruits and vegetables in the diet, immunizations, and acceptable blood pressure, those with dementia are especially susceptible to the negative effects when these components are neglected. Therefore careful attention and aggressive management of symptoms, including depressive symptoms, fatigue, and pre-frailty, are particularly important at this stage.

Early-middle stage dementia is characterized by remaining physical ability juxtaposed with increased cognitive decline. This combination creates the stage for management concerns including wandering, driving impairment, frustration, and negotiations focused on the balance of independence and safety. Opportunities for structured and meaningful engagement can be effective strategies to preempt behavioral and psychological symptoms of dementia. If caregivers have not yet sought training or education programs, this is the stage during which the clinician may recommend focused resources such as the Alzheimer's Association's "50 Activities."[99]

This may also be the stage of disease during which families elect for adjunct caregiving services. Options for supportive care in the community include adult day programs and in-home companion services. For those who are physically mobile, safeguards in the home to alert a caregiver to an exit from the home may be warranted. Emerging technologies to promote meaningful engagement and reminiscence may be helpful at this stage. The SimpleC platform is an example of a daily activity assistive device that combines clinician and family input to prompt engagement in activities as well as communicate with family members and reminisce.[100]

Late-middle stage dementia is characterized by continued dependence for ADLs and decline in communication, often leading to more behavioral and psychological symptoms of dementia. A number of frameworks exist to explain the root causes of the symptoms as well as guide appropriate interventions. Theories include a lowered stress threshold, presence of unmet needs, and behavior as a form of nonverbal communication. Each framework guides the caregiver, both formal and informal, toward a strategy of assessment, diagnosis, planning, intervention, and evaluation—a well-known process to the nurse clinician. Caregivers play a major role in the assessment of behaviors and will serve as the historian for events preceding the behavior, a detailed description of the behavior itself, and what, if anything, reinforces the behavior. Often, the clinician may guide a caregiver through this process, and the input of both the clinician and caregiver yields the most effective intervention to respond to the behavior. The astute clinician must determine at this point whether pharmacological intervention is appropriate. Medications may be helpful in the event that the behavior reflects untreated depression, anxiety, exacerbation of other chronic conditions, insomnia, or psychosis.

The late-middle stage is a highly challenging phase for caregivers as behavioral symptoms peak simultaneously with increasing physical demands. Dementia is a degenerative disorder of the central nervous system. It is often during the late-middle stage that overall physical well-being is affected by dementia, even in the absence of other chronic conditions, such as diabetes, vascular disease, or renal dysfunction. The late-middle stage is also a common phase for repeated falls resulting from even mild knee flexion contractures. Often, dementia coexists with the aforementioned chronic conditions. Lacking self-management may yield many other uncomfortable, bothersome, and potentially life-threatening health problems. Individuals in this stage may have difficulty with personal hygiene in conjunction with refusal of perineal care. This decline in self-management of personal hygiene coupled with age-related declines in immune response and changes in vaginal and urethral structures often results in frequent urinary tract infections.

Late-stage dementia is characterized by continued cognitive and physical decline. Cognition is affected across all domains at this point, although not tested on formal neuropsychological examinations. Language ability is measured by the number of words spoken per day, with the average being seven per day for an affected person entering the late stage. Physical changes are prominent, with a decline in walking ability to the point of chair-bound or bed-bound status; joint contractures are common.[101] It is unclear whether the joint changes are caused by the neurodegenerative process or immobility. Swallowing dysfunction or dysphagia is recognized as a prognostic indicator for 6 months or less of life expectancy, thus it is often the prompt for hospice referral.[102,103] Feeding tubes in the context of late-stage dementia are not recommended.[104]

> **CLINICAL SURVIVAL TIP** Feeding tubes are not recommended in late-stage dementia.

Differentiating Dementia Types

Dementia is best differentiated early in the disease process and is often guided by a detailed symptom history elicited from the affected individual if possible as well as a close observer. By the late-middle to late stage, a universal group of symptoms and signs are shared by all types of dementias. Keep in mind that each individual experiences cognitive impairment

uniquely, and symptom expression is also dependent on premorbid personality traits, comorbid medical conditions, and interaction with one's environment. A guide to the differentiation between dementia types is shown in Table 4.12.

THE OLDER ADULT AS A CAREGIVER

Informal (unpaid) caregivers provide the majority of care for community-dwelling persons affected by dementia. Most caregivers are related to their persons, with 55% of caregivers assisting their parents.[105] In 2020, over 11 million Americans served as informal caregivers for persons living with dementia. The major caregiving task is assistance with ADLs. In 2020, caregivers of persons living with Alzheimer's disease provided an estimated 15.3 billion hours of unpaid care that would cost $256.7 billion if performed by paid personnel. Caregivers' work is not only unpaid, but it also bears a toll on their physical health and psychological and financial well-being. In 2020, 59% of caregivers of persons living with dementia ranked the emotional stress of caregiving as high or very high; 30% to 40% experience depression; and 74% stated they were somewhat or very concerned about their own health.[68] Sixty-six percent of caregivers live with their persons in the community.[106] For care recipients, living at home (rather than in an institutional setting) translates into fewer depressive symptoms, better cognitive performance, higher quality of life, stronger social connectedness, and better performance in ADLs.[107]

Sex Differences Among Caregivers

Caregiver issuers are an important concern for the female patient's health care providers. Most sources estimate that approximately two-thirds of caregivers for older adults are females. Wives more commonly become caregivers for their husbands than vice versa.[68] Daughters constitute over one-third of caregivers of persons living with dementia.[106] This may be an underestimation because many people do not report that they are caregivers.[108]

Compared with male caregivers, females spend more time on caregiving tasks. Daughters spend an average of 102 hours on caregiving monthly, whereas sons average 80 hours.[106] Females are more likely to spend large amount of hours (over 60) caregiving weekly. More than twice as many females than males live with their person and provide care

TABLE 4.12	**Different Dementia Types**
Dementia Type	**Features**
Alzheimer's disease	• Most common type of dementia: 60–80% of all dementias.
	• Most commonly onset is after 75 years of age.
	• Memory loss is the initial symptom.
	• Pathological processes in the brain begin in the hippocampus, hence, short-term memory deficit is most prominent initially.
	• Hippocampal atrophy is evident on radiological imaging.
	• At the early stage, the most common neuropsychiatric symptoms are: depression, anxiety, paranoia, and a lowered threshold for angry outbursts. These symptoms are derived from feelings of uncertainty and an attempt to make sense of an uncertain situation.
	• Two classes of antidementia medications are approved for use in Alzheimer's disease (although they are commonly used in other dementia types): acetylcholinesterase inhibitors and N-methyl-D-aspartate (NMDA) receptor antagonist
	• Acetylcholinesterase inhibitors (donepezil, rivastigmine, galantamine) have been shown to delay progression of the disease and optimize attention by increasing acetylcholine.
	• As many as 22% of those taking acetylcholinesterase will have cardiac arrhythmias (especially bradycardia and syncope), requiring discontinuation.
	• Other common side effects of acetylcholinesterase inhibitors include nausea, diarrhea, and urinary frequency. These may improve with dose reduction and usually diminish with longer duration of therapy.
	• There are questions regarding the length of time for which the medications are effective with a proposed time of 12 months, making the discussion of when to discontinue the medication as relevant as other medication teaching at the time of prescribing.
	• NMDA receptor antagonist (memantine) is the second class of antidementia medications, and memantine is the only drug in this class.
	• Memantine is approved for use in middle stages of Alzheimer's disease and can be prescribed alongside acetylcholinesterase inhibitors. It is well tolerated with the most common adverse reaction of headache.
	• Alzheimer's disease is most common among dementias and it is most well characterized. Thus, most recommendations are based on Alzheimer's framework. It is an important point for a clinician with regard to recommending services, resources, and educational materials, which may or may not be appropriate for non-Alzheimer's dementia types.
Subcortical vascular dementia (vascular dementia)	• Vascular dementia follows a more incremental decline than Alzheimer's disease.
	• The initial symptoms vary greatly depending on the areas of infarction (stroke).
	• A general clue to this diagnosis includes vascular or cerebrovascular disease in the medical history.
	• Word-finding difficulties and gait disturbances early in the disease process are common.
	• A major confounder in the diagnosis of vascular dementia is its frequency of overlap with Alzheimer's disease.
	• Vascular lesions are very common: few Alzheimer's disease cases lack vascular pathology, and in one study there were only 21% of pure Alzheimer's type of dementia, with the rest having both Alzheimer's and vascular type pathology[160]
	• Pharmacotherapy in vascular dementia focuses on optimization of vascular factors. Antidementia medications may be appropriate if the diagnosis is thought to be mixed Alzheimer's and vascular dementia.

TABLE 4.12   Different Dementia Types—cont'd

Dementia Type	Features
Dementia with Lewy Bodies (DLB)	• Occurs more commonly in males and at a younger age than Alzheimer's or vascular dementia. • Affects the brain and body similarly to Parkinson's disease and is commonly diagnosed as such. • Symptoms largely reflect the location of the deposits of Lewy bodies, clumps of alpha synuclein (cortical versus subcortical), and the subsequent depletion of dopamine. • Specific symptom expression and timing drives the diagnosis toward DLB, which is cortical, and thus primarily cognitive, or Parkinson's disease, which is subcortical and primarily motor. • Cognitive testing typically reveals poor visuospatial ability and executive dysfunction. • Other early symptoms include movement disorders such as rapid eye movement (REM) sleep behavior disorder, rigid joints, and slow gait. • Pharmacotherapy in DLB centers around dopaminergic agents (levodopa) and then treatment for the specific symptoms expressed such as depression. Memantine has some benefit. • Antipsychotics should be avoided as the affected brain is highly sensitive to them with deleterious effects. • Although these individuals continue to hallucinate, the visualizations are not necessarily frightening or bothersome. • Agents that increase the available gamma aminobutyric acid (GABA) may be helpful in diminishing excitability that may appear as aggression as GABA soothes overstimulated nerves (e.g., valproic acid, gabapentin). Drug levels and potential organ injury (e.g., liver failure) must be monitored. • A recommendation frequently made to Alzheimer's patients to engage in regular physical activity may not be appropriate: physical activity must be undertaken with great caution for those with characteristic mobility and coordination issues.
Frontotemporal lobar degeneration (FTLD)	• FTLD includes a group of syndromes that can be classified broadly into behavioral and language variants. • Those with the behavioral variant exhibit an impressive level of social disinhibition that is often socially awkward or unacceptable. They may have major family disputes, including estrangement and divorce and encounters with law enforcement early in their disease and before seeking medical care. The disease represents the largest proportion of younger-onset dementias. • Those with the language variant exhibit profound language difficulties early in the disease and in a progressive manner, making communication very challenging. • Atrophy in the frontotemporal lobes is evident on imaging. • With regard to recommendations (which are commonly based on an Alzheimer's framework), recommendation for a support group or therapy for an individual with FTLD may prove more frustrating than helpful with their prominent aphasia.

24 hours a day, 7 days a week.[109] The intensity of round-the-clock caregiving is associated with disease severity. The patient approaching end of life requires more intense care, and this time may be extremely stressful for caregivers. Provision of round-the-clock care disturbs nearly every aspect of a caregiver's life (Fig. 4.3).[109]

Compared with males, females are more likely to become caregivers by default rather than by choice.[110] If females anticipate becoming caregivers for parents, they are better able to transition into their caregiving role when compared with those who take on caregiving tasks unexpectedly.[111]

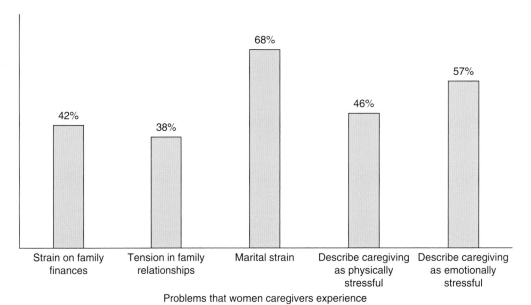

Figure 4.3 Caregiver burden among females who provide round-the-clock care for persons living with dementia. (Data from Alzheimer's Association. 2014 Alzheimer's disease facts and figures. *Alzheimers Dement.* 2014;10[2]:e47–e92.)

> **PATIENT-CENTERED CARE:** Because individuals frequently do not report that they are serving in the role of unpaid caregiver for a relative or friend, always ask whether they are a caregiver. Although caregivers' work is unpaid, this work bears a toll on their physical health, psychological well-being, and finances.

What Is Dementia Caregiving Like?

Caregiving for a person living with dementia has been described as an "unexpected career,"[112] highlighting the extent and nature of changes in personal and professional life that a caregiver must make. The nature of dementia caregiving is likely to contribute to the differences in caregiver burden between females and males. For instance, females are more likely than males to assist their persons with ADLs that include toileting, bathing, managing incontinence, and dressing.[113] Additionally, nearly all dementia patients experience behavioral and psychological symptoms of dementia at some point in the disease trajectory. These symptoms increase caregiver burden. They also can lead to care recipients' institutionalization and increased financial expenditures for families.[114]

Neuromotor disturbance accompanying dementia, such as persistent grasping and paratonia, complicates the caregiver's ability to assist with ADLs,[115] making the work more physically demanding. Moreover, dementia's unpredictable course is likely to be manifested via acute exacerbations (e.g., sudden increase in agitation or aggression) that may prompt the caregiver to reorganize the daily schedule to attend to the care recipient's needs, making planning of other responsibilities difficult. Incidents such as aggression or wandering may cause acute stress for a caregiver, and anticipation of such sudden symptom exacerbation may contribute to the caregiver's chronic stress. Additionally, caregivers frequently must address common comorbidities of dementia such as hypertension, diabetes, and hyperlipidemia.[115]

> **NOT TO BE MISSED**
>
> Behavioral and psychological symptoms of dementia are often the most difficult aspect of the disease for caregivers. Although dementia cannot be cured, these symptoms can be managed in multiple ways. Learn how to manage them pharmacologically and nonpharmacologically.

Positive Aspects of Caregiving

Several population-based studies, not limited to caregivers of persons living with dementia, found that caregivers had increased longevity and significantly decreased mortality compared with noncaregiving controls.[116] Positive aspects of caregiving include: personal and spiritual growth, emotional rewards, relationship strengthening, reciprocity, satisfaction from the sense of role fulfillment and duty, and acquiring mastery and competence in caregiving. In studies not limited to caregivers of persons living with dementia, caregivers frequently report benefits they gain from caregiving and little to no strain.[117] These findings may not be fully applicable to caregivers of persons living with dementia because the latter spend more caregiving hours compared with caregivers of older adults who do not have dementia. Additionally, the total duration of caregiving for persons living with dementia is on average longer relative to total caregiving time for persons with other chronic conditions.[106] This underscores a possible burden increase because of the long duration of dementia caregiving.

Positive aspects of caregiving are likely to be appreciated dissimilarly among caregivers of different ethnicities. For instance, caregiving is associated with less sense of reward among White caregivers compared with Black or Hispanic caregivers.[118] Clinicians should not overlook the burden and stress a caregiver may experience even if she or he is culturally socialized not to show burden (due to filial obligation, reciprocity, or sense of duty toward older relatives). With attention predominantly focused on the dementia patient, clinicians should not overlook caregivers: the "hidden patients."[119] The clinician has a duty to assess the multiple negative effects that caregiving has on the caregiver's physical health and psychological well-being.

> **PATIENT-CENTERED CARE:** Never assume that caregivers of any particular race or ethnicity do not experience caregiver burden. They may not express it overtly, but caregiving is nearly always stressful in numerous ways.

Caregiver Burden

The clinician must assess the positive and negative impact of the role on the caregiver's psychological well-being and physical health. In many areas, female caregivers fare worse than males. Dementia caregiving is associated with stress,[120] depressive symptomatology,[121] anxiety,[122] caregiver burden,[123] decreased health-related quality of life,[124] social isolation,[125] perceived loneliness,[126] and perception of own health as suboptimal.[127] Females are more likely to report marital problems and spending less time with their husbands because of their caregiving responsibilities. Approximately 30% of males and females report feeling isolated as a result of their caregiving role.[109] Several other comparisons between male and female caregivers and the way caregiving affects their psychological well-being differently are summarized in Figure 4.4.

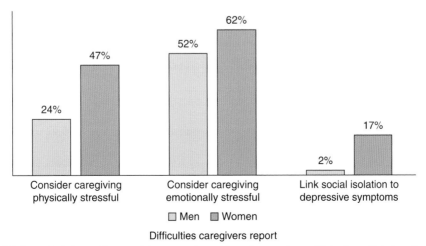

Figure 4.4 Impact of dementia caregiving on male and female caregivers. (Data from Alzheimer's Association. 2014 Alzheimer's disease facts and figures. *Alzheimers Dement.* 2014;10[2]:e47–e92.)

Family obligations that are unrelated to dementia caregiving are likely to exacerbate the female caregiver's stress. For instance, 53% of female caregivers report that they find dementia caregiving more difficult than caring for minor children. Additionally, those who provide simultaneous care for older adults and minor children (sandwich generation caregivers) have a lower quality of life and suboptimal health maintenance behaviors (e.g., less likely to eat a healthy diet or exercise) compared with caregivers without similar responsibilities or noncaregivers.[128] Family conflict is prevalent in caregiving families,[129] and caregivers of individuals with dementia report more family conflict than those of individuals without dementia.[130] The radical change that caregiving onset brings to the family is likely to trigger a new conflict or re-ignite preexisting tensions. Family conflict may stem from three major sources:

- Disagreement about the nature of cognitive impairment, its severity, and required treatment.
- Disagreement about the quality of care that family members other than the caregiver must allocate to the dementia patient.
- Lack of acknowledgment to the primary caregiver from the rest of the family.[131]

The clinician should inquire about psychological climate in the family since the caregiver assumed responsibilities and offer counseling, a support group, or similar interventions. Very often clinicians perform thorough assessments on dementia patients and dedicate all of their time to these patients' needs. Although this is an excellent practice, it may come at the expense of the caregiver who ensures that the person continues living at home rather than in an institution. Caregivers may never disclose stress that they are experiencing and not deem it appropriate to speak about their caregiver burden unless the clinician asks.

Caregiving for a person living with dementia is also financially strenuous. Not only is the caregiver responsible for providing for the patient (which may be more difficult if the patient was working before the illness), but their employment is frequently jeopardized. Work-related difficulties are more pronounced for females compared with males (Fig. 4.5). Other employment-related challenges caused by dementia caregiving include having to leave work early or arrive late, taking leaves of absence, taking a less demanding job, having work performance suffer because of caregiving responsibilities, retiring early, or being forced to turn down a promotion.[109] Being forced to give up employment-associated rewards exacerbates stress, depressive symptoms, and perceived loneliness that female caregivers experience. In light of the financial toll that dementia caregiving takes, a clinician should collaborate with a social worker.

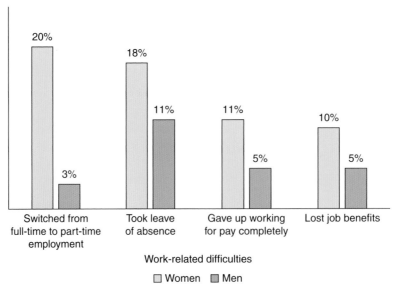

Figure 4.5 Employment difficulties linked to caregiving. (Data from Alzheimer's Association. 2014 Alzheimer's disease facts and figures. *Alzheimers Dement.* 2014;10[2]:e47–e92.)

A social worker may help the caregiver find insurance options, scholarships or "grants" that caregivers may apply for to attend services geared toward caregiving families, and other financial assistance.

Primary Care for Caregivers

Caregivers have added risks to their well-being and physical health that should be considered by their primary care provider. Caregiving is not only related to adverse psychological well-being outcomes, but it also impairs physical health.[132] A caregiver's mental and physical health may be best understood through the interplay between the caregiver's age, chronic conditions, caregiving duties, and social climate. All of these are affected by their caregiving role. Caregivers represent a population that is chronically stressed. Chronic stress is linked to low-grade systemic inflammation,[133] which is an underlying mechanism for multiple chronic conditions including cardiovascular disease,[134] osteoporosis, arthritis, frailty, functional decline,[135] and depression.[136]

Additionally, caregivers' chronic stress may be exacerbated because of their social isolation and associated perceived loneliness. Caregiving duties may lower the priority of maintaining social ties or simply not afford caregivers time for anything but most important responsibilities. Depressive symptoms, common among caregivers,[121] may likewise diminish a caregiver's willingness to socialize. Social isolation among caregivers can have serious implications for their health and must be addressed by the clinician. Social isolation is linked to increased morbidity.[137] Subjective social isolation is linked to pro-inflammatory gene expression,[138] which can lead to an onset of disease of inflammatory pathogenesis, such as cardiovascular disease.[136]

Assessments of the Caregiver's Context and Well-Being

Once a caregiver's status is confirmed, the clinician should assess the caregiver with regard to psychological well-being, physical health, and social context. Assessment may be conducted in a standardized manner, via instruments, or in a semistructured way by asking open-ended questions related to well-being factors that may be compromised.

The questions in Table 4.13 are examples that may be used to begin a discussion if assessment proceeds in an unstructured fashion. More specific questions may be added based on responses (e.g., questions about arthritis or hypertension management if the caregiver mentions these conditions).

In addition to using open-ended questions to assess the caregiver's situation and caregiver burden, several instruments are available. It is beneficial to combine assessment with the use of instrument(s) with a semistructured discussion. An instrument will provide a score that can place the caregiver in a category (e.g., low, moderate, or severe stress) and develop a care plan. An instrument-derived score may confirm concerns that the caregiver revealed in a conversation or may demonstrate, for example, a high level of stress or burden despite the caregiver's claims that he or she lacks any concerns. Table 4.14 provides an overview of commonly used tools.

When using instruments, it is important to remember that participants may be reluctant to disclose their stress, depressive symptoms, or caregiver burden. This may be especially true for Black caregivers who are notably less likely to report caregiver burden compared with White caregivers.[139] Thus every caregiver should be asked about his or her health, well-being, and caregiver burden. Results of questionnaires or answers to discussion questions should not exclude any caregivers from receiving attention.

Interventions for Caregivers

Screening results with the use of the described tools may allow the provider to tailor interventions that may best fit the needs, preferences, and opportunities of individual caregivers. First, merely asking caregivers about their caregiving role may be important for caregivers who may be accustomed to the fact that their person is always at the center of a health care professional's attention. Caregivers may note that they are rarely asked about their own health.

Interventions for caregivers will depend on the combined results of questionnaires and semistructured discussions as well as availability of programs a caregiver may attend. It is critical to validate the stressful nature of caregiving without obscuring its positive aspects, but also without diminishing the degree of burden, stress, and social isolation that caregivers often experience. When selecting interventions for caregivers, it is recommended that caregivers actively participate in planning them. Likewise, it is important to provide opportunities for the patient if he or she is functioning well enough to be involved. Although personalized support is generally

TABLE 4.13   Semistructured Assessment of Health and Well-Being for the Caregiver of a Person Living With Dementia

Domain	Question
Physical health	• Would you like to discuss any health concerns you may be having? • How have you addressed them? • How would you describe your health (e.g., excellent, good, fair, or poor)? • How physically demanding are your caregiving tasks? Does anyone help you with these tasks? • Do you have any chronic pain? Where is your pain? What do you do to treat your pain? • Do you have regular checkups with your primary care provider? • How does caregiving affect your physical health? • What could be done to ameliorate the impact of caregiving on your physical health?
Psychological well-being, caregiver burden	• How stressful is caregiving for you? • What are the most stressful aspects of caregiving for you? • Approximately how many hours every day do you spend caregiving? • Did you have a choice on whether to be a caregiver, or did it happen by default? • What do you do to help curb your stress? • What could be done to help you decrease your stress? • Is there anything related to your person's behaviors or symptoms of dementia that may cause you stress? If so, what do you think could be done to control such symptoms? • Would you like to work with a counselor/therapist now that you are a caregiver?
Social settings	• What is your social support system? • Do you find yourself socially isolated? • Do you find yourself lonely? If so, what causes you to feel this way? • Did relationships in your family change because you became a caregiver? • Does anyone in your family or community help you with caring for your person?
Financial and legal concerns	• Would you like to meet with a social worker to discuss options that you may be eligible for to possibly reduce health care bills for your person? • Would you like information about where to obtain legal advice related to caregiving for a person living with dementia?
Community resources	• Are you using any community resources, such as the Alzheimer's Association, support groups, or educational classes for caregivers? Would you like to receive information about such resources?
Self-care	• What are you doing for self-care? • Do you have an opportunity to participate in any leisure activities? • What can be done to give you respite from caregiving responsibilities?

recommended, multiple group interventions, led by experts or caregivers, have proven successful. In group programs, caregivers often value rapport and mutual support that is established between participants. Caregivers share practical information and empathically listen to others, and many caregivers note a sense of relief from the knowledge that they are not alone in their caregiving experience.[140]

Interventions can be grouped into in-person and telehealth programs. Numerous in-person programs demonstrated their effectiveness in reducing caregivers' stress,[141] depressive symptoms,[142]

anxiety,[143] dysfunctional thoughts,[144] dyadic relationship strain,[145] caregiver burden,[146] and distress caused by care recipients' behavioral and psychological symptoms of dementia.[147] Additionally, these programs help increase caregivers' self-efficacy[148] and caregiving mastery,[145] improve quality of life,[149] including health-related quality of life,[150] improve sleep,[143] increase the use of adaptive coping,[151] and increase the frequency of leisure activities.[144]

Despite the efficacy of in-person programs, their reach is limited, and web-based programs are becoming more prevalent. They allow participation for caregivers in rural

TABLE 4.14 Instruments Used to Assess Dementia Caregivers' Psychological Well-Being[84,123,161]

Instrument	Description	Interpretation of Scores
Zarit Burden Interview[123,161]	• Assesses how the caregiver feels and thinks in relation to caregiving and ways in which caregiving has shifted his or her life. Questions encompass multiple areas of life in relation to caregiving status: caregiver's own health and his or her relationships to other family members and friends, financial well-being, and caregivers' assessment of own performance as a caregiver. • Questions ($N = 22$) are answered on a Likert scale: 0—never, 1— rarely, 2—sometimes, 3—quite frequently, 4—nearly always. Higher score indicates greater caregiver burden.	No clinical cutoff scores.
Revised Memory and Behavior Checklist[91]	• Assesses frequency of behavioral and psychological symptoms of dementia that a care recipient displays (e.g., aggression, agitation, wandering, withdrawal). The scale covers three domains of symptoms: memory, disruption, and depression. • Questions ($N = 24$) assess 24 symptoms: their frequency and distress that they are causing the caregiver. Thus for each behavior (symptom), a caregiver answers two questions: how often a given behavior occurs and how bothersome or upsetting the caregiver finds this behavior. • Questions are answered on a Likert scale. Frequency of the behavior: 0—never occurred, 1—not in the past week, 2—1–2 times in the past week, 3—3–6 times in the past week, 4—daily or more often. Distress that the behavior produces: 0—not at all, 1—a little, 2—moderately, 3— very much, 4—extremely.	No clinical cutoff scores. But review of the answers to this scale (which behaviors occur, how frequently, and how upsetting or bothersome they are to the caregiver) allows the clinician to get a scoping view of the situation the caregiver is dealing with (e.g., predominance of depressive symptoms, aggression, apathy).
Patient Health Questionnaire-9 (PHQ-9)[84]	• Questionnaire that assesses depressive symptomatology. • Nine-item scale, convenient for administration in clinical settings.	Cutoff scores: • 5—mild depression • 10—moderate depression • 15—moderately severe depression • 20—severe depression

areas and urban areas where caregivers may have difficulty commuting. Caregivers who have basic computer and internet skills may participate in online programs because it saves time and resources with simplified logistics and eliminates the need to look for substitute care. Likewise, online programs can afford for building rapport and connectedness as seen in in-person programs.[152]

Numerous interventions for caregivers differ in their format, but all programs are similar in their goal to improve caregivers' psychological well-being, ameliorate adverse outcomes on their mental health, and, possibly, delay the patient's institutionalization. Programs for caregivers can be categorized into counseling, cognitive behavioral therapy, acceptance and commitment therapy, psychoeducation, and environmental programs (Table 4.15).

In sum, females are the primary unpaid caregivers in the United States. It is important for the clinician to inquire and identify informal caregivers.

TABLE 4.15	Summary of Interventions for Caregivers of Dementia Patients	
Approach	**Main Features**	**Examples**
Counseling	• Typically prolonged intervention, may last for the duration of illness. • May involve one or several family members. • Can be professional- or peer-led. • Aims to assist with ongoing and new difficulties in caregiving. • May advise on resources. • Caregivers find the program beneficial and, after the program completion, find behavioral and psychological symptoms of dementia less bothersome.[142] • Leads to reduction in caregivers' depressive symptoms.[164] • Family counseling that relies on telehealth may involve distant relatives[165]	New York University (NYU) Program for Caregivers[142,163-165]
Psychoeducation	• Focus on learning about dementia, its causes, nature, and variation in manifestations • Emphasis on caregiving as a clinical role • Programs are structured as a class: with curricular goals, limited timeline, and expert-led instruction • Learning is of higher priority than emotion processing	Savvy Caregiver Program, Tele-Savvy Caregiver Program (fully remote version)[e]
Cognitive behavioral therapy	• Clarification of thinking patterns that are maladaptive (e.g., self-blame) and replacement of these patterns with realistic thinking based on experience	Numerous cognitive behavioral therapy programs developed in the United States[143,150] and internationally[141]
Acceptance and commitment therapy	• Technique that teaches mindfulness, values, commitment, and ways to cope with irreversible changes	Reported in a study conducted in Spain[144]
Environmental programs	• Modification of the person's immediate environment to decrease behavioral and psychological symptoms of dementia (declutter, reduce noise, simplify the environment)	Home Environmental Skill-building Program (ESP)[168]

NOT TO BE MISSED

Health care professionals should inquire with their adult patients about whether they serve as caregivers, and they should treat female caregivers as patients who require care for their mental and physical health and their social and financial well-being.

KEY POINTS

- Older adults, specifically older females, represent a large and growing segment of the population.
- Age does not equate to disability or disease. Older adults, however, carry the highest risk for multiple chronic conditions (multichronicity), atypical

presentation of illness, and disability stemming from multiple sources and stressors.

- Standardized assessments of common geriatric issues, including mobility, frailty, dementia, medications, and caregiver burden are recommended to optimize the health and well-being of older female patients.
- Aging does not equate to deterioration and irreversible loss. Maintenance of the female patient's quality of life is at the core. Learning about interventions to maintain mobility, independence in ADLs and IADLs, and safety is essential to prevent age-related losses and help females enjoy optimal health.
- Learning about frailty prevention, delay, and interventions to counter frailty may allow female patients

to regain strength that may appear as irreversibly lost.

- Staying up-to-date on geriatric pharmacotherapy guidelines is key to providing quality care without putting patients at risk for inappropriate excessive prescribing or undertreatment resulting from ignorance or ageism.
- Females in general are highly likely to serve as unpaid caregivers for persons living with dementia. Inquiring about the patient's status as a caregiver should be incorporated in every initial visit because individuals are likely to underreport their unpaid labor as caregivers.
- In sum, quality care for older female patients in primary care settings requires clinical acumen in overall primary care and more specialized knowledge of the normal and pathological changes associated with aging. Staying up-to-date on primary care and care for older female patients will allow clinicians to help these patients minimize the impact of aging and add quality to their years of life.

REFERENCES

1. Administration on Aging. *2019 Profile of Older Americans*; 2020. https://acl.gov/sites/default/files/Aging%20and%20Disability%20in%20America/2019ProfileOlderAmericans508.pdf.
2. Carstensen LL, Turan B, Scheibe S, et al. Emotional experience improves with age: evidence based on over 10 years of experience sampling. *Psychol Aging*. 2011;26(1):21–33.
3. Ward BW, Schiller JS. Prevalence of multiple chronic conditions among U.S. adults: estimates from the National Health Interview Survey, 2010. *Prev Chronic Dis*. 2013;10:E65.
4. Song Y, et al. The effect of estrogen replacement therapy on Alzheimer's disease and Parkinson's disease in postmenopausal women: A meta-analysis. *Front Neurosci*. 2020;14:157.
5. Owens IP. Ecology and evolution. Sex differences in mortality rate. *Science*. 2002;297(5589):2008–2009.
6. Hubbard RE, Rockwood K. Frailty in older women. *Maturitas*. 2011;69(3):203–207.
7. Mosca L, Barrett-Connor E, Wenger NK. Sex/gender differences in cardiovascular disease prevention: what a difference a decade makes. *Circulation*. 2011;124(19):2145–2154.
8. Rockwood K, Howlett SE, MacKnight C, et al. Prevalence, attributes, and outcomes of fitness and frailty in community-dwelling older adults: report from the Canadian study of health and aging. *J Gerontol A Biol Sci Med Sci*. 2004;59(12):1310–1317.
9. Postma DS. Gender differences in asthma development and progression. *Gend Med*. 2007;4(suppl B):S133–S146.
10. Centers for Disease Control and Prevention. State-specific 2015 BRFSS prevalence estimates. https://www.cdc.gov/arthritis/data_statistics/state-data-current.htm. Updated May 9, 2017.
11. Centers for Disease Control and Prevention. Cancer rates by race/ethnicity and sex. https://www.cdc.gov/cancer/dcpc/data/index.htm. Page last reviewed June 6, 2022.
12. Centers for Disease Control and Prevention. Prevalence of both diagnosed and undiagnosed diabetes. https://www.cdc.gov/diabetes/data/statistics-report/diagnosed-undiagnosed-diabetes.html. Updated September 30, 2022.
13. Federal Interagency Forum on Aging-Related Statistics. Older Americans 2016: Key Indicators of Well-Being. https://agingstats.gov/docs/LatestReport/Older-Americans-2016-Key-Indicators-of-WellBeing.pdf. Published August 2016.
14. Ormel J, Kempen GI, Deeg DJ, Brilman EI, van Sonderen E, Relyveld J. Functioning, well-being, and health perception in late middle-aged and older people: comparing the effects of depressive symptoms and chronic medical conditions. *J Am Geriatr Soc*. 1998;46(1):39–48.
15. Lakey SL, LaCroix AZ, Gray SL, et al. Antidepressant use, depressive symptoms, and incident frailty in women aged 65 and older from the Women's Health Initiative Observational Study. *J Am Geriatr Soc*. 2012;60(5):854–861.
16. Oksuzyan A, Juel K, Vaupel JW, Christensen K. Men: good health and high mortality. Sex differences in health and aging. *Aging Clin Exp Res*. 2008;20(2):91–102.
17. Studenski S, Perera S, Patel K, et al. Gait speed and survival in older adults. *JAMA*. 2011;305(1):50–58.
18. Centers for Disease Control and Prevention. Falls are Leading Cause of Injury and Death in Older Americans. https://www.cdc.gov/media/releases/2016/p0922-older-adult-falls.html. Updated September 22, 2016.
19. Podsiadlo D, Richardson S. The timed "Up & Go": a test of basic functional mobility for frail elderly persons. *J Am Geriatr Soc*. 1991;39(2):142–148.
20. Wolf SL, Barnhart HX, Kutner NG, McNeely E, Coogler C, Xu T. Reducing frailty and falls in older persons: an investigation of Tai Chi and computerized balance training. Atlanta FICSIT Group. Frailty and injuries: cooperative studies of intervention techniques. *J Am Geriatr Soc*. 1996;44(5):489–497.

21. Centers for Disease Control and Prevention. STEA-DI—Older Adult Fall Prevention. https://www.cdc.gov/steadi/. Updated March 23, 2017.

22. Katz S, Down TD, Cash HR, Grotz RC. Progress in the development of the index of ADL. *Gerontologist*. 1970;10(1):20–30.

23. Lawton MP, Brody EM. Assessment of older people: self-maintaining and instrumental activities of daily living. *Gerontologist*. 1969;9(3):179–186.

24. Graf C. The Lawton instrumental activities of daily living scale. *Am J Nurs*. 2008;108(4):52–62. quiz 62-63.

25. Gallo JJ, Paveza GJ. Activities of daily living and instrumental activities of daily living assessment. In: Gallo JJ, Bogner HR, Fulmer T, Paveza GJ, eds. *Handbook of Geriatric Assessment*. 4th ed. Burlington, MA: Jones and Bartlett Publishers; 2006:193–240.

26. Graf C. Functional decline in hospitalized older adults. *AJN*. 2006;106(1):58–67.

27. Graf C. The Lawton Instrumental Activities of Daily Living Scale. *AJN*. 2008;108(4):52–62.

28. Lawton MP, Moss M, Fulcomer M, Kleban MH. *Multilevel assessment instrument manual for full-length MAI*. North Wales, PA: Polisher Research Institute, Madlyn and Leonard Abramson Center for Jewish Life; 2003.

29. Pearson V. Assessment of function. In: Kane R, Kane R, eds. *Assessing Older Persons, Measures, Meaning, and Practical Applications*. New York: Oxford University Press; 2000.

30. Peel C, Sawyer Baker P, Roth DL, Brown CJ, Brodner EV, Allman RM. Assessing mobility in older adults: the UAB Study of Aging Life-Space Assessment. *Phys Ther*. 2005;85(10):1008–1119.

31. Rockwood K, Song X, MacKnight C, et al. A global clinical measure of fitness and frailty in elderly people. *CMAJ*. 2005;173(5):489–495.

32. Winograd CH. Targeting strategies: an overview of criteria and outcomes. *J Am Geriatr Soc*. 1991;39(9 Pt 2):25S–35S.

33. Rockwood K, Stadnyk K, MacKnight C, McDowell I, Hebert R, Hogan DB. A brief clinical instrument to classify frailty in elderly people. *Lancet*. 1999;353(9148):205–206.

34. Fried LP, Tangen CM, Walston J, et al. Frailty in older adults: evidence for a phenotype. *J Gerontol A Biol Med Sci*. 2001;56(3):M146–M156.

35. Buchner DM, Wagner EH. Preventing frail health. *Clin Geriatr Med*. 1992;8(1):1–17.

36. Bouillon K, Kivimaki M, Hamer M, et al. Measures of frailty in population-based studies: an overview. *BMC Geriatr*. 2013;13:64.

37. Rockwood K, Howlett SE, MacKnight C, et al. Prevalence, attributes, and outcomes of fitness and frailty in community-dwelling older adults: report from the Canadian study of health and aging. *J Gerontol A Biol Sci Med Sci*. 2004;59(12):1310–1317.

38. Hubbard RE, Rockwood K. Frailty in older women. *Maturitas*. 2011;69(3):203–207.

39. Hubbard RE, Lang IA, Llewellyn DJ, Rockwood K. Frailty, body mass index, and abdominal obesity in older people. *J Gerontol A Biol Sci Med Sci*. 2010;65(4):377–381.

40. Lee P-H, Lee Y-S, Chan D-C. Interventions targeting geriatric frailty: a systematic review. *J Clin Gerontol Geriatr*. 2012;3:47–52.

41. Fiatarone MA, O'Neill EF, Ryan ND, et al. Exercise training and nutritional supplementation for physical frailty in very elderly people. *N Eng J Med*. 1994;330(25):1769–1775.

42. Binder EF, Schechtman KB, Ehsani AA, et al. Effects of exercise training on frailty in community-dwelling older adults: results of a randomized, controlled trial. *J Am Geriatr Soc*. 2002;50(12):1921–1928.

43. Morley JE. Anorexia and weight loss in older persons. *J Gerontol A Biol Sci Med Sci*. 2003;58(2):131–137.

44. Villareal DT, Banks M, Sinacore DR, Siener C, Klein S. Effect of weight loss and exercise on frailty in obese older adults. *Arch Intern Med*. 2006;166(8):860–866.

45. Davison KK, Ford ES, Cogswell ME, Dietz WH. Percentage of body fat and body mass index are associated with mobility limitations in people aged 70 and older from NHANES III. *J Am Geriatr Soc*. 2002;50(11):1802–1809.

46. Villareal DT, Chode S, Parimi N, et al. Weight loss, exercise, or both and physical function in obese older adults. *N Engl J Med*. 2011;364(13):1218–1229.

47. Gill TM, Baker DI, Gottschalk M, et al. A prehabilitation program for physically frail community-living older persons. *Arch Phys Med Rehabil*. 2003;84(3):394–404.

48. Artaza-Artabe I, Saez-Lopez P, Sanchez-Hernandez N, Fernandez-Gutierrez N, Malafarina V. The relationship between nutrition and frailty: Effects of protein intake, nutritional supplementation, vitamin D and exercise on muscle metabolism in the elderly. A systematic review. *Maturitas*. 2016;93:89–99.

49. Robinson TN, Wu DS, Pointer L, Dunn CL, Cleveland Jr JC, Moss M. Simple frailty score predicts postoperative complications across surgical specialties. *Am J Surg*. 2013;206(4):544–550.

50. Makary MA, Segev DL, Pronovost PJ, et al. Frailty as a predictor of surgical outcomes in older patients. *J Am Coll Surg*. 2010;210(6):901–908.

51. Centers for Disease Control and Prevention, Merck Institute of Aging & Health. The State of Aging and

Health in America 2004. https://www.cdc.gov/aging/pdf/state_of_aging_and_health_in_america_2004.pdf. Published 2004.

52. Budnitz DS, Lovegrove MC, Shehab N, Richards CL. Emergency hospitalizations for adverse drug events in older Americans. *N Engl J Med.* 2011;365(21):2002–2012.

53. Veronese N, Stubbs B, Noale M, et al. Polypharmacy is associated with higher frailty risk in older people: an 8-year longitudinal cohort study. *J Am Med Dir Assoc.* 2017;18(7):624–628.

54. Gnjidic D, Hilmer SN, Blyth FM, et al. Polypharmacy cutoff and outcomes: five or more medicines were used to identify community-dwelling older men at risk of different adverse outcomes. *J Clin Epidemiol.* 2012;65(9):989–995.

55. Turner JP, Jamsen KM, Shakib S, Singhal N, Prowse R, Bell JS. Polypharmacy cut-points in older people with cancer: how many medications are too many? *Support Care Cancer.* 2016;24(4):1831–1840.

56. Gnjidic D, Hilmer SN, Blyth FM, et al. High-risk prescribing and incidence of frailty among older community-dwelling men. *Clin Pharmacol Ther.* 2012;91(3):521–528.

57. 2019 American Geriatrics Society Beers Criteria® Update Expert Panel. American Geriatrics Society 2019 updated AGS Beers criteria® for potentially inappropriate medication use in older adults. *J Am Geriatr Soc.* 2019;67(4):674–694.

58. Gallagher P, Ryan C, Byrne S, Kennedy J, O'Mahony D. STOPP (Screening Tool of Older Person's Prescriptions) and START (Screening Tool to Alert doctors to Right Treatment). Consensus validation. *Int J Clin Pharmacol Ther.* 2008;46(2):72–83.

59. Gallagher P, Lang PO, Cherubini A, et al. Prevalence of potentially inappropriate prescribing in an acutely ill population of older patients admitted to six European hospitals. *Eur J Clin Pharmacol.* 2011;67(11):1175–1188.

60. Hovstadius B, Petersson G. The impact of increasing polypharmacy on prescribed drug expenditure-a register-based study in Sweden 2005-2009. *Health Policy.* 2013;109(2):166–174.

61. Bourgeois FT, Shannon MW, Valim C, Mandl KD. Adverse drug events in the outpatient setting: an 11-year national analysis. *Pharmacoepidemiol Drug Saf.* 2010;19(9):901–910.

62. Marcum ZA, Amuan ME, Hanlon JT, et al. Prevalence of unplanned hospitalizations caused by adverse drug reactions in older veterans. *J Am Geriatr Soc.* 2012;60(1):34–41.

63. Doan J, Zakrzewski-Jakubiak H, Roy J, Turgeon J, Tannenbaum C. Prevalence and risk of potential cyto-chrome P450–mediated drug-drug interactions in older hospitalized patients with polypharmacy. *Ann Pharmacother.* 2013;47(3):324–332.

64. Crentsil V, Ricks MO, Xue QL, Fried LP. A pharmacoepidemiologic study of community-dwelling, disabled older women: factors associated with medication use. *Am J Geriatr Pharmacother.* 2010;8(3):215–224.

65. Jyrkka J, Enlund H, Lavikainen P, Sulkava R, Hartikainen S. Association of polypharmacy with nutritional status, functional ability and cognitive capacity over a three-year period in an elderly population. *Pharmacoepidemiol Drug Saf.* 2011;20(5):514–522.

66. American Society of Consultant Pharmacists. http://www.ascp.com/.

67. Snyder HM. *Alzheimer's falls more heavily on women than on men.* Scientific American; 2016. https://blogs.scientificamerican.com/mind-guest-blog/alzheimers-falls-more-heavily-on-women-than-on-men/.

68. Alzheimer's Association. *Alzheimer's Disease Facts and Figures*; 2021. https://www.alz.org/alzheimers-dementia/facts-figures.

69. Fitzpatrick AL, Kuller LH, Ives DG, Lopez OL, Jagust W, Bretiner JC, et al. Incidence and prevalence of dementia in the Cardiovascular Health Study. *J Am Geriatr Soc.* 2004;52:195–204.

70. Willis BL, Gao A, Leonard D, Defina LF, Berry JD. Midlife fitness and the development of chronic conditions in later life. *Arch Intern Med.* 2012;172(17):1333–1340.

71. Sachdev PS, Blacker D, Blazer DG, et al. Classifying neurocognitive disorders: the DSM-5 approach. *Nat Rev Neurol.* 2014;10(11):634–642.

72. Bradford A, Kunik ME, Schulz P, Williams SP, Singh H. Missed and delayed diagnosis of dementia in primary care: prevalence and contributing factors. *Alzheimer Dis Assoc Disord.* 2009;23(4):306–314.

73. Alzheimer's Association. 10 Early Signs and Symptoms of Alzheimer's. http://www.alz.org/alzheimers_disease_10_signs_of_alzheimers.asp?type=alzFooter.

74. American Academy of Neurology. Alzheimer's Disease. https://www.neurology.org/collection/alzheimers_disease.

75. Department of Veterans Affairs. Clinical fact sheet: detection of dementia. https://www.prevention.va.gov/docs/0514_VANCP_Dementia_Fact_F.pdf. Updated April 2011.

76. Galvin JE, Sadowsky CH. Practical guidelines for the recognition and diagnosis of dementia. *J Am Board Fam Med.* 2012;25(3):367–382.

77. Sheehan B. Assessment scales in dementia. *Ther Adv Neurol Disord.* 2012;5(6):349–358.

78. Folstein MF, Folstein SE, McHugh PR. Mini-mental state." A practical method for grading the cognitive

state of patients for the clinician. *J Psychiatr Res.* 1975;12(3):189–198.

79. Tariq SH, Tumosa N, Chibnall JT, Perry 3rd MH, Morley JE. Comparison of the Saint Louis University mental status examination and the mini-mental state examination for detecting dementia and mild neurocognitive disorder—a pilot study. *Am J Geriatr Psychiatry.* 2006;14(11):900–910.

80. American Psychiatric Association. *Diagnostic and Statistical Manual of Mental Disorders.* 5th ed. Arlington, VA; 2013.

81. Jette AM, Davies AR, Cleary PD, et al. The Functional Status Questionnaire: reliability and validity when used in primary care. *J Gen Intern Med.* 1986;1(3):143–149.

82. Yesavage JA, Brink TL, Rose TL, et al. Development and validation of a geriatric depression screening scale: a preliminary report. *J Psychiatr Res.* 1982;17(1):37–49.

83. Sheikh JL, Yesavage JA. Geriatric Depression Scale (GDS): recent evidence and development of a shorter version. *Clin Gerontol.* 1986;5:165–173.

84. Kroenke K, Spitzer RL, Williams JB. The PHQ-9: validity of a brief depression severity measure. *J Gen Intern Med.* 2001;16(9):606–613.

85. Alexopoulos GS, Abrams RC, Young RC, Shamoian CA. Cornell Scale for depression in dementia. *Biol Psychiatry.* 1988;23(3):271–284.

86. Desai AK, Schwartz L, Grossberg GT. Behavioral disturbance in dementia. *Curr Psychiatry Rep.* 2012;14(4):298–309.

87. Cummings JL, Mega M, Gray K, Rosenberg-Thompson S, Carusi DA, Gornbein J. The Neuropsychiatric Inventory: comprehensive assessment of psychopathology in dementia. *Neurology.* 1994;44(12):2308–2314.

88. Cummings J. The neuropsychiatric inventory: Assessming psychopathology in dementia patients. *Neurology.* 1997;48(suppl 6):S10–S16.

89. Kaufer DI, Cummings JL, Christine D, et al. Assessing the impact of neuropsychiatric symptoms in Alzheimer's disease: the Neuropsychiatric Inventory Caregiver Distress Scale. *J Am Geriatr Soc.* 1998;46(2):210–215.

90. Kaufer DI, Cummings JL, Ketchel P, et al. Validation of the NPI-Q, a brief clinical form of the Neuropsychiatric Inventory. *J Neuropsychiatry Clin Neurosci.* 2000;12(2):233–239.

91. Teri L, Truax P, Logsdon R, Uomoto J, Zarit S, Vitaliano PP. The revised memory and behavior problems checklist. *Psychol Aging.* 1992;7:622–631.

92. Knopman DS, DeKosky ST, Cummings JL, et al. Practice parameter: Diagnosis of dementia (an evidence-based review). Neurology. 2001;56(9). https://n.neurology.org/content/56/9/1143.

93. Reisberg B, Ferris SH, Anand R, et al. Functional staging of dementia of the Alzheimer's type. *Ann N Y Acad Sci.* 1984;435:481–483.

94. Reisberg B, Ferris SH. Brief Cognitive Rating Scale (BCRS). *Psychopharmacol Bull.* 1988;24(4):629–636.

95. Reisberg B. Functional assessment staging (FAST). *Psychopharmacol Bull.* 1988;24(4):653–659.

96. Reisberg B, Ferris SH, de Leon MJ. Senile dementia of the Alzheimer type: diagnostic and differential diagnostic features with special reference to functional assessment staging. In: Traber J, Gispen WH, eds. *Senile Dementia of the Alzheimer Type.* Vol 2. Berlin: Springer-Verlag; 1985:18–37.

97. Reisberg B, Ferris SH, Shulman E, et al. Longitudinal course of normal aging and progressive dementia of the Alzheimer's type: a prospective study of 106 subjects over a 3.6 year mean interval. *Prog Neuropsychopharmacol Biol Psychiatry.* 1986;10(3-5):571–578.

98. Snow TL. The GEMS®: Brain change model. Positive Approach to Care. https://teepasnow.com/about/about-teepa-snow/the-gems-brain-change-model/.

99. Alzheimer's Association. 50 Activities. https://www.alz.org/help-support/resources/kids-teens/50-activities.

100. SimpleC. http://www.simplec.com/.

101. Wagner LM, Clevenger C. Contractures in nursing home residents. *J Am Med Dir Assoc.* 2010;11(2):94–99.

102. Mitchell SL, Teno JM, Kiely DK, et al. The clinical course of advanced dementia. *N Engl J Med.* 2009;361(16):1529–1538.

103. Mitchell SL. Advanced dementia. *N Engl J Med.* 2015;373(13):1276–1277.

104. American Geriatrics Society Ethics Committee and Clinical Practice and Models of Care Committee. American Geriatrics Society feeding tubes in advanced dementia position statement. *J Am Geriatr Soc.* 2014;62(8):1590–1593.

105. Fisher GG, Franks MM, Plassman BL, et al. Caring for individuals with dementia and cognitive impairment, not dementia: findings from the aging, demographics, and memory study. *J Am Geriatr Soc.* 2011;59(3):488–494.

106. Kasper JD, Freedman VA, Spillman BC, Wolff JL. The disproportionate impact of dementia on family and unpaid caregiving to older adults. *Health Aff (Millwood).* 2015;34(10):1642–1649.

107. Nikmat AW, Hawthorne G, Al-Mashoor SH. The comparison of quality of life among people with mild dementia in nursing home and home care—a preliminary report. *Dementia.* 2015;14(1). 144-125.

108. Cranswick K, Dosman D. *Eldercare: What We Know Today.* Statistics Canada; 2008. http://www.statcan.gc.ca/

pub/11-008-x/2008002/article/10689-eng.htm. Updated November 21, 2008.

109. Alzheimer's Association. 2014 Alzheimer's disease facts and figures. *Alzheimers Dement.* 2014;10(2):e47–e92.

110. Campbell P, Wright J, Oyebode J, et al. Determinants of burden in those who care for someone with dementia. *Int J Geriatr Psychiatry.* 2008;23(10):1078–1085.

111. Pope ND, Kolomer S, Glass AP. How women in late midlife become caregivers for their aging parents. *J Women Aging.* 2012;24(3):242–261.

112. Aneshensel CS, Pearlin LI, Mullan JT, Zarit SH, Whitlatch CI. *Profiles in Caregiving: the Unexpected Career.* San Diego, CA: Academic Press; 1995.

113. Shriver M. *The Shriver Report: A Woman's Nation Takes on Alzheimer's.* Chicago, IL; 2010. https://www.alz.org/news/2010/the-shriver-report-a-woman-s-nation-takes-on-alzh.

114. Souren LE, Franssen EH, Reisberg B. Neuromotor changes in Alzheimer's disease: implications for patient care. *J Geriatr Psychiatry Neurol.* 1997;10(3):93–98.

115. Schubert CC, Boustani M, Callahan CM, et al. Comorbidity profile of dementia patients in primary care: are they sicker? *J Am Geriatr Soc.* 2006;54(1):104–109.

116. Roth DL, Fredman L, Haley WE. Informal caregiving and its impact on health: a reappraisal from population-based studies. *Gerontologist.* 2015;55(2):309–319.

117. Lloyd J, Patterson T, Muers J. The positive aspects of caregiving in dementia: a critical review of the qualitative literature. *Dementia (London).* 2016;15(6):1534–1561.

118. Roth DL, Dilworth-Anderson P, Huang J, Gross AL, Gitlin LN. Positive aspects of family caregiving for dementia: differential item functioning by race. *J Gerontol B Psychol Sci Soc Sci.* 2015;70(6):813–819.

119. Reinhard B, Given B, Petlick NH, Bemis A. Supporting family caregivers in providing care. In: Hughes RG, ed. *Patient Safety and Quality: An Evidence-Based Handbook for Nurses.* Rockville, MD: Agengy for Healthcare Research and Quality; 2008.

120. Corrêa MS, Vedovelli K, Giacobbo BL, et al. Psychophysiological correlates of cognitive deficits in family caregivers of patients with Alzheimer Disease. *Neuroscience.* 2015;286:371–382.

121. Richardson TJ, Lee SJ, Berg-Weger M, Grossberg GT. Caregiver health: health of caregivers of Alzheimer's and other dementia patients. *Curr Psychiatry Rep.* 2013;15(7):367.

122. Iavarone A, Ziello AR, Pastore F, Fasanaro AM, Poderico C. Caregiver burden and coping strategies in caregivers of patients with Alzheimer's disease. *Neuropsychiatr Dis Treat.* 2014;10:1407–1413.

123. Zarit SH, Reever KE, Bach-Peterson J. Relatives of the impaired elderly: Correlates of feelings of burden. *Gerontologist.* 1980;20(6):649–655.

124. Hughes SL, Giobbie-Hurder A, Weaver FM, Kubal JD, Henderson W. Relationship between caregiver burden and health-related quality of life. *Gerontologist.* 1999;39(5):534–545.

125. Nunnemann S, Kurz A, Leucht S, Diehl-Schmid J. Caregivers of patients with frontotemporal lobar degeneration: a review of burden, problems, needs, and interventions. *Int Psychogeriatr.* 2012;24(9):1368–1386.

126. Schulz R, O'Brien AT, Bookwala J, Fleissner K. Psychiatric and physical morbidity effects of dementia caregiving: prevalence, correlates, and causes. *Gerontologist.* 1995;35(6):771–791.

127. Lu YF, Wykle M. Relationships between caregiver stress and self-care behaviors in response to symptoms. *Clin Nurs Res.* 2007;16(1):29–43.

128. Chassin L, Macy JT, Seo DC, Presson CC, Sherman SJ. The association between membership in the sandwich generation and health behaviors: a longitudinal study. *J Appl Dev Psychol.* 2010;31(1):38–46.

129. Gwyther LP. When "the family" is not one voice: conflict in caregiving families. *J Case Manag.* 1995;4(4):150–155.

130. Ory MG, Hoffman 3rd RR, Yee JL, Tennstedt S, Schulz R. Prevalence and impact of caregiving: a detailed comparison between dementia and nondementia caregivers. *Gerontologist.* 1999;39(2):177–185.

131. Pearlin LI, Mullan JT, Semple SJ, Skaff MM. Caregiving and the stress process: an overview of concepts and their measures. *Gerontologist.* 1990;30(5):583–594.

132. Fonareva I, Oken BS. Physiological and functional consequences of caregiving for relatives with dementia. *Int Psychogeriatr.* 2014;26(5):725–747.

133. Miller GE, Murphy ML, Cashman R, et al. Greater inflammatory activity and blunted glucocorticoid signaling in monocytes of chronically stressed caregivers. *Brain Behav Immun.* 2014;41:191–199.

134. Everson-Rose SA, Lewis TT. Psychosocial factors and cardiovascular diseases. *Annu Rev Public Health.* 2005;26:469–500.

135. Kiecolt-Glaser JK, Preacher KJ, MacCallum RC, Atkinson C, Malarkey WB, Glaser R. Chronic stress and age-related increases in the proinflammatory cytokine IL-6. *Proc Natl Acad Sci U S A.* 2003;100(15):9090–9095.

136. Slavich GM, Irwin MR. From stress to inflammation and major depressive disorder: a social signal transduction theory of depression. *Psychol Bull.* 2014;140(3):774–815.

137. Seeman TE. Social ties and health: the benefits of social integration. *Ann Epidemiol.* 1996;6(5):442–451.

138. Cole SW, Hawkley LC, Arevalo JM, Sung CY, Rose RM, Cacioppo JT. Social regulation of gene expression in human leukocytes. *Genome Biol*. 2007;8(9):R189.

139. Fredman L, Daly MP, Lazur AM. Burden among white and black caregivers to elderly adults. *J Gerontol B Psychol Sci Soc Sci*. 1995;50(2):S110–S118.

140. O'Connor MF, Arizmendi BJ, Kaszniak AW. Virtually supportive: a feasibility pilot study of an online support group for dementia caregivers in a 3D virtual environment. *J Aging Stud*. 2014;30:87–93.

141. Aboulafia-Brakha T, Suchecki D, Gouveia-Paulino F, Nitrini R, Ptak R. Cognitive- behavioural group therapy improves a psychophysiological marker of stress in caregivers of patients with Alzheimer's disease. *Aging Mental Health*. 2014;18(6):801–808.

142. Mittelman MS, Roth DL, Coon DW, Haley WE. Sustained benefit of supportive intervention for depressive symptoms in caregivers of patients with Alzheimer's disease. *Am J Psychiatry*. 2004;161(5):850–856.

143. Akkerman RL, Ostwald SK. Reducing anxiety in Alzheimer's disease family caregivers: the effectiveness of a nine-week cognitive-behavioral intervention. *Am J Alzheimers Dis Other Demen*. 2004;19(2):117–123.

144. Losada A, Marquez-Gonzalez M, Romero-Moreno R, et al. Cognitive-behavioral therapy (CBT) versus acceptance and commitment therapy (ACT) for dementia family caregivers with significant depressive symptoms: results of a randomized clinical trial. *J Consult Clin Psychol*. 2015;83(4):760–772.

145. Judge KS, Yarry SJ, Looman WJ, Bass DM. Improved strain and psychosocial outcomes for caregivers of individuals with dementia: findings from Project ANSWERS. *Gerontologist*. 2013;53(2):280–292.

146. Hepburn K, Lewis M, Sherman CW, Tornatore J. The Savvy Caregiver Program: developing and testing a transportable dementia family caregiver training program. *Gerontologist*. 2003;43(6):908–915.

147. Gitlin LN, Corcoran M, Winter L, Boyce A, Hauck WW. A randomized, controlled trial of a home environmental intervention: effect on efficacy and upset in caregivers and on daily function of persons with dementia. *Gerontologist*. 2001;41(1):4–14.

148. Belle SH, Burgio L, Burns R, et al. Enhancing the quality of life of dementia caregivers from different ethnic or racial groups: a randomized, controlled trial. *Ann Intern Med*. 2006;145(10):727–738.

149. Knapp M, King D, Romeo R, et al. Cost effectiveness of a manual based coping strategy programme in promoting the mental health of family carers of people with dementia (the START (STrAtegies for RelaTives) study): a pragmatic randomised controlled trial. *BMJ*. 2013;347:f6342.

150. Gallagher-Thompson D, Gray HL, Dupart T, Jimenez D, Thompson LW. Effectiveness of cognitive/behavioral small group intervention for reduction of depression and stress in non-Hispanic White and Hispanic/Latino women dementia family caregivers: outcomes and mediators of change. *J Ration Emot Cogn Behav Ther*. 2008;26(4):286–303.

151. Kovaleva M, Blevins L, Griffiths PC, Hepburn K. An online program for caregivers of persons living with dementia: lessons learned. *J Appl Gerontol*. 2019;38(2):159–182.

152. Centers for Disease Control and Prevention. The Timed Up and Go (TUG) Test. https://www.cdc.gov/steadi/pdf/TUG_Test-print.pdf.

153. Cesari M, Kritchevsky SB, Penninx BW, et al. Prognostic value of usual gait speed in well-functioning older people—results from the Health, Aging and Body Composition Study. *J Am Geriatr Soc*. 2005;53(10):1675–1680.

154. Studenski S, Perera S, Wallace D, et al. Physical performance measures in the clinical setting. *J Am Geriatr Soc*. 2003;51(3):314–322.

155. Shelkey M, Wallace M. Katz Index of Independence in Activities of Daily Living. *J Gerontol Nurs*. 1999;25(3):8–9.

156. Beasley JM, LaCroix AZ, Neuhouser ML, et al. Protein intake and incident frailty in the Women's Health Initiative observational study. *J Am Geriatr Soc*. 2010;58(6):1063–1071.

157. Borson S, Scanlan JM, Chen P, Ganguli M. The Mini-Cog as a screen for dementia: validation in a population-based sample. *J Am Geriatr Soc*. 2003;51(10):1451–1454.

158. Charlson ME, Pompei P, Ales KL, MacKenzie CR. A new method of classifying prognostic comorbidity in longitudinal studies: development and validation. *J Chronic Dis*. 1987;40(5):373–383.

159. American Geriatrics Society. *Geriatrics Evaluation & Management Tools*. Appropriate Prescribing; 2015.

160. Fernando MS, Ince PG, MRCC Function and Ageing Neuropathology Study Group. Vascular pathologies and cognition in a population-based cohort of elderly people. *J Neurol Sci*. 2004;226(1-2):13–17.

161. Hébert R, Bravo G, Préville M. Reliability, validity and reference values of the Zarit Burden Interview for assessing informal caregivers of community-dwelling older persons with dementia. *Canadian J Aging*. 2000;19(4):494–507.

162. Mittelman MS, Ferris SH, Shulman E, et al. A comprehensive support program: effect on depression in spouse-caregivers of AD patients. *Gerontologist*. 1995;35(6):792–802.

163. Mittelman MS, Ferris SH, Shulman E, Steinberg G, Levin B. A family intervention to delay nursing home placement of patients with Alzheimer disease. A randomized controlled trial. *JAMA*. 1996;276(21):1725–1731.

164. Mittelman MS, Roth DL, Haley WE, Zarit SH. Effects of a caregiver intervention on negative caregiver appraisals of behavior problems in patients with Alzheimer's disease: results of a randomized trial. *J Gerontol B Psychol Sci Soc Sci*. 2004;59(1):P27–P34.

165. Czaja SJ, Rubert MP. Telecommunications technology as an aid to family caregivers of persons with dementia. *Psychosom Med*. 2002;64(3):469–476.

166. Hepburn K, Lewis M, Tornatore J, Sherman CW, Bremer KL. The Savvy Caregiver program: the demonstrated effectiveness of a transportable dementia caregiver psychoeducation program. *J Gerontol Nurs*. 2007;33(3):30–36.

167. Hepburn K, Nocera J, Higgins M, et al. Results of a randomized trial testing the efficacy of Tele-Savvy, an online synchronous/asynchronous psychoeducation program for family caregivers of persons living with dementia. *Gerontologist*. 2022;62(4):616–628.

168. Gitlin LN, Hauck WW, Dennis MP, Winter L. Maintenance of effects of the home environmental skill-building program for family caregivers and individuals with Alzheimer's disease and related disorders. *J Gerontol A Biol Sci Med Sci*. 2005;60(3):368–374.

169. Centers for Medicare and Medicaid Services. Chartbook and Charts. https://www.cms.gov/Research-Statistics-Data-and-Systems/Statistics-Trends-and-Reports/Chronic-Conditions/Chartbook_Charts.

170. Alzheimer's Association. 2014 Alzheimer's disease facts and figures. *Alzheimers Dement*. 2014;10(2):e47–e92.

5

The Well-Woman Visit

Ayanna Gray-Bolden

OBJECTIVES

- Identify the key components of the well-woman visit.
- Review the epidemiological data that supports the components of the well-woman visit.
- Develop a plan of care for the well-woman visit based on history and physical examination, patient education, and counseling.

- Examine how respect for female patients, respect for culture, and respect for the varieties of sexual experiences all work together to assist the provider in providing excellent evidence-based care.

INTRODUCTION

Health promotion and disease prevention have become the hallmark of modern medicine. With health care costs rising and life expectancy increasing, the burden of disease treatment and management has also increased. Because of these factors, proactive management of health rather than reactive disease management is paramount. The Institute of Medicine (IOM) and the Patient Protection and Affordable Care Act (ACA) of 2010 introduced a change in perspective from a framework that is reactive in nature to one that cultivates ideal health and well-being.[1,2]

> *The emphasis over recent years has changed in women's health care; traditional reliance on mainly reactive, consultant-led, hospital-based care has been transformed into a more holistic, proactive, primary care led approach with a goal of involving and educating women throughout their lives aiding*

> *in healthier lifestyle choices. …[Women] deserve care which helps them avoid hospitalization and intervention whenever possible that is provided by community-based carers who understand their needs and aspirations…[3]*

In the 2000s, the *well-women* label replaced what was formerly referred to as the *women's health examination*. Fifty years prior, in 1966, obstetricians were prescribing the first birth control pill, utilization of the Pap test was becoming the gold standard, and present-day mammography methods were progressively advancing. The American College of Obstetricians and Gynecologists (ACOG) fundamental practice guideline book, *Standards for Obstetric-Gynecologic Hospital Services*, reviewed the general physical examination yet generally was centered around obstetrics and reproductive well-being.[4]

By 1996, thirty years later, these practice guidelines evolved to include very specific categories of *primary and preventive care and evaluation and counseling* that were distinguished separately from gynecological services and categorized by age.[4]

Over time, there has been a transition from an emphasis on the Pap and pelvic examination to women's health that cares for the whole woman.

OVERVIEW

The frequency of well-women visits has been the topic of many discussions; in its first set of draft recommendations for the U.S. Health Resources and Services Administration (HRSA), the Women's Preventive Services Initiative (WPSI), established by ACOG, further clarified that there is a need for "at least one annual preventive care visit for women beginning in adolescence and continuing across the lifespan to ensure that women obtain recommended preventive services" as determined by age and risk factors including preconception, and many services necessary for prenatal and interconception care. It is generally recognized that all necessary recommended preventive services, depending on a female patient's health status, health needs, and other risk factors, may require several visits.[4,5]

The conditions addressed in this chapter are not an all-inclusive list, but many of the major issues that must be addressed in the well-woman visit are reviewed.

EPIDEMIOLOGICAL DATA

There are many disease processes that affect the population as a whole but pose very specific threats to females, and specific attention should be paid to disease processes whose incidence rates are increasing, such as women's reproductive organ cancers, breast cancer, diabetes, and cardiovascular disease. It is now widely recognized that disease and other issues affect females very differently than they do males and therefore must be addressed in their own specialized way.

According to the Centers for Disease Control and Prevention (CDC), the top 10 leading causes of death for females include heart disease (number 1), cancer (number 2), stroke (number 4), and diabetes (number 7), all of which can be linked to obesity in many cases.[6] Obesity-related conditions such as heart disease, stroke, type 2 diabetes, and certain types of cancer, are some of the leading causes of preventable death.[7]

Obesity

According to the CDC, obesity affects more than one-third (42.4%) of adults in the United States, and the prevalence of severe obesity was higher in females (11.5%) than in males (6.9%).[8]

Heart Disease and Stroke

Heart disease is the leading cause of death for females and accounts for about 1 of 5 female deaths in the United States, killing close to 300,000 females alone in 2017.[9] Six of 10 people who die from stroke are females.[10]

Diabetes

The CDC reports that greater than 34 million people have diabetes (10.5% of the U.S. population). About 34.5% of adults 18 years of age and older have prediabetes. Type 2 diabetes accounts for 90% to 95% of all diabetes cases. Females account for about one-half of diagnosed cases.[11]

Cervical Cancer

According to the World Health Organization (WHO), cervical cancer is the fourth most common type of cancer in females worldwide, with most cases linked to a sexually-transmitted genital infection with the human papillomavirus (HPV).[12]

Cervical cancer was previously the leading cause of cancer death for females in the United States. The CDC reports that an estimated 12,831 new cases of cervical cancer and 4207 deaths occurred in the United States in 2017.[13] However, in the past 40 years, the number of cases of cervical cancer and the number of deaths from cervical cancer have decreased dramatically since the implementation of widespread cervical cancer screening.[14] Most cases of cervical cancer occur in females who have not been appropriately screened. "Strategies that aim to ensure that all women are screened at the appropriate interval and receive adequate follow-up are most likely to be successful in further reducing cervical cancer incidence and mortality in the United States."[15] The annual well-woman visit provides the opportunity to ensure that appropriate screening is performed as well as offer and administer the HPV vaccine to appropriate candidates.

Breast Cancer

According to the CDC, breast cancer is the most common cancer in females in the United States (not including some kinds of skin cancer), no matter one's race or ethnicity[16]; it is the most common cause of death from cancer among Hispanic females and the second most common cause of death from cancer among Caucasian, Black/African American, Asian/Pacific Islander, and Native American/Alaskan Native females.[17] In 2017, there were 250,520 females diagnosed with breast cancer, and 42,000 died; these numbers continue to rise.[18]

Intimate Partner Violence

According to the CDC, it is estimated that approximately 1.5 million females are raped and/or physically assaulted each year in the United States, and 29 million will be raped and/or physically assaulted at some point in their lifetime. As many as 324,000 pregnant females are affected each year. In addition to the immediate impact, intimate partner violence (IPV) has lifelong consequences beyond injury and death that are both acute and chronic. Victims are more likely to suffer from mental health issues (e.g., depression, anxiety) and engage in habits that are detrimental to their overall health, such as smoking, illegal substance abuse, and heavy/binge drinking. Other health conditions associated with IPV may be a direct result of the physical violence (e.g., bruises, knife wounds, broken bones, traumatic brain injury, back or pelvic pain, headaches) or the result of the impact of IPV on the neurological system (e.g., headaches/migraines), respiratory system (e.g., asthma), cardiovascular/circulatory system, gastrointestinal system (e.g., irritable bowel syndrome), musculoskeletal system (e.g., fibromyalgia/chronic pain syndromes and joint disease), and endocrine and immune systems through chronic stress or other mechanisms.[19]

HISTORY

The well-woman visit should include a very thorough and comprehensive health review and history.

A well-woman visit provides an excellent opportunity to counsel patients about maintaining a healthy lifestyle and minimizing health risks. The periodic well-woman care visit should include screening, evaluation and counseling, and immunizations based on age and risk factors.[20]

> **PATIENT-CENTERED CARE:** Creating and maintaining trust in relationships and being supportive are key to female patients disclosing sensitive information.[19] A level of comfort during the interview can be increased with questions that are asked in an open-ended and nonjudgmental way.

> **CLINICAL SURVIVAL TIP** Consider the verbiage, "Is there any illness that you see your provider for, such as *[provide examples head to toe: head problems like headaches or migraines, neck problems like problems with thyroid, lung problems like asthma, heart problems like high blood pressure, stomach problems like heartburn, muscle problems].*" Medical issues that are also very stable are also often forgotten (e.g., asthma).

Components of a patient history should include the following:
- Medical history
  - Current or past illnesses
  - Hospitalizations
  - Sleep disorders (obstructive sleep apnea)
- Surgical history
  - Past gynecological surgeries
  - Past non-gynecological surgeries
- Gynecological history
  - Cervical cancer screening (CCS) history (normal vs. abnormal)
  - Urogynecological/gynecological issues/illness (e.g., incontinence, fibroids, dysmenorrhea, menorrhagia)
  - Sexually transmitted infection (STI) history, treatment, and sequelae
- Contraceptive history
  - Current method
  - Satisfaction with method
  - Previous methods, including complications, reasons discontinued
- Current medications and allergies
  - Prescription medications
  - Illegal medication use
  - Over-the-counter medications
  - Vitamins
  - Supplements
  - Vaccination history/record review

- Sexual history
  - Respect for the female patient's identity, culture, and religious background is essential to providing the best care possible. Aspects of competent care include awareness of and respect for the varieties of sexual experiences. The following questions found in Box 5.1 can be used to decrease the risk of discouraging some females from providing a complete history or seeking care.
- Menstrual history
  - Age at menarche
  - Last menstrual period
- Menstrual pattern
  - Cycle length
  - Duration of flow
  - Amount of flow
  - Moliminal symptoms: any symptoms, other than bleeding, that precede menstruation
  - Associated pain (dysmenorrhea, mittelschmerz)
  - Intermenstrual bleeding
- Perimenopause/menopause
  - Bleeding pattern
  - Vasomotor symptoms (see Chapter 13)
  - Hormone replacement therapy
- Obstetric history: Describe each pregnancy and the outcome; describe any maternal, fetal, or neonatal complication
- Family history
  - Family members' illnesses should be listed, specifically asking about cardiovascular diseases (hypertension, hyperlipidemia, myocardial infarction, stroke), cancers (making sure to include inherited breast and ovarian cancers), diabetes mellitus, osteoporosis, and other hereditary disorders. The family members who are affected and the age at which each diagnosis was made should be documented.
- Social history
  - Marital or relationship status
  - Level of education

BOX 5.1 Sexual History: Questions to Ensure a Complete Sexual History

General Questions
- Are you currently sexually active? Have you ever been?
- What is your gender? How do you identify? What pronouns do you prefer?

Partners
- How do your partners identify? Do they identify as male, female, or another? or What are the genders of your partners?
- How many partners have you had in the past month? The past 6 months? Your lifetime?
- How satisfied are you with your (and/or your partner's) sexual functioning?
- Has there been any chance in your (or your partner's) sexual desire or the frequency of sexual activity?

Practices
- What type of sexual activities do you participate in? Do you participate in vaginal sex? Oral sex? Anal sex?

Past History/Protection From Sexually Transmitted Diseases and Sexually Transmitted Infections
- Have you ever had any sex-related diseases?
- Do you have, or have you ever had, any risk factors for HIV? (List blood transfusions, needle stick injuries, intravenous drug use, STIs, partners who may have place the patient at risk.)
- Have you ever been tested for HIV? Would you like to be?
- What do you do to protect yourself from contracting HIV?

Pregnancy Plans
- Are you trying to become a parent? Would you like to get pregnant (or father a child)?
- What method do you use for contraception?

Pleasure
- Do you (or your partners) use any particular devices or substances to enhance your sexual pleasure?
- Do you ever have pain with intercourse? Do you have any difficulty with lubrication?
- Do you have any difficulty achieving orgasm?
- Do you have any difficulty obtaining and maintaining an erection?
- Do you have any difficulty with ejaculation?
- Do you have any questions or concerns about your sexual functioning?
- Is there anything about your (or your partner's) sexual activity (as individuals or as a couple) that you would like to change?

Modified from Nusbaum, MR, Hamilton CD. The proactive sexual health history. *Am Fam Physician.* 2022;66(9):1709.

- Occupation
- Alcohol, cigarette, or illegal drug use
- Exercise history
- Diet history
- Nutritional/dietary assessment
  - Further detail can be obtained dependent on patient status (e.g., body mass index [BMI]) and the presence of any relevant medical problems (e.g., diabetes mellitus, any signs of nutritional deficiency).

Review of Systems

All organ systems should be completely reviewed including a systematic gynecological review. Many non-gynecological conditions have associated gynecological symptoms. For example, symptoms that are particularly likely to be associated with gynecological conditions include: a history of significant weight loss or weight gain, excess hair growth (hirsutism), and symptoms of depression.[21]

Breasts

Female patients should be asked about the presence of breast masses, changes in breast shape or appearance, discharge, pain, and any prior history of breast biopsy. When a mass is noted, it is helpful to know how long it has been present and whether it varies in size with the menstrual cycle. Breast discharge should be characterized as *unilateral* or *bilateral* and as *spontaneous* or *elicited,* and the color should be noted.[21-23]

Galactorrhea (a milky discharge), for example, may be unilateral, bilateral, uniductal, and/or multiductal and can be noted in female patients with hyperprolactinemia or hypothyroidism and with the use of certain medications, including oral contraceptives. Unilateral bloody discharge can typically be seen with an intraductal papilloma. Unilateral greenish discharge may be seen with ductal ectasia. Mild cyclic pain is common, related to the hormonal changes of the menstrual cycle. More prolonged or severe pain may be associated with fibrocystic changes.[21,23] Additional details regarding breast health and assessment can be found in Chapter 21.

Assessment of Gastrointestinal Complaints

Female patients should be asked about symptoms of nausea, vomiting, constipation, the need to splint (place pressure on the perineum or on the posterior vaginal wall) to aid in bowel movements, diarrhea, blood in stools, pain with bowel movements, and incontinence of stool or flatus. Female patients with irritable bowel syndrome often report alternating symptoms of constipation and diarrhea that are associated with crampy abdominal pain. Incontinence of stool or flatus may be noted after injuries to the anal sphincter during childbirth or in association with anal or rectovaginal fistulae.[21,23]

Urinary Problems

The urinary system review should include any symptoms of urinary tract infection (dysuria, urinary frequency, urinary urgency, and hematuria), urolithiasis (flank pain and hematuria), and symptoms of urinary incontinence or retention. Urinary incontinence may be experienced with a variety of conditions including urinary tract infections, congenital anomalies, vesicovaginal or ureterovaginal fistulae, cystocele or cystourethrocele, detrusor instability, and various neurologic conditions. Further characterization of the timing of incontinence (e.g., continuously; with activities such as coughing, sneezing, or running; on the way to the bathroom; or with stimuli such as running water) are helpful in management. Factors to consider when addressing urinary retention include causes from compression of the urethra (e.g., leiomyoma or periurethral edema, prior pelvic surgeries) versus incomplete emptying of the bladder (e.g., pelvic floor muscle dysfunction). Female patients should also be asked if there is a current pessary in place for prior pelvic organ prolapse and/or urinary incontinence. Organ prolapse (uterine descensus) can contribute to urinary complaints.[21,23]

Pelvic Pain

Pelvic pain should be dichotomized as *cyclic* (predictably occurring at certain times of the menstrual cycle such as with ovulation or with menses) or *noncyclic.* The mode of onset, character, location, radiation, severity, duration, and exacerbating and relieving factors should be noted. Pain with intercourse (dyspareunia), especially on deep penetration, may be indicative of endometriosis, and other associated symptoms should be noted. Because the reproductive organs are in close proximity to the urinary tract and the gastrointestinal tract, pain that is perceived in the pelvis could potentially be related to one of these organ systems. Pain associated with the abdominal wall musculature, fascia, or nerves often increases with activities such as lifting[21,23] (see the discussion of pelvic pain in Chapter 18).

Review of systems (ROS) questions regarding genital health should also be asked and should include abnormalities of uterine bleeding, symptoms of uterine or vaginal prolapse, quality of vaginal discharge, and the presence of vaginal dryness, lesions, pruritis, burning, and any sexual dysfunction (e.g., dyspareunia). Premenopausal patients should be assessed for abnormalities of intermenstrual interval and menstrual flow, including a lack of bleeding (amenorrhea), short or long intermenstrual interval (polymenorrhea or oligomenorrhea), excessive or prolonged menstrual flow (menorrhagia), and intermenstrual bleeding (metrorrhagia). They also should be asked about the presence of *any* bleeding (postmenopausal bleeding). All female patients should be asked about postcoital bleeding.[21,23]

Female patients with genital tract (uterine or vaginal) prolapse (uterine prolapse, cystocele or cystourethrocele, or rectocele) may be aware of and report pelvic pressure or the presence of tissue at or protruding through the introitus. Female patients with a cystocele or cystourethrocele may note urinary incontinence with activities that increase intraabdominal pressure such as coughing and sneezing, or with athletic activities such as running. Female patients with a rectocele may note constipation and may report the need to splint to facilitate bowel movements.[21,23]

Inquiries should be made about the presence of raised or ulcerative vulvar lesions and any changes in the appearance of lesions that have been present for a period of time.

The patient should be asked about a change or increase in vaginal discharge, and if present, whether there are any associated symptoms such as vulvovaginal pruritus or burning and malodor. Vulvar pruritis or burning could be attributed to contact dermatitis (e.g., from soaps or lotions), vestibulitis, or conditions such as lichen simplex, lichen sclerosus et atrophicus, vulvar intraepithelial neoplasia, and carcinoma of the vulva.

Dryness or decreased vaginal lubrication may be noted when postpartum estrogen levels are low or at the time of menopause, or it may be associated with disorders such as Sjögren syndrome.

Sexual function/dysfunction should also be assessed. Symptoms of sexual dysfunction can fall into several categories including abnormalities of arousal (decreased libido), pain with intercourse (dyspareunia), and inability to achieve orgasm (anorgasmia). Complete vulva health is covered in Chapter 17.[21,23]

> **PATIENT-CENTERED CARE:** At the end of the interview, always be sure to ask whether there are concerns that they would like to discuss that were not addressed previously in the interview.

Screening

In 2016, the HRSA announced the decision to support the WPSI's nine clinical recommendations for screening of the well woman. These recommendations are reviewed and updated annually; in 2021, there were 31 recommendations.[5] These recommendations are categorized by *general health, cancer screening, infectious diseases,* and *specific to pregnancy and postpartum.* The recommendations are not exhaustive (see Figure 5.1 for the complete list of recommendations) but include essential items that should be addressed to promote health over the course of a female patient's lifespan.

Breast Cancer

The WPSI, which is supported by the HRSA, recommends that the average-risk female initiate mammography screening no earlier than 40 years of age and no later than 50 years of age. Screening mammography should occur at least biennially and as frequently as annually. Screening should occur through at least 74 years of age, and age alone should not be a reason to discontinue screening[5] (see the discussion of breast health in Chapter 21 for more details).

Cervical Cancer

In alignment with the American Society for Colposcopy and Cervical Pathology (ASCCP) guidelines, the WPSI (supported by the U.S. Preventive Services Task Force [USPSTF] and the HRSA) recommends cervical cancer screening for average-risk females 21 to 65 years of age. For females 21 to 29 years of age, the WPSI recommends cervical cancer screening using cervical cytology (Pap test) every 3 years. Cotesting with cytology and HPV testing is not recommended for females younger than 30 years of age. Females 30 to 65 years of age should be screened with cytology and HPV cotesting or high-risk HPV testing alone every 5 years or cytology alone every 3 years. Females who are at average risk should not be screened more than once every 3 years.[5,15]

2021 RECOMMENDATIONS FOR WELL-WOMAN CARE

Preventive care visits provide an excellent opportunity for well-woman care including screening, evaluation of health risks and needs, counseling, and immunizations. *Recommendations for Well-Woman Care – A Well-Woman Chart* was developed by the Women's Preventive Services Initiative (WPSI). The Well-Woman Chart outlines preventive services recommended by the WPSI, U.S. Preventive Services Task Force (USPSTF), and Bright Futures based on age, health status, and risk factors. Additional recommendations for immunizations are provided in a separate table from the Advisory Committee on Immunization Practices. Clinical practice considerations, risk assessment methods, and the age and frequency to deliver services are described in the **Clinical Summary Tables** that accompany the chart.

The Well-Woman Chart provides a framework for incorporating preventive health services for women into clinical practice. These services may be completed at a single visit or as part of a series of visits that take place over time. This information is designed as an educational resource to aid clinicians in providing preventive health services for women, and use of this information is voluntary. This information should not be considered as inclusive of all proper treatments or methods of care or as a statement of the standard of care. It is not intended to substitute for the independent professional judgment of the treating clinician. Variations in practice may be warranted when, in the reasonable judgment of the treating clinician, such course of action is indicated by the condition of the patient, limitations of available resources, or advances in knowledge or technology. While every effort is made to present accurate and reliable information, this publication is provided "as is" without any guarantees or warranties of accuracy, reliability, or otherwise, either express or implied. The Chart and Tables are updated annually. The WPSI website (www.womenspreventivehealth.org) has the most up-to-date version of the Chart and Clinical Summary Tables.

PREVENTION SERVICES	AGE (Years) 13–17[a]	18–21[a]	22–39	40–49	50–64	65–75	>75
♥ GENERAL HEALTH							
Alcohol use screening & counseling	●	●	●	●	●	●	●
Anxiety screening	●	●	●	●	●		
CVD & CRC prevention with aspirin[1]					O 50–59		
Blood pressure screening	●	●	●	●	●	●	●
Contraceptive counseling & methods	●	●	●	●	O		
Depression screening	●	●	●	●	●	●	●
Diabetes screening[2]	O	O	O	O	O	O	O
Fall prevention						●	●
Folic acid supplementation[3]	O	●	●	●	O		
Healthy diet & activity counseling[4]	O	O	O	O	O	O	O
Interpersonal & domestic violence screening	●	●	●	●	●		
Lipid screening[5]	O	●	O	●	●		
Obesity screening & counseling	●	●	●	●	●	●	●
Osteoporosis screening[6]					●	●	●
Statin use to prevent CVD[7]					O	O	
Substance use screening & assessment	●	●	●	●	●	●	●
Tobacco screening & counseling	●	●	●	●	●	●	●
Urinary incontinence screening[8]	O	O	O	O	O	O	O
⚕ INFECTIOUS DISEASES							
Gonorrhea & chlamydia screening[9]	●	●	●≤24 O>24	O	O	O	O
Hepatitis B screening[10]	O	O	O	O	O	O	O
Hepatitis C screening (at least once)[11]	O	●	●	●	●	●	●<80
HIV preexposure prophylaxis[12]	O	O	O	O	O	O	O
HIV risk assessment		●	●	●	●		
HIV screening (at least once)	●>15	●	●	●	●	O	O
Immunizations[b]	●	●	●	●	●	●	●
STI prevention counseling[13]	●	●	O	O	O		
Syphilis screening[14]	O	O	O	O	O	O	O
Tuberculosis screening[15]	O	O	O	O	O	O	O
✝ CANCER							
Breast cancer screening[16]				O	●	●	O
Cervical cancer screening		●≥21	●	●	●	●≤65	
Colorectal cancer screening					●	●	
Lung cancer screening[17]					O 55–80	O	O 55–80
Medications to reduce breast cancer risk[18]				O	O	O	O
Risk assessment for *BRCA 1/2* testing[19]		●	●	●	●	●	●
Skin cancer counseling[19]	O	O	O ≤24				

Recommendations from the WPSI and the USPSTF for preventive services for pregnant and postpartum women are also provided in the Well-Woman Chart. Comprehensive recommendations for pregnant and postpartum women can be found in ACOG's practice guidelines and other educational materials.

PREVENTION SERVICES for pregnancy in addition to age-based services listed above.	
⚐ PREGNANCY	
Anxiety screening	●
Bacteriuria screening	●
Breastfeeding counseling, services & supplies	●
Contraceptive counseling & methods	●
Depression screening & preventive interventions[20]	●
Folic acid supplementation	●
Gestational diabetes screening	●
Gonorrhea & chlamydia screening	●
Hepatitis B screening	●
HIV screening (each pregnancy)	●
Interpersonal & domestic violence screening	●
Preeclampsia prevention with low-dose aspirin[21]	O
Preeclampsia screening	●
Rh(D) blood typing	●
Substance use screening & assessment	●
Syphilis screening	●
Tobacco screening & counseling	●

PREVENTION SERVICES for postpartum in addition to age-based services listed above.	
⚐ POSTPARTUM	
Anxiety screening	●
Breastfeeding counseling, services & supplies	●
Contraceptive counseling & methods	●
Depression screening & preventive interventions[20]	●
Diabetes screening after gestational diabetes[22]	O
Folic acid supplementation	●
Interpersonal & domestic violence screening	●
Substance use screening & assessment	●
Tobacco screening & counseling	●

KEY:

● Recommended by the USPSTF (A or B rating), WPSI, or Bright Futures
O Recommended for selected use

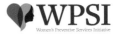

WPSI
Women's Preventive Services Initiative

MEMBERS OF THE ADVISORY PANEL SUPPORT THE WPSI

AMERICAN ACADEMY OF FAMILY PHYSICIANS
STRONG MEDICINE FOR AMERICA

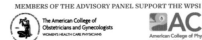

The American College of Obstetricians and Gynecologists
WOMEN'S HEALTH CARE PHYSICIANS

ACP
American College of Physicians
Leading Internal Medicine, Improving Lives

NPWH
NURSE PRACTITIONERS IN WOMEN'S HEALTH
Caring for Women

Figure 5.1 Reprinted with permission from Women's Preventive Services Initiative. Recommendations for well-woman care – a well-woman chart. Washington, DC: ACOG Foundation; 2022. Available at: https://www.womenspreventivehealth.org//srv/htdocs/wp-content/uploads/WellWomanChart.pdf. Retrieved March 17, 2023.

NOT TO BE MISSED

Take care to avoid missing screening guidelines for special populations, such as screening female patients (18 years of age or older) with HIV/AIDS. Screening should be discontinued in female patients who have had a hysterectomy for noncancerous reasons or those who are older than 65 years of age with evidence of adequate negative prior screening results and no history of cervical intraepithelial neoplasia 2 (CIN 2) or higher. Adequate negative prior screening results are defined as three consecutive negative cytology results or two consecutive negative cotest results within the previous 10 years, with the most recent test performed within the past 5 years.[15]

Sexually Transmitted Infections

The CDC recommends minimally testing for chlamydia and gonorrhea annually for sexually active females 15 to 24 years of age and for females 25 years of age and older with risk factors, and more frequently for at risk groups, such as females with more than one partner[5] (see Chapter 15 for full STI screening guidelines).

HPV. High-risk HPV DNA testing in females with normal cytology results. Screening should begin at 30 years of age and should occur no more frequently than every 5 years.[5]

HIV. The WPSI recommends:

…prevention education and risk assessment for human immunodeficiency virus (HIV) infection in adolescents and women at least annually throughout the lifespan. All women should be tested for HIV at least once during their lifetime. Additional screening should be based on risk, and screening annually or more often may be appropriate for adolescents and women with an increased risk of HIV infection.[5]

Hepatitis C. The CDC recommends screening for hepatitis C at least once in the baby boomer population.

NOT TO BE MISSED

Providers should be aware of and follow their state's HIV screening requirements.

Interpersonal and Domestic Violence

Although screening for IPV is recommended by the USPSTF, studies have shown very low screening rates ranging from 2% to 50% of providers stating that they always or almost always screen routinely for IPV.[24]

The USPSTF recommends that clinicians screen female patients of childbearing age for IPV, such as domestic violence, and provide or refer those who screen positive to intervention services. This recommendation also applies to female patients who do not have signs or symptoms of abuse.

! SAFETY ALERT

When interviewing a female patient who may be experiencing IPV, do so when her partner is not in the room. Questions about threats, violence, or abuse can trigger an abuser to escalate the abuse and put the patient in further danger.

The WPSI recommends

…screening adolescents and women for interpersonal and domestic violence at least annually, and, when needed, providing or referring for initial intervention services. Interpersonal and domestic violence includes physical violence, sexual violence, stalking and psychological aggression (including coercion), reproductive coercion, neglect, and the threat of violence, abuse, or both. Intervention services include but are not limited to counseling, education, harm-reduction strategies, and referral to appropriate supportive services.[5]

Providers should also offer ongoing support and review available prevention and referral options.[19,25]

The screening tools in Box 5.2 are tools that the USPSTF evaluated with the most sensitivity and specificity for screening of IPV.[24] Most of the tools listed in Box 5.2 can be found at https://www.cdc.gov/violenceprevention/pdf/ipv/ipvandsvscreening.pdf.

CLINICAL SURVIVAL TIP Patient self-administered or computerized screenings are as effective as clinician interviewing in terms of disclosure, comfort, and time spent screening.[19]

NOT TO BE MISSED

Providers can play a significant role. Creating and maintaining trusting relationships and being supportive is key to female patients disclosing sensitive information.

Providers can inform a patient that IPV is prevalent and has serious health consequences, which is better than just providing information on resources, but may not be better than doing nothing.

Many female patients do not feel comfortable disclosing IPV; by providing education and resources, the patient can still receive the information and use it when it is appropriate. Also, the discussion of safe and healthy relationships is important and can prevent serious abuse from occurring later.[19]

Human and sex trafficking has unfortunately become more prevalent in today's society, requiring providers to become more knowledgeable to help facilitate screening for and identifying potential victims and having the ability to effectively care for victims.

In 2000, the United Nations Convention against Transnational Organized Crime (the Palermo Convention) defined *human trafficking* as:

...the recruitment, transportation, transfer, harbouring or receipt of persons, by means of the threat or use of force or other forms of coercion, of abduction, of fraud, of deception, of the abuse of power or of a position of vulnerability or of the giving or receiving of payments or benefits to achieve the consent of a person having control over another person, for the purpose of exploitation. Exploitation shall include, at a minimum, the exploitation of the prostitution of others or other forms of sexual exploitation, forced labour or services, slavery or practices similar to slavery, servitude, or the removal of organs.[26]

The patient, the patient's relationships, the community, and society at large are four areas in which risk factors can be identified. The risk of trafficking increases at all four levels for those living in poverty. Additional risk factors for being trafficked include runaway or homeless youth, foreign nationals, and victims of domestic violence, sexual assault, war or conflict, and social discrimination.[2] An example screening tool can be found at https://www.ncjrs.gov/pdffiles1/nij/grants/246713.pdf.

The algorithm in Figure 5.2 provides a guide for a stepwise process when caring for female patients and if any red flags for human trafficking are identified.

The National Human Trafficking Hotline (NHTH) is accessible by phone (1-888-373-7888), text messaging (text HELP or INFO to BeFree [233733]), and email (help@humantraffickinghotline.org) and can be used to report trafficking (even if suspected but not disclosed), seek guidance on immediate care, and access social and legal services. The hotline links victims and survivors of trafficking with services and assistance to obtain help and stay safe.[28]

PHYSICAL EXAMINATION

A comprehensive history is the most vital aspect of the well-woman visit. This history can direct which components, if any, of the physical examination will be required for this visit. Shared decision making between the provider and patient refines further the well-woman visit in which healthy behaviors are facilitated and preventive health practices are encouraged.[20]

When a physical examination is needed, the components include the following:[1,21]

- Constitutional and general appearance assessment
- Review of vital signs, weight, weight trends, height, BMI
- General examination of the skin/nails; hair; head, eyes, ears, nose, and throat (HEENT); thyroid gland; heart; lungs; and extremities
- Standard techniques of inspection, auscultation, percussion, and palpation should be used when examining the abdomen. The following techniques aid in assessing the contour of the abdomen, appearance of the skin, quality of bowel sounds, and presence of any abnormalities (e.g., abdominal bruits) and in determining the size of abdominal and pelvic structures such as the liver and any masses or abnormal fluid collections present (e.g., ascites).
- Abdominal and pelvic tenderness can be assessed during percussion and while palpating for any organ enlargement and masses. Any tenderness noted

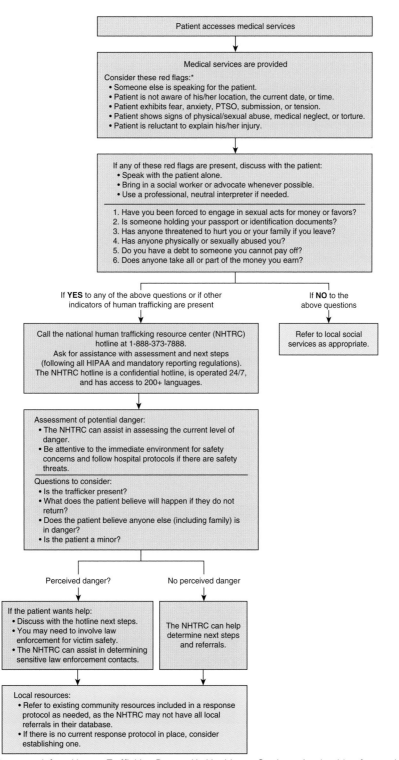

Figure 5.2 Framework for a Human Trafficking Protocol in Healthcare Settings. An algorithm for providing care to trafficked female patients. (Modified from National Human Trafficking Resource Center (NHTRC). (2016, June 7). *Framework for a human trafficking protocol in healthcare settings.* National Human Trafficking Hotline. https://humantraffickinghotline.org/resources/framework-human-trafficking-protocol-healthcare-settings.)

should be further assessed for involuntary guarding and rebound tenderness.

A thorough breast examination should be performed. Components of a complete breast examination are outlined in Box 5.3. Some of the detailed components of the history ROS that are relevant to breast health and assessment should have been obtained previously during the patient interview before assessment and physical examination (see Figure 5.3 for breast examination techniques).

BOX 5.3   Complete Breast Examination

Utilize relevant components of the history/review of systems to reinforce assessment of changes in breast appearance, tissue, and shape. This includes the following:
- Age
- Previous mammography/breast ultrasonography
- Previous breast disease, masses
- Menstrual cycle, menarche, and menopause
- Pregnancies and breastfeeding
- Use of hormonal products
- Surgery of the reproductive system (e.g., oophorectomy)
- Use of alcohol and tobacco

Clinical breast examination:
- Inspection both erect and supine
- Palpating of both breasts in an organized pattern including the area from the clavicle to the mammary ridge, and under the axilla
- Assessment of any accessory breast tissue, such as supernumerary nipples

Abnormalities requiring further assessment and physician consultation:
- Asymmetry of breast contour—mass, indentation or shrinking
- Retraction of breast tissue
- Nipple deviation or retraction (does not include inverted nipples)
- Edema, peau d'orange skin changes
- Firmness or thickening of breast tissue
- Dilated subcutaneous veins not associated with pregnancy and lactation
- Heat or erythema, particularly if localized
- Ulceration or lesions
- Palpable lymph nodes
- Nipple erosion, ulceration, thickening; erythema not associated with breastfeeding or breast sex play
- Nipple discharge or crusting
- Localized granular modularity
- Masses within the breast tissue

From Kriebs J, Gegor C. *Varney's Pocket Midwife.* 2nd ed. Burlington, MA: Jones & Bartlett Learning; 2005: 17–18.

Vertical strip	Circular	Wedge

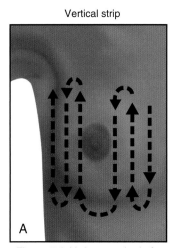
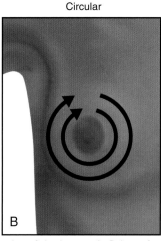
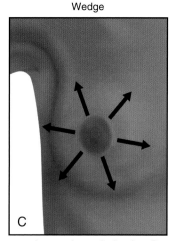

Figure 5.3 Various methods for palpation of the breast. **A,** Palpate from top to bottom in vertical strips. **B,** Palpate in concentric circles. **C,** Palpate out from the center in wedge sections. (Reproduced with permission from Ball JW, Dains JE, Flynn JA, Solomon BS, Stewart RW. *Seidel's Guide to Physical Examination: An Interprofessional Approach.* St. Louis: Elsevier; 2019.)

In reference to Box 5.3, the following are more specific considerations (which should have been obtained previously during the patient interview) when assessing breast health:

- History regarding previous clinical breast examination and imaging (mammography/sonography); documenting the date is important.
- Determining whether self-breast examination is being performed. The ACOG no longer recommends self-breast examination (repetitive inspection for the purpose of detecting breast cancer) in average-risk females, but promotes self-breast awareness (awareness of the shape and feel of the breasts) instead.
- Personal history of breast cancers, personal history of other reproductive cancers, and family medical history of the aforementioned factors are important to review.
- Age of menarche in particular is relevant to breast cancer risk (early onset may increase risk).
- Age of menopause (later onset may increase risk of breast cancer).
- Age of first pregnancy (later first pregnancy may increase risk of breast cancer).
- Duration of breastfeeding (longer duration of breastfeeding may be protective against breast cancer).

For complete details regarding breast health and assessment see Chapter 21.

GYNECOLOGICAL EXAMINATION

The pelvic examination for many female patients can contribute to feeling vulnerable, anxious, exposed, and apprehensive, which may be related to the positioning required to complete the examination. The lithotomy position for female patients can create an "imbalance of power in the patient/provider interaction and can have sexual associations."[21]

Intentions (the provider's unintentional use of words or actions that the patient may find threatening or offensive) and *perceptions* (how the patient may interpret the provider's communication) must be delicately balanced during interactions; the provider may be completely satisfied with how the interaction unfolded, but this may be contrary to how the patient feels. When female patients feel like adequate time is allowed for their visit without feeling rushed and the provider was prepared to answer their questions, it contributes to an overall more positive experience.[21] The following views should be considered in an adult female patient who has never had a prior speculum examination.

"A study of adolescents' views about their first pelvic exams showed that a positive experience was associated with a sense of control during the examination. This depended on a thorough explanation of the procedure before it was undertaken, allowing the patient to participate in decision-making, and receiving assurance that the examination could be discontinued at any point."[29]

> **PATIENT-CENTERED CARE:** A female patient who is at ease with the examination experience may be more likely to spontaneously contribute information that may prove valuable in the evaluation.

> **CLINICAL SURVIVAL TIP:** Consider talking to the patient during the examination as this may increase the patient's level of comfort. Silence may cause the patient to think that something is wrong.

During the examination, it is important to always remember to maintain eye contact as much as possible, explain the next step, and comment on all observations (e.g., "Your vagina looks moist; this is normal."). Incorporating these steps into your examination routine will help the patient feel safer and more relaxed. Figure 5.4 shows an examiner maintaining eye contact while performing a pelvic examination.

> **PATIENT-CENTERED CARE:** Consider offering patients a mirror to view their anatomy as you are performing the examination; this may help them feel more at ease.

> **CLINICAL SURVIVAL TIP:** Good habits: If possible, try to have warm instruments available, and *be as gentle as possible* during the examination. Verbalizing that you will try to be as gentle as possible during the examination and asking patients to let you know if you are doing anything that is uncomfortable or painful often helps them feel more at ease.

During the examination, be sure to be aware of the patient's demeanor, which may indicate anxiety or feeling frightened. Behaviors such as covering or closing eyes, placing hands on shoulders, clasping the hands, using hands to cover the pelvis, putting hands on legs, or using

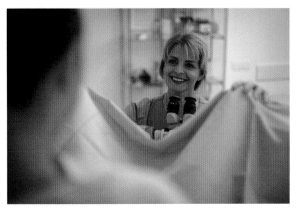

Figure 5.4 Provider maintaining eye contact during a pelvic examination. (Courtesy iStockPhoto.com/Nikola Ilic.)

hands to clutch the table could signal that a more cautious and respectful approach is essential. These signals could also be related to patient discomfort or pain, such as with cervical motion tenderness (CMT), which can be caused by infection such as chlamydia or pelvic inflammatory disease (PID). If any of these signals are identified and there is no concern for presence of inciting pathology, then consider offering strategies to promote relaxation (e.g., breathing exercises). Consider asking probing questions that may help elicit what the patient is feeling (e.g., "What is the most bothersome to you?"). Advise patients of what they may feel during the examination and what the next steps will be in the examination process. Individualization and tailoring the visit to meet each patient's needs should be done with every visit.[21,30]

NOT TO BE MISSED

When age or other health issues are such that a female patient would not choose to intervene on conditions detected during a routine examination, it is reasonable to discontinue pelvic examinations.

Relevant details from the patient's history should be used as a guide for particular observations during the examination.[20] This includes age, menarche, menstrual age, menstrual cycle, perimenopausal symptoms, STIs, recurrent vaginal infections, use of contraceptive or other hormonal products, obstetric experience, and prior gynecological surgery. Examples are as follows:

- Age—Genitourinary symptoms of menopause may cause vaginal atrophy.

- STIs—Increased vaginal discharge or pain on insertion of the speculum or during pelvic examination.
- Obstetric history—Multiparous patients may have soft and redundant vaginal walls, so a larger speculum may be needed to adequately perform the examination.
- Prior gynecological surgery—Patients who are post–total hysterectomy will not have a cervix.

The pelvic examination can be considered to include the entire genitourinary tract. Thus it can include the following:

- Bladder, urethra, and urethral opening
- External genitalia
- Bartholin and Skene glands
- Vagina (vaginal walls, tone, vaginal discharge/odor, lesions)
- Cervix
- Uterus
- Adnexa
- Anus and perirectal area

Inspection of the external genitalia is followed by speculum examination (Fig. 5.5), Pap test, collection of any other necessary cultures as indicated by relevant history, and bimanual evaluation. Rectovaginal examination (Fig. 5.6) is included as needed for adequate assessment of the posterior uterine wall, cul-de-sac, rectovaginal septum, and rectum (e.g., to fully assess a retroverted uterus, more thoroughly investigate pelvic or rectal pain, or check for blood in stool).[22,23]

LABORATORY TESTING/INTERVENTIONS

All laboratory testing should be identified and ordered based on history and physical examination. Testing recommendations should be stratified by the following age and risk factors:

- Urine dipstick (e.g., to assess for the presence of protein, blood, leukocytes)
- Urine cultures as indicated (e.g., if the patient complains of urinary tract infection symptoms)
- Pregnancy testing as indicated by age and history (including LMP); this can be performed as office point-of-care testing using urine if available.
- Cervical cancer screening (formerly known as a *Pap smear*)/HPV screening as indicated. Refer to ASCCP guidelines.
- STI testing as indicated by age and history (e.g., gonorrhea, chlamydia, syphilis, herpes, hepatitis B and C—all based on age and risk factors

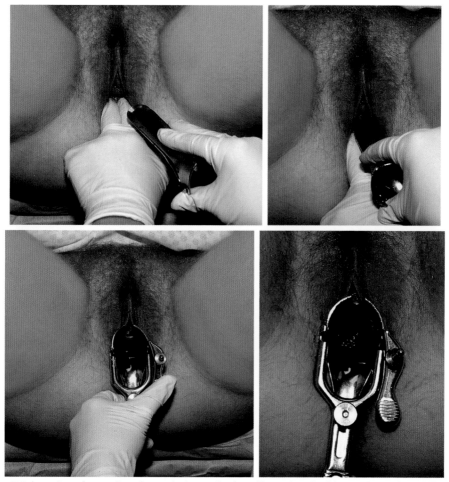

Figure 5.5 Insertion of speculum for vaginal examination. (Reproduced with permission from Wilson SF, Giddens J. *Health Assessment for Nursing Practice.* St. Louis: Elsevier; 2013.)

(see Chapter 15 for information on STI screening guidelines).

- HIV testing as indicated by age, health history, and access to routine health care.
- Vaginal cultures/wet prep if indicated by history and ROS. Patients who present with vaginal discharge should be evaluated for bacterial vaginosis, vulvovaginal candidiasis, and trichomoniasis (see Chapter 15 for information on management guidelines for vaginitis).
- General hematologic screening as indicated by age, health history, and access to routine health care (e.g., complete blood count).
- Any other laboratory tests determined necessary after complete history, ROS, screening, and physical examination (e.g., complete metabolic panel, thyroid-stimulating hormone)
- Order mammogram/bone density testing as indicated by age and history.
- Order laboratory tests as indicated.
- Administer vaccines as appropriate based on vaccination history/record review obtained earlier in the patient interview (for a complete schedule, visit https://www.cdc.gov/vaccines/schedules/hcp/imz/adult.html.)

Pharmacological

Prescribe any medications as appropriate based on history and physical examination. Referral may be indicated if a more specific evaluation is needed. After counseling,

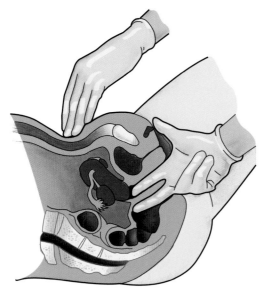

Figure 5.6 Rectovaginal examination. (Reproduced with permission from Ball JW, Dains JE, Flynn JA, Solomon BS, Stewart RW. *Seidel's Guide to Physical Examination: An Interprofessional Approach.* St. Louis: Elsevier; 2019.)

review of the patient's desired method, and review of the appropriateness of the method based on history, female patients should also be prescribed birth control (see Chapter 9 for information on contraception guidelines).

Nonpharmacologic

Review any naturopathic supplementation that may be used as appropriate based on history and physical examination.

NOT TO BE MISSED

Be sure to review the compatibility of naturopathic supplementation with any medications currently being taken (over-the-counter and prescribed).

Education and Counseling

As previously discussed, it is essential to patient relationship, trust, and processing to allow time for education, counseling, questions, and concerns. Physical findings should be reviewed so patients understand their health/disease status.

Education and counseling should address habits/lifestyles that foster general health/wellness and disease

prevention but should also address issues specific to female patients such as health maintenance, contraception, and safe-sex practices. The following is a list of areas to be included in the educational and counseling plan for most female patients.

- Health maintenance—Other areas of health maintenance that are of importance to review with female patients include the following:
  - Diet
  - Calcium, vitamin D, and folic acid intake (specifically in patients of childbearing age)
  - Exercise
  - Use of seatbelts, helmets, sunscreen, and smoke and carbon monoxide detectors
  - Firearms in the home
  - Age-appropriate screenings, such as mammography, CCS schedule (new changes should be reviewed), colonoscopy, bone densitometry, lipid analysis, and glucose.

Immunizations

Box 5.4 provides a brief summary of recommended vaccines for adults 19 years of age and older who meet the age requirement, lack documentation of vaccination, or lack evidence of past infection. For more complete details, refer to the Advisory Committee on Immunization Practices recommendations on the CDC website (https://www.cdc.gov/vaccines/schedules/hcp/imz/adult.html).[31]

Contraception should also be included in education and counseling. The WPSI recommends that adolescent and adult women have access to the "full range of female-controlled contraceptive methods, and access to contraceptive counseling, effective family planning practices, and sterilization procedures as part of contraceptive care. Services include initiation of contraceptive use as well as follow-up care."

The full range of contraceptive methods for females currently identified by the U.S. Food and Drug Administration (FDA) include permanent sterilization, long-acting reversible contraceptives (LARCs), contraceptive injections, short-acting hormonal methods, barrier methods, and emergency contraception.[32] Additionally, instruction in fertility awareness–based methods, including the lactation amenorrhea method, although less effective, should be provided for patients who desire an alternative method.

BOX 5.4   Immunization Recommendations From the Centers for Disease Control and Prevention

- **Influenza**—recommended annually for all ages.
- **Tetanus, diphtheria, and acellular pertussis (Td/Tdap)**—Adults who have not received tetanus and diphtheria toxoids and acellular pertussis vaccine (Tdap) or for whom pertussis vaccination status is unknown should receive one dose of Tdap followed by a tetanus and diphtheria toxoids (Td) booster every 10 years. Tdap should be administered regardless of when a tetanus or diphtheria toxoid–containing vaccine was last received and should also be administered to females in the third trimester of every pregnancy.
- **Human papilloma virus (HPV)**—The number of doses of HPV vaccine to be administered depends on age at initial HPV vaccination.
  - In general, adult females through 45 years of age who have not received any HPV vaccine should receive a three-dose series of HPV vaccine at 0, 1–2, and 6 months.
  - No previous dose of HPV vaccine: Administer three-dose series at 0, 1–2, and 6 months (minimum intervals: 4 weeks between doses 1 and 2; 12 weeks between doses 2 and 3; and 5 months between doses 1 and 3. Repeat doses if given too soon).
  - Age 9–14 years at initiation of HPV vaccination series and received one dose or two doses less than 5 months apart: Administer one dose. Age 9–14 years at initiation of HPV vaccination series and received two doses at least 5 months apart: No additional dose is needed.
- **Measles, mumps, and rubella (MMR)**—One or two doses depending on if indicated and if no prior vaccination—through 64 years of age.
- **Varicella**—Adults without evidence of immunity to varicella (defined later) should receive two doses of single-antigen varicella vaccine (VAR) 4–8 weeks apart, or a second dose if they have received only one dose.
- **Herpes zoster (HZV)**—Adults 50 years of age and older should receive two doses of herpes zoster vaccine, regardless of whether they had a prior episode of herpes zoster.
- **Hepatitis A**—Adults who seek protection from hepatitis A virus infection may receive a two-dose HepA series (Havrix, Vaqta) or the HepA-HepB vaccine (Twinrx).
- **Hepatitis B**—Adults who seek protection from hepatitis B virus infection may receive a two- or three-dose series of single-antigen hepatitis B vaccine (Heplisav-B, HepB) (Engerix-B, Recombivax HB) at 0, 1, and 6 months. Adults may also receive a combined hepatitis A and hepatitis B vaccine (HepA-HepB) (Twinrix) at 0, 1, and 6 months. Acknowledgment of a specific risk factor by those who seek protection is not needed.
- **Pneumococcus**—Age 19–64 years if immunocompromised or at-risk medical conditions; adults 65 years of age and older.
- **Meningococcal vaccine**—if at risk.
- **COVID-19**—Recommended 5 years of age and up. Female patients who seek protection from severe effects of a COVID-19 infection should receive either the mRNA (Pfizer-BioNTech or Moderna) two-injection series or the Johnson & Johnson/Janssen single-injection vaccine. Pregnant patients are advised to avoid the Johnson & Johnson/Janssen vaccine as it carries an increased risk of blood clots with low platelets after vaccination. The mRNA vaccines should be followed up with a booster 5 months after completion of the initial series.

Modified from Centers for Disease Control and Prevention. *Adult Immunization Schedule. Recommendations for Ages 19 Years or Older, United States, 2022.* https://www.cdc.gov/vaccines/schedules/hcp/imz/adult.html)

Sexually Transmitted Infections

The WPSI recommends directed behavioral counseling by a health care provider or other appropriately trained individual for sexually active adolescent and adult women at an increased risk for STIs.[5]

The WPSI recommends that health care providers use the female patient's sexual history and risk factors to help identify those at increased risk of STIs (see the "History" section earlier in this chapter). Risk factors may include age younger than 25 years, a recent history of an STI, a new sex partner, multiple partners, a partner with concurrent partners, a partner with an STI, and lack of or inconsistent condom use. For adolescents and women not identified as high risk, counseling to reduce the risk of STIs should be considered, as determined by clinical judgement.

KEY POINTS

- It is generally recognized that all necessary recommended preventive services, depending on a female patient's health status, health needs, and other risk factors may require several visits.[4,5]
- Creating and maintaining trust in relationships and being supportive is key to female patients disclosing sensitive information.[19]
- Respect for women and respect for culture are both essential to best care. Aspects of competent care include awareness of and respect for the varieties of sexual experiences.[22]
- A woman at ease with the examination experience may be more likely to spontaneously contribute information that may prove valuable in the evaluation.

REFERENCES

1. Conry JA. *Well woman task force: A collaborative initiative hosted by the American College of Obstetricians and Gynecologists.* American College of Obstetricians and Gynecologists; 2014.
2. Conry J, Brown H. Well-woman task force: Components of the well-woman visit. *Obstet Gynecol.* 2015;126(4):697–701.
3. Connolly A, Britton A, eds. *Women's Health in Primary Care.* Cambridge, MA: Cambridge University Press; 2017.
4. Kilgore C. Well-woman care: Reshaping the routine visit. (Women's Health). *Family Practice News.* 2016;46(19):1.
5. Womens' Preventive Services Initiative. *Recommendations for Well Woman Care Clinical Summary Tables*; 2021. https://www.womenspreventivehealth.org/wp-content/uploads/WPSI_ClinicalSummaryTables_2021Updates.pdf.
6. Centers for Disease Control and Prevention. (n.d.). *Leading Causes of Death—Females—All Races and Origins—United States, 2017.* https://www.cdc.gov/women/lcod/2017/all-races-origins/index.htm.
7. Centers for Disease Control and Prevention. (n.d.). *Adult Obesity Facts.* https://www.cdc.gov/obesity/data/adult.html.
8. Hales CM, Carroll MD, Fryar CD, Ogden CL. *Prevalence of Obesity and Severe Obesity Among Adults: United States, 2017–2018.* 2020. NCHS Data Brief No. 360. https://www.cdc.gov/nchs/products/databriefs/db360.htm.
9. Centers for Disease Control and Prevention. (n.d.). *Women and Heart Disease.* https://www.cdc.gov/heartdisease/women.htm.
10. American Heart Association. (n.d.). *Facts, Causes and Risks of Stroke.* https://www.goredforwomen.org/en/about-heart-disease-in-women/facts/facts-causes-risks-and-prevention-of-stroke#:~:text=About%2040%20percent%20of%20stroke,and%2060%20percent%20in%20females.
11. Centers for Disease Control and Prevention. *National Diabetes Statistics Report, 2020.* 2020 https://www.cdc.gov/diabetes/data/statistics-report/.
12. World Health Organization. *Human papillomavirus (HPV) and cervical cancer*; 2020. https://www.who.int/news-room/fact-sheets/detail/human-papillomavirus-(hpv)-and-cervical-cancer.
13. U.S. Cancer Statistics Working Group. *U.S. Cancer Statistics Data Visualizations Tool, Based on 2019 Submission Data (1999-2017): Changes Over Time: Cervix.* U.S. Department of Health and Human Services, Centers for Disease Control and Prevention and National Cancer Institute; www.cdc.gov/cancer/dataviz (released June 2020).
14. Centers for Disease Control and Prevention. (n.d.). *Cervical Cancer Statistics.* https://www.cdc.gov/cancer/cervical/statistics/.
15. Curry SJ. Screening for cervical cancer: U.S. Preventive Services Task Force recommendation statement. *J Am Med Assoc.* 2018;320(7):674–686.
16. Centers for Disease Control and Prevention. (n.d.). *Breast Cancer Statistics.* https://www.cdc.gov/cancer/breast/statistics/.
17. U.S. Cancer Statistics Working Group. U.S. *Cancer Statistics Data Visualizations Tool, Based on 2019 Submission Data (1999-2017): Leading Cancer Cases and Deaths, by Race, Female.* U.S. Department of Health and Human Services, Centers for Disease Control and Prevention and National Cancer Institute; 2017. www.cdc.gov/cancer/dataviz (released June 2020).
18. U.S. Cancer Statistics Working Group. *U.S. Cancer Statistics Data Visualizations Tool, Based on 2019 Submission Data (1999-2017): Changes Over Time: Female Breast.* U.S. Department of Health and Human Services, Centers for Disease Control and Prevention and National Cancer Institute. www.cdc.gov/cancer/dataviz (released June 2020).
19. Agency for Healthcare Research and Quality. *Intimate Partner Violence Screening*; 2015. https://www.ahrq.gov/ncepcr/tools/healthier-pregnancy/fact-sheets/partner-violence.html.
20. Well-woman visit. ACOG Committee Opinion No. 755. *Obstet Gynecol.* 2018;132:e181–e186.

21. Bowdler NC, Elson M. *The gynecologic history and examination.* The Global Library of Women's Medicine; 2009.
22. King TL, et al. *Varney's Midwifery.* 6th ed. Burlington, MA: Jones & Bartlett Learning; 2019.
23. Jarvis C. *Physical Examination and Health Assessment.* 8th ed. St. Louis: Elsevier; 2020.
24. U.S. Preventive Services Task Force. *Final Recommendation Statement: Intimate Partner Violence, Elder Abuse, and Abuse of Vulnerable Adults: Screening;* 2018. https://www.uspreventiveservicestaskforce.org/uspstf/document/RecommendationStatementFinal/intimate-partner-violence-and-abuse-of-elderly-and-vulnerable-adults-screening#bootstrap-panel--3.
25. Intimate partner violence. *ACOG Committee Opinion No. 518;* 2012. https://www.acog.org/clinical/clinical-guidance/committee-opinion/articles/2012/02/intimate-partner-violence.
26. Protocol to prevent, suppress and punish trafficking in persons, especially women. *Resolution 55/25: United Nations Convention Against Transnational Organized Crime, United Nations General Assembly, Resolution 55/25.* 2001. https://www.un.org/en/development/desa/population/migration/generalassembly/docs/globalcompact/A_RES_55_25.pdf.
27. National Human Trafficking Hotline. (n.d.). *The Victims.* https://humantraffickinghotline.org/what-human-trafficking/human-trafficking/victims.
28. National Human Trafficking Hotline. (n.d.). *National Hotline Overview.* https://humantraffickinghotline.org/national-hotline-overview.
29. Oscarsson MG, Benzein EG, Wijma BE. The first pelvic examination. *J Psychosomatic Obstetrics Gynecol.* 2007;28(1):7–12.
30. Seehusen DA, Johnson DR, Earwood JS, et al. Improving women's experience during speculum examinations at routine gynaecological visits: randomised clinical trial. *BMJ.* 2006;333(7560):171–173.
31. Centers for Disease Control and Prevention. *Recommended Adult Immunization Schedule for Ages 19 Years or Older, United States;* 2021. https://www.cdc.gov/vaccines/schedules/hcp/imz/adult.html.
32. U.S. Food and Drug Administration. (n.d.). Birth Control. https://www.fda.gov/consumers/free-publications-women/birth-control.
33. National Human Trafficking Resource Center (NHTRC). *Framework for A Human Trafficking Protocol in Healthcare Settings.* National Human Trafficking Hotline. 2016. https://humantraffickinghotline.org/resources/framework-human-trafficking-protocol-healthcare-settings.
34. Ball JW, Dains JE, Flynn JA, Solomon BS, Stewart RW. *Seidel's Guide to Physical Examination: An Interprofessional Approach.* St. Louis: Elsevier; 2019.
35. Wilson SF, Giddens J. *Health Assessment for Nursing Practice.* St. Louis: Elsevier; 2013.

6

Care Before and Between Pregnancies

Randee L. Masciola

OBJECTIVES

- Develop a plan for to incorporate screening for genetic, medical, psychosocial, and environmental risks into pre-pregnancy and interpregnancy care.
- Apply knowledge of genetic, medical, psychosocial, and environmental risk factors in diagnostic reasoning and management decisions.

- Formulate a reproductive life plan that considers the woman's individual risk factors and reproductive goals.
- Educate women regarding health promotion strategies that optimize maternal and newborn outcomes.

INTRODUCTION

The goal of preconception care is to enhance the female patient's health before pregnancy and to decrease the risk of poor health outcomes for either the patient or the baby.[1] The U.S. Centers for Disease Control and Prevention (CDC) Preconception Work group standardized a working definition of preconception care as "a set of interventions that aim to identify and modify biomedical, behavioral, and social risks to a woman's health or pregnancy outcome through prevention and management."[2] This care occurs during the period before the first pregnancy and continues to the next, as illustrated in Figure 6.1. *Healthy People 2020* reports that preconception care can significantly lower the number of preterm births, low-birth-weight neonates, and birth defects, yet only 30% of females in the United States receive pre-pregnancy health counseling.[3]

Globally the greatest threats of maternal-child health include maternal and child mortality, vertical transmission of human immunodeficiency virus (HIV) and other sexually transmitted infections (STIs), type 2 diabetes,

and cardiovascular disease later in life.[4] The World Health Organization (WHO) supports global preconception care and the positive effect the counseling has on a range of health outcomes. Once pregnancy occurs, it may be too late to implement health modifications or prevention strategies to help avoid certain placental or birth defects. Many medical conditions develop before 6 weeks' gestation, which is usually the time females are typically diagnosed with a pregnancy and see a provider for the first time. This is often too late for optimal health outcomes as many medical conditions affecting the pregnancy are already present (Fig. 6.2).

In addition, over one-half of the 6 million pregnancies in the United States annually are unintended, and most occur without preconception planning.[5] In that so many pregnancies are unintended, preconception care should be included in all primary care and preventive visits during a female patient's reproductive years. Preconception care includes discussing a reproductive life plan, screening for and identifying risks, recommending evidence-based interventions, providing health promotion education, and referring for consultation as indicated.

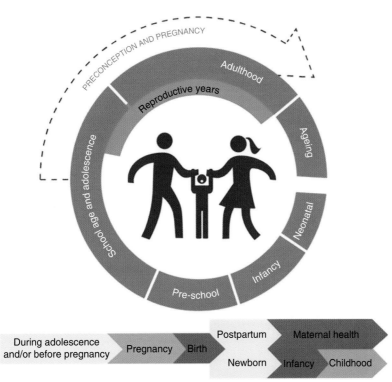

Figure 6.1 Illustration of the period of preconception care. (From Mason E, Chandra-Mouli V, Baltag V, Christiansen C, Lassi ZS, Bhutta ZA. Preconception care: advancing from "important to do and can be done" to "is being done and is making a difference." *Reprod Health*. 2014;11 Suppl 3[Suppl 3]:S8.)

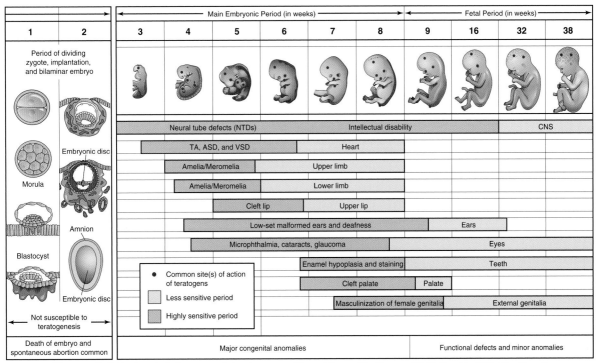

Figure 6.2 Critical periods in prenatal development. (From Moore KL, Persaud TVN, Torchia MG. *The Developing Human*. Elsevier; 2015.)

An easy approach to preconception care is to ask women of reproductive age the *One Key Question* about plans for pregnancy in the next year. This patient-centered method centers on health equity and provides the same support to those who are seeking pregnancy, those who are not seeking pregnancy, and those who are unsure or undecided. More information can be found at https://powertodecide.org/one-key-question.

ASSESSMENT

Preconception care should be a part of every primary and preventive care visit for female patients of reproductive age. The complete health assessment will include a risk assessment as the provider will be identifying risks while performing the thorough health history and physical. At this time, the advanced practice clinician (APC) may identify poor control or untreated or undiagnosed medical conditions, including gaps in health and wellness promotion. Positive findings discovered during the history will guide further laboratory studies, health promotion strategies, interventions, counseling, education, and referrals. In some high-risk situations, preconception collaboration can be initiated between the APC and other members of the health care team including obstetricians and maternal fetal medicine as well as other medical specialists. A list of topics essential to preconception care can be found in Table 6.1.

TABLE 6.1 Topics in Preconceptual Care	
Topic	**Recommendations**
Environmental concerns	Evaluate work related contacts with toxic substances. Workplaces that use chemicals toxic to humans include health care and clinical laboratories, dry cleaners, agriculture, manufacturing plants, and printing plants.
	Evaluate household contacts with toxic substances. Heavy metals, pesticides, and solvents are a few examples.
	Educate patients to avoid consuming mercury found in fish such as shark, king mackerel, swordfish, and tilefish; limit other fish intake such as tuna.
Family history: genetics	Offer screening when a personal or family history of congenital disorders or genetic anomalies exists
	Offer referral to a genetic counselor if screening indicates risk factors.
	Offer testing for carrier status when needed to establish risk to any subsequent pregnancies.
Prescriptions and over the counter drugs	Evaluate prescriptions and over the counter drugs for teratogenic effects
	If patient is taking a drug for chronic disease control, change to safer formulations when available, in the lowest dose that successfully controls the disease.
Mental health illnesses	Evaluate for depression and anxiety.
	Educate patients about the risks of depression that is not treated in pregnancy and the risks related to treatment.
Psychosocial concerns	Perform intimate partner violence screening.
	Assess safety of the patient and give appropriate referrals when needed.
Substance use	Provide screening for alcohol, tobacco, and drug use. Give referrals for patients with alcohol dependence; treatment for tobacco cessation with tobacco dependence; educate patients on the effects of smoking on the fetus and health of the child
	Present short behavioral interventions designed to decrease tobacco, alcohol, and drug use.

Adapted from Farahi N, Zolotor A. Recommendations for preconception counseling and care. *Am Fam Physician.* 2013;88(8):499;506.

BOX 6.1 Genetic Disorders to Screen for During a Verbal History Risk Assessment

- Congenital heart defect
- Cystic fibrosis
- Down syndrome
- Fragile X syndrome
- Hemophilia
- Huntington's chorea
- Intellectual disability
- Muscular dystrophy
- Neural tube defects
- Recurrent miscarriages (more than three)
- Sickle cell disease
- Spina bifida
- Tay-Sachs disease
- Thalassemia

HISTORY

Women who desire pregnancy in the next year warrant further details about preconception care. Healthy lifestyle modifications result in improved pregnancy outcomes. A vital place to start is a thorough history. For patients with or family history of chronic health conditions, this is an ideal time to assess health care to review if adjustments should be made in care. For example, some medications for management of hypertension are contraindicated during pregnancy. Discussions of transition of care for chronic conditions to safer options for pregnancy decreases adverse outcomes. The history should include the following:

Medical/surgical history: Previously diagnosed medical conditions or surgeries related to cardiovascular issues, hypertension, diabetes, depression, and substance abuse

Family history: Genetic disorders (Box 6.1), cancers, cardiovascular disease, infertility, diabetes, and depression

Medications: All medications, including over-the-counter medications, herbs, and supplements.

Immunizations (Table 6.2): Dates for all vaccinations including influenza, rubella (German measles), varicella (chickenpox), Tdap (tetanus, diphtheria, pertussis), tetanus booster, hepatitis B, and HPV (human papillomavirus)

Primary care screening: Cardiovascular risk factors, cervical cancer/pap screening, depression and anxiety, intimate partner violence, obesity, sexual assault, tobacco, marijuana, vaping, alcohol, and illegal and prescription drug use

Gynecological history: Record of abnormal cervical cancer screening and treatment (cone surgery, loop electrosurgical excision procedure [LEEP]/large loop excision of the transformation zone [LLETZ], or any cervical surgery); history of myomectomy; or other gynecologic surgery.

Menstrual history: Cycle length and length of bleeding, noting any intermenstrual bleeding, clots, or heavy bleeding; last menstrual period and last normal menstrual period.

Sexual history (see Table 6.2): Number of past and current partners, sexual practices, STI protection, history of STIs, current use and history of pregnancy prevention strategies (contraception).

Obstetrical history: Record of any previous pregnancy and outcomes, pregnancy attempts, spontaneous or elective abortions, history of pregnancy complications or adverse outcomes, intrapartum and postpartum complications, and neonatal complications.

Social history: Work or environmental hazards, exposures to teratogenic agents (Box 6.2), support networks, diet to include 24-hour recall (asking specifically about calcium, caffeine, and iron-rich foods), exercise, access to care issues, financial concerns, travel history in the past year, cats in household, and gardening.

NOT TO BE MISSED

For patients with or family history of chronic health conditions, the preconception visit is an ideal time to assess health care to review if adjustments should be made in care.

REPRODUCTIVE LIFE PLAN

All female patients of reproductive age should be asked about their reproductive life plan at each health care visit. The Oregon Foundation of Reproductive Health has developed an evidence-based initiative, *One Key Question,* which advocates asking "Would you like to become pregnant in the next year?"[6] at every health-related encounter, including urgent care and emergency department visits.[7] If the patient does not have a reproductive plan, a few minutes to help strategize and

TABLE 6.2 **Infectious Disease Screening and Immunizations in Preconception Care**

Screening/Immunization	Recommendations
Infectious Disease	
Chlamydia[38]	Screen all sexually active women 24 years or younger and in women 25 years or older who are at increased risk for infection.
	Treat infected patients.
Gonorrhea[38]	Screen all sexually active women 24 years or younger and in women 25 years or older who are at increased risk for infection.
	Treat infected patients.
Herpes simplex virus infection	Counsel about the risk of vertical transmission.
Human immunodeficiency virus infection[39]	Screen for HIV infection in adolescents and adults aged 15 to 65 years. Younger adolescents and older adults who are at increased risk of infection should be screened.
	Counsel about the risk of vertical transmission (treatment reduces this risk).
Syphilis[40]	Screen high-risk women.
	Treat infected patients.
Tuberculosis	Screen high-risk women.
	Treat women with active and latent disease before pregnancy.
Immunization	
Hepatitis B[41]	Discuss with provider and vaccinate if high-risk.
	Counsel chronic carriers about prevention of vertical transmission.
Influenza, COVID-19[42]	Vaccinate against the flu by the end of October. Vaccinate against COVID-19.
Measles, mumps, rubella[43]	Screen for immunity.
	Vaccinate all nonimmune women who are not pregnant.
	Counsel patients to avoid pregnancy for 1 month after vaccination.
Tetanus, diphtheria, pertussis[44]	Tetanus vaccination may protect against neonatal tetanus.
	Vaccinate with Tdap during pregnancy (optimal timing is 27 to 36 weeks' gestation) to reduce the risk of neonatal pertussis.
Varicella[45]	Screen for immunity.
	Vaccinate all nonimmune women who are not pregnant.
	Counsel patients to avoid pregnancy for 1 month after vaccination.

Tdap, Tetanus toxoid, reduced diphtheria toxoid, and acellular pertussis.

develop one is a priority. This dialogue would include a nonjudgmental discussion with the patient and ideally her partner regarding their desire and readiness to have a child (or more children) or to not have a child (or another child). If future children are desired, additional conversations should include the optimal number, ideal healthy spacing, timing, age-related potential consequences, and any health promotion strategies and medical interventions that must be implemented before conceiving. It is important that both the provider and patient be aware that this is a fluid plan that could change at any given time. If the female patient states that she does not plan to have children or at least not now, family planning and contraception strategies must be discussed as well as a plan for when pregnancy is desired.

> **CLINICAL SURVIVAL TIP:** Every female patient of reproductive age should be asked the *One Key Question* at every health care visit: "Would you like to become pregnant in the next year?".

REVIEW OF SYSTEMS

A full review of systems is routinely accomplished after the thorough history. Emphasized body systems include

BOX 6.2	**Potential Teratogenic Agents**

- Allergens
- Arsenic
- Cadmium
- Carbon monoxide
- Heavy metals
- Lead
- Mercury
- Pesticides/herbicides/rodenticides
- Radiation
- Secondhand smoke
- Solvents (paint, metal cleaner, furniture stripper)
- Toxic waste

the head, eyes, ears, nose, and throat (HEENT); cardiovascular; respiratory; genitourinary; reproductive; gastrointestinal; lymphatic; neurological; musculoskeletal; and physiological systems.

Physical health assessment includes all aspects of the complete physical examination. The American College of Obstetricians and Gynecologists (ACOG) recommends additional attention to the following systems during the annual well-women examination as the standard of care: thyroid, breast, abdominal, pelvic, and skin examinations.[8] Blood pressure and body mass index (BMI) are critical vital signs. A full gynecological examination should be included with appropriate screening tests.

PRECONCEPTION DIAGNOSTIC TESTING

The goal of preconception testing is to identify any potential medical concerns before conception, avoid complications during the pregnancy, and create a management plan for any identified medical conditions. The most common primary care screening and diagnostic tests for preconception care include hemoglobin/hematocrit, immunity titers, infection screening, and genetic carrier screening. Additional tests may be necessary depending on risk assessment during the health history. For example, if the patient reports symptoms that may suggest diabetes, such as increased thirst, increased urination, and/or frequent yeast infections, a hemoglobin A_{1c} test may be warranted. Likewise, a thyroid-stimulating hormone (TSH) test may be indicated if a patient identifies symptoms of thyroid disease, such as fatigue, temperature intolerance, or hair loss.

Anemia is a common, treatable complication in pregnancy that could be avoided with early identification by a simple and inexpensive hemoglobin blood test. Immunity for rubella and varicella can be confirmed with an antibody screen. If an immunization or a booster should be necessary, it should occur before pregnancy to avoid the potential of teratogenic effects from the vaccine and to avoid the increased risk of poor maternal-child health outcomes from contracting the disease during pregnancy. Required up-to-date primary care screening tests include cervical cancer screening, lipid profile, and STIs. Screening per CDC guidelines for STIs includes HIV, hepatitis B, chlamydia, gonorrhea, syphilis and HIV.[9]

When providing preconception care, APCs should include basic genetic screening, including screening for cystic fibrosis, hemoglobinopathies, and spinal muscular atrophy. Target carrier screening focuses on testing for disorders more common in certain ethnic groups, races or in patients with a family history. An example of this targeted ethnic-based genetic testing would be sickle cell carrier status for African Americans or Tay-Sachs carrier screening for Orthodox Jewish descendants. Expanded carrier screening can also be offered. This could include up to 100 more severe disorders unrelated to race or ethnic background. Genetic counseling is an important component of genetic carrier screening and should be included as part of genetic testing (Table 6.3).

EDUCATION AND INTERVENTIONS

Diet

Diet is an important part of preconception counseling to ensure the health of the mother and fetus. A healthy diet includes fruits and vegetables and limits high-fat food choices. MyPlate, a nutritional model from the U.S. Department of Agriculture (USDA) demonstrates healthy meal choices based on eating healthy portions of a variety of foods from the five food groups (Fig. 6.3).[10] Completing a 24-hour diet recall can be helpful in understanding the female patient's usual nutrition patterns and may provide clues as to food availability and understanding of nutrition choices in line with MyPlate. Hydration is essential for general health, with 6 to 8 glasses of water recommended per day. Many female patients will inquire about the effects of caffeine and artificial

TABLE 6.3	Recommendations for Preconception Testing
Condition	Test
Anemia	Hemoglobin and hematocrit
Immunity titers	Varicella and rubella
Infections	HIV, hepatitis B and C viruses, Zika virus, herpes simplex virus, syphilis
Genetic carrier screening	Cystic fibrosis, Tay-Sachs disease, sickle cell disease
Primary care screening	Cervical cancer and depression

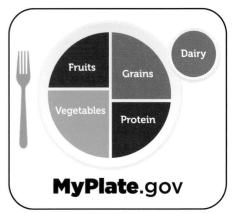

Figure 6.3 MyPlate. (From U.S. Department of Agriculture. [n.d.]. *MyPlate Graphics.* https://www.myplate.gov/resources/graphics/myplate-graphics.)

sweeteners on their health. Because there is minimal evidence currently available, generally it is recommended that caffeine and artificial sweeteners should be used in moderation.

Food safety information is important to discuss during preconception counseling as many women do not seek antepartum care until they are well into their first trimester. Methyl mercury in fish also poses potential risks during pregnancy. High levels of mercury ingestion have been linked to a variety of birth defects. It is found in many bottom-dwelling fish including king mackerel, shark, and orange roughy.[11] Canned tuna fish has a very low mercury content and is recommended no more than two to three times per week, with albacore tuna having a higher mercury content.[11] Raw and uncooked fish as well as raw and undercooked meats should not be consumed because of the increased risk of ingesting parasites or bacteria. Fish is an excellent source of low-fat protein and can be important for the growth and development of the fetus. All fish should not be discouraged from a healthy diet, as it contains omega-3 fatty acids, which have proven to be essential for healthy fetal brain development. Education on safe fish options and quantities as well as excellent resources and up-to-date information are available for providers and patients on the U.S. Food and Drug Administration (FDA) website (https://www.fda.gov/Food/ResourcesForYou/Consumers/ucm393070.htm). Unpasteurized milk, juices, and soft cheeses such as Brie, feta, Camembert, Roquefort, and queso are not recommend because of the risk of *Escherichia coli*, *Listeria*, and *Salmonella* contamination.[12]

Supplements

Adequate supplies of key nutritional elements are essential in preparing for pregnancy (Table 6.4). Some key vitamins and minerals have been shown to have a positive effect on pregnancy outcomes, particularly when they are available at the onset of pregnancy. As female patients prepare for pregnancy, supplementation of key nutrients may be important in optimizing pregnancy outcomes.

Folic Acid

All sexually active female patients of reproductive age are encouraged to take a multivitamin with at least 400 mcg of folic acid. The U.S. Preventive Services Task Force (USPSTF) recommends that all females who are planning or capable of pregnancy take a daily supplement containing 0.4 to 0.8 mg (400 to 800 mcg) of folic acid.[13] Folic acid supplementation initiated at least 1 month before conception can significantly reduce the risks of neural tube defects like spina bifida and anencephaly.[13] Patients with a history of having a child with a neural tube defect are encouraged to take 4 mg to 5 mg of folic acid daily one month before conceiving and through the first 3 months of pregnancy to decrease the risk of neural tube defects in subsequent pregnancies.[46]

! SAFETY ALERT

Methyl mercury in fish also poses potential risks during pregnancy. High levels of mercury ingestion have been linked to a variety of birth defects.

TABLE 6.4 Examples of Food Sources to Add Supplementation in the Diet	
Nutrient	**Food Source for Supplementation**
Folic acid	Dark, leafy green vegetables, dried beans, avocados, lentils, and citrus fruits
Iron	Red meats, spinach, and raisins
Calcium	Milk, yogurt, cheese, orange juice, sardines, green beans, and sunflower seeds

NOT TO BE MISSED

The USPSTF recommends that all females who are planning or capable of pregnancy take a daily supplement containing 0.4 to 0.8 mg (400 to 800 mcg) of folic acid.

Iron

During pregnancy, females need 50% more iron to support the increased blood supply of the placenta and fetus as well as the increased maternal and fetal oxygen needs.[15] The fetus uses the mother's iron reserves for growth and development, commonly leaving the mother depleted. Preconception counseling should include recommending 27 mg of iron a day.[15] Women at risk or who have an identified iron anemia should be counseled on appropriate iron supplementation and foods high in iron to include in their daily diet. Foods high in iron are absorbed better when consumed with vitamin C–rich foods like citrus fruits and tomato sauce.

Calcium

Calcium is another essential element for embryonic growth, and maintaining appropriate consumption can decrease the risk of preeclampsia, preterm birth, and low birth weight.[16] Calcium also helps build strong bones and teeth for the fetus. Supplementation of calcium is only recommended to achieve the recommended daily intake of 1000 mg/day for all females 19 to 50 years of age.[17] The best source of calcium is through diet and can usually be achieved with dairy products and other foods rich in calcium. If supplementation is required, female patients should be instructed to only take 500 mg at a time at breakfast and again at dinner to increase absorption. Calcium supplementation and iron supplementation should not occur at the same time, as they cannot be absorbed adequately when combined. Encourage female patients to take supplements 1 to 2 hours apart.

PATIENT-CENTERED CARE: Consuming iron supplements with ascorbic acid increases the absorption of iron.[18]

Immunization

Women are encouraged to become up-to-date with all vaccinations before trying to conceive. Any identified gaps in their immunization records must be managed as soon as detected. Titers should be drawn to ensure varicella and rubella immunity. If the rubella vaccine is needed, the patient must wait 3 months to become pregnant and abstain from intercourse or use a reliable short-term contraceptive method. The influenza vaccine is recommended annually for preconception and antepartum care. The hepatitis B vaccine is only recommended for high-risk populations, but it may be warranted if any high-risk identifiers were discovered during the history.

Medications

Providers must have a clear understanding of all medications the patient has been prescribed or is taking over the counter, including herbs and supplements. A strong understanding of pregnancy exposure risks is required for both the prescriber and patient. Consider that drug safety can change depending on trimester of exposure; for example, a medication may be safe in the first and second trimesters but have the potential for harm in the third trimester. In December 2014, the FDA set new ground rules and policies for labeling the potential risks of medications during pregnancy and lactation.[19] This new labeling system will replace the old standard five-letter system (A, B, C, D, and X), which was rarely updated after new evidence was established and provided very little detail about the actual risks. The rollout of this revised labeling system has been slow. The new system will provide the patient and prescriber more detailed and specific information about the identified risks to the patient and fetus, information for male and female patients on the potential effects on fertility, and potential risks to a breastfed infant. The revised labeling information will also include contact information for national registries. Patients who have been exposed to medications during preconception, during pregnancy, or while breastfeeding will be encouraged to call and report outcomes so data can be collected on the actual risks.

The decision to take any medication during preconception, pregnancy, or interconception and/or while breastfeeding is an individual decision between the patient and provider, and the risks and benefits related to pregnancy should be discussed. Migraines, epilepsy, anxiety, depression, and diabetes are examples of conditions that are often treated with medications that may place the fetus at risk. Expectant mothers should avoid commonly used over-the-counter medications including aspirin, bismuth subsalicylate, and naproxen. The clinician should stress that even though medications may be available over the counter, they are not necessarily safe during preconception or pregnancy.

! SAFETY ALERT

Expectant mothers should avoid commonly used over-the-counter medications including aspirin, bismuth subsalicylate, and naproxen.

Stabilize Medical Conditions

Diabetes, hypertension, obesity, depression, STIs, and substance use or abuse are all conditions that may affect maternal and fetal health. Modifiable risk factors associated with these conditions should be addressed during preconception screening. Early interventions can modify the disease progress and therefore improve the overall health of the patient and fetus.

Diabetes

Uncontrolled blood sugar can increase the risk of miscarriage, congenital malformations, preterm delivery, and maternal death. [20] Female patients should be screened for diabetes before pregnancy if they are overweight; have a history of polycystic ovarian syndrome, frequent yeast infections, or recurrent miscarriages; or have a strong family history of diabetes. A fasting blood sugar less than 100 mg/dL or a hemoglobin A_{1c} less than 5.6% are typical glycemic targets for high-risk female patients of reproductive age.[21] In patients with a history of gestational diabetes in a previous pregnancy, it is important that they receive postpartum screening and counseling regarding future diabetes risk.

Hypertension

Hypertension screening is routinely completed at the first point of contact with any health care provider. The new American College of Cardiology (ACC) guidelines state that screening blood pressures should be less than 130/80 mm Hg.[22] High blood pressure during pregnancy can result in the following life-threatening complications: preeclampsia, HELLP syndrome (hemolysis, elevated liver enzymes, and low platelet count), premature birth, low birth weight, and placenta abruption.[23] Early diagnoses and identification of chronic or uncontrolled hypertension during preconception care can trigger interventions to decrease poor health outcomes, as one in four chronic hypertensive women will develop preeclampsia during pregnancy.[23] Evidence-based preconception interventions can include medication, increased monitoring, and additional cardiovascular testing to manage the hypertension before conception.

Obesity

Weight and BMI are critical pieces of information for any primary care visit, especially in female patients of reproductive age. Obesity or a BMI greater than 30 kg/m^2 has been linked to complications with maternal health and the health of the fetus during pregnancy, including gestational diabetes, infertility, neural tube defects, preeclampsia, cesarean delivery, and thrombolytic events.[24] Screening for obesity during preconception care and counseling female patients on the benefits of an active lifestyle and healthy eating habits can reduce their risk of developing a chronic illness before and during pregnancy. Interventions should focus on prolonged significant weight loss, including an exercise regime and altered eating habits with nutritional counseling. Screening for underweight is also important as a BMI less than 18.5 kg/m^2 has been linked to personal health concerns and infertility.[24]

Depression

Screening for depression should occur at every visit for every woman. Women who are depressed in pregnancy are at risk for self-medicating with drugs and alcohol, worsening of symptoms and coping mechanisms, and postpartum depression. Using any evidence-based depression screening tool or taking a thorough history to identify depression can easily be performed and allow the opportunity for management of the depression with counseling, medication, or a combination of therapies during the preconception period.

Infections

The CDC recommends that female patients who are candidates for preconception care be screened for the following infections: herpes simplex virus (HSV), gonorrhea, chlamydia, hepatitis B and C viruses, human immunodeficiency virus (HIV), and syphilis.[9] The medications needed to treat many of these infections are teratogenic and ideally would be given before pregnancy to avoid poor health outcomes from the disease or the treatment. Undiagnosed and untreated gonorrhea and chlamydia can lead to pelvic inflammatory disease, which is the leading cause of infertility because of tubal scarring. Early identification of HSV can decrease transmission to the newborn at birth, which can be fatal. HIV can be transmitted to the fetus; however, the risk can decrease to 2% if safe medications are begun preconceptionally.[25] Simple blood tests and urine tests can be utilized to screen for these infections at a primary care or preconception visit. Counseling to avoid sexual risk behaviors, disease prevention, and screening per CDC guidelines are all included in preconception care.

Preconception care includes screening female patients regarding potential exposure for them and their partner to the Zika virus. The Zika virus is spread through infected mosquitos and can be passed from the mother to the unborn child. Exposure to the Zika virus can cause severe birth defects, most commonly macrocephaly and other brain defects.[26] Zika testing is not recommend by the CDC during preconception counseling. Female patients and their families must be educated about travel to areas where there is a risk for acquiring the Zika virus and should be provided resources that update information frequently. Asymptomatic woman who have traveled to an area with the known Zika virus are advised to wait 2 months to plan on conceiving and to use barrier protection during this waiting period. If a male partner travels to an area with known Zika virus, the couple should wait 6 months to plan to conceive and use a barrier method during this waiting period. Symptomatic female patients can have a Zika virus IgM drawn, and symptom management should be implemented. The same waiting period for symptomatic and treated individuals should be

> ### NOT TO BE MISSED
>
> Undiagnosed and untreated gonorrhea and chlamydia can lead to pelvic inflammatory disease, which is the leading cause of infertility because of tubal scarring.

recommended beginning with the onset of symptoms if planning to conceive.[26]

Toxoplasmosis is a parasite found in garden soil, raw meat, and cat feces. The most common activities that can put women at risk are cleaning the litter box and gardening. The clinical manifestations of the disease are flulike systems that often resolve without complications within 5 to 8 days. Immunocompromised pregnant patients may have an increased risk of maternal and fetal complications.[27] Routine preconception screening for toxoplasmosis is not recommend.[27] Education should be provided to women to wear gloves and wash hands thoroughly after cleaning the litter box or gardening and to avoid eating undercooked or raw meats.

Substance Abuse

Substance abuse screening is recommended routinely during well-care or problem primary care visits. Every patient should be asked about history of addiction, tobacco use, alcohol use, and opioid use. Alcohol, an identified teratogen, is one of the leading preventable causes of birth defects and developmental disabilities in the United States and can lead to premature birth, low birth weight, stillbirth, and miscarriage.[28] Leading evidence-based medical organizations agree that all females should be counseled to avoid alcohol if sexually active and not preventing pregnancy. No amount of alcohol is safe, and many birth defects can occur while drinking before a patient may even know she is pregnant. Prenatal exposure to tobacco can lead to increased risk of spontaneous abortion, ectopic pregnancy, low birth weight, sudden infant death syndrome, and preterm birth.[29] Females who smoked before pregnancy have a threefold risk of delivering a baby with a congenital heart defect.[28] It is estimated that eliminating smoking before pregnancy could avoid up to 7% of preterm-related deaths and up to 24% of sudden infant death cases.[4] Ideally patients are counseled on the risks associated with smoking before pregnancy at every visit and should be educated on the maternal and fetal health benefits of not smoking, medication options, treatment programs, and options for augmenting these with intense behavioral counseling for smoking cessation. Opioid use should also be specifically discussed, and resources should be made readily available. Female patients who are identified to be dependent to any substance need immediate referral for appropriate treatment options. A national initiative, Screening, Brief Intervention, and Referral to Treatment (SBIRT), is an evidence-based clinical approach to identify, decrease, and prevent substance abuse and dependency in primary care.[30] A global recommendation by the WHO recommends using the "5 A's" screening tool of *ask, advise, assess, assist,* and *arrange* at every clinical visit to address this area of preconception care.[4]

> **CLINICAL SURVIVAL TIP:** Screening, Brief Intervention, and Referral to Treatment (SBIRT) is an evidence-based clinical approach to identify, decrease, and prevent substance abuse and dependency in primary care and should be engaged at every visit.

MALES AND PRECONCEPTION CARE

Preconception care is also an expectation for male patients at all primary care visits, and they should be asked about their reproductive life plan. If they do not desire children, contraception options should be discussed. Male patients should receive many of the same preconception screens as their female partners. Screening, education, and assessment should include information about STI risk and recommendations to avoid toxic substances, quit smoking, cease using any street drugs or illegal prescriptions, limit alcohol, reach and maintain a healthy weight, have a yearly physical examination to identify any health issues that could affect fertility, report any genetic disease with self or family, screen for mental health and safety, and receive counseling on partner support.[31] Many of the history questions by the provider regarding the male patient's sexual health focus on ensuring quality sperm. Medications, age, surgery on reproductive organs, stress, unhealthy weight, and use of tobacco, drugs, and alcohol can all effect the viability, quantity, and morphology of sperm. [32] Health promotion and disease prevention are standard elements to the well-man visit, and preconception care can easily be incorporated into every visit to promote healthier patients and healthier pregnancies.

INTERCONCEPTION CARE

Interconception care is the care of female patients in between pregnancies. This care can be challenging as these patients often forgo the postpartum appointment, lose insurance coverage after delivery, and have a variety of competing demands.[7] For these reasons, it is critical that providers take every opportunity to discuss interconception care when interacting with female patients of reproductive age at any type of visit. Interconception care occurs at a prime time in a female patient's life to manage issues or conditions identified during pregnancy, promote a healthy lifestyle, and decrease risky health behaviors to improve outcomes in future pregnancies. It is an opportunity to reevaluate the patient's reproductive life plan and discuss interpregnancy intervals. The IMPLICIT (Interventions to Minimize Preterm birth and Low Birthweight Infants using Continuous Improvement Techniques) model focuses on four maternal risk factors that providers can use to counsel mothers during their baby's multiple visits within the first 2 years of life.[7] This model has been successful is incorporating interconception care for the mothers during well-baby visits. The four identified factors can be touched on efficiently and effectively with easy instructions in a very short time frame. These include smoking cessation, depression, multivitamin supplementation with folic acid, and planning pregnancy intervals. Initial results demonstrate strong evidence that female patients are accepting of this education during their child's health care visits and that access to long-acting contraception and folic acid has increased.[7]

SPECIAL POPULATIONS OF WOMEN

Special populations may be at increased risk for fetal or maternal problems and therefore are in greater need of preconception counseling. Such groups include immigrants, survivors of cancer, patients with disabilities, patients older than 35 years of age, and patients with gender identity differences.

> **PATIENT-CENTERED CARE:** The following populations may require additional consideration when providing preconception and interconception care services: cancer survivors, patients with disabilities, patients older than 35 years of age, and patients with gender identity differences.

Immigrants and Refugees

Immigrants and refugees may have limited access to medical care and preconception counseling as a result of factors such as culture, language, or financial barriers. Immigrants and refugees often come from areas that are high risk for tuberculosis and hepatitis B and must receive screening for these conditions.

Cancer Survivors

Cancer survivors will need to consult with their oncology specialist to discuss preconception counseling on fertility preservation options, fertility side effects of medications and treatments, and any long-term medical health risks a pregnancy may trigger. Cancer survivors do not have an increased risk for poor pregnancy outcomes, and most chemotherapy treatments do not increase the risk for birth defects or miscarriage.[33]

Patients With Disabilities

Female patients with disabilities need extensive preconception counseling on any medications and assisted devices needed for their condition. Many of these potential issues should be discussed and a plan formulated to accommodate their special needs. These patients are very capable of having a disability and healthy pregnancy concurrently, and they often need their provider to advocate for administrative, physical, and attitudinal barriers.[33]

Patients Older Than 35 Years of Age

Patients older than 35 years of age should be educated on the additional risks associated with pregnancy after age 35. These patients have an increased risk of infertility. They are also more likely to have medical conditions that can affect pregnancy. Conditions that are associated with advanced maternal age include chromosomal birth defects, preeclampsia, stillbirth, and cesarean delivery.[34]

Patients With Gender Identity Differences

Individuals with gender identity differences including LGBTQ+ patients or questioning patients may need unique preconception care. Additional counseling and resources for this population may include donor sperm, intrauterine insemination, and support networks. Patients with gender identify differences will need all of the other elements of a preconception care visit, but will also need a provider who is an advocate for the many societal barriers within the health care system. Creating an environment of open and honest communication will allow the provider to share necessary information and the patient to be comfortable discussing concerns and fears.

> **PATIENT-CENTERED CARE:** Individuals with gender identity differences including LGBTQ+ patients or questioning patients may need unique preconception care.

REFERRALS

Referrals may be necessary depending on the clinician's practice and clinical experience with preconception care and the level of complexity. All clinicians should have tools for preconception care at their disposal. If a risk is identified or an abnormal screening or diagnostic test is discovered, a referral to a women's health nurse practitioner, certified nurse midwife, obstetrician, or medical specialist may be warranted. Many preventive strategies and the management of uncontrolled medical conditions should be initiated immediately by the primary care provider. High-risk female patients, patients with known genetic risk, or those with complex and multiple risk factors may benefit from a preconception consult with a maternal fetal medicine specialist or geneticist. Referrals to a nutritionist, social services, and mental health services may be warranted depending on history or status.

> **PATIENT-CENTERED CARE:** If a risk is identified or an abnormal screening or diagnostic test discovered, a referral to a women's health nurse practitioner, certified nurse midwife, obstetrician, or medical specialist may be warranted.

CONCLUSION

Preconception care is a universal need for all individuals of childbearing age. Preconception risk assessments and counseling are the responsibility of all health care providers and should be implemented at all primary care and preventive visits. Preconception care should consist of evidence-based screening and interventions that can improve pregnancy outcomes by improving the health of the patient before conception. Clinicians have the potential to be the leaders of preconception risk assessments. Through counseling and education, clinicians will be instrumental in formalizing a reproductive life plan with their patients and strategizing a plan for disease prevention and health promotion to improve maternal-fetal outcomes.

■ KEY POINTS

- Preconception care can have a significant effect on health and wellness outcomes for all females of reproductive age.
- Reproductive life plans are an essential tool for designing individual health and wellness plans for patients.
- A thorough risk assessment is critical to identify areas for evidence-based interventions and education to improve the health of female patients and decrease the risk of poor pregnancy outcomes.
- Nurse practitioners are positioned to be experts in preconception care as they are the leaders in disease prevention and health promotion.

REFERENCES

1. American College of Obstetricians and Gynecologists. ACOG Committee Opinion No. 313, September 2005. The importance of preconception care in the continuum of women's health care. *Obstet Gynecol.* 2005;106(3):665–666.
2. Johnson K, Posner SF, Biermann J, et al. Recommendations to improve preconception health and health care—United States: a report of the CDC/ATSDR Preconception Care Work Group and the Select Panel on Preconception Care. *Morbid Mortal Wkly Rep.* 2006;55(RR-6):1–23.
3. U.S. Department of Health and Human Services, Office of Disease Prevention and Health Promotion. *Healthy People 2020.* Washington, DC; 2016. https://www.healthypeople.gov/.
4. World Health Organization. *Preconception Care: Maximizing the Gains for Maternal and Child Health.* Policy Brief; 2013. https://www.who.int/publications/i/item/WHO-FWC-MCA-13.02.
5. American College of Obstetricians and Gynecologists' Committee on Health Care for Underserved Women. Committee Opinion No. 654: Reproductive life planning to reduce unintended pregnancy. *Obstet Gynecol.* 2016;127(2):e66–e69.
6. Bellanca HK, Hunter MS. One Key Question®: preventive reproductive health is part of high quality primary care. *Contraception.* 2013;88(1):3–6.
7. Fryne DJ. A Paradigm shift in preconception and interconception care: using every encounter to improve birth outcomes. *Zero to Three.* 2017;37:1–10.
8. American College of Obstetricians and Gynecologists. Well-woman visit. Committee Opinion No. 534, August, 2012. *Obstet Gynecol.* 2012;120(1):421–424.
9. American Academy of Pediatrics, American College of Obstetricians and Gynecologists. *Guidelines for Perinatal Care.* 8th ed. Elk Grove Village, IL: AAP; Washington, DC: American College of Obstetricians and Gynecologists; 2017.
10. American College of Obstetrics and Gynecologists. *Nutrition During Pregnancy FAQ001*; 2018. https://www.acog.org/Patients/FAQs/Nutrition-During-Pregnancy#does.
11. U.S. Food and Drug Administration. *Eating Fish: What Pregnant Women and Parents Should Know*; 2017. https://www.fda.gov/Food/ResourcesForYou/Consumers/ucm393070.htm.
12. U.S. Department of Agriculture. *Protect Your Baby and Yourself from Listeriosis*; 2017. https://seafood.oregonstate.edu/sites/agscid7/files/snic/protect-your-baby-and-yourself-from-listeriosis.pdf#:~:text=Listeriosis%20can%20result%20in%20miscarriage%2C%20premature%20delivery%2C%20serious,Service%20www.fsis.usda.gov%20USDA%20Meat%20and%20Poultry%20Hotline%201-888-MPHotlinethermometer.
13. Bibbins-Domingo K, Grossman DC, Curry SJ, et al. Folic acid supplementation for the prevention of neural tube defects: U.S. Preventive Services Task Force Recommendation Statement. *JAMA.* 2017;317(2):183–189.
14. Toriello HV. Policy statement on folic acid and neural tube defects. Policy and Practice Guideline Committee of the American College of Medical Genetics. *Genet Med.* 2011;13(6):593–596.
15. American College of Obstetricians and Gynecologists. (2021a). ACOG Practice Bulletin No. 233. Anemia in Pregnancy. https://www.acog.org/clinical/clinical-guidance/practice-bulletin/articles/2021/08/anemia-in-pregnancy.
16. Hofmeyr GJ, Lawrie TA, Atallah AN, Duley L. Calcium supplementation during pregnancy for preventing hypertensive disorders and related problems. *Cochrane Database Syst Rev.* 2010;8:CD001059.
17. American College of Obstetricians and Gynecologists. Practice Guidelines: ACOG Releases Practice Bulletin on Osteoporosis, 2013. *Am Fam Physician.* 2013;88(4):269–275.
18. National Institutes for Health, Office of Dietary Supplements. (2022). Iron. https://ods.od.nih.gov/factsheets/Iron-HealthProfessional/.
19. Stoffel NU, von Siebenthal HK, Moretti D, Zimmermann MB. Oral iron supplementation in iron-deficient women: how much and how often? *Mol Aspects Med.* 2020;75:100865.
20. Wahabi HA, Alzeidan A, Bawazeer GA, et al. Preconception care for diabetic women for improving maternal and fetal outcomes: a systematic review and meta-analysis. *BMC Pregnancy Childbirth.* 2010;10:63.
21. U.S. Preventive Services Task Force. *Final Recommendation Statement: Abnormal Blood Glucose and Type 2 Diabetes Mellitus: Screening.* https://www.uspreventiveservicestaskforce.org/uspstf/announcements/final-

recommendation-statement-screening-abnormal-blood-glucose-and-type-2-diabetes-mellitus.

22. American College of Cardiology. *New ACC/AHA High Blood Pressure Guidelines Lower Definition of Hypertension*; 2017. http://www.acc.org/latest-in-cardiology/articles/2017/11/08/11/47/mon-5pm-bp-guideline-aha-2017.

23. American College of Obstetricians and Gynecologists. (2021b). ACOG Practice Bulletin No. 230. Obesity in Pregnancy. https://oce.ovid.com/article/00006250-202106000-00038/HTML.

24. Jack BW, Atrash H, Coonrod DV, Moos MK, O'Donnell J, Johnson K. The clinical content of preconception care: an overview and preparation of this supplement. *Am J Obstet Gynecol*. 2008;199(6 suppl 2):S266–S279.

25. U.S. Centers for Disease Control and Prevention. *HIV among pregnant women, infants, and children*; 2018. http://www.cdc.gov/hiv/group/gender/pregnantwomen/index.html.

26. U.S. Centers for Disease Control and Prevention. *CDC expands guidance for travel and testing of pregnant women, women of reproductive age, and their partners for Zika virus infection related to mosquito-borne Zika virus transmission in Miami-Dade, Florida*; 2016. http://emergency.cdc.gov/han/han00394.asp.

27. American College of Obstetricians and Gynecologists. Practice Bulletin No. 151: Cytomegalovirus, parvovirus B19, varicella zoster, and toxoplasmosis in pregnancy. *Obstet Gynecol*. 2015;125(6):1510–1525.

28. Lassi ZS, Imam AM, Dean SV, Bhutta ZA. Preconception care: caffeine, smoking, alcohol, drugs and other environmental chemical/radiation exposure. *Reproductive Health*. 2014;11(suppl 3):S6.

29. Floyd RL, Johnson KA, Owens JR, Verbiest S, Moore CA, Boyle C. A national action plan for promoting preconception health and health care in the United States (2012–2014). *J Womens Health (Larchmt)*. 2013;22(10):797–802.

30. Agerwala SM, McCance-Katz EF. Integrating Screening, Brief Intervention, and Referral to Treatment (SBIRT) into clinical practice settings: a brief review. *J Psychoactive Drugs*. 2012;44(4):307–317.

31. U.S. Centers for Disease Control and Prevention. Preconception health and healthcare: Information for men. 2018;23. https://www.cdc.gov/preconception/men.html.

32. Warner JN, Frey KA. The Well-man visit: addressing a man's health to optimize pregnancy outcomes. *J Am Board Fam Med*. 2013;26(2):196–202.

33. Green DM, Whitton JA, Stovall M, et al. Pregnancy outcome of female survivors of childhood cancer: a report from the childhood cancer survivor study. *Am J Obstet Gynecol*. 2002;187(4):1070–1080.

34. American College of Obstetricians and Gynecologists. *Having a Baby After 35. How Aging Affects Fertility and Pregnancy*; 2020. https://www.acog.org/womens-health/faqs/having-a-baby-after-age-35-how-aging-affects-fertility-and-pregnancy.

35. Mason E, Chandra-Mouli V, Baltag V, Christiansen C, Lassi ZS, Bhutta ZA. Preconception care: advancing from "important to do and can be done" to "is being done and is making a difference. *Reprod Health*. 2014;11 Suppl 3 (suppl 3):S8.

36. Moore KL, Persaud TVN, Torchia MG. *The Developing Human*. Elsevier; 2015.

37. U.S. Department of Agriculture. (n.d.) *MyPlate Graphics*. https://www.myplate.gov/resources/graphics/myplategraphics.

38. U.S. Preventive Services Task Force. (2021, Sept 14). Chlamydia and gonorrhea: Screening. https://www.uspreventiveservicestaskforce.org/uspstf/recommendation/chlamydia-and-gonorrhea-screening#:~:text=The%20USPSTF%20recommends%20screening%20for%20gonorrhea%20in%20all%20sexually%20active,at%20increased%20risk%20for%20infection.

39. U.S. Preventive Services Task Force. (2019, June 11). Human immunodeficiency virus (HIV) infection: Screening. https://www.uspreventiveservicestaskforce.org/uspstf/recommendation/human-immunodeficiency-virus-hiv-infection-screening.

40. U.S. Preventive Services Task Force. (2022, Sept 27). Syphilis infection in nonpregnant adolescents and adults: Screening. https://www.uspreventiveservicestaskforce.org/uspstf/recommendation/syphilis-infection-nonpregnant-adults-adolescents-screening.

41. Centers for Disease Control and Prevention. (n.d.). Vaccines during and after pregnancy. https://www.cdc.gov/vaccines/pregnancy/vacc-during-after.html.

42. Centers for Disease Control and Prevention. (n.d.). Vaccines during and after pregnancy. https://www.cdc.gov/vaccines/pregnancy/vacc-during-after.html.

43. Centers for Disease Control and Prevention. (2022). Adult immunization schedule. https://www.cdc.gov/vaccines/schedules/hcp/imz/adult.html Centers for Disease Control and Prevention. (n.d.). Vaccines before pregnancy. https://www.cdc.gov/vaccines/pregnancy/vacc-before.html#:~:text=Out%20of%20an%20abundance%20of,confirmed%20by%20a%20blood%20test.

44. Centers for Disease Control and Prevention. (2022). Adult immunization schedule. https://www.cdc.gov/vaccines/schedules/hcp/imz/adult.html.

45. Centers for Disease Control and Prevention. (2022). Adult immunization schedule. https://www.cdc.gov/vaccines/schedules/hcp/imz/adult.html Mother to Baby. (2021). Varicella (Chickenpox) vaccine. https://www.ncbi.nlm.nih.gov/books/NBK583013/#:~:text=The%20American%20Academy%20of%20Pediatrics,varicella%20vaccine%20before%20becoming%20pregnant.

46. Centers for Disease Control and Prevention. (n.d.). Folic acid. https://www.cdc.gov/ncbddd/folicacid/recommendations.html

7

Pregnancy

Michele LaMarr-Suggs and Jamille Nagtalon-Ramos

OBJECTIVES:

- Gain a better understanding of the role of the family nurse practitioner in prenatal care
- Learn clinical symptoms of pregnancy and diagnostic measures to confirm pregnancy

- Understand the goals and components of prenatal care including anticipatory guidance and education, screening methods, and diagnostic tests
- Differentiate best practices for management of medical conditions that place pregnancy at risk such as hypertensive disorders and diabetes

---

INTRODUCTION

A healthy pregnancy begins before conception and continues with early and regular antepartum care and the timely recognition and management of problems as they arise. Comprehensive care should begin with an assessment of the pregnant parents' attitude and beliefs (e.g., personal, familial, cultural) toward pregnancy that may affect how they care for themselves and the family and influence the care they seek from the health care team. Nurse practitioners and other obstetrical care providers have an excellent opportunity to provide family-centered, holistic, and supportive care throughout their patient's pregnancy and the postpartum period.

CLINICAL SYMPTOMS AND DIAGNOSIS OF PREGNANCY

A key sign of early pregnancy is amenorrhea, or cessation of menses.[1] When female patients of reproductive age miss a period, pregnancy should be suspected until it is ruled out. The clinician's suspicion should be heightened if the patient reports recent sexual intercourse, especially if contraceptives are not used. However, because no contraceptive method is 100% effective besides abstinence, pregnancy should still be considered

in the setting of amenorrhea, even if the patient was using a form of contraception.

> **CLINICAL SURVIVAL TIP:** All female patients of reproductive age are considered pregnant until a urine or serum pregnancy test rules it out.

Presumptive Signs of Pregnancy

Cessation of menses is one of the presumptive signs of pregnancy. These signs are self-reported by the patient and may be caused by other medical conditions. Taking amenorrhea as an example, although it is a principal sign of pregnancy, it may also be caused by numerous other conditions such as polycystic ovarian syndrome or premature menopause. Other presumptive signs of pregnancy include fatigue, urinary frequency, nausea and vomiting, and breast tenderness.[2]

Probable Signs of Pregnancy

Unlike the presumptive signs that are subjective and reported by the pregnant patient, probable signs of pregnancy are based on the clinical observations of the examiner. These probable signs include the following:

- Positive pregnancy test: detection of human chorionic gonadotropin (hCG) serologically or in the urine
- Abdominal enlargement
- Braxton Hicks contractions: intermittent and irregular uterine contractions that do not lead to cervical change; sometimes referred to as *false labor*
- Chadwick's sign: bluish discoloration of the cervix, vagina, and labia caused by increased blood flow to the area
- Goodell's sign: cervical softening
- Hegar's sign: lower uterine segment softening

Similar to presumptive signs, probable signs alone do not lead to a definitive diagnosis of pregnancy as these may be caused by other medical conditions.[1,2]

Positive Signs of Pregnancy

Positive signs such as auscultation of the fetal heartbeat, visualization of the fetus on ultrasonography, and palpation of fetal movements by the examiner are diagnostic of a pregnancy.[1]

DURATION AND DATING OF PREGNANCY

The estimated date of delivery (EDD) is 280 days or 40 weeks from the beginning of the last menstrual period (LMP) and 266 days from the date of conception. Instead of calendar months, health care providers use lunar months (28 days/4weeks = 1 lunar month) when calculating the gestational age and refer to the dating of pregnancy in weeks. Fertilization usually occurs within 24 hours of ovulation and is predicted by detection of a luteinizing hormone (LH) surge or by ultrasound examination. Roughly only 4% of pregnant patients actually deliver by their EDD. Accurate prenatal assessment is critical in calculating the EDD.

There are now numerous smart phone and web applications that calculate gestational age with the click of a button. On the other hand, Naegele's rule is used to manually calculate gestational age (Box 7.1). The EDD is calculated by counting back 3 months from the LMP and adding 7 days. As an example, if the LMP is January 20, 2022, then the EDD will be October 27, 2023. This method is based on two chief assumptions: (1) the patient has a 28-day menstrual cycle and (2) fertilization occurs on day 14 of the menstrual cycle. Numerous factors may affect the accuracy of the EDD, including (1) variations in menstrual cycle, (2) the fertile window

> **BOX 7.1 Naegele's Rule for Calculating a Due Date in Pregnancy**
>
> Naegele's rule is used to manually calculate a pregnant patient's expected date of delivery.
> First day of last menstrual period (LMP): October 5
> Subtract 3 months: − 3 months
>   = July 5
>   + 7 days
>   = July 12

occurring over a period of days, (3) variations in fertilization and implantation, (4) certainty of LMP, and (5) use of contraception.

Physical examination of uterine size also aids in dating the pregnancy. On physical examination, the pregnant uterus is soft and globular. The size–gestational age correlation is learned by experience and is often described in terms of fruit (e.g., for singleton pregnancies: 6- to 8-week size = plum, 8- to 10-week size = orange, 10- to 12-week size = grapefruit), despite the imprecision of this terminology. The uterus remains a nonpalpable organ in the pelvis until approximately 12 weeks' gestation. After 12 weeks, it is usually able to be palpated abdominally slightly above the symphysis pubis. At approximately 16 weeks, the uterine fundus is palpable midway between the symphysis pubis and the umbilicus, and at approximately 20 weeks it is palpable at the umbilicus. After 20 weeks, the symphysis to fundal height in centimeters should correlate with the week of gestation. In the absence of other dating information, uterine enlargement two fingerbreadths above the umbilicus suggests that the fetus is at a gestational age at the limit of viability if neonatal intensive care is available. Uterine fibroids, uterine position, parity, number of fetuses, and obesity are factors that may affect uterine size or the ability to palpate the uterus and could prohibit accurate assessment.

Ultrasonography is a helpful tool in estimating gestational age. These estimates of gestational age are based on the assumption that the size of the embryo correlates with the age. First-trimester ultrasonography is more accurate than second-trimester ultrasonography in dating gestational age; however, dating by certain LMP is the most accurate method.[3] Limitations in the use of ultrasonography include assessment of multiple gestation, fetal position, fetal anomalies, and biological variation. It is common practice to obtain an early or

BOX 7.2   **Common Known Teratogens**

- Alcohol
- Illicit drugs such as cocaine and heroin
- Testosterone
- Dilantin
- Lithium carbonate
- Methotrexate
- Tetracycline
- Chemotherapeutic agents
- Large amounts of vitamin A
- High levels of ionizing radiation
- Viruses such as cytomegalovirus (CMV), rubella, varicella, and herpes simplex virus (HSV)

first-trimester ultrasound examination to confirm the LMP. The use of ultrasound can be helpful, especially when the LMP, menstrual cycle irregularities, and timing of conception may be uncertain, even in the setting of hormonal contraception use.

NOT TO BE MISSED

First-trimester ultrasonography is more accurate than second-trimester ultrasonography in dating gestational age, but dating by certain LMP is the most accurate method.

TERATOGENS IN PREGNANCY

Teratogens are drugs, chemicals, or even infections that can cause abnormal fetal development (Box 7.2). The use or exposure to possible teratogens can potentially lead to significant birth defects. Teratogens are factors that can alter normal intrauterine development of fetal growth, anatomical structures, physical functioning, and postnatal development. Often teratogens can include environmental exposures, maternal medical disorders, infectious agents, genetic conditions, or drugs. During organogenesis between days 15 and 60, teratogenic agents are more likely to cause major congenital malformations.[4] The embryo is most susceptible to teratogenic agents during periods of rapid cell division. Each organ of an embryo has a critical period during which its development may be disrupted. The type of congenital malformation produced by an exposure depends on which organ is most susceptible at the time of the teratogenic exposure as well as the length and intensity of the exposure.[4]

Commonly used drug classes such as antipsychotics, antiepileptics, antidepressants, angiotensin-converting enzyme (ACE) inhibitors, and other drugs should be prescribed with caution. A detailed and complete patient history is crucial in preventing exposure to the fetus.

NOT TO BE MISSED

During organogenesis between days 15 and 60, teratogenic agents are more likely to cause major congenital malformations.

PRENATAL CARE

The goal of prenatal care is to ensure the health of the infant and minimize maternal risk. Prenatal visits should be a time of ongoing evaluation of the overall well-being of the patient and infant and the recognition and management of maternal/fetal problems. The ultimate goal of prenatal care is to decrease maternal and fetal mortality. Prenatal visits should always incorporate the pregnant patient and her support system in the plan of care. The patient's cultural practices and religious beliefs should be valued, respected, and incorporated into their care. Prenatal care should ideally be initiated within the first trimester.[5] Typical intervals for visits with uncomplicated pregnancies are every 4 weeks until 28 to 30 weeks' gestation, every 2 weeks from 28 to 36 weeks, and then weekly thereafter until delivery. Patients with multiple comorbidities or conditions complicating their pregnancy may require a higher frequency of visits. All pregnant patients are encouraged to inform their health care provider if they experience vaginal bleeding, leakage of fluid from the vagina, or decreased fetal movement (DFM). Signs of preterm labor and signs of preeclampsia will be discussed in detail later in this chapter.

PATIENT-CENTERED CARE: Prenatal visits should always incorporate the patient and her support system in the plan of care. The family's cultural practices and religious beliefs should be valued, respected, and incorporated into their care.

PRENATAL VISITS

Prenatal visits usually occur every 4 weeks until 28 to 30 weeks' gestation, every 2 weeks from 28 to 36 weeks, and then weekly thereafter until delivery. Routine assessments at each prenatal visit typically include the following:

- Measurement of maternal blood pressure (BP) and weight
- Assessment of diet and exercise
- Urine dipstick for protein and glucose
- Assessment of fetal growth, either by measurement of fundal height or by ultrasound evaluation for patients with risk factors for intrauterine growth restriction. Fundal heights are usually measured with a measuring tape beginning at 20 weeks. These measurements should correlate with gestational age within 2 cm above or below. For example, if a patient is at 24 weeks' gestation, the fundal height is expected to be no less than 22 cm and no more than 26 cm. If the fundal height is lower than suspected, consider intrauterine growth restriction, low amniotic fluid volume, or fetal position. If the fundal height

is higher than suspected, consider a large for gestational age fetus. A growth ultrasound examination would be warranted in both cases to assess for gestational diabetes, increased amniotic fluid volume (polyhydramnios), and fetal position.[6]
- Documentation of fetal cardiac activity
- Assessment of the patient's perception of fetal activity (in the second and third trimesters)
- Assessment of fetal presentation (in the third trimester)
- Assessment of significant events since the prior visit, such as recent travel, illness, stressors, or exposure to infection
- See Table 7.1 for a list of laboratory tests, diagnostic tests, and immunizations required in pregnant patients and the trimester in which they should occur.

TABLE 7.1 Laboratory Tests, Diagnostic Tests, and Immunizations Required During Pregnancy

First Trimester	Second Trimester	Third Trimester
Blood type and antibody screen	Maternal serum alpha fetoprotein *(16–22 weeks)*	HIV
Hepatitis B antigen	Anatomy ultrasound examination *(18–22 weeks)*	RPR
Hepatitis C Antigen	1-hour glucose tolerance test *(24–28 weeks)*	Group B streptococcus *(35–37 weeks)*
Rubella immunity	Complete blood count with platelets *(24–28 weeks)*	Gonorrhea and chlamydia
Human immunodeficiency virus (HIV)	Rhogam if Rh negative *(28 weeks)*	Tdap vaccination
Rapid plasma reagin (RPR)		
Pap smear		
Gonorrhea and chlamydia		
Complete blood count with platelets		
Hemoglobin electrophoresis		
Cystic fibrosis		
Sequential screening (trisomies 13, 18, and 21)		
Thyroid-stimulating hormone and free T4 (if applicable)		
Urine culture with sensitivities		
Cell-free DNA *(starting at 10 weeks)*		
Hemoglobin A_{1c}		
Early 1-hour glucose screening (if BMI >30, history of gestational diabetes mellitus or large-for-gestational-age fetus, or other risk factors)		

> **⚠ SAFETY ALERT**
>
> All pregnant patients should be taught about warning signs in pregnancy and encouraged to inform their health care provider if they experience vaginal bleeding, leakage of fluid from the vagina, or DFM.

COMMON LABORATORY TESTS

If pregnancy is suspected, serum hCG levels should be obtained. Additionally, the pregnancy should be confirmed by ultrasound examination to identify intrauterine placement and fetal cardiac activity. A standard obstetrical panel of laboratory tests should be obtained at the first prenatal visit. The tests included in this panel are outlined in the following sections.

Rhesus Type and Antibody Screen

This test will detect antibodies potentially causing hemolytic disease of the newborn. Rh(D)-negative patients without alloantibodies should receive anti-D immunoglobulin if bleeding or trauma occurs at any time during the pregnancy, routinely at 28 weeks and within 72 hours of delivery.[6]

Complete Blood Count Including Platelets

This test detects anemia and provides screening for thalassemia. An MCV less than 80 femtoliters (fL) in the absence of iron deficiency suggests thalassemia; further testing with hemoglobin electrophoresis is indicated.[6]

Cervical Cytology Cancer Screening (Pap Smear Screening)

This test is performed for patients 21 years of age and older who are due for screening based on standard guidelines. For patients 21 to 29 years of age with normal history, cytology alone is recommended every 3 years. For patients 30 years of age and older with normal history, cytology and human papilloma virus (HPV) screening are recommended every 5 years.[7]

Rubella Immunity

Every childbearing patient should have serologic screening for rubella immunity at the first prenatal visit unless they are known to be immune by previous serologic testing. If nonimmune, the patient is advised to avoid exposure to patients with rubella and to receive postpartum

vaccination. MMR vaccinations are live virus vaccines and are contraindicated in pregnancy (see the "Vaccinations in Pregnancy" section later in this chapter.)[6]

> **⚠ SAFETY ALERT**
>
> MMR vaccinations are live virus vaccines and are contraindicated in pregnancy.

Urine Protein

Urine screening for proteinuria, such as with a dipstick, is useful as a baseline for comparison if assessment of renal function is performed later in pregnancy.[6]

Urine Culture

Routine urine culture is recommended because pregnant patients with untreated asymptomatic bacteriuria are at high risk of developing pyelonephritis. Additionally, patients with sickle cell disease or trait and hemoglobin C trait should have a urine culture every trimester because of the risk of bacteriuria.[6]

Gonorrhea and Chlamydia

Vaginal or urine cultures for gonorrhea and chlamydia should be sent at the first prenatal visit for all prenatal patients and again in the third trimester for patients at high risk for infection. The U.S. Centers for Disease Control and Prevention (CDC) recommends screening all pregnant patients 25 years of age and older who are at increased risk for infection (e.g., patients with a new sex partner, more than one sex partner, a sex partner with concurrent partners, or a sex partner who has a sexually transmitted infection). Positive test results should be treated. Patients with a positive test should undergo a test-of-cure 3 to 4 weeks after treatment and be retested 3 to 4 months later.[8]

Human Immunodeficiency Virus

The American College of Obstetricians and Gynecologists (ACOG)[9] supports universal human immunodeficiency virus (HIV) testing of pregnant patients early in each pregnancy using an "opt-out" approach.

Syphilis testing

Serological testing for syphilis is performed at the first visit and again in the second or third trimester, usually with the 28-week laboratory tests.[6]

Hepatitis B Antigen Testing

Hepatitis B antigen screening is recommended to prevent perinatal transmission in all pregnant patients, including those who have been previously vaccinated.[6]

Thyroid Function

Screening for thyroid-stimulating hormone (TSH) and free T4 should be completed in patients with a personal or family history of thyroid disorder or those with symptoms of thyroid disease. Neurological development may be adversely affected in infants born to mothers with hypothyroidism, while maternal hyperthyroidism can lead to fetal and maternal complications.[6]

Type 2 diabetes

For patients who are at increased risk of diabetes, a diagnosis of overt diabetes can be made at the initial prenatal visit if results are as follows:
- Fasting plasma glucose ≥126 mg/dL or
- A_{1c} ≥6.5% using a standardized assay, or
- Random plasma glucose ≥200 mg/dL that is subsequently confirmed by elevated fasting plasma glucose or A_{1c}.

Hepatitis C Antibodies

Pregnant patients who are at high risk for hepatitis C infection should be screened for hepatitis C antibodies.[6]

Toxoplasmosis

The two most common means of acquisition of toxoplasmosis are via environmental exposure (contaminated cat litter boxes or soil) and ingestion of undercooked meat from infected animals. Routine serological screening for toxoplasmosis is not advised in the United States because of its low prevalence and unavailability of standardized assays.[6]

Bacterial Vaginosis

Screening for bacterial vaginosis is not recommended as a routine component of prenatal care.[6]

Trichomonas Vaginalis

Screening for *Trichomonas* is not recommended as a routine component of prenatal care for HIV-negative patients; however, patients with HIV infection should be screened for *Trichomonas* at the first prenatal visit. Symptomatic patients should be evaluated and treated.[6]

Herpes Simplex Virus

Routine screening for herpes simplex virus (HSV) infection in asymptomatic patients is generally not recommended. Patients with a history of HSV 2 should be treated during an outbreak in pregnancy and routinely start suppression with valacyclovir or acyclovir at 36 weeks until delivery.[10,6]

Cytomegalovirus

Routine serological screening for cytomegalovirus (CMV) in asymptomatic patients is not recommended. Testing pregnant patients for CMV is indicated as part of the diagnostic evaluation of mononucleosis-like illnesses, when a fetal anomaly suggestive of congenital CMV infection is detected on prenatal ultrasound examination, or if the patient requests the test.[6]

Zika Virus

In areas with no mosquito-borne Zika virus transmission, health care providers should ask pregnant patients about possible exposure (residence in or travel to an area where mosquito-borne transmission of Zika virus infection has been reported, or unprotected sexual contact with a person who meets these criteria). Testing of pregnant patients who have possible exposure to Zika virus depends on both symptomatology and facts surrounding the possible exposure. Sexual partners of pregnant patients who reside in or are returning from areas endemic for Zika virus are advised to use condoms or abstain from sex throughout pregnancy.[11]

Cystic Fibrosis

Information about cystic fibrosis screening should be available to all couples. Cystic fibrosis carrier screening should be offered, especially to couples who are at increased risk because of Caucasian, European, or Ashkenazi Jewish ancestry.

Fragile X Syndrome

The population at risk includes but is not limited to individuals of either sex with an intellectual disability, developmental delay, or autism.

Hemoglobinopathies

A comprehensive personal and family medical history with emphasis on history of anemia and other hematological disorders should be completed for every patient. Baseline screening includes a complete blood count. An

MCV less than 80 fL in the absence of iron deficiency denotes patients at risk for alpha or beta thalassemia. If a pregnant patient screens positive for a hemoglobinopathy, the patient's partner should be screened as well to determine the risk to the fetus.

- *Beta-thalassemia* occurs with higher frequency in subcontinental ethnic groups, except for Northern Europeans.
- *Alpha-thalassemia* occurs with higher frequency in Chinese, Taiwanese, and Southeast Asian (Thai, Laotian, Cambodian, Vietnamese, Burmese, Malaysian, Singaporean, Indonesian, Filipino) ethnic groups.
- The structural *hemoglobin variants S and C (sickle cell disease)* are most common in African ethnic groups (North Africans, African Caribbeans, African Americans, Black British, and other African ethnicity such as Central and South Americans of partly African ethnicity) and in Greeks, Southern Italians (including Sicilians), Turks, Arabs, and Indians.[6]

> **! SAFETY ALERT**
>
> Ask patients if they own or live with cats. Pregnant patients should not clean or empty litter boxes, as this increases their risk of toxoplasmosis exposure.

GENETIC SCREENING

Ideally, counseling patients of reproductive age about genetic screening should be provided before pregnancy. However, if a patient comes into the office and has not received this type of counseling, a discussion of the risks and benefits of genetic screening and diagnostic testing should be provided. Clinicians should consider referring their obstetrical patients to a genetic counselor to obtain a detailed family history, assess risks for inherited medical conditions, and provide comprehensive counseling.

At the initial prenatal visit, the clinician should discuss the difference between screening and diagnostic testing, the timing, the advantages and disadvantages, and the risk and benefits of each procedure.

During the first trimester (up to 13 weeks and 6 days' gestation), integrated or sequential screening may be offered. A pregnant patient presenting during the second trimester may be offered quadruple screening, cell-free DNA (cfDNA), and an ultrasound examination.

Genetic counseling and diagnostic testing should be offered to patients with increased risk of aneuploidy with their first-trimester screening. Prenatal patients found to have abnormal first-trimester screening results may also have an increased risk for fetal loss before 24 weeks' gestation, fetal demise, preterm birth, or low birth weight.

DIAGNOSTIC TESTING

Pregnant patients may choose to have diagnostic testing for aneuploidy as the next step after receiving abnormal genetic screening results or in place of screening tests. Two options are available for diagnostic testing:

- Chorionic villus sampling (CVS): Performed between 10 and 13 weeks' gestation, and under ultrasound guidance, a small sample of placental tissue is removed either transabdominally or transcervically.[12] Patients must be comprehensively counseled on the risks and benefits of this testing before the procedure. Risk includes a pregnancy loss rate of 1 in 455.
- Amniocentesis: Performed between 15 and 20 weeks' gestation, a sample of amniotic fluid is removed with ultrasound guidance. Risks associated with this procedure include a pregnancy loss rate of 0.1% to 0.3%, vaginal spotting, and amniotic fluid leakage.[12]

GESTATIONAL DIABETES MELLITUS

Gestational diabetes mellitus (GDM) is found in 86% of all diabetes cases in pregnancy. Diet-controlled GDM is considered class A1.[13,14] GDM class A2 is the category used when medication is needed for glycemic control.[13] GDM is prevalent among African American, Native American, Pacific Islander, and Hispanic patients.[13] The risk for GDM is increased in patients who are older and obese. Having GDM places the pregnant patient at an increased risk for comorbidities such as preeclampsia. Additionally, the risk for cesarean delivery is higher for patients with GDM. Infants born to mothers with GDM have heightened risks for hypoglycemia, increased bilirubin, macrosomia, shoulder dystocia, and trauma at birth.[13] It would be prudent for the clinician to discuss with their patients diagnosed with GDM that they are at an increased risk for developing type 2 diabetes later in life and take the opportunity to discuss nutrition and exercise.[13]

TABLE 7.2 Diagnostic Criteria for Gestational Diabetes Mellitus		
Timing	Carpenter and Coustan Conversion of Plasma or Serum Glucose Level in mg/dL	National Diabetes Data Group Conversion of Plasma Level in mg/dL
Fasting	95	105
1 hour	180	190
2 hours	155	165
3 hours	140	145

American Diabetes Association. Classification and Diagnosis of Diabetes. *Diabetes Care 2017*; 40 (Suppl. 1):511–524.

The U.S. Preventive Services Task Force (USPSTF) recommends screening all pregnant patients for GDM. Typically, screening is performed between 24 and 28 weeks' gestation.[13,15] Patients who are at high risk for type 2 diabetes are those who are overweight or obese and have additional risk factors such as a diagnosis of GDM with a previous pregnancy. These patients should be offered early screening for GDM for the current pregnancy at the first prenatal visit. The screening widely used in the United States consists of two steps. The first step is the administration of a 50-g oral glucose solution and testing of glucose levels after 1 hour. If the results of this initial step are above the normal range for the laboratory, the patient then proceeds to the second step, which includes administration of a 100-g oral glucose solution.[13] This second step requires four venous samplings of glucose levels: fasting before administration of glucose solution, and then at 1 hour, 2 hours, and 3 hours after ingestion of the glucose solution. If results for this second step shows two or more abnormal values, a diagnosis of GDM can be made.[13,15] Table 7.2 demonstrates the diagnostic criteria for GDM. At this point in the patient's care, the clinician may choose to refer the patient to a diabetologist who specialize in caring for pregnant patients diagnosed with diabetes.

HYPERTENSION IN PREGNANCY

There are four major hypertensive disorders that occur in pregnant patients:

- **Preeclampsia-eclampsia:** Preeclampsia is the syndrome of new onset of hypertension and proteinuria or new onset of hypertension and end-organ dysfunction with or without proteinuria, most often after 20 weeks' gestation in a previously normotensive patient. Eclampsia is diagnosed when seizures have occurred.[16]
- **Chronic (preexisting) hypertension:** Chronic (preexisting) hypertension is diagnosed when systolic pressure ≥140 mm Hg and/or diastolic pressure ≥90 mm Hg before pregnancy and is present before the 20th week of pregnancy *or* persists longer than 12 weeks postpartum.[11]
- **Chronic hypertension with superimposed preeclampsia:** Chronic hypertension with superimposed preeclampsia is diagnosed when a patient with chronic hypertension develops worsening hypertension with new-onset proteinuria or other features of preeclampsia (including elevated liver enzymes, low platelet count, right upper quadrant pain, and headache).[11]
- **Gestational hypertension:** Gestational hypertension is diagnosed when elevated BP (taken on two occasions, at least 4 hours apart) is first detected after 20 weeks' gestation in the absence of proteinuria or other diagnostic features of preeclampsia.[16]

The decision to treat hypertension during pregnancy should consider the risks and benefits for both the patient and fetus. Hypertension can be categorized as follows:

- Severe hypertension: systolic BP ≥160 mm Hg and/or diastolic BP ≥110 mm Hg
- Moderate hypertension: systolic 150 to 159 mm Hg, diastolic 100 to 109 mm Hg
- Mild hypertension: systolic 140 to 150 mm Hg, diastolic 90 to 100 mm Hg

Poorly controlled blood pressures have been associated with intrauterine growth restriction, preterm delivery, stillbirth, and maternal risks including placental abruption, stroke, superimposed preeclampsia, pulmonary edema, and cesarean delivery.[11]

All antihypertensive drugs cross the placenta. Severe hypertension is usually always managed with medication to prevent maternal stroke. Mild and moderate hypertension may be managed with medications if the patient becomes symptomatic. Many drugs are used to treat this condition both in the oral and or parenteral form. Commonly used medications include methyldopa, labetalol, nifedipine, and hydralazine. ACE inhibitors, angiotensin II receptor blockers (ARBs), direct renin inhibitors, mineralocorticoid receptor antagonists, spironolactone, and nitroprusside should be avoided. The indications for initiating antihypertensive drugs in patients with mild to moderate hypertension in pregnancy without evidence of target organ damage who have not previously been treated or who have discontinued therapy are not clear. Neither the patient nor the fetus appears to be at risk from mildly elevated BP during pregnancy (systolic <150 mm Hg, diastolic <100 mm Hg). It is not clear whether patients with moderately elevated BP levels (systolic 150 to 160 mm Hg or diastolic 100 to 109 mm Hg) have similar benign outcomes. Patients with chronic hypertension who are normotensive or mildly hypertensive on medication may continue their therapy or have their antihypertensive agents tapered and/or stopped during pregnancy, with close monitoring of the maternal BP response.

Laboratory evaluation of pregnant patients with preexisting hypertension or development of preeclampsia includes baseline urinalysis, creatinine, 24-hour urine protein, liver function studies (AST, ALT, LDH), and uric acid to assess for kidney function. An electrocardiogram should be obtained for patients with a history of chronic hypertension. Patients with a history of preeclampsia in a previous pregnancy are encouraged to start low-dose aspirin therapy daily before 16 weeks' gestation.[11] Antepartum evaluation is directed toward early diagnosis of preeclampsia and measures to decrease the risk of intrauterine growth restriction. During prenatal visits, patients should routinely have their BP checked, urinalysis or dipstick testing for proteinuria, fundal height measurements, and ultrasound examinations with Doppler studies to measure placental blood flow. When there is a high concern for intrauterine growth restriction or uteroplacental vasculopathy, nonstress tests or biophysical profiles may be recommended in the third trimester. To date, there have been no studies supporting the ideal timing of delivery for patients with chronic hypertension. The ACOG suggests the following approach for patients with chronic hypertension: 38 to 39 6/7 weeks' gestation for patients not requiring medication, 37 to 39 6/7 weeks for patients with hypertension controlled with medication, and 36 to 37 6/7 weeks for patients with severe hypertension that is difficult to control. For patients with superimposed preeclampsia or other pregnancy complications, the timing of delivery should be decided on a case-by-case basis based on the type and severity of these complications.

NOT TO BE MISSED

Laboratory evaluation of pregnant patients with preexisting hypertension or development of preeclampsia includes baseline urinalysis, creatinine, 24-hour urine protein, liver function studies (AST, ALT, LDH), and uric acid to assess for kidney function.

EVALUATION OF FETAL WELL-BEING

Fetal Movement Counts

Fetal movement can begin as early as 7 weeks' gestation but is often not felt by the nulliparous patients until 16 to 22 weeks and as early as 13 weeks in parous patients.[6] The first signs of movement are usually described by patients as "flutters." Until the patient can feel movement, pregnancy can be a time of concern for fetal well-being and provoke anxiety. Forty percent of pregnant patients report DFM at some point in their pregnancy. Maternal perception of fetal movement is reassuring for pregnant patients, while DFM is a common reason for concern. Fetal movement counting (FMC), also commonly referred to as *fetal kick counting* (FKC), is a form of fetal surveillance that can provide early detection of a compromised fetus. DFM requires prompt evaluation and management. Fetal movement increases throughout the day, with peak activity usually late at night. Because of this phenomenon, patients should be discouraged from counting while they are busy and active during the day and instead monitor during the evenings, after a meal, or while resting in bed. The frequency of fetal movement in a normal pregnancy is probably constant throughout the third trimester; however, the quality of perceived movements changes. Early recognition of DFM provides opportunities for identifying fetuses that may be compromised and could benefit from an intervention such as delivery to prevent fetal injury or death.

FKC is a way to quantify the assessment of fetal activity. The minimum number of maternally perceived fetal movements consistent with fetal well-being is termed the *alarm limit*. Various methods for defining an alarm limit have been proposed. The following are four examples of thresholds for reassurance of fetal well-being:[6]

- Perception of least 10 fetal movements over up to 2 hours when the patient is at rest and focused on counting (Cardiff *count to 10* method)
- Perception of at least 10 fetal movements during 12 hours of normal maternal activity
- Perception of at least 4 fetal movements in 1 hour when the patient is at rest and focused on counting
- Perception of at least 10 fetal movements within 25 minutes in pregnancies 22 to 36 weeks' gestation and 35 minutes in pregnancies 37 or more weeks' gestation

Although the Cardiff count-to-10 method is the most widely used method in practice, the practice has also faced scrutiny from clinicians because further studies have shown that the amount of time to obtain 10 movements varied greatly among pregnant patients. A decrease in fetal movement may be caused by fetal sleep cycles, maternal use of sedatives, and maternal smoking. Poor maternal perception of fetal activity is another reason for maternal report of DFM. Anterior placentas can also diminish the quality of fetal movement felt by the patient. Maternal assessment of fetal activity is a beneficial screening tool for fetal status; therefore further evaluation is necessary in patients reporting DFM. Patients who report a perceived decrease in fetal activity should be advised to come to the office or triage unit for a non-stress test (NST).[17]

> **CLINICAL SURVIVAL TIP:** Maternal assessment of fetal movement is a valuable and beneficial tool for fetal status. The patient's perception of a decrease in fetal activity warrants further evaluation.

WEIGHT GAIN IN PREGNANCY

Gaining the appropriate amount of weight in pregnancy is important for healthy outcomes for both the pregnant patient and the infant (Fig. 7.1). Too little weight gain has been linked to premature labor and delivery and intrauterine growth restriction. Excessive weight gain can be linked to maternal diabetes, preeclampsia, fetal macrosomia, increased risk for cesarean delivery, and delayed maternal weight loss after delivery. Weight gain in pregnancy is dependent on the patient's pre-pregnancy weight and current body mass index (BMI). Tables 7.3 and 7.4 show the recommended weight gain in pregnancy for both singleton and twin pregnancies. These recommendations are based on the patients' pre-pregnancy BMI (Box 7.3).

Maternal weight gain during pregnancy can be attributed primarily to increases in maternal body water and fat. On average, weight gain at term is distributed as follows:[18]

- Fetus: 7 to 8 lb (3.2 to 3.6 kg)
- Fat stores: 6 to 8 lb (2.7 to 3.6 kg)

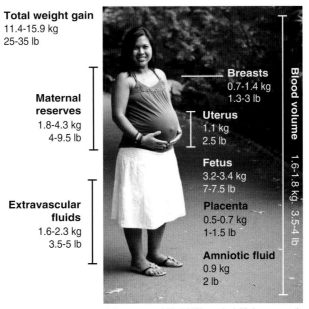

Total weight gain
11.4-15.9 kg
25-35 lb

Maternal reserves
1.8-4.3 kg
4-9.5 lb

Extravascular fluids
1.6-2.3 kg
3.5-5 lb

Breasts
0.7-1.4 kg
1.3-3 lb

Uterus
1.1 kg
2.5 lb

Fetus
3.2-3.4 kg
7-7.5 lb

Placenta
0.5-0.7 kg
1-1.5 lb

Amniotic fluid
0.9 kg
2 lb

Blood volume 1.6-1.8 kg 3.5-4 lb

Figure 7.1 Total weight gain. (Courtesy of Todd Westphal / Ishootamerica.com.)

TABLE 7.3   **Institute of Medicine Recommendations for Weight Gain for a Single-Gestation Pregnancy Based on Pre-Pregnancy Body Mass Index (2009)**

Pre-Pregnancy Weight/BMI	Recommended Total Weight Range
Underweight (BMI less than or equal to 18.5)	28–40 lb
Normal weight (BMI 18.5–24.9)	25–35 lb
Overweight (BMI 25–29.9)	15–25 lb
Obese (BMI greater than 30)	11–20 lb

BMI, Body mass index.
Institute of Medicine and National Research Council. 2009. *Weight Gain During Pregnancy: Reexamining the Guidelines.* https://doi.org/10.17226/12584. Adapted and reproduced with permission from the National Academy of Sciences, Courtesy of the National Academies Press, Washington, D.C.

TABLE 7.4   **Institute of Medicine Recommendations for Weight Gain for a Twin Pregnancy Based on Pre-Pregnancy Body Mass Index (2009)**

Pre-Pregnancy Weight/BMI	Recommended Total Weight Range
Normal weight (BMI 18.5–24.9)	37–54 lb
Overweight (BMI 25–29.9)	31–50 lb
Obese (BMI greater than 30)	25–42 lb

BMI, Body mass index.
Institute of Medicine and National Research Council. 2009. *Weight Gain During Pregnancy: Reexamining the Guidelines.* https://doi.org/10.17226/12584. Adapted and reproduced with permission from the National Academy of Sciences, Courtesy of the National Academies Press, Washington, D.C.

BOX 7.3   **Body Mass Index Classification**

Body mass index (BMI) is a measure of body fat based on height and weight. BMI classification is as follows:
- Underweight = BMI less than 18.5
- Healthy weight = BMI 18.5–24.9
- Overweight = BMI 25–29.9
- Obese = BMI greater than 30
- Morbidly obese = BMI greater than 40

- Increased blood volume: 3 to 4 lb (1.4 to 1.8 kg)
- Increased fluid volume: 2 to 3 lb (0.9 to 1.4 kg)
- Amniotic fluid: 2 lb (0.9 kg)
- Breast enlargement: 1 to 3 lb (0.45 to 1.4 kg)
- Uterine hypertrophy: 2 lb (0.9 kg)
- Placenta: 1.5 lb (0.7 kg)

Regardless of BMI, dieting and intentional weight loss in pregnancy are not recommended. Unintentional weight loss in pregnancy is not uncommon as long as the fetus is growing well; however, weight monitoring is advisable. Gaining weight slowly and steadily is best. It is not uncommon to lose weight, especially in the first trimester.

NUTRITION IN PREGNANCY

During pregnancy, there is rapid fetal growth and development and maternal physiological change. Adequate intake of macronutrients and micronutrients during pregnancy promotes these processes, while malnutrition can be associated with adverse pregnancy outcomes. Therefore it is important to evaluate, monitor, and, when appropriate, make changes to improve maternal nutrition both before and during pregnancy. Caloric intake is a key nutritional factor in determining birth weight. Patients of normal weight with a singleton pregnancy must increase their daily caloric intake by 340 and 452 additional kcal/day in the second and third trimesters, respectively, for appropriate weight gain, but do not need to increase energy intake in the first trimester.[19] Recommendations should be individualized based on physical activity, age, weight, and height. The key components of healthy eating during pregnancy include appropriate fetal and maternal weight gain; appropriate vitamin and mineral supplementation; avoidance of alcohol, tobacco, and other illicit substances; and safe food handling and preparation. Most pregnant patients in the latter two trimesters will require between 2200 and 2900 kcal/day, although calorie needs can vary widely, and this should be assessed individually.[20] An easy way to demonstrate to patients how to distribute these caloric needs throughout the day are through food group serving sizes (Box 7.4).

Protein is essential for healthy fetal growth. The Institute of Medicine recommends 1.1g/kg/day of protein. Foods rich in protein include low-fat and lean meats, beans, legumes, nuts, and eggs. Protein-rich dietary supplements should be discouraged as meal replacements.

> ### BOX 7.4 Food Group Serving Ranges Required to Meet Caloric Requirements in Pregnancy (2200 to 2900 kcal/day)
>
> Fruits: 2 to 2.5 cups
> Vegetables: 3 to 3.5 cups
> Grains: 6 to 10 oz
> Protein: 6 to 7 oz
> Dairy: 3 cups

Daily recommended carbohydrate requirements increase to 175 g/day in pregnancy.[21] The focus should be on consuming several servings of whole foods (fruits, vegetables, and whole grains); highly processed carbohydrates should be minimized to help manage weight gain. Pregnant patients should be counseled to ingest whole grain bread and pastas. Sugary beverages like soda and juices should be minimized. Fiber intake of 28 g/day is recommended for pregnant patients, which, along with adequate fluid intake, may help prevent or reduce constipation. At least 64 fluid ounces of water is recommended daily. Caffeine is safe in small amounts. Consuming fewer than 200 mg of caffeine daily is recommended in pregnancy.[22]

Careful evaluation of diet should be completed to ensure adequate dietary sources of micronutrients such as iron, calcium, vitamin D, folate, and iodine. At a minimum, the daily supplement should contain key vitamins/minerals that are often not met by diet alone, such as pregnancy:[21]

- Iron: 27 mg daily
- Calcium: 1000 mg daily for pregnant and breastfeeding patients older than 18 years of age and 1300 mg daily for teenage girls up to 18 years of age
- Folate: At least 0.4 mg daily (0.6 mg daily in the second and third trimester)
- Iodine: 150 mcg daily
- Vitamin D: 200 to 600 international units daily

In addition to these key ingredients, pregnant patients must get adequate amounts of vitamins A, E, C, and B as well as zinc.

Folic acid, also known as *folate,* is a B vitamin that is important for pregnant patients. Before pregnancy and during pregnancy, patients need 400 mcg of folic acid daily to help prevent major birth defects of brain and spine called *neural tube defects.*[23] Current dietary guidelines recommend that pregnant patients get at least 600 mcg of folic acid daily from all sources. It may be difficult to get the recommended amount of folic acid from food alone. For this reason, all pregnant patients and all patients who may become pregnant should take a daily vitamin supplement that contains folic acid. Patients with a personal or family history of spina bifida are encouraged to take 4 mg of folic acid daily.[23] Dietary sources of folic acid include fortified foods, citrus fruits, green leafy vegetables, nuts, and liver.

NOT TO BE MISSED

Before and during pregnancy, patients need 400 mcg of folic acid daily to help prevent major birth defects of the brain and spine called *neural tube defects.*

Iron is used to make a substance in red blood cells that carries oxygen to the maternal organs and tissues. During pregnancy, patients need about double the amount of iron as nonpregnant patients. This extra iron helps provide more blood to supply oxygen to the fetus. The daily recommended dose of iron during pregnancy is 27 mg, which is found in most prenatal vitamin supplements.[21] Iron-rich foods include lean red meats, poultry, fish, dried beans and peas, iron-fortified cereals, and prune juice. Iron also can be absorbed more easily if iron-rich foods are eaten with vitamin C–rich foods, such as citrus fruits and tomatoes.[21]

Fetal skeletal development requires about 30 g of calcium during pregnancy, primarily in the last trimester. The Recommended Dietary Allowance (RDA) for elemental calcium is 1000 mg per day in pregnant and lactating patients 19 to 50 years of age (1300 mg for girls 14 to 18 years of age).[6] The dietary recommendation for calcium is the same for nonpregnant patients of the same age. Calcium-rich foods include green leafy vegetables such as spinach and kale, broccoli, sardines, milk, cheese, and yogurt. Vitamin D works with calcium to help fetal skeletal development. Vitamin D also is essential for healthy skin and eyesight. All patients, including those who are pregnant, need 200 to 600 international units of vitamin D per day. Good sources are milk fortified with vitamin D and fatty fish such as salmon. Exposure to sunlight also converts a chemical in the skin to vitamin D.

Omega-3 fatty acids are a type of fat found naturally in many kinds of fish and have been found to aid in brain development. It is recommended that patients eat at least two servings (about 8 to 12 ounces per serving)

BOX 7.5   Listeriosis

Listeriosis is a type of food-borne illness caused by bacteria. Listeriosis can cause mild, flulike symptoms such as fever, muscle aches, and diarrhea, but it also may not cause any symptoms. Listeriosis can lead to miscarriage, stillbirth, and premature delivery. To help prevent listeriosis, avoid eating the following foods during pregnancy:

- Unpasteurized milk and foods made with unpasteurized milk
- Refrigerated pâté and meat spreads
- Refrigerated smoked seafood
- Raw and undercooked seafood, eggs, and meat

---

of fish per week.[24] While pregnant or breastfeeding, patients should limit servings of certain types of fish (such as albacore [white] tuna) that may contain concerning amounts of mercury. Some types of fish have higher levels of mercury than others. Mercury has been linked to birth defects. Fish and shellfish such as shrimp, salmon, catfish, and pollock should be chosen over shark, swordfish, king mackerel, or tilefish, which have the highest level of mercury concentrations.

Although common, the use of herbal preparations in pregnancy should be discouraged. Most of these supplements are not regulated by the U.S. Food and Drug Administration (FDA), and their effects have not been thoroughly studied in pregnant subjects. Herbal preparations can interact with commonly prescribed medications and lead to dangerous side effects.

Foodborne illnesses can cause maternal disease as well as congenital disease, miscarriage, premature labor, and fetal death. According to the CDC,[25] listeriosis is a rare foodborne illness that affects pregnant patients at 10 times the rate of others (Box 7.5). To reduce this risk, pregnant patients are advised to take the following precautions:

- Wash food thoroughly before eating, cutting, or cooking.
- Consume only meat, fish, and poultry that are fully cooked. Do not eat sushi made with raw fish (cooked sushi is safe). Food such as beef, pork, or poultry should be cooked to a safe internal temperature.
- Avoid unpasteurized dairy products and fruit/vegetable juices.
- Wash hands, food preparation surfaces, cutting boards, dishes, and utensils that come in contact

with raw meat, poultry, or fish with hot, soapy water. Countertops can be sanitized by wiping with a solution of 1 teaspoon liquid chlorine bleach per quart of water and leaving it to dry for 10 minutes.

EXERCISE IN PREGNANCY

In a healthy normal pregnancy, exercise does not increase the risk of complications. In fact, at least 30 to 60 minutes of moderate aerobic activity at least 3 to 4 days of the week is recommended in pregnancy.[6] Exercise in pregnancy is not recommended for childbearing/pregnant patients with the following conditions:

- Certain types of heart and lung diseases
- Cervical insufficiency or cerclage
- Pregnancy with twins, triplets, or multiples with risk factors for preterm labor
- Placenta previa after 26 weeks' gestation
- Preterm labor or ruptured membranes (water has broken) during this pregnancy
- Preeclampsia or pregnancy-induced high BP
- Severe anemia

Patients should be advised to discontinue exercise if any of the following symptoms occur, which could be an indication of a potential problem: vaginal bleeding, painful contractions, leakage of amniotic fluid, dyspnea, dizziness, headache, chest pain, muscle weakness, or calf pain. Dehydration is a risk associated with prolonged or intense exercise. Patients should be advised to hydrate before, during, and after periods of exercise. Yoga is a form of exercise that is often recommended for pregnant patients and relieves common pregnancy discomforts such as round ligament pain. Additionally, practicing yoga or other meditation-based routines helps encourage the practice of mindfulness, which promotes relaxation, especially during the phases of labor.

ANTENATAL DEPRESSION

Antenatal depression is associated with poor outcomes for both the mother and infant. It has been associated with spontaneous abortion, bleeding, operative deliveries, preterm birth, and abnormal infant and child development.[26] Pregnant patients should be assessed at least once during pregnancy and again in the postpartum period for depression and anxiety symptoms using a validated screening tool. Depression screening usually is initiated at the first prenatal visit. Multiple screening tools exist, but the Edinburgh Postnatal Depression Scale is the most commonly used assessment. This questionnaire takes less than 5 minutes to administer and is very easily scored. Antenatal depression is one of the greatest factors for developing postpartum depression. Patients with a history of depression before and during pregnancy should be monitored closely during the postpartum period. Pregnant patients with depressive symptoms may be safely treated with pharmacotherapy. The most commonly prescribed antidepressants in pregnancy are selective serotonin reuptake inhibitors (SSRIs). Drugs in this category include citalopram, escitalopram, fluoxetine, fluvoxamine, paroxetine, and sertraline. Despite antidepressants crossing the placenta and the fetal blood-brain barrier, many studies have reaffirmed the general safety of SSRIs and that antidepressants pose little teratogenic risk.[27]

Untreated depression during pregnancy has adverse fetal outcomes such as risk for prematurity, low birth weight, and intrauterine growth restriction.[28,29] Moreover, untreated depression puts the mother in a higher risk of maternal morbidity, including suicide ideation and attempts as well as postpartum depression.[30] Nurse practitioners providing obstetrical care should discuss the risks and benefits of treating depression with their pregnant patients. Collaboration with more experienced nurse practitioner and medical colleagues and/or referral of the patient to mental health services in the community can be considered if needed.

NOT TO BE MISSED

Pregnant patients should be assessed for depression and anxiety symptoms using a validated screening tool at least once during pregnancy and again in the postpartum period.

INTIMATE PARTNER VIOLENCE IN PREGNANCY

Intimate partner violence (IPV) is the term used to describe actual or perceived risks of physical, psychological, or sexual harm by a past or current partner. Examples of this type of violence include physical force or threats used to cause persuasion or coercion with the intent to harm, injure, or cause death. Sexual violence includes the use of force to compel a sexual act, a sexual act with a person who is unable to consent, or abusive sexual contact. IPV, especially sexual and physical assaults, are often underreported. A U.S. survey found that 24% of women and 12% of men acknowledged a lifetime threatened or completed physical or sexual IPV. Worldwide, the lifetime prevalence of physical or sexual IPV in women ranges from 6% to 62%. IPV was a factor in approximately 20% of U.S. homicides, with greater than one-half of the female victims of all homicides killed by an intimate partner.[31]

IPV often begins or escalates during pregnancy and pregnancy can result from reproductive coercion when IPV is already occurring. Risk factors for IPV include being a young female, alcohol or drug use, being less educated, and family history or prior exposure to violence. In pregnancy, IPV often leads to perceived or actual medical problems and pregnancy complications including hypertension; vaginal bleeding; severe nausea, vomiting, or dehydration; kidney infection or urinary tract infection; preterm delivery; low-birth-weight infant; and an infant requiring care in the intensive care unit.[32] Additionally, abruption, fetal fractures, premature labor, and perinatal death have also been associated with IPV.[32] The risk for postpartum depression is twofold to threefold in females who have experienced psychological or physical abuse during pregnancy.[32] All pregnant patients should be screened at the initial prenatal visit, during each trimester, and in the postpartum period.

CLINICAL SURVIVAL TIP: IPV often begins or escalates during pregnancy. All pregnant patients should be screened at the initial prenatal visit, during each trimester, and in the postpartum period.

VACCINATIONS IN PREGNANCY

The risks for vaccinating pregnant patients are mainly theoretical. There is no current evidence that vaccinating patients with inactivated virus or bacterial vaccines or toxoids have lead to harm to the fetus. Because there may be a theoretical risk to the fetus from the administration of live vaccines, the CDC recommends the avoidance of live, attenuated virus, and live bacteria vaccines during pregnancy.[33]

- **COVID-19:** Although safety data on the COVID-19 vaccine in pregnancy is limited, pregnant patients are at an increased risk for serious illness from COVID-19. The risks of exposure to the COVID-19 virus must be weighed against the benefits and risks of the vaccine.[34]

- **Hepatitis A:** Although the safety of hepatitis A vaccine has not been established, the theoretical risk to the developing fetus is deemed to be low; therefore, providers should weigh the risks of the vaccination against the mother's risk of Hepatitis A exposure.

- **Hepatitis B:** Pregnant patients who have had more than one sex partner during the previous 6 months, recent or current illicit injection drug use, or has a partner who has tested for Hepatitis BsAg are at an increased risk for Hepatitis B infection should be offered vaccination. Hepatitis B vaccination does not pose a risk to the developing fetus.

- **HPV:** The HPV vaccine is contraindicated for pregnant patients. If the three-dose series has begun, the remaining vaccinations should be delayed until the postpartum period.

- **Inactivated influenza:** Because of the increased risk for severe and complicated influenza for pregnant patients, the CDC recommends that all patients who are pregnant or planning to become pregnant during the influenza season should be vaccinated.

- **Live, attenuated influenza vaccine (LAIV):** This type of influenza vaccine should be avoided in pregnancy.

- **Measles, mumps, rubella (MMR):** The MMR is a type of vaccine that contains a live virus. Administration of the MMR vaccine should be avoided in pregnancy and offered in the postpartum period. Because of the theoretical risk to the fetus associated with a live vaccine, patients should be counseled to avoid pregnancy for 28 days after vaccination.

- **Meningococcal (MenACWY or MPSV4):** The CDC states that if indicated, pregnancy should not preclude vaccination with MenACWY or MPSV4. Moreover, patients who become pregnant at the time of MenACWY vaccination should alert their health care provider to be enrolled in the vaccine manufacturer's vaccination registry.

- **Meningococcal (MenB):** The use of MenB vaccines in pregnant and lactating patients has not been studied in a randomized controlled clinical trial. Unless a patient is at increased risk for contracting meningococcus, vaccination with MenB should be avoided in pregnant and lactating patients.

- **Pneumococcal conjugate (PCV13):** The Advisory Committee on Immunization Practices (ACIP) has not published recommendations for the use of PCV13 during pregnancy.

- **Pneumococcal polysaccharide (PPSV23):** The PPSV3 vaccine should be avoided in pregnancy because the safety of the vaccine has not been evaluated.

- **Polio (IPV):** Unless a patient is at increased risk for polio, IPV should be avoided in pregnancy because of theoretical risks to the fetus.

- **Tetanus, diphtheria, and pertussis (Tdap) and tetanus and diphtheria (Td):** The CDC recommends administration of the Tdap vaccine for pregnant patients during each pregnancy regardless of whether or not they have received the vaccine previously. The most beneficial time to provide the vaccine is between 27 and 36 weeks' gestation. This period allows for the patient to build an antibody response and pass antibodies to the infant.

- **Varicella:** This vaccine contains a live virus and should be avoided in pregnancy because of theoretical risks to the fetus. Patients of childbearing age should be counseled to avoid pregnancy for 4 weeks after administration of the varicella vaccine.

Visit the CDC website (https://www.cdc.gov/) for recommendations for travel vaccines such as anthrax, Japanese encephalitis, rabies, typhoid, smallpox, and yellow fever.

> **❗ SAFETY ALERT**
>
> Vaccination with live viruses may pose a risk of harm or death to the fetus and must be avoided in pregnancy.

CHILDBIRTH PREPARATION

Beginning as early as the second trimester, pregnant patients should be encouraged to start exploring and documenting their ideal birth experience in preparation for delivery. A review of personal expectations, cultural practices, and support systems should be included in this discussion. Patients should be the leader of this discussion and should be encouraged to advocate for the birth experience desired and gain the knowledge and support they need to make informed decisions that are right for them. Many structured educational programs exist to assist in childbirth education, which often includes the basic anatomy and physiology of labor and birth and simple strategies (typically relaxation and breathing) to cope with the pain of contractions. The components of childbirth preparation include the following:

- The normal, natural physiologic process of labor and birth
- Factors that facilitate normal physiologic labor, including allowing labor to start on its own, providing freedom of movement, and avoiding supine positions during the second stage
- Signs of labor and distinguishing prodromal labor from active labor
- When and how to call the health care provider
- What to expect in the hospital, policies, and resources
- Ways that laboring patients find comfort; the importance of labor support
- The role of pain in labor
- Prevention and management of possible complications of labor (e.g., prolonged labor, nonreassuring fetal heart rate)
- Routine interventions
- Newborn issues (e.g., circumcision, choosing a pediatrician, infant needs and capabilities, the importance of keeping mother and baby together, rooming-in)
- The importance of breastfeeding, how to prepare and get started breastfeeding

Benefits of childbirth education include fewer visits to labor and delivery for assessment, decreased use of epidural anesthesia, reduced elective inductions, and increased breastfeeding rates. Continuous labor support from loved ones or trained professionals such as nurses and doulas have been linked to a slight reduction in the length of labor and improvement in maternal satisfaction. A list of recommended childbirth preparation resources can be found in Box 7.6.

> **PATIENT-CENTERED CARE:** Pregnant parents should have a birth experience that encompasses their cultural values and beliefs, includes their support system, and considers their personal expectations.

PRETERM LABOR AND BIRTH

Preterm labor is one of the most common reasons for hospitalization of pregnant patients. Detection of patients who experience true preterm labor requires detailed evaluation and interventions such as tocolysis,

> **BOX 7.6 Resources for Childbirth Preparation**
>
> Besides in-person courses, numerous programs, websites, videos, and books exist to help prepare patients for labor. Patients should be encouraged to pursue information from reputable, evidence-based sources. The following are a few suggested sources from the author:
> - Penny Simpkins labor videos
> - *The Official Lamaze Guide: Giving Birth with Confidence*
> - *Ina May's Guide to Childbirth*
> - *Our Bodies, Ourselves Pregnancy and Birth Book*
> - March of Dimes
> - Lamaze International (www.lamaze.org)
> - Childbirth Connection (www.childbirthconnection.org)
> - American College of Nurse-Midwives (www.midwife.org)
> - Coalition for Improving Maternity Services (www.motherfriendly.org)

antenatal steroid therapy, group B streptococcal infection prophylaxis, and intravenous administration of magnesium sulfate for neuroprotection.[17] Betamethasone is the most commonly used antenatal steroid and is administered intramuscularly in two separate doses 12 hours apart. Magnesium sulfate is usually given to gravid patients between 24 and 32 weeks' gestation to provide neuroprotection against cerebral palsy and other motor dysfunctions in the fetus.

Educating patients about the warning signs and symptoms of preterm labor is essential. Signs of true labor regardless of gestational age include uterine contractions accompanied by rapid cervical changes that include dilation, effacement, and softening. Often a shortened cervix on ultrasound examination may be the first indicator of triggered preterm labor. Early symptoms include menstrual-like cramping that may be mild and increasing in intensity at least 4 to 6 times per hour, low backache, vaginal pressure, vaginal bleeding, and possible leakage of amniotic fluid. The greatest risk factor for preterm labor is having had a history of preterm labor or delivery in a previous pregnancy. Additional risk factors include multiple gestation, cervical shortening, infection, and substance abuse.[6] Nulliparous patients should be educated on warning signs throughout the course of prenatal care. Evaluation of preterm labor should include the following:

- Review of the patient's past and present obstetrical and medical history and assessment of gestational age
- Evaluation of signs and symptoms of preterm labor
- Assessment of maternal vital signs (temperature, BP, heart rate, respiratory rate)
- Review of the fetal heart rate pattern
- Assessment of contraction frequency, duration, and intensity
- Examination of the uterus to assess firmness, tenderness, fetal size, and fetal position
- Cervical assessment using a nonlubricated speculum. Lubricants may interfere with tests on vaginal samples. The goals of this examination are to determine cervical dilation. Cervical dilation greater than 3 cm with progressive cervical change supports the diagnosis of preterm labor.
- Cervicovaginal fluid specimen evaluation if fetal fibronectin (fFN) testing is desired after transabdominal ultrasound examination. If a speculum is unavailable, a blind cervical sweep can be performed. Semen, digital cervical examination lubricant, and blood can give false-positive results. If a cervical examination occurs it should be *after* the fFN.
- Evaluation for intact or ruptured fetal membranes. Preterm premature rupture of membranes (PPROM) often precedes or occurs during preterm labor.
- Assessment for uterine bleeding. Bleeding from placental abruption or placenta previa can trigger preterm labor.
- Laboratory evaluation should include culture for group B streptococcus (if not collected within the previous 5-week period); urine culture to rule out bacteriuria, which can increase the risk of preterm labor; drug screening due to links with cocaine use and placental abruption; and fFN in patients between 24 and 34 weeks' gestation with cervical dilation <3 cm.

fFN is a protein present at the decidual-chorionic interface of the placenta. Disruption of the interface caused by infection, bleeding, or contractions releases fFN into the vaginal secretions. This release enables the presence of fFN to be used as a predictor of preterm labor. fFN tests can often be unreliable and have been shown to not significantly reduce rates of hospitalization, steroid use, or preterm delivery. The results of fFN testing are reported as positive or negative. Positive results correlate with an increased risk for delivery within 7 days. If the fFN test is positive, interventions are usually implemented to reduce morbidity but may be institution specific. If fFN testing is negative, patients are usually monitored for observation and discharged after 4 to 6 hours in the absence of progressive cervical change. Patients should be followed by health care providers within 1 week of discharge and should be educated on the warning signs and when to seek follow-up if they are experiencing additional symptoms. Use of sonographic cervical length and fFN determinations to differentiate true labor from false labor in preterm symptomatic patients is supported by the ACOG and the Society for Maternal-Fetal Medicine, although high-quality evidence of efficacy is not available.

Preterm birth refers to a delivery that occurs before 37 weeks' gestation. In the United States, preterm births are highest among patients younger than 20 years of age and older than 35 years of age and among non-Hispanic Black females, followed by American Indian or Alaskan Natives, Hispanics, non-Hispanic whites, and Asian or Pacific Islanders.[17] It may or may not be preceded by preterm labor and is the leading cause of neonatal death within the first 21 days of life. Preterm births are classified by gestational age, birth weight, and initiating factor and are outlined as follows:

- Gestational age
  - World Health Organization
    - Moderate to late preterm: 32 to <37 weeks
    - Very preterm: 28 to <32 weeks
    - Extremely preterm: <28 weeks
  - CDC
    - Late preterm: <37 weeks
    - Preterm : 34 to 36 weeks
    - Early preterm: <34 weeks
- Birth weight
  - Low birth weight (LBW): <2500 g
  - Very low birth weight (VLBW): <1500 g
  - Extremely low birth weight (ELBW): <1000 g
- Initiating factor: spontaneous or iatrogenic
  - Spontaneous: Caused by preterm labor or preterm rupture of membranes
  - Iatrogenic: Caused by maternal or fetal issues including preeclampsia, placenta previa, placental abruption, intrauterine growth restriction, and multiple gestation

Because of the risk of preterm birth in subsequent pregnancies of patients with a history of preterm birth, preventive measures are key. Several medical options are available including cerclage placement, pessary use, and vaginal or intramuscular progesterone supplementation.

KEY POINTS

- A healthy pregnancy begins before conception and continues with early and regular antepartum care and the timely recognition and management of problems as they arise.
- When a patient of reproductive age misses a period, pregnancy should be suspected until it is ruled out.
- All patients are encouraged to inform their health care provider if they experience vaginal bleeding, leakage of fluid from their vagina, or DFM.
- Good nutrition, exercise, and avoidance of teratogens all lead to a healthy pregnancy.
- Testing for communicable diseases and infections can prevent negative outcomes for both the mother and fetus.
- Screening and early treatment of diabetes and hypertensive disorders in pregnancy are key components in prenatal care.
- IPV often begins or escalates during pregnancy. Screening for IPV is critical to keeping pregnant patients safe.
- Vaccines that do not contain live, attenuated virus or live bacteria may be given during pregnancy.
- Childbirth education prepares patients and their families for the birthing process and can result in fewer visits to labor and delivery for assessment, decreased use of epidural anesthesia, reduced elective inductions, and increased breastfeeding rates.
- Educating patients about the warning signs and symptoms of preterm labor is an essential part of prenatal care.

REFERENCES

1. Cunningham FG, Leveno KJ, Bloom SL, et al. *Williams Obstetrics*. 25th ed. McGraw Hill Professional; 2018.
2. Nagtalon-Ramos J. *Maternity-Newborn Nursing Care: Best Evidence-Based Practices*. Philadelphia: FA Davis; 2013.
3. Napolitano R, Dhami J, Ohuma EO. Pregnancy dating by fetal crown-rump length: a systematic review of charts. *Br J Obstetr Gynecol*. 2014;121(5):556.
4. Conley JM, Richards SM. Teratogenesis. *Earth Systems and Environmental Sciences*. 2008:3528–3536.
5. Kilpatrick SJ, Papile LA, Macones GA, eds. *Guidelines for Perinatal Care*. 8th ed. American Academy of Pediatrics; 2017.
6. King TL, Brucker MC, Jevitt CM, Osborne K. *Varney's Midwifery*. 6th ed. Burlington, MA: Jones & Bartlett Learning; 2018.
7. Perkins RB, Guido RS, Castle PE, et al. 2019 ASCCP risk-based management consensus guidelines for abnormal cervical cancer screening tests and cancer precursors. *J Lower Genital Tract Dis*. 2020;24(2):102–131.
8. Workowski KA, Bolan GA. Sexually transmitted diseases treatment guidelines, 2015. *MMWR Recommendation Rep*. 2015;64(3):55–68.
9. American College of Obstetricians and Gynecologists. ACOG Committee Opinion No. 752: Prenatal and perinatal human immunodeficiency virus testing. *Obstet Gynecol*. 2018b;132(3):e138–e142.
10. American College of Obstetricians and Gynecologists. Management of genital herpes in pregnancy: ACOG Practice Bulletin, Number 220. *Obstetr Gynecol*. 2020a;135(5):e193–e202.
11. American College of Obstetricians and Gynecologists. ACOG Practice Bulletin No. 203: Chronic hypertension in pregnancy. *Obstet Gynecol*. 2019a;133(1):e26–e50.
12. Driscoll DA, Simpson JL, Holzgreve W, Otano L. Genetic screening and prenatal genetic diagnosis. In: Gabbe SG, Niebyl JR, Simpson JL, et al., eds. *Obstetrics: Normal and Problem Pregnancies*. 7th ed. Philadelphia: Elsevier; 2016.
13. American College of Obstetricians and Gynecologists. ACOG Practice Bulletin No. 190: Gestational diabetes mellitus. *Obstet Gynecol*. 2018a;131(2):e49–e64.
14. Landon MB, Catalano PM, Gabbe SG. Diabetes mellitus complicating pregnancy. In: Gabbe SG, Niebyl JR, Simpson JL, et al., eds. *Obstetrics: Normal and Problem Pregnancies*. 7th ed. Philadelphia: Elsevier; 2016.
15. U.S. Preventive Services Task Force. Final Recommendation Statement: Gestational Diabetes Mellitus, Screening. https://uspreventiveservicestaskforce.org/uspstf/announcements/final-recommendation-statement-screening-gestational-diabetes.
16. American College of Obstetricians and Gynecologists. Gestational hypertension and preeclampsia: ACOG Practice Bulletin, Number 222. *Obstet Gynecol*. 2020c;135(6):e237–e260.
17. Gabbe SG, Niebyl JR, Simpson JL, Anderson GD. *Obstetrics: Normal and Problem Pregnancies*. 7th ed. New York: Churchill Livingstone; 2016.
18. Truong YN, Yee LM, Caughey AB, Cheng YW. Weight gain in pregnancy: does the Institute of Medicine have it right? *Am J Obstet Gynecol*. 2015;212(3):362. e1–e8.
19. Elliott-Sale KJ, Graham A, Hanley SJ, Blumenthal S, Sale C. Modern dietary guidelines for healthy pregnancy; maximising maternal and foetal outcomes and limiting excessive gestational weight gain. *Eur J Sport Sci*. 2019;19(1):62–70.
20. Ellis E. *Healthy Weight During Pregnancy*; 2019. https://www.eatright.org/health/pregnancy/prenatal-wellness/healthy-weight-during-pregnancy.

21. Korminiarek, M. A. & Rajan, P. (2016). Nutrition recommendations in pregnancy and lactation. Medical Clinics in North America, 100(6), 1199–1215.

22. March of Dimes. (n.d.a). *Caffeine in Pregnancy*. https://www.marchofdimes.org/pregnancy/caffeine-in-pregnancy.aspx.

23. March of Dimes. (n.d.b). *Folic Acid*. https://www.marchofdimes.org/pregnancy/folic-acid.aspx.

24. American College of Obstetricians and Gynecologists. FAQ: *Nutrition During Pregnancy;* 2021. https://www.acog.org/womens-health/faqs/nutrition-during-pregnancy.

25. Centers for Disease Control and Prevention. (n.d.a). Listeria (Listeriosis). https://www.cdc.gov/listeria/index.html#:~:text=An%20estimated%201%2C600%20people%20get,people%20with%20weakened%20immune%20systems.&text=Pregnant%20women%20are%2010%20times,to%20get%20a%20Listeria%20infection.

26. Benatar S, Cross-Barnet C, Johnson E, Hill I. Prenatal depression: Assessment and outcomes among Medicaid participants. *J Behav Health Services Res.* 2020;47(3):409–423.

27. Stewart DE. Clinical practice. Depression during pregnancy. *New Engl J Med.* 2011;365(17):1605–1611.

28. Andersson L, Sundström-Poromaa I, Wulff M, Aström M, Bixo M. Neonatal outcome following maternal antenatal depression and anxiety: a population-based study. *Am J Epidemiol.* 2004;159(9):872–881.

29. Dayan J, Creveuil C, Herlicoviez M, et al. Role of anxiety and depression in the onset of spontaneous preterm labor. *Am J Epidemiol.* 2002;155(4):293–301.

30. Chan J, Natekar A, Einarson A, Koren G. Risks of untreated depression in pregnancy. *Can Family Phys.* 2014;60(3):242–243.

31. Centers for Disease Control and Prevention. (n.d.b). Violence Prevention. https://www.cdc.gov/violenceprevention/intimatepartnerviolence/fastfact.html.

32. Silverman JG, Decker MR, Reed E, Raj A. Intimate partner violence victimization before and during pregnancy among people residing in 26 U.S. states: Associations with maternal and neonatal health. *Am J Obstet Gynecol.* 2006;195(1):140–148.

33. Centers for Disease Control and Prevention. *Guidelines for Vaccinating Pregnant Women;* 2016. https://www.cdc.gov/vaccines/pregnancy/hcp-toolkit/guidelines.html.

34. American College of Obstetricians and Gynecologists. COVID-19 Vaccination Considerations for Obstetric-Gynecologic Care. Practice Advisory, December 2020; 2020b. https://www.acog.org/clinical/clinical-guidance/practice-advisory/articles/2020/12/covid-19-vaccination-considerations-for-obstetric-gynecologic-care.

8

Postpartum and Lactation Care

Jamille Nagtalon-Ramos and Kelly Convery

OBJECTIVES

- Understand the female anatomy and physiology in relation to the changes that occur in the puerperium period.
- Diagnose the most common postpartum complications, and identify the recommended management/treatment strategies.
- Understand the anatomy and physiology of the breast and how it relates to the changes during pregnancy and lactation.
- Understand normal breastfeeding behavior in infants, and identify normal postpartum lactation expectations for new postpartum patients.

- Identify and treat common challenges and complications relating to lactation.
- Have a working understanding of the way medications pass into breastmilk, and identify resources available for clinicians regarding medications and breastmilk.
- Have a working knowledge of the challenges and role of lactation in common specialty pediatric populations.

POSTPARTUM

The puerperium period, also known as the *postpartum period,* is the first 6 to 12 weeks after a childbearing patient gives birth. In this crucial time of healing, the patient's body goes through anatomical, physiological, and hormonal changes to return to its pre-pregnancy state. Much emphasis in the care of the childbearing patient is placed on the preconception period, pregnancy, and delivery of the infant. Childbearing patients in the postpartum period, who are caring for themselves and their infant, lacking sleep, and dealing with lactation challenges, also must figure out their changing bodies and fluctuating hormones on their own as the postpartum visit is typically not scheduled until 4 to 6 weeks after delivery. As of 2020, the rate of maternal deaths in the United States was 23.8 for every 100,000 live births.[12] This number is more than double compared with most other high-income countries such as Canada (8.6),

the Netherlands (3), the United Kingdom (6.5), and Sweden (4.3).[1] Over one-half of these maternal deaths occur between the first day after the birth of the infant to 1 year after delivery.[1,2] Along with the high mortality rate, the morbidity associated with pregnancy is also of great concern. The U.S. Centers for Disease Control and Prevention (CDC) estimates that 50,000 women are affected by severe morbidity related to both diagnosed and undiagnosed pre-pregnancy conditions.[3] Obstetrical providers play a vital role in providing excellent care for postpartum patients. This chapter will discuss changes during this period and the role of the clinician in managing the care of the postpartum patient.

Changes in Anatomy and Physiology
Cardiovascular System
In a healthy pregnancy, a woman's plasma volume increases by 1250 mL, about 50% from pre-pregnancy levels (2600 mL).[4] Blood loss after the birth of the infant

and expulsion of the placenta decreases the plasma volume by 1000 mL.[5] At around the 1-week mark postdelivery, blood volume returns to pre-pregnancy levels.[6] Previous studies showed that cardiac output only remained elevated for 48 hours after delivery and returned to normal within 10 days postpartum.[7] However, more recent studies have shown that cardiac output may continue to be elevated for 1 year.[8]

Vagina and Cervix

The vagina and the vaginal outlet, which increased dramatically in size during the delivery of the infant, gradually decreases during puerperium; however, the tissues may not return to their pre-pregnancy state.[6] As early as the third week, reformation of the vaginal rugae occurs, but not to the same extent as before pregnancy.[6] Similarly, the cervix also goes through a rapid change of size from becoming thick during pregnancy, thinning out and shortening during effacement in the intrapartum period, and regressing to normal size in the first week postpartum.[5,6]

Uterus

After the birth of the infant and expulsion of the placenta, the contracted uterus weighs approximately 1000 g and is normally found at the level of the umbilicus. Uterine involution commences by the second day postpartum.[6] By 1 week postpartum, the uterus weighs approximately 500 g, and by 2 weeks postpartum, the uterus weighs about 300 g and has contracted back into the pelvis.[5,6] By 6 weeks postpartum, the uterus has returned to its normal size (Fig. 8.1).

Lochia

Vaginal discharge after birth (also known as *lochia*) is the result of the sloughing of decidual tissue from the uterus. In the first few days of the puerperium, this discharge is referred to as *lochia rubra,* for the deep, dark red color. This vaginal discharge turns into a pale, pink color, referred to as *lochia serosa,* on the third or fourth day postpartum. The vaginal discharge that persists for up to 8 weeks postdelivery is yellowish white in color as a result of the mixture of fluid and leukocytes and is referred to as *lochia alba.*

Urinary Tract

The renal pelvis and ureters, which were dilated in pregnancy, return to their normal state between the second

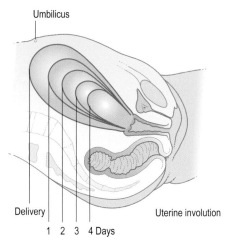

Figure 8.1 Uterine involution during the first week after delivery. (From Symonds IM, Arulkumaran S. *Essential Obstetrics and Gynaecology.* Elsevier; 2019.)

and eighth week postpartum.[6] Studies have not shown that infant weight or an episiotomy had an effect on bladder function, but epidural anesthesia use and prolonged labor may have a temporary effect.[5]

Hair Loss

The hair cycle consists of three phases: growth *(anagen),* involution *(catagen),* and resting *(telogen)* phases and typically lasts about 3 to 5 years.[9] During pregnancy, the increased levels of estrogen allows for hair to remain in a prolonged anagen phase, giving the gravid woman a full head of hair.[10] As a result of shifting hormones in the postpartum period, hair goes through the next phase of the cycle, the catagen phase.[10] This transient diffuse loss of hair in which the postpartum woman finds much hair falling out at the same time is referred to as *telogen gravidarum.*[10]

Thyroid Function

Triiodothyronine (T3) and thyroxine (T4) are vital thyroid hormones that increase in pregnancy by almost 50% and return to normal within 4 weeks after delivery.[6,11] In countries that are deficient in iodine, the thyroid gland increases in size by 20% to 40%; on the other hand, in countries with sufficient iodine, the thyroid gland grows by 10%.[11] The thyroid gland steadily returns to its pre-pregnancy size by 12 weeks.[6]

Both hypothyroidism and hyperthyroidism may have an impact on lactation and the milk-ejection reflex; therefore for women who are experiencing lactation problems with no other reasons found, the American Thyroid Association recommends assessment of thyroid-stimulating hormone levels.[11]

> **CLINICAL SURVIVAL TIP:** The American Thyroid Association has a detailed compilation of their newest guidelines for the diagnosis and management of thyroid disease in pregnancy and postpartum. The guidelines can be accessed at: http://online.liebertpub.com/doi/full/10.1089/thy.2016.0457.

Weight Loss

As many postpartum patients are often eager to lose their pregnancy weight immediately after giving birth, health care providers can take the opportunity to provide nutrition and exercise education and recommendations for these willing patients. There is an estimated 11- to 13-lb weight loss during birth attributed to the infant, placenta, amniotic fluid, and blood loss, along with an additional 2 to 4 lb resulting from the increased diuresis during this period of hormonal changes.[6] Most postpartum patients will likely achieve their pre-pregnancy weight by 3 months postpartum by making healthy food choices and engaging in exercise; however, it may take some patients up to 6 months to lose all the weight they gained during pregnancy.[5] Women who gained more than the recommended weight for the pregnancy (>35 lb) will likely retain about 11 lb of their pregnancy weight.[5]

Care in the Postpartum Period

This section is focused on the care of the postpartum patient who has been discharged from the hospital.

The Postpartum Follow-Up Visit

According to the American College of Obstetricians and Gynecologists (ACOG), only 60% of females attend their postpartum follow-up visit.[12] This visit is typically scheduled for 4 to 6 weeks after the birth of the infant; new recommendations based on ACOG's Presidential Task Force on Redefining the Postpartum Visit and the Committee on Obstetric Practice is to schedule a visit within the first 3 weeks of delivery and continue ongoing care thereafter.[12] Waiting longer for postpartum follow-up after the birth of an infant obliges the patient to determine how to deal with possible postpartum blues, fluctuating hormones, potential breastfeeding difficulties, pain secondary to uterine involution, perineal laceration/episiotomy,

and surgical incision without expert guidance. The ACOG recommends earlier postpartum follow-up, particularly for female patients who have pregnancy complications such as gestational hypertension.[12]

At the postpartum visit, the health care provider should review the patient's antepartum, intrapartum, and immediate postpartum records. During this review, particular attention should be paid to chronic conditions, pregnancy complications, type of delivery, birth complications, infant health status, postpartum laboratory values, and significant events in the immediate postpartum period. For example, if a patient had a postpartum hemorrhage, the health care provider should note the estimated blood loss, complete blood count at discharge (particularly the patient's hemoglobin, hematocrit, and platelet levels), if the patient needed blood transfusions, and/or intravenous iron. The data gathered from this review should inform the provider on issues, problems, or concerns that need follow-up. The components of the postpartum visit are listed in Box 8.1.

> **PATIENT-CENTERED CARE:** New parents may face dealing with changes and/or complications of the postpartum period without guidance when follow-up visits are scheduled 6 weeks after delivery. Scheduling a follow-up visit at 3 weeks can assist these new postpartum patients in coping with new changes and early identification of complications.

> **! SAFETY ALERT**
> If the patient has Rh-negative blood type and the infant's blood type is Rh-positive, the patient should receive a 300-mcg dose of Rho(D) immune globulin (RhoGAM) typically within the first 72 hours postdelivery. This intramuscular injection is used to prevent Rh isoimmunization, which is the development of antibodies in the Rh-negative patient after exposure to the Rh-positive blood of the infant.

Postpartum Complications

Postpartum Hemorrhage. Postpartum hemorrhage is defined as "cumulative blood loss of greater than or equal to 1,000 mL or blood loss accompanied by signs or symptoms of hypovolemia within 24 hours after delivery."[13] Secondary postpartum hemorrhage occurs after the first 24 hours after birth and up to 12 weeks

BOX 8.1 Components of Postpartum Care

Mood and emotional well-being
- Screen for postpartum depression and anxiety with a validated instrument[1,2]
- Provide guidance regarding local resources for mentoring and support
- Screen for tobacco use; counsel regarding relapse risk in postpartum period[3]
- Screen for substance use disorder and refer as indicated[4]
- Follow-up on preexisting mental health disorders, refer for or confirm attendance at mental health-related appointments, and titrate medications as appropriate for the postpartum period

Infant care and feeding
- Assess comfort and confidence with caring for newborn, including
  - feeding method
  - child care strategy if returning to work or school
  - ensuring infant has a pediatric medical home
  - ensuring that all caregivers are immunized[5]
- Assess comfort and confidence with breastfeeding, including
  - breastfeeding-associated pain[6]
  - guidance on logistics of and legal rights to milk expression if returning to work or school[7,8]
  - guidance regarding return to fertility while lactating; pregnancy is unlikely if menses have not returned, infant is less than 6 months old, and infant is fully or nearly fully breastfeeding with no interval of more than 4–6 hours between breastfeeding sessions[9]
  - review theoretical concerns regarding hormonal contraception and breastfeeding, within the context of each woman's desire to breastfeed and her risk of unplanned pregnancy[7]
- Assess material needs, such as stable housing, utilities, food, and diapers, with referral to resources as needed

Sexuality, contraception, and birth spacing
- Provide guidance regarding sexuality, management of dyspareunia, and resumption of intercourse
- Assess desire for future pregnancies and reproductive life plan[10]
- Explain the rationale for avoiding an interpregnancy interval of less than 6 months and discuss the risks and benefits of repeat pregnancy sooner than 18 months
- Review recommendations for prevention of recurrent pregnancy complications, such as 17α-hydroxyprogesterone caproate to reduce risk of recurrent preterm birth, or aspirin to reduce risk of preeclampsia
- Select a contraceptive method that reflects patient's stated needs and preferences, with same-day placement of LARC, if desired[11]

Sleep and fatigue
- Discuss coping options for fatigue and sleep disruption
- Engage family and friends in assisting with care responsibilities

Physical recovery from birth
- Assess presence of perineal or cesarean incision pain; provide guidance regarding normal versus prolonged recovery[12]
- Assess for presence of urinary and fecal continence, with referral to physical therapy or urogynecology as indicated[13,14]
- Provide actionable guidance regarding resumption of physical activity and attainment of healthy weight[15]

Chronic disease management
- Discuss pregnancy complications, if any, and their implications for future childbearing and long-term maternal health, including ASCVD
- Perform glucose screening for women with GDM: a fasting plasma glucose test or 75 g, 2-hour oral glucose tolerance test[16]
- Review medication selection and dose outside of pregnancy, including consideration of whether the patient is breastfeeding, using a reliable resource such as LactMed
- Refer for follow-up care with primary care or subspecialist health care providers, as indicated

BOX 8.1   Components of Postpartum Care—cont'd

Health maintenance
- Review vaccination history and provide indicated immunizations, including completing series initiated antepartum or postpartum[17]
- Perform well-woman screening, including Pap test and pelvic examination, as indicated[18]

Abbreviations: ASCVD, arteriosclerotic cardiovascular disease; GDM, gestational diabetes mellitus; LARC, long-acting reversible contraceptive.

References
1. Screening for perinatal depression. Committee Opinion No. 630. American College of Obstetricians and Gynecologists. *Obstet Gynecol.* 2015;125:1268–1271.
2. Earls MF. Incorporating recognition and management of perinatal and postpartum depression into pediatric practice. Committee on Psychosocial Aspects of Child and Family Health American Academy of Pediatrics. *Pediatrics.* 2010;126:1032–1039.
3. American College of Obstetricians and Gynecologists. Tobacco and nicotine cessation toolkit. Washington, DC: American College of Obstetricians and Gynecologists; 2016.
4. Opioid use and opioid use disorder in pregnancy. Committee Opinion No. 711. American College of Obstetricians and Gynecologists. *Obstet Gynecol.* 2017;130:e81–e94.
5. American Academy of Pediatrics. Protect infants against pertussis: cocooning through Tdap vaccination. Washington, DC: AAP. Available at: https://www.aap.org/en-us/Documents/immunization_protect_infants_against_pertussis.pdf. Retrieved January 23, 2018.
6. Berens P, Eglash A, Malloy M, Steube AM. ABM Clinical Protocol #26: persistent pain with breastfeeding. *Breastfeed Med.* 2016;11:46–53.
7. Optimizing support for breastfeeding as part of obstetric practice. Committee Opinion No. 658. American College of Obstetricians and Gynecologists. *Obstet Gynecol.* 2016;127:e86–e92.
8. Breastfeeding in underserved women: increasing initiation and continuation of breastfeeding. Committee Opinion No. 570. American College of Obstetricians and Gynecologists. *Obstet Gynecol.* 2013;122:423–428.
9. Centers for Disease Control and Prevention. Lactational amenorrhea method. In: US medical eligibility criteria (US MEC) for contraceptive use. Atlanta (GA): CDC; 2017.
10. Reproductive life planning to reduce unintended pregnancy. Committee Opinion No. 654. American College of Obstetricians and Gynecologists. *Obstet Gynecol.* 2016;127:e66–e69.
11. Immediate postpartum long-acting reversible contraception. Committee Opinion No. 670. American College of Obstetricians and Gynecologists. *Obstet Gynecol.* 2016;128:e32–e37.
12. MacArthur C, Winter HR, Bick DE, Lilford RJ, Lancashire RJ, Knowles H, et al. Redesigning postnatal care: a randomised controlled trial of protocol-based midwifery-led care focused on individual women's physical and psychological health needs. *Health Technol Assess.* 2003;7:1–98.
13. Prevention and management of obstetric lacerations at vaginal delivery. Practice Bulletin No. 165. American College of Obstetricians and Gynecologists. *Obstet Gynecol.* 2016;128:e1–e15.
14. Urinary incontinence in women. Practice Bulletin No. 155. American College of Obstetricians and Gynecologists. *Obstet Gynecol.* 2015;126:e66–e81.
15. American College of Obstetricians and Gynecologists. Obesity toolkit. Washington, DC: American College of Obstetricians and Gynecologists; 2016.
16. Gestational diabetes mellitus. ACOG Practice Bulletin No. 190. American College of Obstetricians and Gynecologists. *Obstet Gynecol.* 2018;131:e49–e64.
17. American College of Obstetricians and Gynecologists. Immunization for women. Washington, DC: American College of Obstetricians and Gynecologists; 2017.
18. Conry J, Brown H. Well-Woman Task Force: Components of the Well-Woman Visit. *Obstet Gynecol.* 2015;126:697–701.

Reprinted with permission from Optimizing postpartum care. ACOG Committee Opinion No. 736. American College of Obstetricians and Gynecologists. *Obstet Gynecol.* 2018;131:e140–e150.

postpartum.[13] Secondary hemorrhage may result from uterine atony caused by retained placenta or products of conception, endometritis, or a bleeding disorder such as von Willebrand disease. Uterine ultrasound evaluation is recommended to determine the presence of intrauterine tissue. Management may include uterotoxic agents, antibiotic therapy, and/or removal of uterine tissue by curettage. Although rare, patients should be counseled for the possibility of a uterine hysterectomy.

Before discharge, the clinician should provide education regarding signs and symptoms of hypovolemia and monitor for increased lochia and passage of clots. Education should also include how to contact the health care team for further evaluation.

Postpartum Infection. A cardinal sign of a puerperal infection is a fever greater than or equal to 100.4°F (38°C) after the first 24 hours postdelivery and before 11 days postpartum. Differential diagnoses include infection of the uterus (endometritis), urogenital tract, kidney (pyelonephritis), incision, perineal laceration/episiotomy, breasts (mastitis), and lungs (pneumonia).

Postpartum Depression. Perinatal depression may be diagnosed any time during pregnancy and up to 1 year after the birth of the infant.[14] With one in seven female patients affected by perinatal depression and mood disorders, the effects on these patients and their families can be distressing. The ACOG recommends that clinicians use a validated tool to screen all pregnant patients at least once during pregnancy and the postpartum period.[14]

NOT TO BE MISSED

The Edinburgh Postnatal Depression Scale (EPDS) is a 10-question screening tool developed in 1987 to assist in identifying possible symptoms of depression in the postpartum period. Although the EPDS is not a diagnostic tool, it is a screening tool aimed at identifying female patients who may benefit from further assessment and follow-up with a mental health professional. An example of the EPDS and scoring can be accessed at: http://www.fresno.ucsf.edu/pediatrics/downloads/edinburghscale.pdf.

LACTATION

Breastmilk offers many unique and lifelong benefits for childbearing parent and infants. For infants, breastmilk provides protection against illness and a decreased risk of ear infections, lower respiratory infections, obesity, asthma, allergies, and certain types of cancer. For women, breastfeeding reduces the risk of type 2 diabetes as well as breast and ovarian cancer.[15]

BOX 8.2   Breastfeeding Resources for Providers

- American College of Obstetricians and Gynecologists: https://www.acog.org/clinical/clinical-guidance/committee-opinion/articles/2021/02/breastfeeding-challenges
- American Academy of Pediatrics Breastfeeding Residency Curriculum: https://www.aap.org/en/learning/breastfeeding-curriculum/
- Academy of Breastfeeding Medicine: http://www.bfmed.org/
  - Breastfeeding protocols: https://www.bfmed.org/protocols
- American Academy of Family Physicians Breastfeeding Toolkit: https://www.aafp.org/family-physician/patient-care/prevention-wellness/birth-control-pregnancy-childbirth/breastfeeding/toolkit.html
- U.S. Centers for Disease Control and Prevention. The CDC Guide to Strategies to Support Breastfeeding Mothers and Babies: https://www.cdc.gov/breastfeeding/resources/guide.htm
  - *The CDC Guide to Strategies to Support Breastfeeding Mothers and Babies* (PDF of the whole booklet): https://www.cdc.gov/breastfeeding/pdf/BF-Guide-508.PDF
- LactMed (National Institutes of Health Toxicology Data Network) https://toxnet.nlm.nih.gov/newtoxnet/lactmed.htm. The LactMed smartphone app is available for free.
  - Android: https://play.google.com/store/apps/details?id=gov.nih.nlm.sis.lactmed&hl=en
  - iTunes: https://itunes.apple.com/us/app/lactmed/id441969514?mt=8
- Massachusetts Breastfeeding Coalition: https://massbreastfeeding.org/
- Office on Women's Health: https://www.womenshealth.gov/breastfeeding/
- The Surgeon General's Call to Action to Support Breastfeeding: https://www.surgeongeneral.gov/library/calls/breastfeeding/calltoactiontosupportbreastfeeding.pdf
- U.S. Department of Agriculture. Women, Infant, and Child Breastfeeding program: https://www.fns.usda.gov/wic/breastfeeding-priority-wic-program
- Zipmilk: http://www.zipmilk.org/

In 2020, the U.S. Department of Health and Human Services published the *Healthy People 2030* national health goals; one of these goals targeted increasing the number of breastfed infants in the United States.[16] Along with these government efforts, professional organizations like the American Academy of Pediatrics (AAP) offer additional guidance for families and providers. The AAP currently recommends exclusive breastfeeding until 6 months of age and then continued complementary breastfeeding after the initiation of solids for at least 1 year or thereafter for as long as the patient and infant mutually desire.[17]

As a provider for females of childbearing age, the likelihood of caring for a lactating patient is higher than ever. U.S. breastfeeding rates are on the rise.[18] In practices that also treat children, clinicians have the unique opportunity to care for the complete breastfeeding dyad. As rates of breastfeeding continue to increase, it is vital for providers to have a strong understanding of the physical changes to the breasts during pregnancy and lactation. Box 8.2 provides breastfeeding resources for providers. It is also important for providers to be aware of special considerations during lactation regarding medications, complications, and certain pediatric populations.

> **PATIENT-CENTERED CARE:** In practices that also treat children, clinicians have the unique opportunity to care for the complete breastfeeding dyad.

Anatomy and Physiology

Breast development begins in the first month of gestation. Two lines of glandular tissue appear from thigh to axilla on bilateral sides of the developing fetus. Throughout pregnancy, this glandular tissue, also known as the *milk lines,* will mature into the mammary ducts, areola, and nipples; thus the structural anatomy of the breast is present but will remain nonfunctional until puberty.

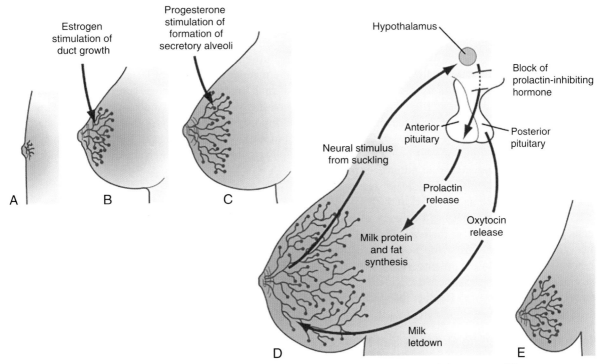

Figure 8.2 Hormonal control of development of the breast and mammary ducts. **(A)** Newborn; **(B)** young adult; **(C)** adult; **(D)** lactating adult; and **(E)** adult after the cessation of lactation. (From Carlson, BM. (2019). The reproductive system. In: Carlson BM, ed. *The Human Body.* Academic Press; 2019: 373–396. https://doi.org/10.1016/b978-0-12-804254-0.00014-4.)

It is important to note that this fetal breast development happens for both males and females. Consequently, supernumerary nipples along the milk line may be present on both males and females during physical assessment. During lactation or certain hormonal conditions, these supernumerary nipples may even excrete small amounts of milk.

At the onset of puberty in females, estrogen, progesterone, and other hormones work to further mature the breasts and prepare the breast tissue for full functionality during lactation. The small alveolar buds and immature duct system grow and proliferate under the hormones of puberty. New connective tissue develops, and adipose tissue is deposited as the breasts grow larger with time. These changes in breast tissue can be assessed using the Tanner staging system (see Fig. 2.11).

Pregnancy heralds the next developmental changes in the breasts. The hormones of pregnancy prompt the mammary epithelium to differentiate into lactocytes, the milk-making cells of lactation. As more alveoli develop, the breasts become larger. By 16 to 20 weeks' gestation, the breasts can secrete the first type of milk, known as *colostrum*. Most of the breast development in pregnancy happens in the first two trimesters, although breast development can continue until the third trimester (Fig. 8.2).

It is important to note that many hormones regulate and control the development of the breasts for lactation during pregnancy and beyond. These hormones range from sex and thyroid hormones to glucocorticoids such as cortisol and insulin. For the purposes of this chapter, only basic endocrine function will be reviewed; however, in the event of known thyroid, adrenal, or pituitary dysfunction, potential effects on breast development and lactation should be monitored closely.

Following the detachment and delivery of the placenta, an abrupt decrease in the levels of progesterone and other hormones signals the next developmental shift for the breasts. In the presence of these decreased hormones, prolactin levels increase, and further hormones such as insulin work together to signal the onset of copious milk production or secretory activation.

Normal Breastfeeding and Milk Supply

For most childbearing/lactating individuals, secretory activation or "milk coming in" occurs between 2 and 4 days postpartum.[19] It tends to happen faster for lactating patients who have breastfed previously. In these early days, actual milk production is driven largely by hormones; however, the frequent removal of milk from the breasts as well as the stimulation of suckling at the nipple is now understood to play a role in the total overall volume of milk production a lactating individual will achieve.[20] Frequent feeds or pumping sessions stimulate the development of prolactin receptor sites within the mammary gland. With more prolactin receptors available, an increased activation of lactocytes will occur. During secretory activation, there is an increase in fluid in the lactiferous ducts as well as increased blood volume and vascularization. As a result, the breasts grow larger and may feel warm with signs of diffuse redness. This is known as *engorgement* and may be accompanied by feelings of tightness or slight discomfort that may last for up to 5 days. During engorgement, the most important goal is removal of milk from the breast to provide comfort to the patient and decrease the risk of mastitis.[21]

Most lactating individuals proceed through engorgement with no complications; however, if milk is not flowing easily or stagnation of milk occurs within the ducts (causing palpable hardened areas of the breasts), patients will develop an increased risk of mastitis, which is a cellulitis of the breast tissue (Fig. 8.3).

After engorgement, the breasts enter a stage of mature milk production and supply. This is considered the maintenance phase of lactation. Hormonal control of milk production becomes autocrine and local to the breast tissue. Put simply, milk supply is driven by local hormones in the lactocytes that respond to the filling and emptying of the breast. The more frequently and fully emptied the breast becomes, the more milk will be

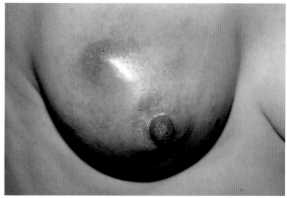

Figure 8.3 Mastitis of the breast. (From Garden OJ, Parks RW. *Principles and Practice of Surgery*. St. Louis: Elsevier; 2018.)

produced. When the breasts are not emptied and infant feedings become less frequent, the total milk volume will decrease over time.[23]

Another important component of lactation is the role of oxytocin on the milk ejection reflex (also known as the *let-down reflex*). Each alveolus in the breast is surrounded by myoepithelial cells that contract in the presence of oxytocin to push milk out to the milk ducts. Small muscles along the ducts similarly contract, increasing pressure and moving the milk out to trickle from the nipple.[22] Oxytocin is released in response to suckling and in response to the sight, smell, and cry of an infant. One of oxytocin's other vital functions is to cause contractions in the uterus that help with the involution of the womb following delivery.

Risk Factors for Delayed or Low Milk Production

Because of the importance of hormones in the early development and onset of lactation, health conditions that affect any of the hormones of lactation may influence onset of milk production and overall milk supply. For example, normal insulin levels are known to play an important role in secretory activation. Consequently, diabetic patients, especially those with insulin resistance or uncontrolled blood sugar, are at increased risk of delayed or compromised milk production.[24] Untreated thyroid or pituitary problems may also negatively affect milk production. Similarly, females with polycystic ovarian syndrome (PCOS) or infertility suffer from more general hormonal dysfunction and are at increased risk for lactation issues.[20] Retained placenta fragments will prevent the full onset of secretory activation, and rarely, oxygen deprivation from severe postpartum hemorrhage may result in pituitary injury. This rare complication is known as *Sheehan syndrome*.

Besides hormone-based conditions, nearly any maternal illness or scenario that inhibits early removal of milk from the breast may inhibit the establishment of milk production and supply. This includes patients who receive large volumes of fluids in labor as the breasts swell with generalized edema and compete for space with the onset of milk during engorgement.[25]

Past breast or chest surgeries may also affect milk production. Nerves around the nipple and along the ribs that are severed during chest and heart surgeries can prevent the let-down response or milk ejection. This is also seen in cases of breast reduction surgery in which the nipple is removed and then reattached. Breast reduction surgery also removes both breast tissue and milk ducts. Conversely, breast augmentation is routinely done by placing implants behind the pectoral muscles, which helps preserve the breast and nipple anatomy; however, it is important to ask patients with breast augmentation about their presurgery breast size and shape.

Breast and Nipple Variations

Anatomy of breasts and nipples vary as a result of many factors such as race and ethnicity. The normal variations of the female breast should not impede breastfeeding; however, certain features may be cause for concern. For example, profound asymmetry in breast shape/size may be concerning for a breast defect known as *hypoplastic breast tissue* in which the glandular tissue necessary for milk production fails to develop.[26] Depending on the degree of absent tissue, patients may experience a compromised milk supply. Assessing the breasts before pregnancy helps screen for possible lactation complications in the future.

Much like breast anatomy, nipples vary considerably in size and shape. Walker describes five basic types of nipples:[27]

- The common nipple typically protrudes outward from the areola's surface at rest and becomes more erect upon stimulation. When suckling, an infant can easily grasp the nipple and bring it to the junction of the hard and soft palates, thus achieving a deep latch.
- The inverted-appearing nipple may seem recessed at first glance, but this nipple type becomes erect with stimulation, allowing for the infant to latch with minimal difficulty.
- A flat nipple does not protrude much from the areola and does not become erect, even after stimulation. An infant may encounter difficulty in grasping a flat nipple and drawing it forward into the mouth to achieve a deep latch.
- A retracted nipple may appear to be protruding outward, but it actually retracts upon stimulation. This type of nipple may also result in latching challenges for the infant.

The areola is the center, pigmented part of the breast that surrounds the nipple and varies widely in size, shape, and color. During pregnancy, the areola darkens significantly to provide a visual aid for the infant to locate the nipple. On the surface, small bumps indicate the location of Montgomery glands. These are sebaceous glands that provide natural lubrication to the nipple and areola during breastfeeding. It is important to instruct patients not to rub or cleanse their nipples and areola directly with harsh soaps as this can dry the sensitive skin and lead to increased cracking or trauma.

Normal Infant Feeding Behavior

Infants eat often in the first few weeks following delivery, generally at least 8 to 12 times a day. Lactating patients should be instructed to "watch the baby, not the clock" and to feed whenever an infant is showing hunger cues. Feeding duration and frequency can change based on the time of day and infant alertness. Most newborns tend to sleep longer stretches during the day and eat more frequently at night. They may even "cluster" feed (eat frequently for a 2- to 3-hour stretch). All of this serves to match with a lactating patient's natural prolactin surges and to help establish a milk supply. As long as an infant is having six to eight wet diapers per day and gaining weight, feeding behaviors can vary widely among infants and should be treated as normal.

After a few weeks, breastfeeding should be well established. Infants may start to sleep longer stretches at night and drop to eating 8 times a day. However, the occasional frequent feeding bursts may be connected to growth spurts or an increase in milk volume demand and should be expected. There is no set time to expect breastfeeding infants to sleep through the night. It depends on several factors, including the ability of the infant's liver to maintain blood sugar levels.

As previously mentioned, the AAP recommends exclusive breastfeeding until 6 months of age and then continued complementary breastfeeding after the initiation of solids for at least 1 year or thereafter for as long as the patient and infant mutually desire.[17]

Latching and Common Positions

The first step in a successful latch is teaching lactating patients to recognize hunger cues. Crying is considered a late sign of hunger. Sleeping infants first show early feeding cues when they start to demonstrate rapid eye movement right before waking. A quiet but alert infant who is licking her lips or making smacking/sucking noises is showing early hunger cues. Before fussing, an infant may root back and forth or start sucking on her hands. Babies latch easiest when in this calm, alert state.

To physically latch an infant, the infant is placed in a comfortable hold that allows both the patient and infant visibility of the breast/areola. The patient is instructed to tap the infant's nose and upper lip with her nipple. Once the infant opens wide and begins rooting, the patient rolls the nipple and areola into the infant's mouth. Most of the patient's areola should be inside the infant's mouth, and audible swallowing should begin within 1 minute or so of latching. The infant's lips should be flanged, and the tongue should cover the lower gumline (Fig. 8.4). With a deep latch, the nipple sits at the junction of the

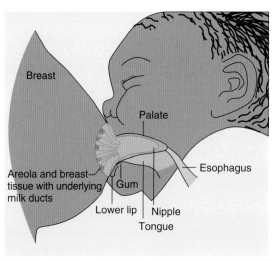

Figure 8.4 Infant latched onto the breast correctly. (From Perry, S., et al. [2014]. *Maternal child nursing care* [5th ed.]. Elsevier/Mosby.)

hard and soft palate. It is important that the infant does not latch directly on the nipple as this may cause tissue trauma and interfere with milk transfer.

Different breastfeeding holds can be used based on the patient's anatomy, circumstances, and comfort level. The most common holds include the following:

- **Cradle hold** (Fig. 8.5): While sitting straight up, instruct the patient to cradle the infant in her arm with the infant's head resting comfortably in the bend

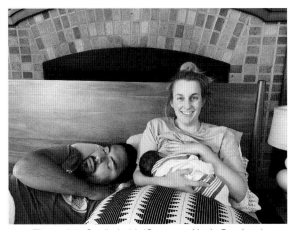

Figure 8.5 Cradle hold. (Courtesy Alexis Ramirez.)

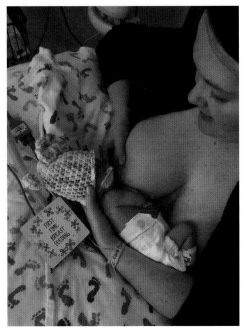

of her elbow. The infant's whole body is facing the patient. This hold is commonly used and comfortable for most lactating patients.

- **Cross-cradle or transitional hold** (Fig. 8.6): While sitting straight up, instruct the patient to cradle the infant along the opposite arm from the breast she is using. The infant's head is supported with the palm of the patient's hand at the base of the infant's head. This allows for more control of the infant's head during the latching process. This hold is ideal for infants who are premature and more likely hypotonic.
- **Football or clutch hold** (Fig. 8.7): While sitting straight up, instruct the patient to hold the infant at her side (like tucking a football under the arm). The infant should be at the patient's waist level, and the infant's head should be at the level of the nipple. The infant's head is supported by the patient's palm placed at the base of the head. This hold is good for lactating patients who had a cesarean delivery, have large breasts, or have inverted nipples.
- **Side-lying hold** (Fig. 8.8): Assist the patient to lie on her side with the infant positioned parallel to her body and facing her. The patient may hold her breast to guide the nipple into the infant's mouth or use her hand to guide the infant's head to her breast. This hold is good for patients who had a cesarean delivery as it keeps the infant's weight off the incision.

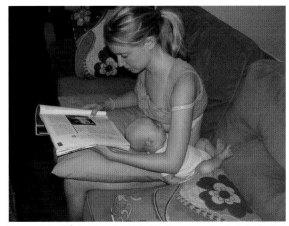

Figure 8.6 Cross-cradle or transitional hold. (Courtesy Kari Fredricks.)

Figure 8.7 Football or clutch hold. (Courtesy Beth Gribbin Kangas.)

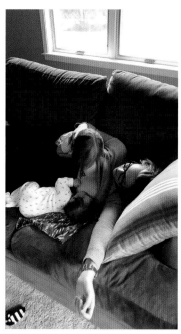

Figure 8.8 Side-lying hold. (Courtesy Kate Turner.)

Troubleshooting Common Lactation Challenges

Nipple Pain/Trauma

When a lactating patient reports nipple pain, the first step is determining the cause. Although there may be very mild soreness as the infant learns in the first few days of life, persistent nipple pain should always be of concern and requires further assessment. Ask the patient the following questions:

- Does the infant have a deep and correct latch?
- Does the patient have a history of Reynaud syndrome? If so, the patient could experience a vasospasm of the nipple when the infant stops suckling and her skin is exposed to the cooler air.
- Does the infant have a visible case of ankyloglossia or tongue-tie?
- Is the patient unlatching the infant incorrectly by forgetting to break the suction first?

If the patient was previously breastfeeding without issue but now has new onset pain with no other signs of mechanical latching issues, infections such as yeast or dermatitis should be ruled out. Ask the patient the following questions:

NOT TO BE MISSED

Recognizing Ankyloglossia or Tongue-Tie[24]

Tongue-tie commonly refers to a condition in which the lingual frenulum (the membrane that connects the bottom of the tongue to the floor of the mouth) limits mobility of the tongue. An infant may also have a labial frenulum tie (the membrane that connects the inside of the upper lip to the upper gums). Tongue-ties often run in families.

The tongue plays an important role in latching. To achieve a deep latch, the infant's tongue should extend past their lower gumline to draw the patient's nipple and areola fully into the mouth. Although not all tongue-ties affect breastfeeding, a patient who reports persistent pain despite the outward appearance of a good latch could indicate trouble with latching mechanics within the infant mouth.

To diagnose a tie, visualize the infant's mouth as follows:

- Does the tongue extend past the lower gumline?
- Does it form a heart shape and roll up at the sides?
- Refer to a health care provider who is familiar with diagnosing ankyloglossia and performing frenotomy/frenulectomy/frenuloplasty.
- Options for treating tongue-tie are based on the type and severity of the tie:
  - Frenotomy: "Snipping" can be performed without anesthesia in the outpatient office; this is usually suited for thin ties located toward the anterior of the mouth.
  - Frenulectomy and frenuloplasty: This more involved surgical procedure generally requires referral to a pediatric eye, ear, nose, and throat specialist or a pediatric dentist. The procedure may involve laser treatment. It is suited for more involved, thicker ties, especially when located deeply posterior.

- Is the patient experiencing burning, shooting pain that radiates into her breast?
- Because yeast favors growing in a dark, damp environment, consider asking if the patient frequently leaks milk or wears nursing pads.
- To assess if the patient is more prone to irritation and possible microabrasions for bacteria to enter, ascertain if the patient has sensitive skin at baseline. Does the patient have eczema in other parts of her body?
- Is there any new redness, dry skin, or flaking on the skin or areola?
- Does the patient have a clogged nipple pore or bleb?

Treatment/Management

For general nipple soreness, creams like lanolin help keep the skin moisturized and prevent cracking and breakdown. If there is visible breakdown like blisters or cracks, hydrogel pads work well to protect the skin as well as support healing.

If a mild nipple infection is suspected, medicated creams such as Dr. Jack Newman's All-Purpose Nipple Ointment may be prescribed to cover both superficial fungal and bacterial infections.[28]

Candida Infection of the Breast

A candida infection of the breast should be considered if the lactating patient is experiencing breast pain that feels deep and is radiating within the breast. This sharp pain is typically accompanied by affected nipples that are shiny or flaky (Fig. 8.9). Topical treatment of candida of the breast using miconazole or clotrimazole is initially used. These topical treatments are preferred over nystatin cream because they have been shown to have less resistance to *Candida* species.

There is a lack of studies that investigate the effects of topical antifungal agents, but lactation experts believe that these treatment regimens are unlikely to be of concern during breastfeeding. Patients should be instructed to apply topical antifungal medication after a feeding. Before the next feeding, excess residue of the medication should be removed. If there are cracks and fissures noted on the nipples, a topical antibiotic ointment such as mupirocin and bacitracin should be added to the treatment plan. Like the topical antifungals, visible residual of the medication should be removed before each feeding and reapplied after completion of each feeding session.

Gentian violet is another alternative to treating candida infection of the breast. Although inexpensive, this therapy is messy and temporarily stains the infant's mouth and the lactating patient's nipples and breasts. Gentian violet is diluted in water and applied to the inside of the infant's mouth before feeding once a day for 3 to 4 days.

If the topical therapies fail, oral antifungal medication should be considered. The treatment plan includes oral fluconazole 400 mg the first day followed by 200 mg per day for 14 days.

Clogged Ducts

It is possible for milk ducts within the breast to become sluggish and clogged. Oftentimes this results from milk stasis caused by pressure on or within a full breast. Clogged ducts feel like small, firm pebbles or marbles beneath the skin. Patients can often pinpoint the exact location based on pain and discomfort. To treat a clogged duct, encourage the patient to do continuous massage on the clog while breastfeeding or pumping. It should eventually breakdown and milk will start flowing again.

To prevent clogging of the ducts, encourage patients to avoid underwire bras, especially in the first few weeks of breastfeeding. Purse straps may also contribute to clogs if worn for long periods across the breasts. Some lactating patients are simply prone to clogs despite their best efforts to prevent them. Lecithin supplements have been shown to be a relatively safe and effective intervention for chronic clogged ducts.[29] Lecithin is a natural fat emulsifier that helps decrease the viscosity of breast milk and hopefully allow it to move easier through the ducts.

Flat/Inverted Nipples

Expert opinion for the treatment of flat/inverted nipples varies greatly. A systematic review of the treatment of a benign inverted nipple by Hernandez Yenty and colleagues[30] found that no superior treatment technique for nipple inversion was identified. Some providers recommend routine screening before and during pregnancy for patients with flat/inverted nipples.

One type of device used to treat flat/inverted nipples is the breast shell. These shells are dome-shaped and made of soft plastic. They are placed inside the bra between feedings to stretch underlying tissue and draw the nipple out. Breast shells have fallen out of favor with

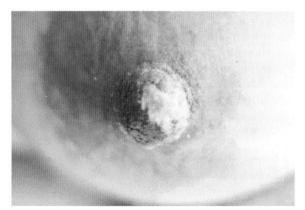

Figure 8.9 Candida infection of the breast. (Courtesy J. Newman, MD, FRCPC, Hospital for Sick Children, Toronto.)

most health care providers and lactation consultants because of the lack of evidence for their effectiveness; however, some may still utilize this treatment plan.

The Hoffman technique can be manually performed by the lactating patient on her own breasts to treat flat/inverted nipples. The patient places the thumbs on the base of the nipple (of note, not the base of the areola) and pushes inward toward the chest while at the same time moving the thumbs away from each other. This technique is thought to break adhesions and loosen the nipple and cause eversion.

If the patient has a breast pump available, she can use the pump to draw the nipple out before feeding. The breast pump can also be used between feedings to break adhesions within the breast tissue and loosen the nipple.

If the aforementioned techniques do not work to evert the nipple, a nipple shield can be used to help with latching the infant. The nipple shield should be used under the guidance of a lactation consultant. It is important that a proper latch be achieved with the shield, and the patient should be supported with establishing milk production.

Mastitis

Mastitis is an infection of the breast that most often occurs within the first 6 weeks after delivery. It may affect up to 20% of lactating women.[31] The diagnosis of mastitis can be made clinically when a patient presents with complaints of flulike symptoms along with a bright, triangle-shaped, red area on the breast. The redness generally moves out from the nipple and develops with an accompanying fever >101.3°F (38.5°C).

Conservative management for mastitis includes effective and frequent milk removal. The patient should be instructed to massage her breasts before and during the feeding and to massage from the clogged area of the breast toward the nipple. Anti-inflammatory analgesics such as ibuprofen may be prescribed for pain relief. If mastitis is not relieved after 12 to 24 hours of conservative management, antibiotics should be prescribed to avoid further complications. Outpatient therapy for nonsevere mastitis include dicloxacillin 500 mg orally four times daily or cephalexin 500 mg orally four times daily. In the presence of beta-lactam hypersensitivity, clindamycin 300 to 450 mg orally three times daily may be used. The length of therapy typically lasts 10 to 14 days.

Mastitis may prompt patients to cease breastfeeding. Providers should proactively provide reassurance that breastfeeding with mastitis is safe and may continue, even

with the analgesic and antibiotics prescribed. Additionally, because the most vital component of the treatment plan is the effective and frequent removal of milk, acute cessation of breastfeeding may lead to further engorgement, milk stasis, and development of an abscess.

If a well-defined hardened, erythematous area is noted on the breast, abscess should be considered as a top differential diagnosis. Depending on the clinician's experience and comfort in possible serial surgical drainage of the abscess, consider referring to a breast specialist.

Who Should Avoid Breastfeeding?

As per the CDC,[32] breastfeeding should be avoided entirely in the following circumstances:

- An infant with diagnosed galactosemia, a rare genetic metabolic disorder (newborns are tested for this condition immediately following delivery)
- A lactating patient in the following circumstances:
  - Infection with human immunodeficiency virus (HIV)
  - Infection with human T-lymphotropic virus (HTLV)
  - Taking antiretroviral medications
  - Infection with untreated, active tuberculosis
  - Using or dependent on illicit drugs
  - Taking prescribed chemotherapy agents
  - Undergoing radiation therapy; however some nuclear medicine treatments may only require short term breastfeeding cessation

Other conditions that may affect breastfeeding include active herpes lesions on the nipple or areola and cracked and bleeding nipples for hepatitis C–positive patients. In both cases, the CDC recommends emptying the breasts using a handheld or electronic pump and dumping the pumped milk (known commonly as *pump and dump*). This process allows for maintenance of the milk supply until treatment and/or healing are completed. As this short list indicates, there are very few maternal or infant conditions that result in a total contraindication of breastfeeding.

! SAFETY ALERT

Other conditions that may affect breastfeeding include active herpes lesions on the nipple/areola as well as cracked and bleeding nipples for hepatitis C–positive patients.

Medication Use During Lactation

For years, the prevailing attitude regarding medications and breastfeeding was to avoid them at all costs. The paradigm has shifted in light of a large and growing body of research surrounding the use of medications during lactation. Dr. Thomas Hale is one of the foremost researchers on the subject and maintains a website and text summarizing medication risk.[33] There is now more guidance than ever for clinicians weighing medication choices with their patients.

One of the best free resources for providers is LactMed, a site maintained by the National Institutes of Health (NIH).[34] LactMed is a database dedicated to best practice recommendations regarding medications and breastfeeding. The NIH also offers the LactMed database in the form of an easy-to-use smart phone application that can be readily accessed by providers.

CLINICAL SURVIVAL TIP: Texas Tech University's Infant Risk Center and the University of Rochester's Human Lactation Center offer hotlines for health care providers to answer questions or concerns regarding the latest recommendations and research on medication use and breastfeeding.
- Infant Risk Center—Provider Hotline: (806) 352-2519; www.infantrisk.com
- Human Lactation Center—Provider Hotline: (585) 275-0088; https://www.urmc.rochester.edu/childrenshospital/neonatology/lactation.aspx

---

It is important to remember that medications in lactation do not necessarily follow the same guidelines as medications in pregnancy. The transfer of medications into breast milk depends on many different factors. With the overwhelming evidence regarding the benefit of human milk to both infants and childbearing parents, it is prudent to carefully consider the risks and benefits of a medication before simply assuming that a patient is unable to breastfeed.

Medications enter breastmilk by crossing from the capillaries of the maternal bloodstream through the lipid bilayer of the mammary alveoli and into the milk. Although diffusion is the driving force for medication entry into human milk, the following important factors affect the amount that enters:[32]
- Lipid solubility
- pH (breastmilk is more acidic than blood)
- Molecular size
- Protein-binding capacity
- Oral bioavailability
- Half-life
- Dose

As a rule, drugs with shorter half-lives are more compatible with lactation, as they are less likely to concentrate over time in an infant. Additionally, drugs with a large molecular weight or high affinity for protein binding are more likely to have trouble crossing the lipid bilayer of the mammary alveoli and into milk.

The oral bioavailability of a drug also plays a large role. Medications present in breast milk must still be absorbed through the infant's intestinal tract. A medication that is not orally bioavailable will likely be destroyed in the infant gut before it ever reaches the infant.

The age of the infant also plays an important role in medication decisions. Premature infants are the most vulnerable to medications, while older children who are also eating solid foods are the least susceptible. Medication administration can be planned around feedings based on the half-life of the drug.

The aforementioned is admittedly a simplification of a complex process; however, the important point to remember is that medication use during pregnancy does not necessarily require cessation or avoidance of breastfeeding without further investigation of the drug's pharmacokinetics.

▌ KEY POINTS

- The postpartum period is a time of change and healing in which new patients are faced with coping with numerous changes and new demands.
- Women undergo many changes to their anatomy and physiology after giving birth and returning to a near pre-pregnancy state.
- Postpartum hemorrhage, infection, and depression are complications in the puerperium that the clinician must be able to recognize and treat or refer for treatment.
- As rates of breastfeeding increase in the United States, it is important that the clinician is well-versed in the needs of the lactating patient and can provide assistance if problems arise.
- There are very few contraindications to breastfeeding for either the lactating patient or the infant.

REFERENCES

1. Tikanen R, Gunja MZ, FitzGerald M, Zephyrin L. *Issue Briefs: Maternal Mortality and Maternity Care in the United States Compared to 10 Other Developed Countries;*

2020. https://www.commonwealthfund.org/publications/issue-briefs/2020/nov/maternal-mortality-maternity-care-us-compared-10-countries.

2. Kleppel L, Suplee PD, Stuebe AM, Bingham D. National initiatives to improve systems for postpartum care. *Matern Child Health J.* 2016;20(S1):66–70.

3. U.S. Centers for Disease Control and Prevention. *Severe Maternal Morbidity in the United States.* https://www.cdc.gov/reproductivehealth/maternalinfanthealth/severematernalmorbidity.html.

4. Hytten F. Blood volume changes in normal pregnancy. *Clin Haematol.* 1985;14(3):601–612.

5. Isley MM, Katz VL. Postpartum care and long-term health considerations. In: Gabbe SG, Niebyl JR, Simpson JL, et al., eds. *Obstetrics: Normal and Problem Pregnancies.* 7th ed. Philadelphia: Elsevier; 2016:499–516.

6. Corton MM, Leveno K, Bloom S, Hoffman B. *Williams Obstetrics.* 24th ed. New York: McGraw Hill Education; 2014.

7. Robson SC, Dunlop W, Hunter S. Haemodynamic changes during the early puerperium. *Br Med J (Clin Res Ed).* 1987;294(6579):1065.

8. Clapp JF, Capeless E. Cardiovascular function before, during, and after the first and subsequent pregnancies. *Am J Cardiol.* 1997;80(11):1469–1473.

9. Habif TP. Hair diseases. In: *Clinical Dermatology: A Color Guide to Diagnosis and Therapy.* 6th Rev. ed. Elsevier; 2016:923–959.

10. Malkud S. Telogen effluvium: a review. *J Clin Diagn Res.* 2015;9(9):WE01.

11. Alexander EK, Pearce EN, Brent GA, et al. 2017 guidelines of the American Thyroid Association for the diagnosis and management of thyroid disease during pregnancy and the postpartum. *Thyroid.* 2017;27(3):315–389.

12. Hoyert, D. L. (2022). *Maternal mortality rates in the United States,* 2020. [PDF]. https://www.cdc.gov/nchs/data/hestat/maternal-mortality/2020/E-stat-Maternal-Mortality-Rates-2022.pdf.

13. American College of Obstetricians and Gynecologists. Postpartum hemorrhage. Practice Bulletin Number 183. *Obstet Gynecol.* 2017;130(4):e168–e186.

14. American College of Obstetricians and Gynecologists. ACOG Committee Opinion No. 757: Screening for Perinatal Depression. *Obstet Gynecol.* 2018;132(5):e208–e212.

15. National Institute of Child Health and Human Development. *What Are the Benefits of Breastfeeding?*; 2017. https://www.nichd.nih.gov/health/topics/breastfeeding/conditioninfo/Pages/benefits.aspx.

16. U.S. Department of Health and Human Services. (n.d.) Healthy People 2030. *Infants: Increase the proportion of infants who are breastfed exclusively through age 6 months—MICH-15.* https://health.gov/healthypeople/objectives-and-data/browse-objectives/infants/increase-proportion-infants-who-are-breastfed-exclusively-through-age-6-months-mich-15.

17. American Academy of Pediatrics. Breastfeeding and the use of human milk. *Pediatrics.* 2012;129(3):e827–e841.

18. Centers for Disease Control and Prevention. (n.d.). *Results: Breastfeeding rates.* https://www.cdc.gov/breastfeeding/data/nis_data/results.html.

19. Pang WW, Hartmann PE. Initiation of human lactation: secretory differentiation and secretory activation. *J Mammary Gland Biol Neoplasia.* 2007;12(4):211–214.

20. Riordan J. *Breastfeeding and Human Lactation.* 5th ed. Burlington, MA: Jones & Bartlett; 2015.

21. Alekeev NP, Vladimir II, Nadez TE. Pathological breast engorgement: prediction, prevention, and resolution. *Breastfeeding Med.* 2015;10(4):203–208.

22. Neville MC, Morton J. Physiology and endocrine changes underlying human lactogenesis II. *J Nutrition.* 2001;131(11):3005S–3008S.

23. Hale TW, Hartmann PE. *Textbook of Human Lactation.* Amarillo, TX: Hale; 2007.

24. Mannel R, Martens PJ, Walker M, eds. *Core Curriculum for Lactation Consultant Practice.* 3rd ed. Burlington, MA: Jones & Bartlett; 2013.

25. Chantry CJ, Nommsen-Rivers LA, Peerson JM, Cohen RJ, Dewey KG. Excess weight loss in first-born breastfed newborns relates to maternal intrapartum fluid balance. *Pediatrics.* 2011;127(1):e171–e179.

26. Huggins K, Petok E, Mireles O. Markers of lactation insufficiency: A study of 34 mothers. In: *Current Issues in Clinical Lactation.* Jones & Bartlett; 2000:25–35.

27. Walker M. The nipple and areola in breastfeeding and lactation: Anatomy, physiology, problems and solutions. *Clinics in Human Lactation.* Vol 7. Amarillo, TX: Praeclarus Press; 2017.

28. Newman J, Pitman T. All-purpose nipple ointment. In: *Dr. Jack Newman's Guide to Breastfeeding.* Toronto: HarperCollins; 2009.

29. Scott CR. Lecithin: it isn't just for plugged milk ducts and mastitis anymore. *Midwifery Today.* 2005;76:26–27.

30. Hernandez Yenty QM, Jurgens WJFM, van Zuijlen PPM, de Vet HCW, Verhaegen PDHM. Treatment of the benign inverted nipple: A systematic review and recommendations for future therapy. *Review.* 2016;29:P82–P89.

31. Amir LH. ABM clinical protocol #4: Mastitis. *Breastfeeding Med.* 2014;9(5):239–243.

32. Centers for Disease Control and Prevention. (n.d.). *Contraindications to breastfeeding or feeding expressed milk to infants.* https://www.cdc.gov/breastfeeding/breastfeeding-special-circumstances/Contraindications-to-breastfeeding.html.

33. Hale TW, Rowe HE. *Medications and Mothers' Milk.* 17th ed. New York: Springer; 2017.

34. National Institutes of Health. *LactMed: Drugs and Lactation Database*; 2017. https://www.ncbi.nlm.nih.gov/books/NBK501922/.

9

Contraception

Stacy Selbert and Lisa L. Ferguson

OBJECTIVES

- Identify the current contraceptive methods approved for use in the United States.
- Apply the U.S. Medical Eligibility Criteria for Contraceptive Use and the identification of appropriate candidate use for a selected method.

- Utilize the tiered system approach in contraceptive method effectiveness for contraceptive counseling.
- Develop a plan for recognition and management of the side effects of contraception.
- Develop a plan of care to meet the contraceptive needs of special populations.

INTRODUCTION

The use of contraception is listed as one of the 10 great public health achievements of the 20th century.[1] Use of effective contraception allows one, especially females, to control their family planning desires while working toward their personal, educational, and career goals. This can help individuals achieve independence, equity, and be a productive member of society. In the United States, approximately 90% of individuals approve the widespread use of contraception.[2] It is estimated that greater than 99% of females 15 to 44 years of age who have ever had sexual intercourse have used at least one method of contraception, and 62% of reproductive-age females are currently using a contraceptive method.[3]

Just under one-half (45% or 2.8 million) of the 6.1 million pregnancies in the United States are unintended. In recent years, the unintended pregnancy rate has declined, although it is still higher than in many other developed nations. Of these pregnancies, 40% end in abortion.[4] Of the births resulting from these pregnancies, 68% are paid for by public insurance programs.[5] It is estimated that the total U.S. government expenditure for births and care through the first year of life is $21 billion annually. This includes prenatal care, delivery,

hospitalizations, abortions, miscarriages, and social support systems such as the Women, Infants, and Children (WIC) Nutrition Program.[5] This recent decline in unintended pregnancies may be attributed to the increasing use of long-acting reversible contraceptives (LARCs).[6] The decline is disproportionate to females with means versus those without because of cost and a lack of insurance in some populations. This can include an increase in short interpregnancy interval.[7] According to Pimental et al., if the interval between pregnancies is less than 18 months, the adverse outcome risk is increased.[9] With modern contraception availability in 2016, it is estimated that for every $1 spent on providing effective contraception, there could be a savings of $4.83 to the government.[9]

There is a need for a variety of contraceptive options. It is estimated that the average female will change her contraceptive method 3.4 times throughout her reproductive life span, which is approximately 35 years from menarche to menopause.[10] Reasons for this are numerous and include cost, access, acceptability to the user and/or partner, relationship changes, and real or perceived side effects.

As clinicians, it is our responsibility to help educate patients about contraceptive options so they can make the best decision for themselves based on their health history, lifestyle, and acceptability of the method along with the potential side effects, noncontraceptive benefits, and individual psychological and social factors. Despite the reason for the current office visit, the clinician may ascertain what measures male and female patients are taking to prevent an unintended pregnancy and achieve their personal reproductive life plan. The following questions may be asked at each visit:

- What method of contraception are you using?
- Are you satisfied with this method?
- If not, are you aware of your contraceptive choices?

NOT TO BE MISSED

The best contraceptive for any couple is the one they use correctly and consistently and one that is acceptable to both individuals in the relationship.

OVERVIEW OF CONTRACEPTION

The goal of contraception is to prevent the oocyte and sperm from uniting, resulting in fertilization. This can be accomplished in several ways: hormonally, mechanically, and behaviorally. Hormonal contraception can be oral, intramuscular, intrauterine, vaginal ring, subdermal implant, or transdermal patch. Mechanical contraception is accomplished via use of barriers that prevent the egg and sperm from meeting. Behavioral contraception is via avoidance of times of higher fertility or withdrawal of the penis before ejaculation. No method of contraception is 100% effective except for abstinence. However, some methods are more effective than others. Effectiveness of a method is determined by measuring the number of unplanned pregnancies that occur during a specified period of exposure and use of a contraceptive method.[11] Only 5% of unintended pregnancies result from consistent use of contraception. The other 95% are from inconsistent use or no use.[13] The effectiveness (or efficacy) of a method is how well it works to produce a desired result when the method is used exactly as prescribed, without accounting for user error (Fig. 9.1).

When discussing contraceptive options, it is recommended that methods are presented in order of effectiveness with the most effective methods being first and then proceeding in descending order to the least effective.[12] Based on the World Health Organization (WHO), the methods can be presented in tiers (see Fig. 9.1). This

is how the method information will be presented going forward in this chapter.

CLINICAL SURVIVAL TIP The Reproductive Health National Training Center provides resources for educating the clinician in family planning and adolescent/women's health issues. Visit rhntc.org for information on their resources.

When discussing contraceptive options, multiple models exist to guide the clinician. These models range along a spectrum from nondirective (in which the patient is counseled about various options without any opinion or influence from the provider) to directive (in which the patient is counseled about contraception according to provider preference such as ranked tiers in order of efficacy).[14] The shared decision-making model values both the provider and the patient as experts. The provider is the clinical expert, while the patient is the expert in his or her values, preferences, and experiences.

PATIENT-CENTERED CARE The shared decision-making model provides a patient-centered approach to choosing which contraception is right for the patient.

Knowledge is key. The way in which information is presented can determine how that information is used and retained. Contraceptive counseling is important to the patient's ability to choose and succeed in the use of their contraceptive method. This should begin with establishing rapport. Studies have shown that a warm welcome conveying a sincere open and inviting rapport at the start of the visit is related to continuation of the chosen contraceptive method.[17] Next, discover whether the patient has a need for this counseling. Simply ask if the patient if she would like to discuss contraception or prevention of pregnancy at this visit. This question may open an opportunity for preconception counseling, discussed further in Chapter 6. Once the need for contraception has been established, assess the patient's medical history (discussed later) for potential contraindications or the need to address the safety of some methods during counseling. The process of method selection can now begin. Box 9.1 provides critical components of effective counseling within the shared decision-making

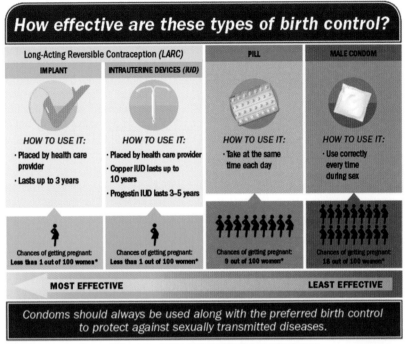

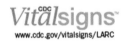

Figure 9.1 The order of effectiveness of contraception. (From Trussell J., Contraception, May 2011; www. cdc.gov/reproductivehealth/UnintendedPregnancy/Contraception.htm.)

BOX 9.1 **Stages of Contraceptive Counseling in Shared Decision Making**

- Begin the conversation. Using questions that relate that the patient's decisions will be respected.
- Assist in identifying preferences.
- Discuss the characteristics of methods of contraception.
- Facilitate decision making.
- Select the method.

Modified from Dehlendorf C. *Contraception: Counseling and Selection.* UpToDate; 2022. https://www.uptodate.com/contents/contraception-counseling-and-selection?search=https:%2F%2Fwww.uptodate.com%2Fcontents%2Fcontraception-counseling-and-selection&source=search_result&selectedTitle=1~150&usage_type=default&display_rank=1.

model for choosing a contraceptive method. Ideally, a patient should leave an appointment with her contraceptive method of choice. If she cannot get her method of choice the same day, a bridge method should be given until her method of choice can be provided.

FOCUSED HISTORY AND PHYSICAL EXAMINATION

To provide contraception in a safe manner, a focused medical history and physical examination should be done. Part of the history collection is conducting a sexual health assessment. There are **"five P's"** that can be gathered:[12]

- **Practices:** the type of sexual activity the patient is engaging in (vaginal, anal, or oral sex).
- **Pregnancy prevention:** past and current contraceptives use, when was the last act of intercourse and was protection used, and what contraceptive method the patient is interested in.
- **Partners:** number and gender of partners.
- **Protection from sexually transmitted infections (STIs):** condom use and whether there are partners for whom condoms are used and partners for whom condoms are not used.
- **Past STI history:** patient and partner's history of STIs. This is a good opportunity to inform that if

TABLE 9.1[14]   Recommendations for History and Assessment by Method

Method	History	Assessment
IUDs	Liver disease, breast cancer, cervical dysplasia	Date of LMP, bimanual examination, and cervical inspection. If screening for sexually transmitted infections has not been performed per screening guidelines, it can be done at the time of insertion. Baseline weight and BMI can be helpful for monitoring users over time but are not required.
Implant	Liver disease, breast cancer	Date of LMP. No physical examination needed. Baseline weight and BMI can be helpful for monitoring users over time but are not required.
Combined hormonal contraception	Medical conditions: hypertension, hyperlipidemia, diabetes, seizure disorder, history of venous thrombus embolus, breast cancer, cervical cancer, ovarian cancer, endometrial cancer, liver disease, migraine headache, smoking status, and age	Blood pressure is required. Baseline weight and BMI can be helpful for monitoring users over time but are not required.
Injectables	Hypertension, hyperlipidemia, diabetes	No physical examination needed. Baseline weight and BMI can be helpful for monitoring users over time but are not required.
Progestin-only contraception	Hypertension, hyperlipidemia, diabetes	IUD: bimanual examination and cervical inspection
Barrier methods: diaphragm, cervical cap		Bimanual examination and cervical inspection

BMI, Body mass index; *IUD,* intrauterine device; *LMP,* last menstrual period.

there is a past history of an STI, there is a higher likelihood of one in the future.

There are few physical assessments that need to be made.[13] The only time a pelvic examination is needed before contraceptive initiation is with an intrauterine device (IUD) insertion. Blood pressure measurement is required before starting combined hormonal contraception.[12] Table 9.1 shows the information needed before you can prescribe methods of contraception.

Next, medical eligibility for a method should be determined. The *U.S. Medical Eligibility Criteria for Contraceptive Use (U.S. MEC),* an evidence-based report, guides clinicians in determining the safety of a method both for initiation and continuation of use. Various criteria including medical conditions and medication use are listed. There are many modalities to access this report: printed, electronic, and apps for Android and iOS along with quick reference charts that are colored-coded.[14] The *U.S. MEC* full report, which offers these modalities

can be found at https://www.cdc.gov/reproductivehealth/contraception/mmwr/mec/summary.html. Table 9.2 provides information on this guide.

> **CLINICAL SURVIVAL TIP** A summary table of the U.S. MEC can be found at https://www.cdc.gov/reproductivehealth/contraception/pdf/summary-chart-us-medical-eligibility-criteria_508tagged.pdf.

METHODS OF CONTRACEPTION

See Figure 9.1 for an overview of the methods of contraception.

Tier 1 Methods

Tier 1 methods include the following reversible and nonreversible devices:
Reversible: contraceptive implant and IUDs (LARCs)
- Nexplanon: a progestin-only single implant
- Paragard T380A: a non-hormonal, copper IUD

Category	Recommendation
MEC 1	Indicates a condition for which no restrictions exist for use of the contraceptive method.
MEC 2	Indicates a condition for which the advantages of using the method generally outweigh the theoretical or proven risk; generally can be used, although careful follow-up might be required.
MEC 3	Indicates a condition for which the risks, proven or theoretical, of using the method outweigh the advantages; generally can be used, although careful follow-up might be required.
MEC 4	Indicates the conditions that represent an unacceptable health risk if the method is used.

TABLE 9.2[13,14] **Categories of Medical Eligibility Recommendation**

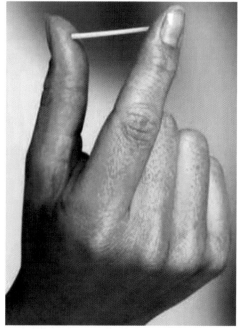

Figure 9.2 Nexplanon device. (From Melmed S, Polonsky KS, Larsen PR, Kronenberg H. *Williams Textbook of Endocrinology.* 13th ed. Philadelphia: Elsevier; 2016.)

- Kyleena: A 19.5-mg levonorgestrel IUD
- Liletta: A 52-mg levonorgestrel IUD
- Mirena: A 52-mg levonorgestrel IUD
- Skyla: A 13.5-mg levonorgestrel IUD

Nonreversible: permanent sterilization.

The effective rate is the same (<1% failure rates) for both the reversible and nonreversible methods.

LARCs

There are many advantages to the LARC methods. After insertion, LARCs require no user responsibility. They are effective for at least 3 to 10 years depending on the particular method. They are cost-effective. LARC benefits are so great that several professional societies and government entities, including the American College of Obstetricians and Gynecologists (ACOG), the U.S. Centers for Disease Control and Prevention (CDC), the National Association of Nurse Practitioners in Women's Health (NPWH), and the American Academy of Pediatrics (AAP) recommend these as first-line methods for all females regardless of parity and age.[13,14,16,19] Despite these recommendations, current use of LARCs in the United States is low and is estimated to be 18%. This is up from 2.4% in 2002.[20] Some of the barriers to use have been high up-front cost and untrained or misinformed providers, leading to issues with access and lack of patient knowledge of these methods. Among females who are given many different contraceptive choices without cost being a problem, 67% of would chose a LARC method.[6]

Implant. Nexplanon, a progestin-only subdermal contraceptive implant, is the only contraceptive implant currently approved for use in the United States. It does not contain estrogen. It consists of a single, radiopaque, rod-shaped implant containing 68 mg of etonogestrel placed under the skin of the medial upper arm. At 4 cm long, Nexplanon is approximately the size of a matchstick and is latex free (Fig. 9.2).

The mechanisms of action include suppression of ovulation, increased viscosity of the cervical mucus, and alterations within the endometrium. It is considered the most effective reversible contraceptive available, with a typical use failure rate of 0.1%. Nexplanon is effective for at least 3 years. Fertility return is considered to be rapid following implant removal, which can be done at any time before the end of the third year of use. It may be immediately replaced by a new implant at the time of removal if continued contraceptive protection is desired.[20]

Insertion and removal are considered to be simple, in-office procedures. A clinician must obtain training in the insertion and removal procedures by the manufacturer. To inquire about training, contact the company.[20]

Nexplanon's most common side effect is irregular bleeding caused by atrophy of the endometrium. It is usually transient and lasts no more than 90 days. However, some patients experience frequent bleeding, leading them to discontinue use. Nexplanon is contraindicated in patients using CYP3A-inhibiting or CYP3A-inducing medications, as it can decrease the effectiveness of the implant or decrease the effectiveness of the concurrently using medications.

Intrauterine Devices. IUDs are one of the most common contraceptive methods used worldwide. The failure rate is <1% after 1 year. Use in the United States has been gaining popularity in the past decade. Currently, there is one non-hormonal IUD and four hormonal IUDs on the market. The newer IUDs are on a *T*-shaped frame with a monofilament string. This design has proven to be much safer than the IUDs used in the late 1960s and 1970s (Fig. 9.3).

Recent studies have shown that IUD use does not increase the rate of pelvic inflammatory disease (PID) or tubal occlusion that could result in infertility and chronic pelvic pain.[13] There are many modalities to be trained in the insertion and removal of an IUD. Manufacturers have provided detailed written, graphic, and multimedia presentations.[21-25] Training is also offered at continuing education venues. Trusted mentors and academic centers are other ways to gain training.

Copper Intrauterine Devices. The non-hormonal IUD is known as the *Copper-T 380A* or *Paragard*. It is a latex-free, polyethylene, *T*-shaped device wrapped in copper wire. It is approved for at least 10 years of use, although there is evidence of effectiveness for 12 years.[16] Given the extended time frame of use and cost, it is the cheapest prescriptive method. Copper ions that act as a natural spermicide are released and cause an inflammatory change of the endometrium. The mechanisms of action are thought to be interference with sperm transport, thus decreasing fertilization and preventing implantation. It is immediately effective for contraception after placement. Given that this not a hormonal method, the patient should expect a monthly menses. Use of the Paragard can result in a longer, heavier, and potentially more painful menses.[21] However, use of nonsteroidal anti-inflammatory drugs (NSAIDs) during this time often alleviates these symptoms.

Hormonal IUDs. There are four hormonal IUDs containing a levonorgestrel reservoir on a *T*-shaped frame. They vary depending on amount of levonorgestrel, size of frame, diameter of insertion tube, and approved duration of use (Table 9.3). They are approved for 3 to 5 years of use. There is evidence that the 52-mg levonorgestrel-containing IUDs may be effective for 7 years of use.[16] The mechanism of action includes thickening of cervical mucous, endometrial lining changes, and inhibition of sperm survival. Ovulation is sometimes suppressed but can also occur. Irregular bleeding is the most common side effect, especially during the first 3 to 6 months. It is usually light but can be persistent. However, amenorrhea rates increase thereafter, making this a desired noncontraceptive benefit for many users. In addition, the levonorgestrel IUDs can help with menorrhagia, dysmenorrhea, and protection of the endometrium from unopposed estrogen. Ovarian cysts >3 cm can occur, however they usually resolve spontaneously.

Long-Acting Reversible Contraceptive Initiation. Same-day LARC insertion is preferred. This means that when a patient chooses either an IUD or implant, all efforts should be made for the patient to receive their LARC method before leaving that appointment. When a patient must return to the office for a contraceptive method, this presents an increased inconvenience that may result in loss of work time, transportation issues, and childcare issues, decreasing the likelihood that she will return and possibly conceiving during that time.[26]

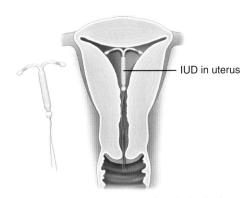

IUD in uterus

Figure 9.3 Placement of an intrauterine device in the uterus. (From LaFleur DS, LaFleur-Brooks M, Levinsky D. *Exploring Medical Language: A Student-Directed Approach.* St. Louis: Elsevier; 2022.)

TABLE 9.3 [17,21-25] **Comparison of Intrauterine Devices**

Brand Name	TCu-38A	LNG IUD	LNG IUD	LNG IUD	LNG IUD
	ParaGard	*Mirena*	*Liletta*	*Kyleena*	*Skyla*
Description	T-shaped polyethylene frame with approximately 176 mg of copper wire coiled along the vertical stem and a 68.7-mg collar on each side of the horizontal arm	T-shaped polyethylene frame with a steroid reservoir containing 52 mg of LNG; releases approximately 20 mcg per day, decreasing to one-half of this value after 5 years	T-shaped polyethylene frame with a drug reservoir containing 52 mg of LNG packaged within a sterile inserter; releases approximately 18.6 mcg per day, decreasing to 12.6 mcg per day at 3 years	T-shaped polyethylene frame with a steroid reservoir containing 19.5 mg of LNG; releases approximately 17.5 mcg per day, decreasing to 7.4 mcg per day after 5 years	T-shaped polyethylene frame with a steroid reservoir containing a total of 13.5 mg of LNG; releases approximately 14 mcg per day after 25 days, decreasing to 5 mcg per day after 3 years
Duration of approved use	10 years	5 years	4 years (study ongoing)	5 years	3 years
Efficacy	>99%	>99%	>99%	>99%	>99%
Size of device	32 mm horizontally and 36 mm vertically	32 mm both horizontally and vertically	32 mm both horizontally and vertically	28 mm horizontally and 30 mm vertically	28 mm horizontally and 30 vertically
Diameter of insertion tube	3.65 mm	4.4 mm	4.5 mm	3.8 mm	3.8 mm
Color of removal threads	White	Brown	Royal blue	Blue	Brown
Most common side effects	Menstrual bleeding alterations (heavier and longer periods) Cramping after insertion and/or during periods Painful sexual intercourse Urticarial allergic skin reaction Vaginitis Device expulsion	Menstrual bleeding alterations (spotting and lighter periods) Cramping after insertion Abdominal or pelvic pain Ovarian cysts Headache or migraine Acne Depressed or altered mood Device expulsion	Menstrual bleeding alterations (spotting and lighter periods) Cramping after insertion Abdominal or pelvic pain Ovarian cysts Headache or migraine Acne Depressed or altered mood Device expulsion Vaginal/vulvovaginal infection	Menstrual bleeding alterations (spotting and lighter periods) Cramping after insertion or during periods Vulvovaginitis Abdominal or pelvic pain Acne or seborrhea Ovarian cysts Headache Nausea Device expulsion	Menstrual bleeding alterations (spotting and lighter periods) Cramping after insertion or during periods Vulvovaginitis Abdominal or pelvic pain Acne or seborrhea Ovarian cyst Headache Nausea Device expulsion

Continued

TABLE 9.3[17,21-25]   **Comparison of Intrauterine Devices—cont'd**

	TCu-38A	LNG IUD	LNG IUD	LNG IUD
Effect on bleeding patterns	Often, increased amount and duration of bleeding; approximately 50% increase in blood loss	Unpredictable, with frequent light bleeding for the first 3 months. By 3 to 6 months, usually dramatically reduced bleeding. Amenorrhea in about one-third of users after 12 months	During first 3 to 6 months, bleeding and spotting may increase, and bleeding may be irregular. Thereafter, the amount of bleeding and spotting decreases, but bleeding may remain irregular.	Spotting and irregular or heavy bleeding during the first 3 to 6 months. By 3 months, periods may be shorter, lighter, or both. Cycles may remain irregular, become infrequent, or cease.
Special benefits	Can be used as emergency contraception; prevents pregnancy when inserted up to 5 days after unprotected intercourse. Contains no hormones; a good contraceptive choice for female patients who cannot or prefer not to use estrogen. Can use while breastfeeding. No pill to take daily	Budget-friendly. Can use while breast-feeding. No pill to take daily. May reduce period cramps and make period lighter. Good contraceptive choice for female patients who cannot or prefer not to use estrogen	Can use while breast-feeding. No pill to take daily. May reduce period cramps and make period lighter. Good contraceptive choice for female patients who cannot or prefer not to use estrogen	Can use while breast-feeding. No pill to take daily. May reduce period cramps and make period lighter. Good contraceptive choice for female patients who cannot or prefer not to use estrogen

See product labeling for a full description of contraindications and other prescribing information. (Liletta inserter diameter, Bob Starr, Medicines360, Personal Communication, November 2016.)

LNG, Levonorgestrel; *TCu-38A*, Copper-T 380A.

PATIENT-CENTERED CARE A LARC can be started on the day the patient chooses this option, as long as pregnancy can be ruled out through a urine or serum hCG level, preventing the need to return to the office to begin contraception.

A LARC method can be inserted at any time in the menstrual cycle when a pregnancy can be reasonably ruled out (Table 9.4).

If pregnancy cannot be ruled out, the patient should be bridged with another method and an appointment scheduled for insertion after 2 to 4 weeks and negative urine pregnancy test results[13] (Fig. 9.4). There is no need to wait for the onset of menses. IUD insertion at the time of menses is not associated with ease of placement.

NOT TO BE MISSED

The following are relative and absolute contraindications with LARC use.

Absolute contraindications for LARC initiation:[14]
- IUDs
  - Currently pregnant
  - Current purulent cervicitis, gonorrhea or chlamydia

TABLE 9.4 When to Start Using Specific Contraceptive Methods

Contraceptive Method	When to Start (if Provider Is Reasonably Certain That the Patient Is Not Pregnant)	Additional Contraception (Backup) Needed	Examinations or Tests Needed Before Initiation[1]
Copper-containing IUD	Anytime	Not needed	Bimanual examination and cervical inspection[2]
Levonorgestrel-releasing IUD	Anytime	If >7 days after menses started, use backup method, or abstain for 7 days.	Bimanual examination and cervical inspection[2]
Implant	Anytime	If >5 days after menses started, use backup method, or abstain for 7 days.	None
Injectable	Anytime	If >7 days after menses started, use backup method, or abstain for 7 days.	None
Combined hormonal contraceptive	Anytime	If >5 days after menses started, use backup method, or abstain for 7 days.	Blood pressure measurement
Progestin-only pill	Anytime	If >5 days after menses started, use backup method, or abstain for 2 days.	None

[1]Weight (BMI) measurement is not needed to determine medical eligibility (or any method of contraception because all methods can be used or generally can be used among obese female patients. However, measuring weight and calculating BMI at baseline might be helpful for monitoring any changes and counseling women who might be concerned about weight change perceived to be associated with their contraceptive method.

[2]Most women do not require additional STD screening at the time of IUD insertion if they have already been screened according to the CDC's STD Treatment Guidelines (http://www.cdc.gov/std/treatment). If a patient has not been screened according to guidelines, screening can be performed at the time of IUD insertion, and insertion should not be delayed. Patients with purulent cervicitis, current chlamydial infection, or gonorrhea should not undergo IUD insertion. Patients who have a very high individual likelihood of STD exposure (e.g, those with a currently infected partner) generally should not undergo IUD insertion. For these patients, IUD insertion should be delayed until appropriate testing and treatment occurs.

BMI, Body mass index; IUD, intrauterine device; STD, sexually transmitted disease.

Modified from Centers for Disease Control and Prevention. Appendix B: When To Start Using Specific Contraceptive Methods. Recommendations and Reports. 2013;62(RR05);55–55. https://www.cdc.gov/mmwr/preview/mmwrhtml/rr6205a3.htm

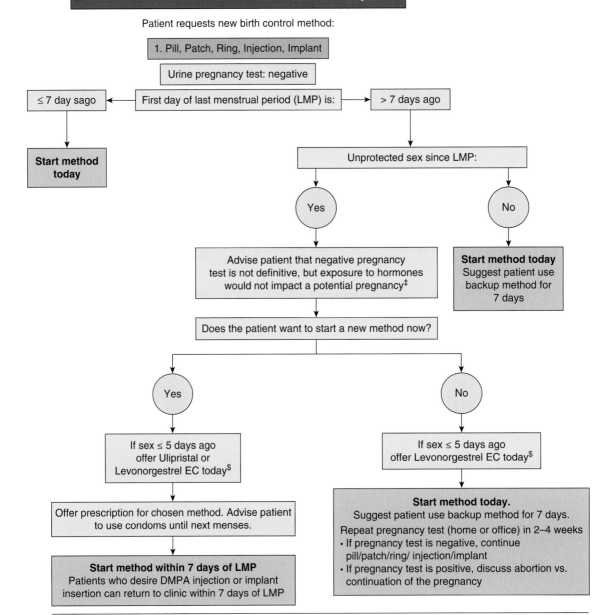

QUICK START ALGORITHM for hormonal contraception‡

Patient requests new birth control method:

1. Pill, Patch, Ring, Injection, Implant

Urine pregnancy test: negative

≤ 7 day sago ← First day of last menstrual period (LMP) is: → > 7 days ago

Start method today

Unprotected sex since LMP:

Yes / No

Advise patient that negative pregnancy test is not definitive, but exposure to hormones would not impact a potential pregnancy‡

Start method today Suggest patient use backup method for 7 days

Does the patient want to start a new method now?

Yes / No

If sex ≤ 5 days ago offer Ulipristal or Levonorgestrel EC today$

If sex ≤ 5 days ago offer Levonorgestrel EC today$

Offer prescription for chosen method. Advise patient to use condoms until next menses.

Start method today. Suggest patient use backup method for 7 days. Repeat pregnancy test (home or office) in 2–4 weeks
• If pregnancy test is negative, continue pill/patch/ring/ injection/implant
• If pregnancy test is positive, discuss abortion vs. continuation of the pregnancy

Start method within 7 days of LMP Patients who desire DMPA injection or implant insertion can return to clinic within 7 days of LMP

‡ Based on select practice recommendations – Benefits of starting contraceptive likely exceed risk of early pregnancy.
$ Patients should wait 5 days after taking Ullipristal before starting a hormonal method. It is not recommended for quick start.

 RHEDI

Figure 9.4 Quick start guide for starting contraception. (From Rhedi. *Quick Start Algorithms.* [n.d.]. https://rhedi.org/quick-start-algorithms/.)

- PID within the past 3 months
- Postpartum or postabortion sepsis within the past 3 months
- Unexplained vaginal bleeding
- Current breast, cervical, or endometrial cancer
- Distorted uterine cavity
- Recent gestational trophoblastic disease with persistent β-HcG levels
- Wilson's disease (for the Cu-IUD)
- Subdermal contraceptive implant initiation:
  - Currently pregnant
  - Current breast cancer

Aseptic technique is key with IUD placement to decrease overall infection occurrence. The risk of PID is greatest in the first 20 days after insertion.[13] If cervicitis is noted at the time of placement, IUD insertion should be withheld and cervicitis treatment initiated. Screening for gonorrhea and chlamydia can occur at the time of placement based on CDC recommendations. Patients can be offered oral NSAIDs before insertion to help with post-insertion cramping, although there is no evidence that it helps to decrease pain with insertion, Perforation of the uterus is a potential complication and thought to occur in 1 in 1000 insertions. This can necessitate surgery.

After insertion, it is recommended that the patient return for a string check to determine possible partial or complete expulsion. Expulsion rates are highest within the first month of placement, although the overall expulsion rate is very low, ranging from 3% to 11%.[19,27] The post-insertion string check is also an opportunity to address questions or concerns and to review warning signs of when the patient needs to report problems with the use of the IUD. Patients can check for the presence of the strings if comfortable, otherwise, it can be done by a provider at the annual well-woman examination. If strings are not easily visualized, a cytobrush at the endocervix gently rotated can help expose IUD strings that can curl into the os. If that technique is unsuccessful, then an ultrasound should be obtained to confirm fundal placement. If still not seen, an x-ray of the pelvis can determine if it is in the body, but it does not verify correct placement. If it is determined that the IUD is present but no longer in the correct place, it should be removed to prevent further complications and possible pregnancy.

Although IUDs are highly effective in preventing pregnancy, it can still occur. If so, the location of the pregnancy should be determined by a transvaginal and pelvic ultrasound. There is a higher incidence of ectopic pregnancy with IUD use than without, remembering the overall pregnancy rate is <1%.[13] If an intrauterine pregnancy is diagnosed, the IUD should be removed as soon as possible within the first trimester. Leaving the IUD in place increases the risk of spontaneous and septic abortion.

> **CLINICAL SURVIVAL TIP** If strings are not easily visualized, a cytobrush at the endocervix gently rotated can help expose IUD strings that can curl into the os.

Sterilization

Female Sterilization. Female sterilization is the second most common method of contraception used in the United States. Female patients who are finished with childbearing are appropriate candidates. There is no age requirement. However, for public health programs such as Medicaid, the minimum age is 21. Also, consents may need to be signed for at least 30 days before the procedure is performed, and the patient may need to be reconsented if greater than 90 days has lapsed since the initial consent was obtained. Female sterilization is considered a permanent method, although there are reports of reversal, though with low success rates. There are several techniques to accomplish sterilization. Most involve some form of a segment of fallopian tube being removed and closure of the remaining tube ends by cautery or clips. This can occur immediately after a caesarean delivery or other abdominal surgery. It can also occur via laparotomy or laparoscopy. Tubal occlusion techniques have been utilized via hysteroscopy.

Male Sterilization. Male sterilization is known as *vasectomy*. The vas deferens is clipped, cut, or tied to interrupt passage from the testicle. It is less invasive than female sterilization and usually performed in an outpatient setting. It is considered permanent. However, it does have a higher rate of reversal than that of female sterilization. A 3-month follow-up is needed to ensure that the semen no longer contains sperm. Thus couples must use an alternative form of contraception until clearance is given by a clinician.

Tier 2 Methods

These methods are highly effective (>99.1%) with perfect use. However, more user responsibility is required. Thus the overall effectiveness rates are lower, at approximately 91% to 93% on average or 7 to 9 pregnancies per 100 females in a year.[31] These methods are also known as *refillables* and include contraceptive pills, the patch, the ring, and injectables. Depending on the method, they are used daily, weekly, monthly, or every 3 months. They can contain some combination of estrogen and/or a progesterone.

Progesterone mechanisms of action include suppression of luteinizing hormone (which suppresses ovulation), thickening of cervical mucous, and alteration of fallopian tube peristalsis, which inhibits sperm movement and thinning of the endometrial lining. Estrogen mechanisms of action include suppression of follicle-stimulating hormone (FSH) and maturation of a follicle as well as potentiation of the progesterone effect. Estrogen helps decrease irregular bleeding that can be caused by progesterone. Return to fertility is quickly achieved with discontinuation of use. There can be some risk associated with the use of estrogen-containing methods, such as venous thromboembolism (VTE), but they are safer than a pregnancy and the risks it can bring.[28] There are also many non-contraceptive benefits including oligomenorrhea, amenorrhea, relief of dysmenorrhea, decrease in acne, and protection against ovarian and endometrial cancers, bone loss, PID, and fibrocystic breast disease. A 1-year supply (up to 13 cycles) should be prescribed.[13,18] Off-label extended-cycle use for continuous contraceptive coverage can also be utilized. This will eliminate a scheduled withdrawal bleed for users.

Combined Oral Contraceptives

Combined oral contraceptives (COCs) contain both progesterone and estrogen in various dosage formulations in order to help minimize side effects and potential risks. Progestins used include norethindrone, levonorgestrel, norgestrel, desogestrel, drospirenone, norgestimate, ethynodiol diacetate, and dienogest. Two types of estrogen are currently approved for use: ethinyl estradiol and estradiol valerate (Table 9.5). They are packaged in several different dosing sequences. The most common is 21 days of hormone-containing tablets followed by 7 placebo tablets. Other formulations include 24 days of active pills followed by 4 placebo tablets and extended-cycle use containing eight-four active pills followed by 7 placebo tablets. Extended-cycle oral contraceptives can

TABLE 9.5[13]   Differences in Estrogen Doses

µcg of Ethinyl Estradiol	Benefits	Concerns
≥50	Cycle control/high efficacy	↑ VTE/EE side effects
30/35	Cycle control/high efficacy	EE side effects/↓ side effects
20	↓ EE side effects/ high efficacy	↑ Breakthrough bleeding, spotting

be desirable to help decrease the frequency of bleeding episodes. Oral contraceptives must be taken at the same time daily to maximize effectiveness. Ideally, a 1-year supply of pills should be authorized at the visit. Common side effects include nausea, breast tenderness, and irregular bleeding, which may resolve after the first 2 to 3 months of use.

Timing recommendations are as follows:[13]

- Combined hormonal contraceptives can be initiated at any time if it is reasonably certain that the patient is not pregnant (validated through urine or serum hCG level before initiation of COCs)
- A dose is considered late when <24 hours have elapsed since the dose should have been taken.
- A dose is considered missed if ≥24 hours have elapsed since the dose should have been taken.

Backup contraception recommendations are as follows:[13]

- If combined hormonal contraceptives are started within the first 5 days since menstrual bleeding started, no additional contraceptive protection is needed.
- If combined hormonal contraceptives are started >5 days since menstrual bleeding started, the patient must abstain from sexual intercourse or use additional contraceptive protection for the next 7 days.

Progesterone-Only Oral Contraceptives

Progesterone-only pills (POPs) are an alternative method for patients in whom COCs are contraindicated. They contain 28 days of 0.35-mg of norethindrone only.

Another name for POPs is the *mini-pill.* No placebo tablets are needed. A tablet is taken at the same time daily, and they are even more time-sensitive than COCs. There is no scheduled withdrawal bleed; however, many patients will experience vaginal bleeding with POP use.

Timing recommendations are as follows:

- POPs can be started at any time if it is reasonably certain that the patient is not pregnant (must be validated as previously discussed)

Backup contraception recommendations are as follows:[13]

- If POPs are started within the first 5 days since menstrual bleeding started, no additional contraceptive protection is needed.
- If POPs are started >5 days since menstrual bleeding started, the patient must abstain from sexual intercourse or use additional contraceptive protection for the next 2 days.

A dose is considered missed if it has been >3 hours since it should have been taken.[13]

- Take one pill as soon as possible.
- Continue taking pills daily, one each day, at the same time each day, even if it means taking two pills on the same day.
- Use backup contraception (e.g., condoms), or avoid sexual intercourse until pills have been taken correctly on time for 2 consecutive days.
- Emergency contraception (EC) should be considered (with the exception of ulipristal acetate (UPA) if the patient has had unprotected sexual intercourse.

Vaginal Ring

There is one contraceptive ring available in the United States. The NuvaRing became available in 2001. It is a flexible, clear ring containing a combination of etonogestrel and ethinyl estradiol (Fig. 9.5). The ring is placed into the vagina for 3 weeks and then removed for 1 week and disposed of. A new ring is placed 7 days after removal, and the cycle is repeated. There is enough hormone for 28 days of protection if it is not removed per the 21-day package instructions. Therefore the patient only needs to think about it monthly. However, a good practice would be to check for its presence after intercourse. The most common side effects can include vaginal tissue irritation, headache, and mood changes.

If the NuvaRing is out of the vagina for more than 3 continuous hours:

- During weeks 1 and 2: Contraceptive efficacy may be reduced. The patient should reinsert the ring as soon as she remembers. A barrier method such as condoms with spermicide must be used until the ring has been used continuously for 7 days.
- During week 3: The patient should discard this ring. One of the following two options should be chosen:
  - Insert a new ring immediately. Inserting a new ring will start the next 3-week use period. The patient may not experience a withdrawal bleed from her previous cycle. However, breakthrough spotting or bleeding may occur.
  - Insert a new ring no later than 7 days from the time the previous ring was removed or expelled, during which time the patient may have a withdrawal bleed. This option should only be chosen if the ring was used continuously for at least 7 days before inadvertent removal/expulsion.

In either case, a barrier method such as condoms with spermicides must be used until the new ring has been used continuously for 7 days.[29]

Patch

A transdermal contraceptive method is also an option (Fig. 9.6). It is a combination of norelgestromin and ethinyl estradiol. It is used for a 28-day cycle and is changed weekly for 3 weeks. Week 4 is a patch-free week. Then a new patch is placed, and the cycle is repeated. The patch can be placed on the outer arm, lower abdomen, or buttocks. There may be a decrease in contraceptive effectiveness in females greater than 198 pounds, and these patients must be counseled appropriately. There is also a "black box" warning regarding an increased risk of VTE in females with a BMI greater than or equal to 30 kg/m^2 and serious cardiovascular events in females older than 35 years of age who smoke with use. Per the package insert, estrogen exposure is approximately 60% higher than a typical 35-mcg COC. The most common side effects include breast symptoms; headache; nausea and vomiting; dysmenorrhea; vaginal bleeding; mood, affect, and anxiety disorders; and application site irritation.[30]

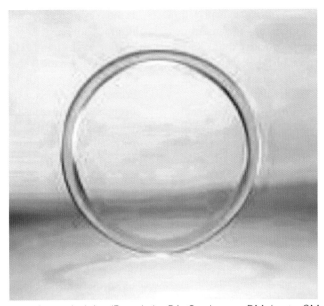

Figure 9.5 The contraceptive vaginal ring (From Lobo RA, Gershenson DM, Lentz, GM, Valea FA. *Comprehensive Gynecology.* 7th ed. Philadelphia: Elsevier; 2017.)

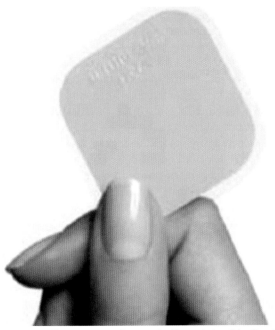

Figure 9.6 The contraceptive patch. (From Lobo RA, Gershenson DM, Lentz, GM, Valea FA. *Comprehensive Gynecology.* 7th ed. Philadelphia: Elsevier; 2017.)

If the patch has been off or partially off, recommendations are as follows:

- For less than 1 day, it should be reapplied. If the patch does not adhere completely, the patient should apply a new patch immediately. (No backup contraception is needed, and the patch-change day will stay the same.)
- For more than 1 day or if the patient is not sure for how long, the patient may not be protected from pregnancy. To reduce this risk, the patient should apply a new patch immediately and start a new 4-week cycle. The patient will have a new patch-change day and must use a non-hormonal backup method for the first 7 days.[30]

> **! SAFETY ALERT**
>
> The transdermal contraceptive patch contains a black-box warning that this form of contraception is contraindicated in females with a BMI greater than or equal to 30 kg/m² and females older than 35 years of age who smoke (because of increased risk of VTE).

Injectable

There are two available injectables. Both contain depo-medroxyprogesterone acetate (DMPA). One formulation is 150 mg given intramuscularly, and the other is 104 mg given subcutaneously. The interval between injections is the same: every 3 months or 11 to 13 weeks. There is a bolus effect, which then slowly decreases. There can be some reversible bone loss associated with long-term use >2 years. However, it is not recommended that bone density screenings routinely be ordered. Therefore it is not recommended for use longer than 2 years unless there are no alternative methods available. There are reports of a delay in return to fertility up to 1 year and in rare cases up to 3 years. The most common side effects include dysfunctional uterine bleeding, headache, amenorrhea, injection site reactions, and weight gain. Bleeding can improve, and many users become amenorrheic.[31]

Generic Products

Many contraceptives have generic formulations. Most of the time, patients tolerate the generic versions without side effects. Generic formulations may have a significantly lower cost. It is recommended that the clinician check with local pharmacies to learn cash prices. Some offer a limited formulary for $9 per month.

Drug-Drug Interactions

Interactions between the contraceptive method and other medications or supplements can occur. This can lead to a difference in the amount of drug the patient receives and may require a dose adjustment. This applies especially to some antiretrovirals, anticonvulsants, antimicrobials, and psychotropic medications.[14,32] Boxes 9.2 and 9.3 list the drugs that can cause interaction and may require a dose adjustment. Refer to the *US MEC* for a complete explanation.

Tier 3 Methods

Tier 3 methods are attainable without a health care provider's authorization. These methods are the least effective. The pregnancy rate is 18 or more per 100 females per year.[13]

BOX 9.2   Drug Interactions Requiring an Increase in Estrogen Dose[32]

Cytochrome P450 3A4 (CYP3A4) enzyme inducers decrease the effectiveness of estrogen and progesterone, thus decreasing contraceptive effectiveness. Consider increasing the contraceptive dose to at least 30 mcg of estrogen.
- Aminoglutethimide
- Barbiturates
- Bexarotene
- Bosentan
- Carbamazepine
- Dexamethasone
- Efavirenz
- Ethosuximide
- Felbamate
- Fosphenytoin
- Griseofulvin
- Modafinil
- Nafcillin
- Nevirapine
- Oxcarbazepine
- Phenobarbital
- Phenytoin
- Primidone
- Rifabutin
- Rifampin
- Rifapentine
- St. John's wort
- Topiramate

BOX 9.3   Drug Interactions Requiring an Increase in Medication Dose[32]

There is no P450 induction of enzymes and no decrease in EE/progestin levels for these neuro/anticonvulsants. The dose of Lamotrigine may need to be adjusted to maintain seizure control.
- Gabapentin
- Lamotrigine
- Levetiracetam
- Valproate

Barrier Methods

Male Condom. The male condom is applied over the erect penis to prevent semen from being deposited into the female body. It is placed before penetration and must be kept on through full withdrawal of the penis from the vagina. The base of the condom must be held against the penis as it is withdrawn after ejaculation before the penis softens. They are made from natural rubber latex, polyurethane, and natural or lambskin material. Some are packaged with lubricants and/or spermicide. Additional water-based lubricants can be used in conjunction with a condom. Oil-based lubricants should not be used, as they can weaken the condom causing it to break, thus increasing the risk of an unintended pregnancy or STI. Condoms are the only contraceptive method that helps prevent STIs. They are easily obtainable at many stores and do not require a prescription. They come individually packaged and sealed with air inside. If the package seems deflated or the seal is broken, it should not be used. Excessive heat exposure can also damage the package.

> ### NOT TO BE MISSED
>
> A new condom must be used with every new act of intercourse, be it vaginal, anal, or oral. The overall failure rate is 13%.[34]

Internal Condom. The internal condom, or female condom, is placed into the vagina before penis insertion. It is made of a thin, lubricated polyurethane pouch that fits inside the vagina and extends externally covering the vulva (Fig. 9.7). An inner ring within the condom is located at the base. It is squeezed and advanced all of the way inside the vagina for proper placement. There is an external ring that is twisted after the penis is removed to enclose the semen as the condom is removed. It can be placed up to 8 hours before intercourse. A new female condom is used with each act of intercourse. Like male condoms, additional water-based lubricants can be used, and oil-based lubricants should never be used. A male and female condom never should be used in conjunction, as this can increase friction, causing one or both to break. They are available over the counter and cost more than male condoms. The female condoms has a failure rate of 21%.[34,35]

Diaphragm. The diaphragm is a barrier method that covers the cervix, preventing the sperm from fertilizing the egg. There is one brand available in the United States: the Caya contoured diaphragm (Fig. 9.8). It is a single-size, latex-free device that fits most females (those who would have used a 65-mm to 80-mm traditional latex diaphragm. A prescription is required.

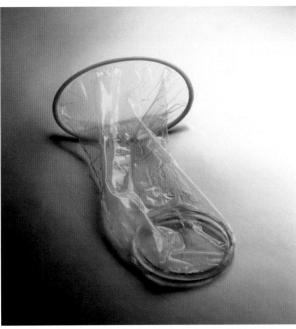

Figure 9.7 The female condom. (From Beksinska M, Smit J, Joanis C, Usher-Patel M, Potter W. Female condom technology: new products and regulatory issues. *Contraception.* 2011;83[4]:316–321.)

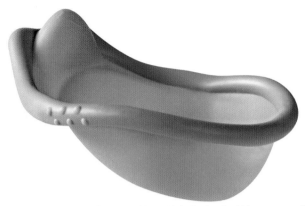

Figure 9.8 Caya diaphragm. (Courtesy Kessel Medintim GmbH. www.medintim.de.)

There are three ways for patients to obtain this diaphragm: through a mail order pharmacy, independent pharmacy, or provider's office. It is placed up to 2 hours before intercourse and must remain in place for at least 6 hours afterward. The diaphragm should never remain in the vagina for greater than 24 hours. Caya diaphragms should always be used with water-soluble contraceptive gels and water-based lubricants. They are not compatible with silicone-based lubricants and gels and thus should not be used together. Additional spermicide is needed with each act of intercourse while the diaphragm is in place. To learn more, visit: http://www.hpsrx.com.[36]

Contraindications include the following:
- Absolute contraindications
  - Application in the first 6 weeks after childbirth
  - Previous use of a size 60-mm, 85-mm, or larger diaphragm
  - Acute or chronic-recurrent urinary tract infections
  - Infections of the genital organs and the true pelvis
  - Cystocele with obliteration of the retropubic niche in the vagina
  - Weakly formed or absent retropubic niche
- Relative contraindications
  - Marked and/or fixed retroversion/retroflexion
  - Psychological or somatic difficulties with application

Cervical Cap. The cervical cap is a soft cup with a round rim that fits snugly around the cervix, preventing sperm from entering (Fig. 9.9). It is placed in the vagina before intercourse and must remain in place for

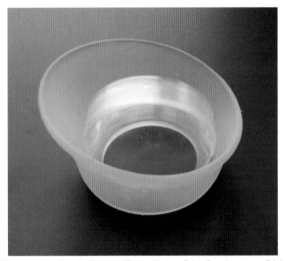

Figure 9.9 Cervical cap. (From Lobo RA, Gershenson DM, Lentz, GM, Valea FA. *Comprehensive Gynecology.* 7th ed. Philadelphia: Elsevier; 2017.)

at least 6 hours and no more than 48 hours. The FemCap brand is available in the United States. This is a reusable cervical cap made of non-allergenic, durable, surgical-grade silicone. It requires fitting by a health care provider and a prescription. It is available in three different sizes depending on vaginal delivery history. If a patient has had a vaginal delivery, the cervical cap may not be the best method as the cervix can be larger, preventing the cap from fitting as well against the cervix. It is obtained in the same manner as the diaphragm: mail order pharmacy, independent pharmacy, or a provider's office. Spermicide use is required and placed at the rim immediately before placement. However, it is not necessary to use more spermicide during the 48 hours it can remain in place. Clinical trials show that, when used in conjunction with spermicide, this noninvasive, non-hormonal contraceptive device is over 92% effective in the prevention of pregnancy.[37,38]

Sponge. The contraceptive sponge is another barrier method marketed under the Today Sponge. It is a soft, disposable polyurethane foam sponge that contains 1000 mg of nonxynol-9 spermicide. It is available over the counter without a prescription. This method is considered 89% to 91% effective. It works in three ways: the nonxynol-9 kills sperm, the sponge blocks the cervical opening, and the sponge traps and absorbs the sperm. Individually packaged, the sponge is wet with water, placed into the vagina, and pushed all of the way to the cervix. It must be placed before intercourse and remain in place for at least 6 hours afterward. It is effective for 24 hours and must be removed before 30 hours. Condoms can be used in conjunction to increase effectiveness and decrease sexually transmitted infection risk.[39,40]

Spermicide. Spermicides are chemicals that kill sperm, preventing the opportunity for the egg and sperm to meet. They are available over the counter without a prescription and come in several different forms: cream, foam, jelly, tablet, suppository, or film. A spermicide is placed into the vagina up to 1 hour before intercourse and should remain in place for at least 6 hours afterward. As a sole birth control method, it is approximately 72% effective. Used with other methods, effectiveness increases. Nonoxynol-9 can be an irritant to the vaginal tissue and could increase the risk of contracting HIV if a partner is positive.[41]

Fertility Awareness–Based Methods

Fertility awareness–based methods help identify times during the reproductive cycle when pregnancy is most likely to occur. By learning the physiologic signs of ovulation or keeping track of fertile windows, pregnancy can be prevented. If a couple avoids intercourse around the most fertile time or uses a barrier method during this time, a pregnancy is less likely. There are different ways to help predict the timeframe to avoid. Table 9.6 provides an interpretation of the parameters of these methods.

Emergency Contraception

If a patient has unprotected sexual intercourse or was underprotected, she should be offered EC. *Underprotected intercourse* refers to when a method has a known failure rate, such as a condom breaking or slipping off. EC can be oral or by placement of a copper IUD. The copper IUD is the most effective method of EC covering for the prior 5 days. Ella (Ulipristal acetate) can be taken orally for up to 96 hours. A prescription from a health care provider is required. Plan B, levonorgestrel, is available over the counter and can be used up to 120 hours after unprotected intercourse. The ideal timeframe for initiation of Plan B is within 72 hours of unprotected intercourse because the effectiveness diminishes after 72 hours. Some retailers keep the over-the-counter medications either in a locked, plastic container or behind the pharmacy counter in attempt to prevent theft. This means a patient would have to ask a store employee for the method, which could be a deterrent to taking it and risk an unintended pregnancy. The closer to the act of unprotected sexual intercourse the oral dose is taken, the more effective it is. In the summer of 2016, the CDC issued revised recommendations for initiation of contraception after using oral EC.[13]

TABLE 9.6[13,42,43] Fertility Awareness–Based Methods	
Basal Body Temperature Method (BBT)	Note body temperature every morning before getting out of bed (temperature increases 0.4°F around ovulation)
Cervical mucous method (Creighton or Billings Method)	Note the amount and texture of cervical mucous. Around ovulation, mucous becomes clear and slippery.
Calendar method (or rhythm method)	Chart menstrual cycle on a calendar or app for ideally 12 prior months. Keep track of fertile days based on length of cycle.
Standard day method (cycle beads)	Identifies a fixed fertile window based on colored beads that correspond to days in the cycle.

NOT TO BE MISSED

Initiation of Regular Contraception After Emergency Contraception

Ulipristal acetate (UPA)

- Advise the patient to start or resume hormonal contraception no sooner than 5 days after use of UPA, and provide or prescribe the regular contraceptive method as needed. For methods requiring a visit to a health care provider, such as DMPA, implants, and IUDs, starting the method at the time of UPA use may be considered; the risk that the regular contraceptive method might decrease the effectiveness of UPA must be weighed against the risk of not starting a regular hormonal contraceptive method.
- The patient must abstain from sexual intercourse or use barrier contraception for the next 7 days after starting or resuming regular contraception or until her next menses, whichever comes first.
- Any nonhormonal contraceptive method can be started immediately after the use of UPA.
- Advise the patient to have a pregnancy test if she does not have a withdrawal bleed within 3 weeks.

Levonorgestrel and Combined Estrogen and Progestin ECPs

- Any regular contraceptive method can be started immediately after the use of levonorgestrel or combined estrogen and progestin ECPs.[13]
- The patient must abstain from sexual intercourse or use barrier contraception for 7 days.
- Advise the patient to have a pregnancy test if she does not have a withdrawal bleed within 3 weeks.

SPECIAL POPULATIONS AND SELECTED MEDICAL CONDITIONS

Special Populations

Adolescents

Adolescents are known to use some of the least effective methods and use them inconsistently, making them among the highest-risk group for unintended pregnancy.[7] Also, there is a high risk of short interpregnancy interval. Health care providers are seen as trusted sources by teens.[16] Thus it is imperative that open, repeated conversations take place at each encounter with these patients. One framework that can be used with an adolescent is GATHER.[44] Research has shown that the more elements of GATHER that are used, the more effective the counseling is and the more satisfied the patient is (Table 9.7).[7]

Confidentiality must be assured. Most states do not require parental permission to evaluate a minor for contraception, however open discussions about sexual and reproductive health with parents or other trusted adults is encouraged. Office encounters with teens include information about all contraceptive methods, STIs, and abstinence. It should be stressed that abstinence is an effective way to prevent an unintended pregnancy and STIs. Per recommendations by the ACOG and the AAP, LARC use is safe and can be offered as first-line contraceptive methods to all teens until proven otherwise.[16]

Transmasculine Patients

Existing research finds that many clinicians and transmasculine (TM) patients falsely believe there is no risk of pregnancy when they are no longer having menses or are on testosterone treatments. Several studies have record rates of unplanned pregnancies among transmasculine patients, even within those who have previous or current testosterone use. Therefore it is important that TM patients are offered individualized and comprehensive counseling on contraception that takes into account future fertility desires. Considerations regarding contraception for the TM population remain the same as those for cisgender females, although there exist TM-specific concerns to address. A discussion of the TM-specific concerns regarding contraception is beyond the scope of this chapter, however, an excellent article by Krempasky et al. provides guidance for the clinician on choosing a contraceptive method based on the varied issues experienced by the TM patient.[43]

Postpartum

Initiation of contraception after delivery has changed in recent years. Previously, health care providers commonly advised patients to avoid sexual intercourse for at least 6 weeks postpartum. Now, IUDs can be placed post–placental delivery along with implants and the injection being provided before discharge from the hospital. An issue is that many female patients do not return for a postpartum visit, or they resume sexual intercourse before the visit. This can contribute to an unplanned short interpregnancy interval, placing the patient and pregnancy at risk. Thus postdelivery contraception should be discussed throughout the pregnancy. In addition, if sterilization is desired, procedure consents may

TABLE 9.7[44]	**GATHER Framework**				
GREET	**ASK**	**TELL**	**HELP**	**EXPLAIN**	**RETURN**
Assure Privacy	Inquire about friend's behavior	Use visual aids to discuss options	Summarize options	Keep it short and simple	Make follow-up appointment
Discuss confidentiality	Use open-ended questions	Avoid "should"	Ask for teen's decision	Repeat the information	Anchor experience to external event
Interview alone	Show active listening	Ask permission to give advice	Repeat the plan back to the teen	Check understanding	Make reminder call

need to be signed 30 days before the delivery for publicly funded insurance programs to cover it.

Risks in the postpartum period are higher. IUD expulsion happens at a slightly higher incidence. Perforation of the uterus can also occur. Estrogen-containing contraception is contraindicated in the first 4 weeks postpartum because of a higher risk of VTE (MEC category 4).[14]

> **PATIENT-CENTERED CARE** IUDs can be placed post–placental delivery along with implants and the injection being provided before discharge from the hospital.

Lactation

Lactation itself can be a method of contraception. The lactational amenorrhea method is a temporary contraception from birth to 6 months postpartum if continuous breastfeeding occurs. During this time, ovulation is suppressed. For maximum effectiveness, breastfeeding, not pumping, should occur every 4 hours during the day and every 6 hours at night.[46] Once menses resumes, other methods of contraception should be used.[13,47] Estrogen is known to decrease milk production. Breastfeeding for the first year of life is recommended by the AAP, the WHO, and the ACOG.[48] New medical eligibility guidelines were released in 2016 regarding use of estrogen- containing methods and time from delivery. If less than 21 days from delivery, estrogen-containing methods are considered MEC category 4. Going forward, use ranges from MEC category 2 to category 3 depending on other maternal factors.[13]

Age Older Than 35 Years

If using an estrogen-containing method, turning 35 years of age and smoking tobacco increases the risk of VTE. Thus alternative methods should be used based on number of cigarettes smoked per day. Better yet, smoking cessation should be discussed and encouraged for overall health benefit. This conversation should be occurring *no later than* when the patient is in her early thirties.[13]

> **! SAFETY ALERT**
>
> The combination of age 35 and greater, taking exogenous estrogen, and cigarette smoking exponentially increases a patient's risk for VTE.

Perimenopause

The average age of menopause in the United States is 51 years of age. The ability to become pregnant decreases at around 45 years of age. However, because these are averages, the upper limits may still be a few years past 45 and 51 years of age, respectively. Perimenopausal females are in the second-highest age group for unintended pregnancies behind adolescents. Females may think their ability to get pregnant is decreased and may decrease the use of contraception, leading to a pregnancy. Advanced maternal age and pregnancy present risks to both the mother and baby. Also, as females age, more comorbidities may occur, and specific contraceptive method use may be prohibited.[13]

Medical Conditions

Preexisting medical conditions may further increase health risk if an unintended pregnancy were to occur (Box 9.4). Sometimes treatments for these conditions are teratogenic, leading to poor pregnancy outcomes. Thus it is imperative that the need for highly effective contraception is discussed, encouraged, and documented in the medical chart.

Some medical conditions and use of certain contraceptive methods may not be compatible or may increase

BOX 9.4   Conditions Associated with Increased Risk for Adverse Health Events As a Result of Pregnancy[14]

- Breast cancer
- Complicated valvular heart disease
- Cystic fibrosis
- Diabetes: insulin dependent, with nephropathy, retinopathy, or neuropathy, or other vascular diseases or >20 years' duration
- Endometrial or ovarian cancer
- Epilepsy
- Hypertension (>160/100)
- History of bariatric surgery within the past 2 years
- HIV: not clinically well or not receiving antiretroviral therapy
- Ischemic heart disease
- Gestational trophoblastic disease
- Hepatocellular adenoma and malignant liver tumors
- Peripartum cardiomyopathy
- Schistosomiasis with fibrosis of the liver
- Severe (decompensated) cirrhosis
- Sickle cell disease
- Solid organ transplantation within the past 2 years
- Stroke
- Systemic lupus erythematosus
- Thrombogenic mutations
- Tuberculosis

TABLE 9.8[14]   Medical Conditions that Complicate Contraceptive Use*

Medical Conditions	Contraceptive Method Use Cautions
Migraine headaches with aura	Estrogen use could increase the risk of VTE.
Prior venous thromboembolism (VTE)	Estrogen use could increase the risk of further VTE.
Seizure disorders	Anti-epileptic medications may be less effective with use of estrogen.
Obesity	Contraceptive method may be less effective based on weight and body mass index (BMI).
Breast cancer	If it is estrogen or progesterone receptor positive, then the corresponding containing contraceptive would be prohibited.

*This is not an inclusive list.

the risk of further medical complications. Reference of the U.S. Medical Eligibility Criteria for Contraceptive Use is recommended. https://www.cdc.gov/mmwr/volumes/65/rr/rr6503a1.htm. The MEC rating should be documented in the medical record. Some of the conditions and cautions are listed in Table 9.8.

PATIENT EDUCATION AND COUNSELING

Reproductive Life Plan

It is important to know what patients are thinking when it comes to a possible pregnancy and when it may be desired. This will help guide you and may prevent incorrect assumptions. Patients themselves may not have even considered the subject or verbalized it to anyone. By discussing it at a patient visit, it may be a perfect opportunity for the patient to begin a contraceptive method and prevent an unintended pregnancy.

- If the patient does not want a child at this time and is sexually active, then offer contraceptive services.

- If the patient desires pregnancy testing, then provide testing and counseling.
- If the patient wants to have a child now, then provide services to help the patient achieve pregnancy.[13]

Compliance

If having intercourse, the best contraceptive method is one that is going to be used correctly and consistently and is acceptable to both individuals in the relationship. Patients must be aware of the requirements on their part to maximize a methods effectiveness. If patients are not adherent, then they need to be aware of other options available.

Protection From Sexually Transmitted Infections

There is no contraceptive method that prevents sexually transmitted infections 100% except abstinence. Condoms come close and should be advocated for those who have new partners, multiple partners, or high-risk sexual activity. Dual-method use is when a condom is used in conjunction with a tier 2 or tier 3 method and should be encouraged.

By promoting contraceptive use, family planning is being provided to patients, partners, families, communities, and society. Couples are able to work toward their desired goals and aspirations instead of facing an unplanned pregnancy, options, and long-term commitments they may not be ready or prepared for. Conversations initiated with patients by health care providers can help normalize the subject matter, possibly allowing for more patient disclosure and identification of issues that may otherwise not be mentioned. With many method choices and highly effective methods available, safe, consistent contraceptive use should be possible, thus allowing for planned pregnancies instead of unplanned pregnancies. If future pregnancy is desired, LARC should be the first-line method readily offered as it comprises the most effective reversible methods for all females.

KEY POINTS

- The ability to control if or when one will begin a family is a fundamental right for females and families.
- Listening to the patient's needs and desires and offering careful counseling on medically appropriate methods of contraception are key practices in providing contraceptive care.
- There are many available methods of contraception that are tailored to the needs of most female and male patients.
- The best method of birth control is the one that will be used consistently and correctly.

REFERENCES

1. U.S. Centers for Disease Control and Prevention. *Achievements in Public Health, 1900–1999: Family Planning.* 1999. https://www.cdc.gov/mmwr/preview/mmwrhtml/mm4847a1.htm.
2. Roper Center for Public Opinion Research. (n.d.). *Public Attitudes About Birth Control.* Cornell University. https://ropercenter.cornell.edu/public-attitudes-about-birth-control.
3. Guttmacher Institute. *Contraceptive Use in the United States by Demographics*; 2021. https://www.guttmacher.org/fact-sheet/contraceptive-use-united-states.
4. Sawhill SV, Guyot K. *Preventing Unplanned Pregnancy: Lessons from the States.* The Brookings Institution; 2019. https://www.brookings.edu/research/preventing-unplanned-pregnancy-lessons-from-the-states/.
5. National Conference of State Legislatures. *Preventing Unplanned Pregnancy*; 2021. https://www.ncsl.org/research/health/preventing-unplanned-pregnancy.aspx.
6. Troutman M, Rafique S, Plowden TC. Are higher unintended pregnancy rates among minorities a result of disparate access to contraception? *Contracept Reprod Med.* 2020;5:16.
7. Guttmacher Institute. *Powerful Contraception, Complicated Programs: Preventing Coercive Promotion of Long-Acting Reversible Contraceptives*; 2021a. https://www.guttmacher.org/gpr/2021/05/powerful-contraception-complicated-programs-preventing-coercive-promotion-long-acting.
8. Todd N, Black A. Contraception for adolescents. *J Clin Res Pediatr Endocrinol.* 2020;12(suppl 1):28–40.
9. Pimental J, Ansari U, Omer K, et al. Factors associated with short birth interval in low- and middle-income countries: a systematic review. *BMC Pregnancy Childbirth.* 2020;20(1):156.
10. Guttmacher Institute. *Publicly Supported Family Planning Services in the United States*; 2019. https://www.guttmacher.org/fact-sheet/publicly-supported-FP-services-US#:~:text=Altogether%2C%20the%20services%20provided%20at,state%20governments%20of%20%2412%20billion.
11. Frederiksen B, Ranji U, Salganicoff A, Long M. *Women's Sexual and Reproductive Health Services: Key Findings from the 2020 KFF Women's Health Survey*; 2021. https://www.kff.org/womens-health-policy/issue-brief/womens-sexual-and-reproductive-health-services-key-findings-from-the-2020-kff-womens-health-survey/.
12. World Health Organization. *Family Planning/Contraception Methods*; 2020. https://www.who.int/news-room/fact-sheets/detail/family-planning-contraception.
13. Guttmacher Institute. *Contraceptive Effectiveness in the United States*; 2020. https://www.guttmacher.org/fact-sheet/contraceptive-effectiveness-united-states#:~:text=Effectiveness%20estimates%20vary%20across%20different,based%20on%20moderate%2Dquality%20studies.
14. American College of Obstetricians and Gynecologists' Committee on Health Care for Underserved Women, Contraceptive Equity Expert Work Group, and Committee on Ethics. Patient-Centered Contraceptive Counseling: ACOG Committee Statement Number 1. *Obstet Gynecol.* 2022;139(2):350–353.
15. Gavin L, Moskossky MS, Carter M, et al. Providing quality family planning services: recommendations of CDC and the U.S. Office of Population Affairs. *MMWR.* 2014;63(RR-4):54.
16. Wu JP, Pickle S. Extended use of the intrauterine device: a literature review and recommendations for clinical practice. *Contraception.* 2014;89(6):495–503.

17. Dehlendorf C. *Contraception: Counseling and Selection*. UpToDate; 2022. https://www.uptodate.com/contents/contraception-counseling-and-selection?search=https:%2F%2Fwww.uptodate.com%2Fcontents%2Fcontraception-counseling-and-selection&source=search_result&selectedTitle=1~150&usage_type=default&display_rank=1.

18. Curtis KM, Jatlaoui TC, Tepper NK, et al. US selected practice recommendations for contraceptive use; 2016. *MMWR Recommend Rep.* 2016;65(4):3–68.

19. Curtis KM, Tepper NK, Jatlaoui TC, et al. US medical eligibility criteria for contraceptive use; 2016. *MMWR Recommend Rep.* 2016;65(3):1–103.

20. Guttmacher Institute. *Contraceptive Use in the United States by Method*; 2021b. https://www.guttmacher.org/fact-sheet/contraceptive-method-use-united-states.

21. Menon S, Committee on Adolescence. Long-acting reversible contraception: specific issues for adolescents. *Pediatrics.* 2020;146(2):e2020007252.

22. American College of Obstetricians and Gynecologists. *Adolescents and Long-Acting Reversible Contraception: Implants and Intrauterine Devices*; 2018. Committee Opinion 735 https://www.acog.org/clinical/clinical-guidance/committee-opinion/articles/2018/05/adolescents-and-long-acting-reversible-contraception-implants-and-intrauterine-devices#:~:text=Because%20adolescents%20are%20at%20higher%20risk%20of%20STIs%2C%20obstetrician%E2%80%93gynecologists,risk%20of%20STIs%2C%20including%20HIV.

23. Organon Global Inc. *Highlights of Prescribing Information.* Nexplanon; 2021. https://www.organon.com/product/usa/pi_circulars/n/nexplanon/nexplanon_pi.pdf.

24. Cooper Surgical. *Highlights of Prescribing Information.* Paragard; 2020. https://www.paragard.com/wp-content/uploads/2018/10/PARAGARD-PI.pdf.

25. Allergan. *Highlights of Prescribing Information.* Liletta; 2019. https://www.accessdata.fda.gov/drugsatfda_docs/label/2019/206229s008lbl.pdf.

26. Bayer Healthcare Pharmaceuticals. *Highlights of Prescribing Information.* Skyla; 2018. https://www.accessdata.fda.gov/drugsatfda_docs/label/2018/203159s010lbl.pdf.

27. Bayer Healthcare Pharmaceuticals. *Highlights of Prescribing Information.* Mirena; 2020. https://www.accessdata.fda.gov/drugsatfda_docs/label/2020/021225s040lbl.pdf.

28. Bayer Healthcare Pharmaceuticals, Inc. *Highlights of Prescribing Information.* Kyleena; 2021. https://www.accessdata.fda.gov/drugsatfda_docs/label/2021/208224Orig1s002lbl.pdf.

29. Bergin A, Tristan S, Terplan M, Gilliam ML, Whitaker AK. A missed opportunity for care: two-visit IUD insertion protocols inhibit placement. *Contraception.* 2012;86(6):694–697.

30. Barbieri RL. How common is IUD perforation, expulsion, and malposition?. *OBG Manag.* 2022;34(4):8–9, 13–14, 16, 22.

31. Britton LE, Alspaugh A, Greene MZ, McLemore MR. An evidence-based update on contraception. *Am J Nurs.* 2020;120(2):22–23.

32. Allen RH. *Combined Estrogen-Progestin Oral Contraceptives: Patient Selection, Counseling, and Use.* UpToDate; 2022.

33. Merck & Co., Inc. *Highlights of Prescribing Information.* NuvaRing; 2020. https://www.nuvaring.com/static/pdf/nuvaring-pi.pdf.

34. Mylan Pharmaceuticals Inc. *Highlights of Prescribing Information.* Xulane; 2022. https://dailymed.nlm.nih.gov/dailymed/fda/fdaDrugXsl.cfm?type=display&setid=f7848550-086a-43d8-8ae5-047f4b9e4382.

35. Pfizer Inc. *Highlights of Prescribing Information. Depo-SubQ Provera*; 2019. https://www.accessdata.fda.gov/drugsatfda_docs/label/2019/021583s016,%20s024,%20s029lbl.pdf.

36. Dickey RP, Seymour ML. *Managing Contraceptive Pill Patients.* 17th ed. Fort Collins, CO: EMIS, Inc. Medical Publishers; 2021.

37. Centers for Disease Control and Prevention. (n.d.). *Contraception.* https://www.cdc.gov/reproductivehealth/contraception/.

38. HPSRx Enterprises Inc. (n.d.). *Caya Guidelines for Healthcare Professionals.* https://www.caya.us.com/wp-content/uploads/2022/04/Caya-Guidelines-for-Healthcare-Providers-Medintim.pdf.

39. FemCap, Inc. (n.d.). *Frequently Asked Questions: How Effective Is FemCap?* https://femcap.com/new/faq/.

40. Mayer Labs. (n.d.). *Today Sponge. Health professionals.* http://www.todaysponge.com/healthcareprofessionals.html.

41. World Health Organization. (n.d.). *Nonoxynol-9 Ineffective in Preventing HIV Infection.* https://www.who.int/news/item/28-06-2002-nonoxynol-9-ineffective-in-preventing-hiv-infection.

42. Association of Reproductive Health Professionals. Fertility Awareness Methods. *Health Matters Fact Sheets.* 2009. https://www.arhp.org/health-matters-fact-sheets/.

43. Krempasky C, Harris M, Abern L, Grimstad F. Contraception across the transmasculine spectrum. *Am J Obstet Gynecol.* 2020;222(2):134–143.

44. Sridhar A, Salcedo J. Optimizing maternal and neonatal outcomes with postpartum contraception: impact on breastfeeding and birth spacing. *Matern Health, Neonatol Perinatol.* 2017;3:1.

45. Meek JY. *Infant benefits of breastfeeding.* UpToDate; 2022. https://www.uptodate.com/contents/infant-benefits-of-breastfeeding#!.

10

Reproductive Options Counseling

Alison Hathaway and Annelle Taylor

OBJECTIVES

- Develop a plan for best practices in reproductive options counseling and decision assessment using a patient-centered approach, including patient history and physical examination.
- Describe three alternatives in options counseling:
  - Pregnancy continuation and parenting
  - Pregnancy continuation and adoption
- Abortion
- Devise a counseling plan for follow-up care for each option.
- Identify important abnormal pregnancy presentations.
- Integrate the role of options counseling into the patient visit.

Reproductive options counseling fosters nonbiased, patient-centered care that is comprehensive with respect to the full spectrum of possible pregnancy decisions, including pregnancy continuation, adoption, and abortion. Nearly one-half of all pregnancies in the United States are unintended[1]; the clinician must develop the appropriate skills to assist patients faced with both planned and unplanned pregnancies. In this chapter, we will review best practice reproductive options counseling methods and an outpatient care plan that supports patients in what can be a challenging—yet common—life experience.

REPRODUCTIVE OPTIONS COUNSELING FOR UNINTENDED PREGNANCY

Each year, approximately 45% of all pregnancies in the United States are unintended.[2] An unintended pregnancy refers to a pregnancy that was either not currently planned but may be desired in the future (*mistimed*, 27% of pregnancies) or one that was unintentional and undesired in the future (*unwanted*, 18% of pregnancies)[2]. An *intended* pregnancy is one that is planned and/or desired at the time that it occurred. In 2011, 42% of unintended pregnancies ended in abortion, while 58% ended in birth, miscarriages excluded.[2]

Before 1973, the adoption rate for infants born to never-married pregnant individuals younger than 45 years of age was 8.7%.[3] Following the national legalization of abortion in the United States, the adoption rate declined significantly; between 1996 and 2002, only 1% of infants born to never-married pregnant individuals younger than 45 years of age were placed for adoption.[3] Statistics show that 2% to 3% of teen pregnancies result in adoption.[4] The unintended pregnancy rate in the United States is significantly higher than in other developed countries,[2] highlighting the importance of reproductive options counseling in a patient-centered care model.

With the reversal of *Roe v. Wade* on June 24, 2022, more than one-half of U.S. states are certain or likely to ban abortion.[5] The shifting legal landscape for abortion care at the state level will affect the clinician's scope of practice and patient access to life-saving care. In 2020, the maternal mortality rate for Black women was 2.9 times higher than for non-Hispanic White women in the United States[6]; this disturbing statistic highlights how communities of color will be disproportionately affected by being forced to carry unwanted pregnancies to term. Awareness of health care disparities and systemic racism is necessary for clinicians to address inequalities and improve patient outcomes.

In addition, understanding that pregnant patients possess varied sexual orientations and gender identities is crucial; the clinician should ask patients their pronoun preference before assuming gender identity—this inclusive practice recognizes that transgender men, nonbinary, and gender nonconforming individuals have pregnancies and deserve to be informed about their range of options when it comes to unintended pregnancy. Clinicians must be vigilant and inclusive, keep abreast of state laws, and support patients to receive essential, high-quality health care.

> **PATIENT-CENTERED CARE:** The unintended pregnancy rate in the United States is significantly higher than in other developed countries,[2] highlighting the importance of reproductive options counseling in a patient-centered care model.

A health care visit that includes a positive pregnancy test requires that the clinician engage in reproductive options counseling, medical assessment and evaluation, patient education, and appropriate referrals. Reproductive options counseling is the first step in offering support, information, and counseling that allows patients to make the best decision for themselves and their family (Fig. 10.1). Before offering complete options counseling, it is important that the clinician participate in a values clarification exercise themselves; this practice helps identify possible internal and external biases and the effect they potentiate on the counseling offered to patients that is meant to be free from predisposition.

VALUES CLARIFICATION

Values clarification is a method that allows for examination of the implicit biases and judgments all humans possess, which stem from their varied life experiences and worldview.[7] During a values clarification activity, clinicians are presented with different clinical scenarios to encourage self-reflection regarding internal

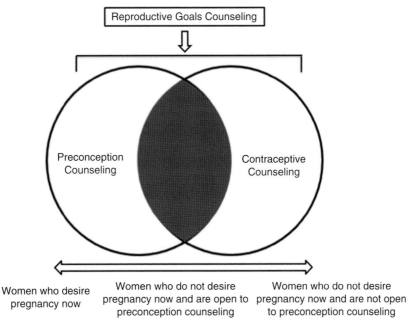

Patient-Centered Family Planning Care

Figure 10.1 Model of reproductive counseling. (From Callegari LS, Aiken AR, Dehlendorf C, Cason P, Borrero S. Addressing potential pitfalls of reproductive life planning with patient-centered counseling. *Am J Obstet Gynecol.* 2017;216[2]:129–134.)

BOX 10.1   Example Questions for Values Clarification Exercise

- How do you feel about a person who has had one abortion?
- How do you feel about a person who has had ten abortions?
- How do you feel about a teenager who has dropped out of high school and is having her second child?
- How do you feel about a 35-year-old married, working professional having her fifth child?

BOX 10.2   Example Questions for Establishing Patient Pregnancy Intention

- What were you hoping the results of your pregnancy test would be?
- How are you feeling about your result today?
- Does anyone know that you're here or that you might be pregnant?
- What thoughts or feelings are you having at this moment?
- What has it been like for you since you found out you were pregnant?
- Do you have any thoughts about what you would like to do with this pregnancy?

---

prejudices they might have internalized that could affect patient counseling (Box 10.1).

Questions are used to start an internal investigation into one's personal belief system. There are no "right" or "wrong" answers. These inquiries are constructive in that they reveal what scenarios may challenge the clinician's individual principles. Clinicians are asked to acknowledge their internal biases and, through conscious awareness, prevent them from affecting the counseling offered to patients. Participating in values clarification ensures that the visit is focused wholly on the patient's unique experience, thereby allowing for a decision-making process that is entirely the patient's own.

CLINICAL SURVIVAL TIP: An excellent resource for a values clarification workshop can be found here: https://www.reproductiveaccess.org/wp-content/uploads/2014/12/values_clarification-workshop.pdf.

Pregnancy, abortion, and adoption are complex, often politicized and polarizing topics. To provide patients with a safe and open space to express themselves, it is imperative that clinicians recognize their own biases and leave them outside the examination room.

ESTABLISHING PATIENT INTENTION REGARDING PREGNANCY AND INITIATING OPTIONS COUNSELING

When a patient presents to the health care setting with a positive pregnancy test, it is critical that the clinician not assume what the result means for the patient. The skilled clinician will observe the patient's affect, listen attentively, and follow the patient's lead to determine the clinical course of action and management plan.

Although a positive pregnancy test might be a joyous occasion for one patient, it could be unwelcome, difficult news for another patient. It is important that the clinician explore pregnancy intention with questions that allow each patient to express herself (Box 10.2).

Pregnancy has the potential to bring up varied feelings for the patient; it is the understanding clinician's job to support the gamut of emotional responses to better allow the patient a decision-making process that offers resolution. As Alissa Perrucci points out in her seminal work on decision assessment and counseling, "The patient has the answer to [their] dilemma; the counselor serves as facilitator and guide."[7]

Patients have three principal choices when faced with a pregnancy: (1) continue the pregnancy and parent; (2) continue the pregnancy and place the baby for adoption; (3) terminate the pregnancy by medication or procedural abortion. Many patients will already know what they plan to do. Other times, it may be challenging for a patient to reach a decision, and several visits and more extensive counseling may be required. It is up to the clinician to provide counseling and care in a manner that allows for full deliberation and self-determination on the part of the patient.

When a patient decides to continue the pregnancy and parent, it will be necessary to provide initial prenatal recommendations and a referral if the current setting does not provide prenatal care. The initial prenatal visit involves advising the patient to start taking prenatal vitamins to ensure adequate folic acid, calcium, and iron intake; reviewing any current medications to confirm the absence of teratogens; and educating patients to avoid alcohol and tobacco products, including secondhand smoke. The clinician must consider if there are laboratory tests that need to be drawn and if imaging is needed to confirm gestational age. A brief explanation of genetic testing options should be discussed. Because of increased rates of intimate partner violence during pregnancy, it is necessary to confirm that the patient is in a safe living situation. Most initial prenatal visits occur before or around 12 weeks, so helping the patient find a provider and establish prenatal care quickly is needed. If a patient is uninsured, underinsured, or undocumented, connecting her to resources and insurance enrollment programs in a timely manner is crucial.

! SAFETY ALERT

Because of the increased rate of intimate partner violence during pregnancy, it is necessary to confirm that the patient is in a safe living situation.

When a patient decides to continue a pregnancy with the intention of placing the baby for adoption, the same plan of action for prenatal care should be initiated with additional referrals to adoption agencies that will guide the patient regarding the appropriate legal processes. It is important that the provider's health care setting have some established adoption agencies to recommend to the patient seeking adoption. Although the prenatal care provider is not involved in arranging the adoption process or protocol, it is essential that the provider check in with the patient throughout the pregnancy because patients may change their mind at any time during the pregnancy and decide to parent, or they may experience a range of emotions necessitating additional counseling and/or therapy. It is crucial to recognize that the patient can reverse the decision to adopt before or at the time of the birth and that this scenario should be written into the legal clause they devise with their adoption agency and lawyer. It is also important to note that it is uncommon for birth parents to change their minds regarding their adoption decision once the child has been officially placed with their adoptive family.[8] The adoption agency should be able to fully inform the adopting parents of their particular agency's statistics surrounding the rate of planned adoptions that remain with the birth parents or are returned to the birth parents because of a change of intention.

All-Options is an organization that maintains a national phone line that offers counseling and support for decision making around pregnancy, parenting, adoption, and abortion. They provide resources for adoption agencies that may be helpful to both patients and providers on their website: https://www.all-options.org/resources/.

CLINICAL SURVIVAL TIP:
All-Options is an organization that maintains a national phone line that offers support for decision making and options counseling to discuss pregnancy, adoption, and abortion: https://www.all-options.org/resources/.

When a patient decides to terminate a pregnancy, there are two options for abortion: medication or an in-clinic procedure. The patient's gestational age, personal preference, and geographic location may all affect which type of abortion is suitable. Medication abortion is approved by the U.S Food and Drug Administration (FDA) for use up to 70 days (10 weeks) from the last menstrual period (LMP); however, it can be safely used off-label for later gestations. Depending on the state, an in-clinic procedure may be offered up to 20 weeks, 24 weeks, or rarely into the third trimester.[9] Regulations are based on state laws, so it is important to check the scope of abortion provision in the individual provider's state of practice. With the Supreme Court decision reversing *Roe v. Wade* in June 2022, the legal landscape for abortion access in the United States is changing. Abortion funds are available to help patients travel and obtain accommodations if they must leave their home state to terminate their pregnancy. The National Network of Abortion Funds is an organization that helps decrease financial and logistical barriers to accessing abortion care: https://abortionfunds.org/. Because of the increasingly hostile landscape for patients seeking an abortion, it is crucial that the clinician be aware of supportive resources for patients.

NOT TO BE MISSED

Regulations are based on state laws, so it is important to check the scope of abortion provision in the individual provider's state of practice. If the patient is 10 weeks or less from the LMP, comprehensive abortion options counseling should be done. Although both medication and in-clinic abortion are safe and effective options for terminating an early pregnancy, patients often have a strong preference for one or the other. According to the Guttmacher Institute, medication abortion accounted for 54% of all abortions in the United States in 2020; this number will likely increase as in-clinic abortion access decreases with the overturning of *Roe v. Wade*.

Nurse practitioners are well-equipped to provide medical and in-clinic abortion services with proper training. Between 2007 and 2013, a California-based, multisite study evaluated outcomes when first-trimester aspiration abortion was provided by nurse practitioners, midwives, and physician assistants in comparison with physicians; the study concluded that nurse practitioners, midwives, and physician assistants have the same safety and patient satisfaction results as their physician colleagues.[10] This seminal study laid the groundwork for increased scope of practice, delivering clinical evidence that nurse practitioners can be excellent abortion providers.[10] According to the UCSF Bixby Center for Global Reproductive Health, nurse practitioners, midwives, and physician assistants are now safely dispensing mifepristone-misoprostol and/or providing aspiration abortion care in nearly one-third of the states.[11]

In the United States, medication abortion involves sequential administration of two drugs—mifepristone and misoprostol—to halt embryonic development and induce uterine contractions so the patient may pass the pregnancy at home. Depending on the state, nurse practitioners may or may not be permitted to dispense mifepristone within their scope of practice. In countries outside the United States, the regimen for medication abortion varies. See Table 10.1 for more information.

In the United States, patients typically take mifepristone in the clinic, which has antiprogesterone activity to stop the pregnancy from growing. The patient then goes home and takes misoprostol, which induces uterine cramping and bleeding.[12] In some states, the patient must return to the clinic to receive the misoprostol. With the expansion of telehealth, mifepristone and misoprostol can both be taken in the patient's home. Evidence supports that self-managed medication abortion using online telemedicine is a safe option for most patients.[13] Analgesia and antinausea medication should be offered to alleviate uncomfortable side effects (cramping pain, diarrhea, and nausea are common). The benefits of medication abortion are that it usually avoids the need for instrumentation of the uterus and an invasive procedure. In addition, some patients feel it is more natural and appreciate that they can end their pregnancy in a private space.

Patients who elect medication abortion should have a follow-up assessment to confirm that the pregnancy has ended. Typical questions at follow-up address quantity and duration of bleeding, pregnancy symptoms (nausea, breast tenderness), and any signs of infection (fever, pain, abnormal discharge, heavy bleeding). Follow-up care management options include but are not limited to an in-office ultrasound examination to confirm

TABLE 10.1 Medication Abortion Regimens		
Mifepristone + misoprostol (initial FDA-approved regimen in 2000)	Mifepristone 600 mg PO given in office, followed by misoprostol 800 mcg (buccally or vaginally) 72 hours later given in office; follow-up visit in 2 weeks	Used up to 49 days from LMP Efficacy rate: 96%-99% Increased cost, more office visits, more gastrointestinal side effects from higher dose of mifepristone
Mifepristone + misoprostol (updated evidence-based FDA-approved regimen since 2016)	Mifepristone 200 mg PO followed by misoprostol 800 mcg (buccally or vaginally) 24–48 hours later	Used up to 70 days from LMP Efficacy rate: 96%–99% Recommended by the ACOG, NAF, and WHO
Methotrexate + misoprostol	Methotrexate 50 mg orally or IM injection + misoprostol 800 mcg (vaginally) 3–7 days later	Used up to 63 days from LMP Efficacy rate: >90%[18] Not recommended by the WHO because of teratogenicity if it fails
Misoprostol only	Misoprostol 800 mcg (sublingually or vaginally) for up to three repeat doses Q 3–12 hours	Used up to 84 days from LMP per WHO guidelines Utilized when no access to mifepristone/standard care Efficacy rate: 80.4%–88%

ACOG, American College of Obstetricians and Gynecologists; IM, intramuscular; LMP, last menstrual period; NAF, National Abortion Federation; PO, by mouth; WHO, World Health Organization.

expulsion of the gestational sac, a follow-up phone call and a low-sensitivity pregnancy test 2 weeks later, or a questionnaire over e-mail accompanied by a high-sensitivity pregnancy test 1 month after the medication abortion. Recent research developments offer additional safe and effective modalities for medication abortion provision and aftercare; protocols have evolved beyond the FDA-approved regimen.

For some patients, the idea of a medication abortion may be scary or unpleasant; they may have concerns about heavy bleeding or seeing the pregnancy tissue during the process. There is a small possibility that the medication abortion will be ineffective; approximately 0.4% to 3% of patients will experience a continuing pregnancy[14]; if this occurs, the patient will require additional medical intervention or an in-clinic procedure.[12] For these reasons and more, some patients will elect to terminate their pregnancy with an in-clinic procedure rather than medication.

Aspiration abortion is an in-clinic procedure that involves dilating the cervix, inserting a sterile cannula into the uterus, and applying gentle suction to remove pregnancy tissue.[12] Following the abortion procedure, the provider reviews the products of conception (POC) to confirm that all pregnancy tissue has been removed; patients do not need to schedule an additional follow-up visit unless they develop a fever, heavy bleeding, abnormal vaginal discharge, severe pelvic pain, or symptoms consistent with an ongoing pregnancy. Aspiration abortion is used during the first trimester of pregnancy, typically takes less than 10 minutes to perform, and has a very low complications rate (<0.1%).[12] The potential complications include hemorrhage, pelvic infection, cervical injury, uterine perforation, hematometra, adverse reaction to anesthesia, and incomplete evacuation of the uterus.[12] In present-day developed countries, the risk of death from a legally induced abortion is negligible; an abortion performed in a safe setting is less dangerous than receiving a penicillin injection or carrying a pregnancy to term.[12] Patients with access to safe, legal abortion will rarely have medical issues that require additional follow-up. In contrast, a major global health concern is that millions of women lack access to safe, legal abortion, and approximately 47,000 women will die each year as a result.[12]

Most patients undergoing an aspiration abortion will experience menstrual-like cramps and bleeding.[12] Pain is often a concern for patients; it is important to counsel on analgesia and sedation options—from local to general anesthesia—depending on preference and clinical setting. Many patients will decide to terminate their pregnancies with an in-clinic procedure because they feel it is timely and definitive. They may also find reassurance in a medical procedure that is directly managed by their health care provider; thus it is important that clinicians be familiar with their local abortion resources if these services are not provided at their clinical site. The ability to offer referrals and resources is paramount when supporting the patient through all pregnancy experiences and decisions. Abortion Finder offers an expansive directory of certified abortion service providers in the United States: https://www.abortionfinder.org/.

> **! SAFETY ALERT**
>
> The ability to offer referrals and resources is paramount when supporting the patient through all pregnancy experiences and decisions.

For patients beyond the first trimester, cervical preparation is necessary before their abortion. Patients may need to go into the office the day before their procedure to have osmotic dilators placed inside their cervix. Because of the increased level of cervical expansion necessary for dilation and evacuation (D&E) abortions, it is useful to advise patients at or beyond 16 weeks from their LMP that a 2-day procedure may be warranted. Parity, medical history, and provider training may all be factors that affect decision making around cervical preparation to achieve adequate dilation. Osmotic dilator insertion can cause discomfort and cramping; if available, patients should be offered analgesia and sedation to decrease discomfort during placement. When a patient returns for the D&E procedure the next day, the provider may or may not use misoprostol for additional cervical preparation.

The D&E procedure begins with the provider removing osmotic dilators from the patient's cervix while performing a bimanual examination. Following removal, mechanical dilation is used to open the cervix further. After dilation is complete, suction may be applied to remove amniotic fluid. Forceps are then utilized to extract the pregnancy and placental tissues. Following extraction, suction is used again to remove blood and residual tissue and to promote uterine contractions. Although not necessary, many providers prefer to perform D&E procedures under ultrasound guidance.[12] After the procedure, the provider may give additional uterotonic agents to decrease bleeding risk.

Following an in-clinic abortion, pregnancy symptoms such as breast tenderness, nausea, and fatigue should resolve within 1 week. Patients can expect their menses to return within 6 weeks of the procedure. If pregnancy symptoms persist or if a period has not returned after 6 weeks, the patient should return for a follow-up visit.

NOT TO BE MISSED

If pregnancy symptoms persist or if a period has not returned after 6 weeks following an aspiration or D&E abortion, the patient should return for a follow-up visit.

PATIENT-CENTERED CARE: Contraceptive counseling should occur at any visit related to pregnancy decision making. Patient-centered contraceptive counseling can begin by asking the patient what contraceptive methods they have heard about, what they know about different methods, what they have used in the past, and what has worked well for them. Determining if the patient has had any past negative experiences can be useful in excluding certain options and choosing one that will be successful for them in the future.

Although long-acting reversible contraceptives (LARCs) such as intrauterine devices (IUDs) and implants may be the provider method of choice, the clinician must be alert to each patient's individual needs and values. It is important that clinicians listen and support the patient's decision to use or not use contraception, regardless of what they think is "right" for them. The clinician must be aware that vulnerable communities and people of color have a long history of reproductive oppression in the United States, including forced sterilization and insertion of LARCs against their will. Although IUDs have a lower failure rate than birth control pills, some patients may not feel comfortable with having a device inside their body, or they may prefer having the control to start and stop a daily pill when they choose. A patient's bodily autonomy and right to make her own decision about contraception must be respected and honored.

Listening to and allowing patients to express themselves helps the clinician support and guide them toward a decision that is truly their own. If the patient has received little

information in the past, it will be helpful to give a brief overview of contraceptive options, how they are taken, and the general risks and benefits. Medication abortion patients should leave with their contraceptive method of choice unless they select an IUD, which can be inserted at their follow-up visit. For in-clinic abortion patients, all contraceptive methods can be provided that day, including IUDs and implants. Although it may take up to 6 weeks to have a normal period, post–medical and in-clinic abortion patients can ovulate within 1 to 2 weeks of a procedure; thus thorough education and timely initiation of a contraceptive method is encouraged for improved outcomes and prevention of future unintended pregnancies.

NOT TO BE MISSED

Patient-centered contraceptive counseling can begin by asking patients what contraceptive methods they have heard about, what they know about different methods, what methods they have used in the past, and what has worked well for them. Determining if the patient has had any past negative experiences can be useful in excluding certain options and in choosing one that will be successful for them in the future.

FOCUSED HISTORY AND PHYSICAL EXAMINATION

For patients who present with a positive pregnancy test, an initial evaluation should include determination of gestational age and confirmation of the pregnancy intentions of the patient.

Confirmation of Pregnancy

Confirmation of pregnancy includes a urine pregnancy test and/or in-clinic ultrasonography if available and depending on patient history. Consider a serum pregnancy test for quantitative beta-human chorionic gonadotropin (b-hCG) levels if the patient has an empty uterus on the ultrasound examination and/or any symptoms concerning for ectopic pregnancy. This quantitative b-hCG test should be repeated in 48 hours and monitored as indicated.

Establishing Gestational Age

Establishing gestational age includes the following:
- Ask the patient the following: "When was your last menstrual period?" This question should be followed

by a brief menstrual history: "Was your last period normal for you? Are your periods regular/do they come monthly?" If the patient's periods are irregular, the LMP is less likely to be useful in determining gestational age.

- Calculate the LMP. Calculating the LMP is a practical tool for assessing likely gestational age to gauge the necessity for any immediate prenatal care tests and evaluations or to determine what abortion options are available to the patient. To quickly calculate gestational age based on LMP, use a medical app on your smart phone or a pregnancy wheel. Naegele's rule[15] can be used to calculate the estimated due date:

$$\text{LMP} - 3 \text{ months} + 7 \text{ days} + 1 \text{ year}$$
$$= \text{Estimated Date of Delivery (EDD)}$$

Clarification of Patient Intention

The next series of questions should focus on allowing the patient to confirm, define, and/or deliberate, if needed, regarding their intentions for this pregnancy. These questions should be asked in a nonjudgmental manner that allows patients to feel comfortable expressing themselves.

- Ask the patient the following: "Now that we have established that you are pregnant, how are you feeling? Are there any questions or concerns that you have? Were you seeking pregnancy at this time? Do you know what you would like to do with this pregnancy? What information can I offer to help guide you? Would you like more time to think about your options?"
- Create a nonjudgmental space for patients to completely consider their pregnancy intention. This allows for validation of the patient's thoughts and feelings. By establishing an unbiased clinical setting, the clinician encourages patient-centered reflection and exudes impartial support so patients can make the best decision for themselves and their families.
- Following establishment of gestational age and patient intention, the clinician should proceed with the history and physical examination.

Essential History and Screening

- Information gained from the patient's history allows the clinician to better determine the extent of physical examination, laboratory tests, and imaging that

must be performed or ordered at this visit. It also allows the clinician to determine if high-risk, specialty consult, or referral must be considered.

- As with any visit, it is important to ask about past and current medical history— particularly past pregnancy and gynecological history—in order to determine if there are any particular risk factors for this patient that must be assessed now or noted for future visits. Ask if there is a history of prior pregnancy or pregnancy with risk factors including gestational diabetes, gestational hypertension, or preeclampsia. Ask if there is any history of abnormal pregnancy, such as ectopic or molar pregnancy. Ask about prior cesarean and vaginal deliveries as well as a history of abortion, miscarriage, or preterm delivery. Ask if the patient has any current health conditions, particularly chronic conditions that require taking medications. Common chronic medical conditions include diabetes, hypertension, human immunodeficiency virus (HIV), bipolar disorder, depression, and hepatitis B and C. Also ask about past and current tobacco, alcohol, and drug use. Confirm vaccination history and whether the patient is up to date with immunizations. Ask about current or prior sexually transmitted infections. Obtaining the patient's past and current medical history will guide the care plan. See Box 10.3 for obstetrical history and Box 10.4 for focused history.
- Confirm and assess any medications the patient might be taking, particularly if contraindicated in pregnancy. If uncertain, consult the provider. Advise

---

BOX 10.3 Obstetrical History: GP(TPAL)

G = Number of gestations (the number of times a patient has been pregnant)
P = Number of live births
T = Number of full-term births (>37 weeks gestation)
P = Number of preterm births (<37 weeks gestation)
A = Number of spontaneous and/or therapeutic abortions
L = Number of living children
Example 1: A patient who has been pregnant 5 times, had 2 abortions, 2 full-term births, and 1 preterm delivery, with 3 living children would be written: G5P2123.
Example 2: A patient who has been pregnant once with twins and had a full-term delivery would be written: G1P1002.

BOX 10.4 Focused History

- LMP and gestational age
- Menstrual history
- OB/GYN History (including miscarriage, abnormal pregnancy, cesarean delivery)
- Past medical/surgical history
- Family history
- Current medications
- Allergies
- STI/HIV Status
- Drug/alcohol use
- Mental health history
- Social history
- Interpersonal violence (IPV) screening
- Targeted ROS (Constitutional, GYN, Psych)

patients not to take any medications, including over-the-counter and herbal medications, without discussing it with their prenatal provider. For patients with concerns about possible exposures during their pregnancy, MotherToBaby offers scientific information and fact sheets to help parents understand if they may have had an at-risk medical or environmental exposure: https://mothertobaby.org/.

- Confirm any allergies.
- Ask about potential social stressors including factors that place the patient at risk for emotional, economic, or physical strain. Ask about current housing status and economic resources. Confirm food and housing stability. Offer social support services if there are concerns for scarcity. Ask about current or prior history of abuse. Ask the patient if they feel safe in her living situation and if they have experienced any physical or emotional abuse or threat of abuse. Offer social work resources or referrals as indicated. If the patient reports current abuse, a more immediate plan is needed including possible involvement of law enforcement. Know your local domestic violence resources and clinic protocols for mediating current acts of violence and violent threats. Make sure you are in compliance with mandatory reporting laws, with special consideration to minors.
- Assess for depression and anxiety using the Patient Health Questionnaire-4 (PHQ4) to determine if further evaluation or referral for therapy is indicated. For patients who are already in established psychiatric care, ask about medications, and advise that

they call their current mental health provider to alert them of their pregnancy status and for follow-up care if they are planning to continue the pregnancy. If the patient demonstrates signs of severe depression or anxiety and/or any suicidal or homicidal ideation, it is important to have a clinical plan in place for immediate referral, assessment, and evaluation, including potential emergency department transfer.

- Ask about Rh factor if known. If the patient is Rh-negative, ask about any bleeding to date. Consider an early Rhogam injection as indicated.
- Perform a review of systems with attention to pregnancy-related symptoms. Ask about urinary frequency, breast tenderness, nausea, vomiting, fatigue, pelvic pain, bleeding, and mood changes. A limited review of systems may be done, but it is very important to ask about any pelvic pain, cramping, vaginal bleeding including spotting, and/or shoulder pain that has occurred since the patient's LMP; these questions are useful in highlighting any red flag symptoms that might indicate risk for spontaneous abortion, ectopic pregnancy, and/or other abnormal pregnancies.
- Offer a brief synopsis of genetic testing options so the patient can elect the preferred tests and make a decision regarding testing at a follow-up appointment. A multitude of options exist. Some patients will select all testing options, while others will elect no testing, and others might request that the clinician help them in their decision-making process. A referral to a genetic counselor might be necessary for patients who are undecided or who have higher-risk histories such as prior pregnancies with genetic abnormalities, children born with genetic differences, a maternal or paternal family history of genetic abnormalities, and/or advanced maternal age (usually considered to be 35 years of age and older). The specific genetic testing options during pregnancy will depend on what is available in the provider's health care setting, but four general options exist:
  - No genetic testing.
  - First-trimester screening combines a nuchal translucency ultrasound examination and blood testing to screen for trisomy 21 (Down syndrome) and trisomy 18. The ultrasound examination is performed between weeks 11 and 14 along with a blood test. A second blood test, also know as *the triple screen or maternal serum alpha-fetoprotein*

screen, is then performed between weeks 15 and 22 but is most accurate between 16 and 18 weeks; this tests for genetic issues including neural tube defects and spina bifida. Patients who are beyond 14 weeks can elect the QUAD screening blood test to be drawn between 15 and 22 weeks, but this is less accurate than the first-trimester ultrasound screening plus the triple screen blood test.

- Noninvasive prenatal screening (NIPS) offers more extensive aneuploidy screening for Down syndrome, trisomy-18, trisomy-13, and other genetic abnormalities including triploidy and microdeletion without the invasive technique of the following option. In addition, this testing reveals the chromosomal sex of the fetus.
- Chorionic villi sampling (CVS) and amniocentesis are diagnostic procedures used to detect genetic abnormalities in the fetus. Both options are invasive and involve taking a sample from the placenta or the amniotic fluid with a needle or catheter. Whereas the previous genetic testing options give percentages of risk for genetic outcomes, these options give definitive results but bear a slightly increased risk for miscarriage. CVS is performed during weeks 10 to 12, and amniocentesis is performed during weeks 15 to 22.

Physical Examination

- Consider the patient history when determining if this visit necessitates a pelvic examination. If the patient complains of pelvic pain, bleeding, dysuria, or malodorous and/or itchy vaginal discharge, a pelvic examination should be part of the clinician's management plan. See Box 10.5 for physical examination,

---

BOX 10.5 Physical Examination/Lab Tests/Diagnostics

- Urine pregnancy test
- Blood pressure
- Transvaginal or abdominal ultrasound examination
- Possible pelvic examination
- Hemoglobin/hematocrit
- Rh factor
- STI/HIV screening
- Possible quantitative b-HCG testing
- Prenatal laboratory panel

---

laboratory tests, and diagnostics used when evaluating the pregnant patient.

- If the patient reports an LMP consistent with a gestational age of 11 to 12 weeks or more and wishes to hear the fetal heart tones, listening for a fetal heart rate can be performed; however, consider that listening to the fetal heart rate might be inappropriate for an unwanted pregnancy, and it is important to ask patients for their preference.

The Use of Ultrasonography in Early Pregnancy to Assess for Gestational Age and Abnormal Pregnancy

- Depending on the clinical setting, an ultrasound examination may be offered to confirm that the pregnancy is located inside the uterus, determine gestational age, and to assess for viability. It is important to ascertain whether the patient would like to see the ultrasound scan or not, be informed about multiple gestations, or receive a copy of the ultrasound scan. One patient may be elated to see the 4-millimeter embryo within her early gestational sac; another patient may feel the exact opposite, wishing to move through the clinical assessment as quickly as possible.
- Although it is not necessary to perform an ultrasound examination before providing reproductive options counseling, it can contribute useful information to the clinical picture. For example, for patients who are certain that they do not want to continue the pregnancy and their LMP was around 10 weeks ago, an ultrasound examination will determine if they are still a candidate for medication abortion.
- Consider that ultrasonography might show a multiple-gestation pregnancy. If the patient does not wish to continue the pregnancy, it is important to confirm before the ultrasound examination whether or not the patient would like to know about multiple gestations. If the patient wishes to continue the pregnancy, either for the purpose of parenting or for adoption, have resources ready to counsel the patient. In many settings, multiple pregnancies are managed by either high-risk obstetrics or an obstetrician/gynecologist, so clinicians should be aware of the policy, plans, and procedures surrounding multiple-gestation pregnancies in their health care setting. Just as a positive pregnancy test might elicit different emotional responses from different patients,

so might the revelation of a multiple-gestation pregnancy. The supportive clinician should be ready to engage in options counseling should this finding prompt indecision or an array of emotions from the patient.

- If a patient is 5 weeks from the LMP, the provider should expect to see a gestational sac with a yolk on transvaginal ultrasonography. If the urine pregnancy test is positive and the uterus appears empty on ultrasonography, the patient is diagnosed with a pregnancy of unknown location (PUL). A PUL can be an early pregnancy that is too small to be seen, a resolving spontaneous abortion, or an ectopic pregnancy.

- Miscarriage or spontaneous abortion is an involuntary loss of pregnancy that occurs before 22 completed weeks of pregnancy. It should be suspected in an early pregnancy that presents with bleeding or that cannot be located on ultrasonography. It is very common and occurs in 10% to 20% of known pregnancies, most commonly in the first trimester.[16] Suggestive ultrasound findings along with significantly down-trending serial quantitative b-hCG levels aid in the diagnosis of miscarriage.

- An ectopic pregnancy occurs when the pregnancy develops outside the uterine endometrial cavity; the most common location for ectopic pregnancy is the fallopian tube.[17] Ectopic pregnancy can lead to tissue rupture, internal bleeding, and death; suggestive symptoms or risk factors for ectopic pregnancy are not to be missed. Risk factors for ectopic pregnancy include prior ectopic pregnancy, tubal surgery, prior genital infections (especially chlamydia), IUD use at the time of pregnancy diagnosis, and smoking. A patient who presents with an early pregnancy whose location has not been confirmed and significant pelvic pain and/or bleeding requires a more immediate ultrasound examination to confirm pregnancy location. Patients with a suspected ectopic pregnancy should be assessed with quantitative b-hCG levels and referred for a diagnostic pelvic ultrasound examination and/or emergent management depending on their symptoms and presentation. If an intrauterine pregnancy cannot be confirmed on ultrasonography when the b-hCG level reaches 1500 to 2000 mU/mL, it should raise increased suspicion for an ectopic pregnancy. The vigilant clinician will always consider ectopic pregnancy as a

potential diagnosis as it can quickly become a medical emergency with a significant risk of morbidity and mortality.

- Additional pregnancy abnormalities that can be determined though ultrasonography include anembryonic gestation, hydatidiform mole, and intrauterine fetal demise. Anembryonic gestation is defined as a pregnancy in which the gestational sac has a mean diameter of greater than or equal to 25 mm but contains no embryo. A molar pregnancy is a chromosomally abnormal pregnancy that has the potential to become malignant; these pregnancies are often described as having a "beehive" or "cluster of grapes" appearance on ultrasonography. An intrauterine fetal demise is defined in most states as demise of a previously confirmed viable fetus at ≥20 weeks of gestation and/or weight of ≥500 g.

- The clinician should always consider the possibility of abnormalities in an early pregnancy whose location and presentation has yet to be confirmed on ultrasonography, particularly if a patient presents with a positive pregnancy test and significant vaginal bleeding and/or severe pain. Although cramping and spotting are quite common in early pregnancy, more significant pain or bleeding or a combination of the two should alert the clinician to consider further evaluation for abnormalities. It should also be noted that many ectopic and abnormal pregnancies are asymptomatic and that ultrasonography is the diagnostic tool of choice for confirming a viable intrauterine pregnancy and/or ruling out other abnormalities.

NOT TO BE MISSED

Ectopic pregnancies can lead to tissue rupture, internal bleeding, and death; suggestive symptoms or risk factors for ectopic pregnancy are not to be missed.

POPULATION-SPECIFIC CONSIDERATIONS FOR PATIENTS WITH SPECIAL NEEDS, RISK FACTORS, OR SPECIAL SITUATIONS

A patient's own physical conditions, developmental delays, chronic health issues, genetic disorders, family history, and mental health have the potential to add an additional layer of complexity to options counseling. Patients with health conditions will likely consider the risk for their own health and for that of the fetus; they might be concerned about the possibility that the child may be born with similar health conditions. Diabetic patients might consider the risk of pregnancy both for themselves and the fetus. Patients with a learning disability might wonder if their child will face the same challenges they had in school. Patients who are currently treated with psychotropic medications for bipolar disorder might debate the risk versus benefit of medication continuation for stability of their condition versus stopping medications for fear of potential fetal harm. Patients with cerebral palsy might wonder if their child would be born with this condition. In addition to the complex psychosocial factors affecting their decision to continue the pregnancy, adopt, or terminate, patients with one or more health conditions might need additional counseling or resources to make the best decision for themselves, their families, and their futures.

Beyond the medical issues that may complicate pregnancy and/or abortion, there are additional psychosocial factors that may cause issues for pregnant patients seeking reproductive options counseling. Prior history of mental health disorders, history of physical and/or sexual abuse, and patients with low self-worth or a limited sense of control over their lives may be at risk for poor coping.[7] The clinician should seek to understand their patient's multi-faceted life circumstances and provide guidance to identify supportive individuals, while also referring the patient to additional community resources as needed.

NOT TO BE MISSED

- Reproductive options counseling must be comprehensive, nonbiased, and patient-centered care; the clinician should understand that systemic racism and lack of inclusivity can negatively affect patient outcomes.
- A health care visit that includes a positive pregnancy test requires that the clinician engage in reproductive options counseling, medical assessment and evaluation, patient education, and appropriate referrals.

■ KEY POINTS

- A positive pregnancy test result does not always entail a streamlined or predictable visit format; establishing pregnancy intention and exploring pregnancy options with each patient is critical.
- Well-prepared clinicians will enlist comprehensive reproductive options counseling into their armory of clinical tools.
- Clinicians should engage in values clarification exercises to prevent their own internal biases and judgments from affecting the clinical care they provide.
- Using inclusive language and asking patients for preferred pronouns and gender identity creates an inclusive space for all patients.
- Patient-centered advocacy methods must be utilized to empower pregnant patients to make the best decision for themselves, whether it involves continuation, adoption, or abortion.

REFERENCES

1. Abbas D, Chong E, Raymond EG. Outpatient medical abortion is safe and effective through 70 days gestation. *Contraception*. 2015;92(3):197–199.
2. Guttmacher Institute. *Unintended Pregnancy in the United States*; 2019. https://www.guttmacher.org/fact-sheet/unintended-pregnancy-united-states
3. Jones J. Adoption experiences of women and men and demand for children to adopt by women 18–44 years of age in the United States, 2002. *Vital Health Stat*. 2008;23(27):1–36.
4. Planned Parenthood Federation of America. Pregnancy and Childbearing Among U.S. Teens. July 2014. https://www.plannedparenthood.org/uploads/filer_public/56/25/5625151f-3aac-4fcb-a861-1ab8ddb64a48/pregnancychildbearing_070814.pdf
5. Guttmacher Institute. U.S. Supreme Court Overturns Roe v. Wade; 2022. https://www.guttmacher.org/news-release/2022/us-supreme-court-overturns-roe-v-wade.
6. U.S. Centers for Disease Control and Prevention. *Maternal Mortality Rates in the United States, 2020*; 2020. https://www.cdc.gov/nchs/data/hestat/maternal-mortality/2020/E-stat-Maternal-Mortality-Rates-2022.pdf.
7. Perrucci AC. *Decision Assessment and Counseling in Abortion Care*. Lanham, Maryland: Rowman & Littlefield Publishers, Inc; 2012.

8. Adamec C. *The Adoption Option Complete Handbook: 2000–2001*. Rocklin, California: Prima Lifestyles; 1999.

9. Guttmacher Institute. *An Overview of Abortion Laws*; 2022. https://www.guttmacher.org/state-policy/explore/overview-abortion-laws

10. UCSF Bixby Center for Global Reproductive Health. *The Abortion Provider Toolkit*; 2018. https://aptoolkit.org/nurse-practitioners-midwives-and-physician-assistants-as-abortion-providers/history-of-providing-comprehensive-health-care-including-abortion-care/.

11. UCSF Bixby Center for Global Reproductive Health. *The Abortion Provider Toolkit*; 2018. https://aptoolkit.org/advancing-scope-of-practice-to-include-abortion-care/state-abortion-laws-and-their-relationship-to-scope-of-practice/#state-laws.

12. World Health Organization. *Safe Abortion: Technical and Policy Guidance for Health Systems*. 2nd ed. Geneva, Switzerland: World Health Organization; 2012.

13. Aiken ARA, Romanova EP, Morber JR, Gomperts R. Safety and effectiveness of self-managed medication abortion provided using online telemedicine in the United States: a population based study. *Lancet Reg Health Am*. 2022;10: 100200.

14. Grossman D, Grindlay K. Alternatives to ultrasound for follow-up after medication abortion: a systematic review. *Contraception*. 2011;83(6):504–510.

15. Dutton LA, Densmore JE, Turner MB. *The Efficient Midwife*. Sudbury, Massachusetts: Jones & Bartlett Publishers; 2010.

16. Alberman E. *Spontaneous Abortions: Epidemiology*. London: Springer London; 1992.

17. Bouyer J, Coste J, Fernandez H, Pouly JL, Job-Spira N. Sites of ectopic pregnancy: a 10 year population-based study of 1800 cases. *Hum Reprod*. 2002;17(12): 3224–3230.

18. World Health Organization. *Safe Abortion: Technical and Policy Guidance for Health Systems*. 2nd ed. Geneva, Switzerland: World Health Organization; 2012. https://apps.who.int/iris/bitstream/handle/10665/70914/9789241548434_eng.pdf.

11

Sexual Health Assessment

Lorraine Byrnes

OBJECTIVES:

At the completion of this chapter the reader will be able to:
- Describe the theoretical and conceptual models of sexual response for females and males.
- Conduct a comprehensive sexual health history with individuals seeking health care.
- Conduct a comprehensive physical assessment in relation to sexual health, sexual dysfunction, and sexual complaints.
- Develop a plan of care based on assessment findings.
- Refer patients for treatment of complex sexual dysfunction.

INTRODUCTION

Sexuality and sexual health are essential to well-being and quality of life for most, if not all, humans. *Sexuality* is defined as the sexual habits and desires one has, the capacity of humans to have erotic experiences, and the attractions, responses, and feelings we have toward others. Sexuality is a complex concept that is integral to our experience as humans and touches on biological, psychological, emotional, and environmental factors. A sexual history is an integral part of a thorough and comprehensive physical examination and serves as the starting point to address sexual health and dysfunction. This chapter provides an evidence-based comprehensive guide to collecting a sexual history from individuals along with recommendations for maintaining sexual health and treating sexual complaints. This chapter does not provide an in-depth overview of treating sexual dysfunction, but resources and references are included for further knowledge development.

UNDERSTANDING SEXUAL RESPONSE: THEORETICAL AND CONCEPTUAL FRAMEWORKS

Masters and Johnson, regarded as pioneers in the study of human sexual response, developed the four-phase sexual response cycle (1966).[1] This cycle was based on research conducted at the Kinsey Institute. The four phases are conceptualized to occur in a linear manner (Fig. 11.1).

- Phase 1: Excitement. This phase may last minutes to hours and includes an increased heart and respiratory rate, muscle tension, flushing of skin, and increased blood flow to the genitalia resulting in an erection in the male and increased vaginal lubrication in the female.
- Phase 2: Plateau. This phase extends from phase 1 to the brink of orgasm. Physical characteristics include retraction of the testicles and clitoris, increasing muscle tension, and increased blood pressure, heart rate, and respiratory rate.
- Phase 3: Orgasm. This is the shortest phase and may last only a few seconds. This phase consists of involuntary muscle contractions, a sudden forceful release of sexual tension, contraction of the genitalia, and a flushing of the skin.
- Phase 4: Resolution. This phase includes a sense of well-being, enhanced intimacy, and perhaps some fatigue. Females are capable of a quicker recovery and return to the orgasmic phase. Males need time to recover (the refractory period) before they can again reach orgasm. The length of this refractory

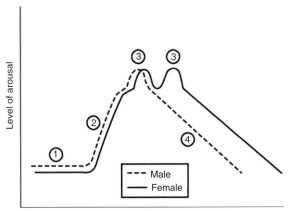

Figure 11.1 Four-phase sexual response cycle. (From *Textbook of Primary Care Medicine*. Third Edition, Elsevier.)

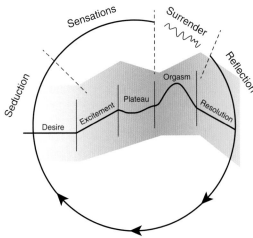

Figure 11.2 Circular model of female sexual response. (Reprinted with permission from *The Female Patient*. 2002;27:39-44. ©2002, Frontline Medical Communications Inc.)

period is dependent on age and general health. For more information about Masters and Johnson, visit: https://kinseyinstitute.org/collections/archival/masters-and-johnson.php

Whipple and Brash-McGreer (1997)[21] developed an alternate model of human sexual response that is circular and postulates that sexual response for females is differentiated by the addition of a phase that includes seduction, which also encompasses desire. Whipple and Brash-McGreer believed that if the sexual experience was pleasurable and satisfying for the female, then there

was an increased likelihood of the experience being repeated (Fig. 11.2).

Rosemary Basson (2001)[3] postulates that the goal of sexuality for females is not orgasm but physical and emotional satisfaction. Basson's model of human sexual response is based solely on females and is nonlinear. It emphasizes the importance of intimacy, sexual stimulation, and a satisfactory relationship. This conceptual model may help clinicians who are working with female patients explore issues around sexual response (Fig. 11.3).

> **PATIENT-CENTERED CARE:** These conceptual models of sexual response are representations to share with patients and can be utilized to describe sexual response and help identify sexual dysfunction when it is present. Each model conceptualizes sexuality from a different perspective, and each can help providers and patients understand the complexity of sexual response and explore clinical solutions.

DEVELOPING COMFORT AND EXPERTISE WITH ASSESSING SEXUAL HEALTH

Fully understanding human sexual response is critically important to addressing the sexual complaints that patients bring to the primary care setting. The ability to conduct a comprehensive sexual health interview enables the clinician to explore and examine the patient's perception of the problem, understanding of

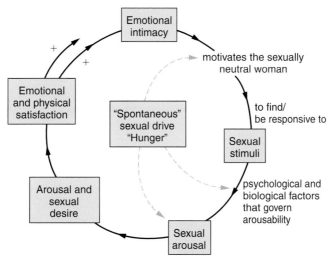

Figure 11.3 Nonlinear model of female sexual response. (From Basson R. Female sexual response: the role of drugs in the management of sexual dysfunction. *Obstet Gynecol.* 2001;98[2]:350–353.)

sexual function, and other factors contributing to sexual health or sexual dysfunction. Sexual activity should be consensual and pleasurable, but these concepts are often absent from the sexual health assessment.

A comprehensive sexual history should be taken at the initial visit and updated annually and when the patient presents with concerns or signs and symptoms of a sexually transmitted infection (STI) or sexual dysfunction.

> **CLINICAL SURVIVAL TIP:** Conducting a sexual history is an opportunity to not only learn about your patient's sexuality and sexual behaviors but identify risky behaviors and gaps in knowledge and to share information about maintaining sexual health.

Individuals, including health care providers, may not be comfortable discussing sexuality, sexual practices, and other sexual information. Health care providers should approach the topic in a nonjudgmental manner and develop the skills necessary to put patients at ease as the interview progresses. Providers should inform patients that this information and all information collected as part of the health encounter will remain confidential and is being collected to develop a comprehensive plan of care. The goals of the sexual health assessment should include an assessment of satisfaction with sexual response, questions or issues with sexual identity and orientation, and risky behaviors including inconsistent use of contraceptives

when pregnancy is not a goal and behaviors/practices that may cause physical and/or psychological trauma or increase the risk of infection. Sexual complaints are not uncommon in the primary care setting, and most can be treated without referral to a specialist.

SEXUAL ORIENTATION

Sexual orientation is often defined by sexual preference. As part of the sexual health assessment we ask our patients the following questions:
- Who do you have sex with?
  or
- Do you have sex with males, females, or both?

We ask these questions, as providers, not to be intrusive but to assess the potential for risk and exposure to preventable diseases like STIs. Patients may prefer not to be assigned or labeled with a sexual orientation or sexual preference, but they may feel very comfortable using terms such as *bisexual, heterosexual, pansexual, asexual, transgender, lesbian, homosexual, gay,* or *same-sex relationship.* Explore with your patients the terms they are comfortable using, and make a notation in the health record for continued use.

> **PATIENT-CENTERED CARE:** Sexual preference may by dynamic and vary as the individual experiences different stages of life.

CONDUCTING A SEXUAL HEALTH ASSESSMENT

The PLISSIT model (permission, limited information, specific suggestions, intensive therapy) is a framework for counseling patients with sexual/behavioral problems.[4,5] The model begins with an exploration of sexual questions, problems, and/or issues in a nonjudgmental manner by seeking permission to engage. The PLISSIT model can be used as a framework for initiating the sexual health assessment in which the clinician seeks permission to inquire and explore sexual health in a nonjudgmental manner, gathers information based solely on the presenting concern, and makes recommendations to improve sexual health and reduce sexual risk. This may be in the form of health education and counseling, referral for sex therapy, or referral to an expert clinician who specializes in the problem.

NOT TO BE MISSED

A quick primer on initiating the PLISSIT model into a primary care practice (Palmisano, 2017) can be found at: https://www.psychiatryadvisor.com/home/practice-management/plissit-model-introducing-sexual-health-in-clinical-care/

Surveys, questionnaires, and devices can assist in the data collection process. Questionnaires can be mailed to patients before clinical encounters or can be completed in the waiting room using paper and pencil or as part of the electronic health record. Utilization of reliable and valid screening instruments to assess sexual health and sexual dysfunction can also assist with time management for the patient and clinician.

The Female Sexual Function Index (FSFI) is a 19-item Likert scale instrument that helps assess the domains of arousal, orgasm, satisfaction, and pain among females.[6] The FSFI is a self-report measure that has been validated among females with female orgasmic disorder (FOD) and hypoactive sexual desire disorder (HSDD). The FSFI has also been tested in a sample of females who have sex with females, and it was found to be reliable and valid.[7] The FSFI is available free of charge at: https://www.nva.org/wp-content/uploads/2015/01/FSFI-questionnaire2000.pdf.

The Sexual Health Inventory for Men (SHIM) is a five-item Likert scale instrument used to assess erectile dysfunction. It is available free of charge at: http://www.rohbaltimore.com/SHIM.pdf.

Anatomical models can provide a visual guide when exploring sexual questions or concerns that patients may have. Patients may be unfamiliar with their own anatomy and may need assurance that their genitalia are normal. An anatomical model can help explain the structure and function of the genitalia. A large hand mirror is an inexpensive investment that will allow patients to view their own genitalia while you point out and name the structures and their function.

Lastly if you, as the provider, are uncomfortable asking questions about sexuality, the patient may sense it. Practicing and role-playing the encounter with a trusted colleague will help address discomfort before you introduce sexual assessment into your clinical toolbox. The National Coalition for Sexual Health has made available a series of videos discussing the role of the health care provider to address potential discomfort when taking a sexual health history. These are available at: https://nationalcoalitionforsexualhealth.org/tools/for-healthcare-providers.

Additional Assessment Resources

A Guide to Taking a Sexual History, published by the U.S. Centers for Disease Control and Prevention (CDC) and available at https://www.cdc.gov/std/treatment/sexual-history.pdf, provides a comprehensive framework for conducting a sexual history. This guide is structured around the five *P*s: *p*artner(s) *p*ractice(s), *p*rotection from STIs, *p*ast history of STIs, and *p*revention of pregnancy. The guide was developed to assess the risk for STIs, but it can serve as a foundation for assessing sexual function, sexual dysfunction, and sexual concerns or issues that your patients may have.

Sexual Health and Your Patients: A Providers Guide, published by The National Coalition for Sexual Health and available at https://nationalcoalitionforsexualhealth.org/tools/for-healthcare-providers/asset/Provider-Guide_May-2022.pdf, is a comprehensive guide to sexual health history taking. This guide builds on the work of the CDC and adds a sixth *P*, *p*leasure, to be assessed and provides both the rationale and sample questions for assessing sexual pleasure as part of the sexual history.

ASSESSMENT OF THE FEMALE PATIENT: A GENERAL OVERVIEW

A sexual health assessment should be part of the female patient's comprehensive annual examination. Sexuality, sexual orientation, and sexual response can be assessed during the review of systems. Asking questions in simple, direct language and making eye contact with patients will help put them at ease. Begin the sexual history by asking the following screening questions:

- Have you been sexually active during this past year?
- Do you have sex with males, females, or both?
- How many sex partners have you had this past year?

Then ask the following screening questions to assess sexual function:

- Do you have concerns about your sexual function?
- Do you have concerns about sexual satisfaction or sexual desire?

Studies have shown that females may have difficulty initiating a discussion about sexual dysfunction with a health care provider or their sexual partner.[8-11] Therefore, it is extremely important to address this issue on an annual basis. Additional areas to assess may include sexual pleasure, pain during sex, and any other dysfunction or concern experienced by the patient. Dysfunction can be categorized as physical (e.g., vaginismus) or psychological (anorgasmia).[12] Suggest exploring whether the problem is lifelong or acquired and specific or generalized.

The clinician may ask the following focused questions:

- Does the problem always occur, or is it specific to a partner or circumstances?
- Did the problem always exist, or did it occur as a result of an illness, surgery, accident, or use of a medication?

A physical examination should be conducted at baseline and when a patient presents with a sexual concern or complaint. Consider utilizing an anatomical model to assess the patient's knowledge of her own anatomy and function of her genital structures. The patient can visualize and ask questions about structures and function in a nonthreatening environment. If an anatomical model is not available, it is fairly easy to draw a two-dimensional representation on paper and then review it with the patient (Fig. 11.4). Box 11.1 demonstrates selected sexual conditions and available therapies.

PATIENT-CENTERED CARE: Consider utilizing an anatomical model to assess the patient's knowledge of her own anatomy and function of her genital structures. The patient can visualize and ask questions about structures and function in a nonthreatening environment.

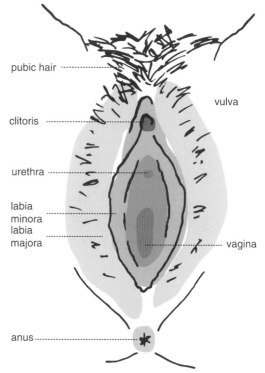

Figure 11.4 Example of a simple two-dimensional drawing of the vulva. (Image reproduced from *The Labia Library* https://www.labialibrary.org.au/ with permission of the copyright holder Women's Health Victoria Inc.)

ASSESSING FEMALE ORGASMIC DISORDER

According to the *Diagnostic and Statistical Manual of Mental Disorders,* 5th edition, text revision *(DSM-5-TR),* the diagnosis of female orgasmic disorder (FOD) must meet certain diagnostic criteria. The criteria include infrequent, delayed, or absent orgasms and a decrease in the intensity of orgasms. The symptoms must cause significant distress and have been present 75% to 100% of time the patient engages in sexual activity for a minimum of 6 months.

FOD can be classified as *specific* (occurs only with certain situations, partners, and/or stimulation) or *generalized* (not limited to the aforementioned factors). FOD can be lifelong (the problem has existed since sexual activity was initiated) or acquired (the problem began after normal orgasmic experiences). The prevalence of FOD has been estimated to range from 10% to 42% of the female population in the United States, but it is dependent on age, culture, and other factors.

BOX 11.1   **Selected Sexual Conditions and Available Therapies**

Sexual Condition	Therapy
Low libido	• Identification of contributing medications (e.g., selective serotonin reuptake inhibitors, antihypertensive medications) and consideration of an alternative or lower dose, if possible • Referral to a sex therapist • Rx: flibanserin or bremelanotide • Off-label use of testosterone
Vaginal dryness	• Sexual activity on a regular basis to promote blood flow • Vaginal lubricants and/or moisturizers • Localized estrogen therapy: vaginal tablet, ring, or cream
Difficulty achieving orgasm	• Sex therapy • Use of a vibrator • Off-label use of sildenafil
Pain	• Lubricants and/or moisturizers • Topical estrogen • For postmenopausal women: ospemifene (selective estrogen receptor modulator) • Vaginal dilators • Sex therapy • Physical therapy

Physiological factors include spinal cord injury, multiple sclerosis, the use of medications including selective serotonin reuptake inhibitors (SSRIs), and genitourinary syndrome of menopause (GSM). Psychological factors include anxiety, fear of pregnancy, or the experience of sexual assault including forced sexual activity or the experience of sexual abuse as a child.

Treatment is largely determined by the cause and is tailored to the individual patient. For female patients with FOD related to sexual inexperience, education focuses on anatomy and physiology, and sexual response may be a starting point and an end point. Clinicians may refer female patients to a sex therapist or a therapist with training and certification in sexual issues as an option when time and/or reimbursement issues exist. If the cause of FOD is related to medications, an adjustment may be made if warranted. Female patients

with histories of abuse, trauma, persistent psychiatric disorders, or relationship issues can be comanaged with a qualified therapist.

ASSESSING FEMALE SEXUAL INTEREST/AROUSAL DISORDER

In 2013, the authors of the *DSM-5* merged the diagnosis of *female sexual arousal disorder* with *hypoactive sexual desire disorder* into one diagnosis: *female sexual interest/arousal disorder.* The *DSM-5-TR* defines female sexual interest/arousal disorder (FSIAD) as a lack of or significantly reduced interest in sex and includes, at minimum, three of the following: absent or reduced initiation of sexual activity, absent or reduced sexual fantasies or thoughts, unresponsiveness to a partner's attempt to initiate sexual activity, absent or reduced excitement or pleasure from sexual activity, and absent or reduced sensation in the genitalia during sexual encounters. The symptoms must cause significant distress to the individual and be present for 6 months or longer. The prevalence of FSIAD has been estimated to be as high as 30% of females in the United States. Risk factors for developing FSIAD include the following:

- Negative attitudes about sex and sexuality
- Medical conditions including endocrine disorders
- Medications known to negatively affect libido
- Substance misuse or abuse
- Physical and/or emotional abuse
- Relationship and/or communication problems

In an effort to develop an effective treatment plan, it is important to determine the etiology of the problem and if the condition is lifelong or acquired. Referring a patient for individual or couples therapy is often the first step to treat FSIAD.

Bremelanotide and flibanserin are currently the only medications specifically developed for the treatment of FSIAD that are approved by the U.S. Food and Drug Administration (FDA). Both are indicated for premenopausal female patients with low libido that causes significant distress. Female patients using flibanserin must be counseled to refrain from the use of alcohol, as severe hypotension and syncope are likely to result. For more information on flibanserin, visit: https://addyihcp.com/. For more information on bremelanotide, visit: https://vyleesipro.com/?utm_source=dtc_vyleesi&utm_medium=website&campaign=sticky_header.

Testosterone is not FDA approved in the United States as pharmacotherapy to treat FSAID, but studies have found that when used alone or with sildenafil, buspirone, or bupropion, testosterone increases sexual desire and/or satisfaction compared with placebo.[13,14] For a more comprehensive review of the use of testosterone among females, refer to the Global Consensus Position Statement on the Use of Testosterone Therapy for Women at https://academic.oup.com/jcem/article/104/10/4660/5556103?login=false.

> ## ⚠ SAFETY ALERT
>
> Female patients who are prescribed flibnaserin must be counseled against alcohol consumption, as the concomitant use of flibanserin and alcohol can cause severe hypotension and syncope.

ASSESSING GENITOPELVIC PAIN/ PENETRATION DISORDER

Dyspareunia is the term used to describe painful sexual intercourse related to physical or psychological causes. However, pain may also be experienced when attempting to insert a tampon, a contraceptive ring, or a finger. Determining the cause of the pain is critical to developing a plan of care. Pain is often described as burning or stabbing. The pain can be concentrated in one area or be diffuse.

Explore with the patient when the pain occurs. Is the pain experienced when penetration is attempted? Is penetration possible with lubrication? Is there sufficient time given to foreplay? Using the sexual response model, you can provide education about female response time and that lubrication generally occurs during the excitement phase if given sufficient time. Demonstrate the use of lubricants and, if possible, have samples available in your office.

> **PATIENT-CENTERED CARE:** Determining the cause of dyspareunia is critical to developing a plan of care. Pain is often described as burning or stabbing. The pain can be concentrated in one area or be diffuse. Explore with the patient when the pain occurs.

Does the patient experience vaginismus? Vaginismus is the occurrence of involuntary muscle spasms in the vaginal musculature that can lead to pain and difficulty with penetration. Female patients with vaginismus may never have experienced any type of penetration.

Has the patient experienced trauma or injury to her genitalia? Inquire about childhood injuries, birth injuries, and any history of genital surgery. Has the patient had female circumcision? Explore with your patient any history of congenital malformation. The patient may have been born with an imperforate hymen or vaginal agenesis in which the vagina was not fully formed and developed.

Vulvodynia is defined as chronic vulvar pain without an identifiable etiology and is divided into two subtypes: generalized and localized. Localized vulvodynia occurs in response to pressure to the vestibule and is localized to a particular spot. When assessing vulvodynia, it is helpful to use an anatomical model and ask the patient to locate the point of pain she experiences before conducting a physical examination. Gynecological examinations can provoke localized vulvodynia, therefore it is very important to discuss the reason for the examination before beginning. The exact cause of vulvodynia remains unknown, but contributing factors include elevated levels of inflammatory substances in the vulva, genetic susceptibility, pelvic floor weakness or spasm, injury or irritation to the nerves that connect the spinal cord to the vulva, and possibly an increase in the number and/or sensitivity of pain-sensing nerve fibers in the vulva. Symptoms may be exacerbated by tight clothing, tampon insertion, sexual intercourse, prolonged sitting, exercise, and bathing.

Diagnosis of vulvodynia may take time, and it is important to have a referral source for complicated cases. STIs and other infections should be ruled out by collecting cultures. A cotton swab test is conducted in which the clinician gently applies pressure to the vulva in a methodical manner and asks the patient to describe and rate any pain or discomfort experienced. A vulvoscope can be used to examine suspicious areas, and biopsies can be taken and sent to the laboratory.

Treatment of vulvodynia is based on the causative factor(s). Irritants are eliminated from use. Topical anesthetics and/or hormones may be effective, and medications including tricyclic antidepressants (TCAs), serotonin-norepinephrine reuptake inhibitors (SNRIs), and anticonvulsants (gabapentin) have been found to be effective in some sample groups.

Because vulvodynia often adversely affects sexual functioning, it is important to either provide counseling or refer the patient to a therapist with experience in this area. A physical therapist with expertise in treating pain disorders should be part of every clinician's referral network. More information about vulvodynia can be found at the National Vulvodynia Association website: www.nva.org.

NOT TO BE MISSED

Gynecological examinations can provoke localized vulvodynia, therefore it is very important to discuss the reason for the examination before beginning.

SEXUALITY AND PREGNANCY

Female patients often seek information from health care providers during pregnancy about the developing fetus and how to maintain their own health. Sex during pregnancy is a topic that may not be adequately addressed, and myths persist about sex and the potential for harm to the baby. Generally, oral, vaginal, manual, and anal sex is safe during pregnancy if there have been no or few complications. Assure your patients that the fetus cannot be harmed during intercourse. It is important to clarify with the patient and her partner what type of sex they are having. Ask direct, specific questions in a supportive, nonjudgmental manner.

Couples may engage in their usual sexual activities if the pregnancy is without complications. The pregnant patient should be the "guide" as to what is comfortable for her sexually, especially as the pregnancy progresses. Sexual positions may need to be adjusted with the patient lying on her side or assuming the "top" position for penetrative intercourse.

Female patients with a history of preterm labor may be advised to avoid penetrative intercourse during the pregnancy. However, the patient may participate in sexual activity if she avoids penetration. Patients with certain conditions, including placenta previa, unresolved or undiagnosed vaginal bleeding, confirmed diagnosis of ruptured membranes, or suspicion of ruptured or leaking membranes, should be counseled along with their partners to refrain from penetrative sex.

! SAFETY ALERT

Patients with certain conditions, including placenta previa, unresolved or undiagnosed vaginal bleeding, confirmed diagnosis of ruptured membranes, or suspicion of ruptured or leaking membranes, should refrain from penetrative sex.

Explore with the patient how she could engage sexually that would be satisfying to her and her partner. Kissing, touching, and verbal expressions of love, intimacy, and desire can be explored as a substitute if penetrative sex must be avoided. The pregnant patient can engage in sex by giving and/or receiving oral or manual sex.

Patients should be cautioned not to have sex if they experience vaginal spotting or bleeding or if they suspect that their membranes have ruptured.

Some providers encourage the use of sexual intimacy at the beginning of labor to increase the output of maternal oxytocin. This increased output could potentially increase the frequency of uterine contractions and reduce the need for artificial interventions. Birth in the United States is increasingly medicalized, and this may discourage a couple from engaging in expressions of sexual intimacy. Although there are no evidence-based studies on the use of partner or self-stimulation during labor, many anecdotal stories exist. If there are no contraindications including vaginal bleeding, placenta previa, or intrauterine growth restriction, it is acceptable to encourage the laboring woman to engage in sexual activity. Kissing, caressing, nipple stimulation, touch as tolerated to the genitalia, massage, and verbal expressions of love and support should be encouraged during labor. Provide privacy for the couple that wants to engage in this activity during labor and birth.

SEXUALITY AND THE POSTPARTUM PERIOD

A sexual health assessment is a key component of the postpartum visit, as sexual dysfunction is fairly prevalent in the postpartum period.[15] Important contributions have been made to sexuality and the postpartum period, but many gaps exist, and much of the information we provide to female patients is anecdotal.[16,17]

Refraining from sexual activity is often recommended in the postpartum period for up to 8 weeks, but there is little scientific evidence or studies available to support this time frame. Clinicians can explore the resumption of sexual activity with patients at the postpartum visit. To help patients make informed decisions, inquire about the status of lochia, healing of the perineum or surgical scar, method of birth, and complications during the birth and/or postpartum period. Ask about the desire to resume sexual activity using the PLISSIT model.

Female patients who have experienced a surgical birth or perineal trauma may need a longer period for sufficient healing, both physically and psychologically. Consider scheduling a brief postpartum visit or call during the first 2 weeks to assess recovery, adjustment, and healing and to answer questions the patient may have about postpartum recovery.

Assess sleep, sleep quality, breastfeeding, and maternal mood, as they can be contributing factors to sexual dysfunction during this period. Providing support and education can help each patient resume and maintain sexual health. Referral to a sex therapist and a physical therapist who specializes in sexual health should be considered for female patients with new sexual concerns including pain or relational problems.

SEXUAL ASSESSMENT OF THE LGBTQIA+ PATIENT

The *LGBTQ+* community has the same basic health care needs as the general population but faces significant barriers to accessing health care, including real or perceived homophobia, discrimination, and stigma. Studies have shown that negative attitudes toward the *LGBTQ+* community persist among health care providers.[18-20] The Gay and Lesbian Medical Association (GLMA) recommends creating a safe and welcoming environment for all patients, emphasizing confidentiality, providing sensitivity training for health care providers and staff, and creating or adapting sex-neutral health care intake forms and educational materials. It is estimated that approximately 45% of lesbian and bisexual females have not disclosed their sexual orientation to their health care provider.

The Fenway Institute provides a comprehensive guide entitled *Taking a Sexual History with Sexual and Gender Minority Individuals* (Thompson, 2020): https://fenwayhealth.org/wp-content/uploads/6.-Taking-an-Affirming-Sexual-History.pdf.

SEXUAL ASSESSMENT OF THE POSTMENOPAUSAL WOMAN

Menopause is diagnosed after menses have ceased for 1 full year. It is a normal physiological event in a female's life. Females may experience a variety of symptoms including vaginal dryness or loss of lubrication, pain or discomfort with intercourse, burning with urination, hot flashes, diminished libido, difficulty sleeping, night sweats, fatigue, weight gain, and poor self-image.

The physical changes related to menopause include thinning of the vaginal mucosa, decreased sexual response and pleasure, bone loss, skin laxity, and hair loss. Changes and loss of the sex hormones, estrogen, progesterone, and testosterone negatively affect the postmenopausal patient's ability to become aroused, lubricate, and experience orgasm as she may have previously. This can cause significant distress.

A thorough sexual assessment of the postmenopausal patient should be conducted annually and should include questions about previous sexual experiences of desire, arousal, ability to lubricate, and ability to achieve orgasm. The PLISSIT model is very effective in this situation.

The North American Menopause Society (NAMS) offers a free online module to develop clinical expertise in sexual health and menopause: www.menopause.org/for-women/sexual-health-menopause-online.

CONCLUSION

Sexuality is a challenging and complex subject for clinicians. Training opportunities are available through the National Organization of Nurse Practitioners in Women's Health (NPWH). This organization presents a 3-day intensive sexual health course biannually. The course brings experts in sexual health together to share state of the science information about sexuality. A separate workshop on vulvoscopy is also offered at additional cost. NPWH also offers a mobile app to be used at the point of care with sexual health content.

The International Society for the Study of Women's Sexual Health (ISSWSH) cohosts the biannual training and offers an interdisciplinary course on female sexual health. ISSWSH also offers a Fellowship designation for interdisciplinary specialists in female sexual health.

The NAMS offers courses, certification, and online continuing education modules for menopause-specific topics. An app is available with sexual health content from the NAMS website: www.menopause.org/for-women/sexual-health-menopause-online.

■ KEY POINTS

- Understanding the conceptual models of sexual response can assist with understanding the symptoms of and diagnosing sexual dysfunction in patients.

- The clinician should develop both comfort and expertise in discussing sexual health with patients.
- Factors that negatively affect individuals with regard to sex and sexuality are complex and can be multifactorial.
- Patients should have a sexual health screening at each visit, capturing changes since the last visit and prompting them to discuss a topic they may not normally broach themselves.
- Sexuality for individuals spans their lifetime, and attention should be paid to its evaluation regardless of age or sexual orientation.

REFERENCES

1. Masters WH, Johnson VE. *Human Sexual Response.* Boston: Little, Brown; 1966.
2. Whipple B. Women's sexual pleasure and satisfaction. A new view of female sexual function. *Female Patient.* 2002;27:39–44.
3. Basson R. Female sexual response: the role of drugs in the management of sexual dysfunction. *Obstet Gynecol.* 2001;98(2):350–353.
4. Albaugh J, Kellogg-Spadt S. Sexuality and sexual health: the nurse's role and initial approach to patients. *Urol Nurs.* 2003;23(3):227–229.
5. Annon J. *The Behavioral Treatment of Sexual Problems.* Honolulu: Enabling Systems; 1974.
6. Rosen R, Brown C, Heiman J, et al. The female sexual function index (FSFI): a multidimensional self-report instrument for the assessment of female sexual function. *J Sex Marital Ther.* 2000;26(2):191–208.
7. Boehmer U, Timm A, Al Ozonoff Potter J. Applying the female sexual functioning index to sexual minority women. *J Women's Health (Larchmont).* 2012;21(4):401–409.
8. Faubian S, Rullo J. Sexual dysfunction in women: a practical approach. *Am Family Physician.* 2015;40(2):281–288.
9. Nappi RE, Kingsberg S, Maamari R, Simon J. The CLOSER (CLarifying Vaginal Atrophy's Impact on SEx and Relationships) survey: implications of vaginal discomfort in postmenopausal women and in male partners. *J Sex Med.* 2013;10(9):2232–2241.
10. Reiter S. Barriers to effective treatment of vaginal atrophy with local estrogen therapy. *Int J Gen Med.* 2013;6:153–158.
11. Chism LA. Overcoming resistance and barriers to the use of local estrogen therapy for the treatment of vaginal atrophy. *Int J Womens Health.* 2012;4:551–557.
12. Wincze J, Weisberg R. *Sexual Dysfunction: A Guide for Assessment and Treatment.* 3rd ed. New York: Guilford Press; 2015.
13. Van Rooji K, Poels S, Bloemers J, et al. Toward personalized sexual medicine (part 3): testosterone combined with a serotonin1A receptor agonist increases sexual satisfaction in women with HSDD and FSAD, and dysfunctional activation of sexual inhibitory mechanisms. *J Sex Med.* 2012;10:824–837.
14. Poels S, Bloemers J, von Rooik K, et al. Toward personalized sexual medicine (part 2): testosterone combined with a PDE5 inhibitor increases sexual satisfaction in women with HSDD and FSAD, and a low sensitive system for sexual cues. *J Sex Med.* 2013;10:810–823.
15. Khajehel M, Doherty M, Tilley PJ, Sauer K. Prevalence and risk factors of sexual dysfunction in postpartum Australian women. *J Sex Med.* 2015;12(6):1415–1426.
16. O'Malley D, Higgins A, Smith V. Postpartum sexual health: a principle-based concept analysis. *J Adv Nurs.* 2015;71(10):2247–2257.
17. Leeman LM, Rogers RG. Sex after childbirth: postpartum sexual function. *Obstet Gynecol.* 2012;119(3):647–655.
18. Richardson BP, Ondracek AE, Anderson D. Do student nurses feel a lack of comfort in providing support for Lesbian, Gay, Bisexual or Questioning adolescents: what factors influence their comfort level? *J Adv Nurs.* 2017;73(5):1196–1207.
19. Rowe D, Ng YC, O'Keefe L, Crawford D. Providers attitudes and knowledge of lesbian, gay, bisexual, and transgender health. *Fed Practit.* 2017;34(11):28–34.
20. Dorsen C, Van Devanter N. Open arms, conflicted hearts: nurse-practitioner's attitudes towards working with lesbian, gay and bisexual patients. *J Clin Nurs.* 2016;25(23–24):3716–3727.
21. Whipple, B. and Brash-McGreer, K. (1997) Management of Female Sexual Dysfunction. In: Sipski, M.L. and Alexander, C.J., Eds. *Sexual Function in People with Disability and Chronic Illness. A Health Professional's Guide*, Aspen Publishers, Inc., Gaithersburg, 3716–3727.
22. Palmisano B. PLISSIT Model: Introducing Sexual Health in Clinical Care-Psychiatry Advisor. Psychiatry Advisor. Published December 17, 2018. https://www.psychiatryadvisor.com/home/practice-management/plissit-model-introducing-sexual-health-in-clinical-care/
23. Thompson J. Taking a Sexual History with Sexual and Gender Minority Individuals.; 2020. https://fenwayhealth.org/wp-content/uploads/6.-Taking-an-Affirming-Sexual-History.pdf

RESOURCES

American Association of Sexuality Educators, Counselors and Therapists (AASECT): www.aasect.org.

Center for Research & Education on Gender and Sexuality: Summer Institute on Sexuality: https://cregs.sfsu.edu/.

Gay and Lesbian Medical Association (GLMA): www.glma.org.

International Society for the Study of Women's Sexual Health (ISSWSH): www.isswsh.org.

National Association of Nurse Practitioners in Women's Health (NPWH): www.npwh.org.

National Coalition for Sexual Health: https://nationalcoalitionforsexualhealth.org.

North American Menopause Society: www.menopause.org.

The Guide to Getting it On: www.guidetogettingiton.com.

The National Lesbian, Gay, Bisexual and Transgender Health Education Center: https://www.lgbthealtheducation.org/.

The National LGBTQIA+ Health Education Center: https://www.lgbtqiahealtheducation.org/.

The National Vulvodynia Association: www.nva.org.

12

LGBTQ Health Assessment

Ginny Cassidy-Brinn and Simon Adriane Ellis

OBJECTIVES

- Discuss historical context and key sexual orientation and gender identity concepts.
- Identify barriers to health care for lesbian, bisexual, and queer females and transgender and non-binary individuals.
- Discuss sexual, reproductive, and preventive health needs of lesbian, bisexual, and queer females and transgender and non-binary individuals.
- Describe appropriate physical examination techniques and communications strategies when working with lesbian, bisexual, and queer females and transgender and non-binary individuals.
- Describe medical management of gender-affirming therapy.
- Discuss the unique aspects of care for lesbian, bisexual, queer, transgender, non-binary, and questioning adolescents and young adults.

Introduction

In recent years, support for the rights of lesbian, gay, bisexual, and queer (LGBQ) as well as transgender and non-binary (TNB) individuals has increased dramatically in the United States. However, LGBQ and TNB individuals still experience health care discrimination and encounter health care providers who have little knowledge of their needs. Additionally, LGBQ and TNB communities continue to experience documented health disparities. This chapter will help primary care providers deliver clinically and culturally proficient care to their LGBQ and TNB patients, with a focus on meeting the care needs of lesbian, bisexual, and queer (LBQ) females and TNB individuals. Of note, the terms *LGBQ* and *TNB* are used throughout this chapter rather than the more traditional term *LGBTQ* in order to appropriately address the distinct care needs of these two populations.

LGBQ and TNB individuals make up a significant portion of the population, and whether or not they recognize it, most if not all primary care providers serve members of these communities. About 99% of the counties in the United States contain same-sex couples.[1] There are approximately 10 million LGBQ and TNB adults in the United States; rates of LGBQ and TNB identification are higher in females than in males and in Generation Z individuals.[2] One estimate of the number of LBQ females in the United States is 7 million.[3] An estimate of TNB individuals in the United States is 1.6 million.[4]

NOT TO BE MISSED

LGBQ and TNB individuals make up a significant portion of the population, and whether or not they recognize it, most if not all primary care providers serve members of these communities.

Estimates vary widely because national surveys with large data sets rarely ask about sexual orientation or gender identity.[5] Of those that do ask, most only count individuals who live together in same-sex relationships. In 2019, the U.S. Census Bureau included same-sex family data, including those who are married and those who cohabitate, in their annual America's Families and Living Arrangements surveys for the first time. Additionally, in July 2021, they added questions about sexual orientation and gender identity to this survey.[6] Soon, it will be possible to get an accurate estimate of the number of LGBQ and TNB individuals in the United States.

HISTORICAL PERSPECTIVE

The invisibility of LGBQ and TNB individuals in research grew out of societal values that defined heterosexuality and traditional gender roles as normative, thus framing sexual orientation and gender diversity as immoral and pathological rather than as a normal variation in human experience. Throughout the 20th century, being LGBQ or TNB was a criminal offense, and psychiatric diagnoses designated LGBQ and TNB individuals as mentally ill.[7] Public policies based on these laws and psychiatric concepts have affected all aspects of LGBQ and TNB individuals' lives including employment, career advancement, parental rights, housing, and health care.[7]

In the mid-20th century, despite the constant threat of police violence,[7] LGBQ and TNB individuals began forming support groups and finding places to meet while usually keeping their identities secret from the larger society.[7] Some of these groups began to publicly advocate against LGBQ discrimination. As protests became more widespread and LGBQ movements gained strength, public interest and sympathy began to increase. In general, advocacy and acceptance during this time were focused primarily on LGBQ individuals; advocacy for the rights of TNB individuals often lagged behind significantly or was overshadowed by more mainstream LGBQ groups.

At the same time as LGBQ and TNB movements brought issues of discrimination into the public discourse, mainstream scientific research began to broaden to include LGBQ populations. New research supported LGBQ advocates' assertion that LGBQ behaviors were normal and should not be treated as mental illnesses. Eventually, in the late 1980s, the American Psychological Association (APA) discontinued the diagnosis of homosexuality as a disease and, along with the American Public Health Association (APHA), publicly advocated for removal of all laws about same-sex sexual behavior.[8,9]

Diagnosis of TNB identity as a mental illness has persisted much longer. In 1980, the APA added the two diagnoses of *transsexualism* and *gender identity disorder* as psychosexual disorders to the *Diagnostic and Statistical Manual of Mental Disorders III (DSM III)*.[10] The diagnosis of the psychosexual disorder of transsexualism from a mental health provider was a prerequisite for any gender-affirming care such as medical or surgical treatment to change an individual's appearance to be more congruent with their gender identity.[10]

In 1994, transsexualism was removed from the *DSM*, and only the *gender identity disorder* diagnosis remained. Many TNB individuals and their advocates saw this as progress, although the new diagnosis implied pathology. However, a mental health diagnosis was still necessary to support efforts to obtain insurance coverage for gender-affirming care by asserting medical necessity.[7] To remove the pathological connotations of the diagnosis *gender identity disorder*, the diagnosis *gender dysphoria* replaced it in the *DSM 5* in 2013.[10] A diagnosis of gender dysphoria describes the clinically significant distress that some individuals experience as a result of incongruence between their sex assigned at birth and their gender identity.

This effort to move gender variance out of the realm of pathology has carried over from the *DSM* to the *International Classification of Diseases (ICD)*. In contrast with the DSM, the ICD catalogues diagnoses for medical and surgical health care. In 2018, ICD-11 renamed *transsexualism* to *gender incongruence* and moved this diagnosis from *Mental and Behavioral Disorders* to *Conditions Related to Sexual Health*. This change allows the ICD-11 to follow the trajectory of the *DSM*, focusing on the "experience of incongruence between experienced gender and assigned sex," rather than considering TNB identity a mental health disorder.[11]

Over time as the public dialogue about sexual orientation and gender identity continued, LGBQ and TNB communities began to be more open about their identities. As the visibility of these communities continues to grow, public opinion toward LGBQ and TNB individuals has become more positive. Over time, court decisions, laws, and public policy have become more favorable to LGBQ and TNB rights. However, positive developments have usually been followed by waves of anti-LGBQ and TNB legislation. It remains to be seen how further developments on the local, state, and federal level will influence LGBQ and TNB health and access to care.

SEXUAL ORIENTATION AND GENDER IDENTITY: KEY CONCEPTS

The concepts of sex, sexual orientation, and gender identity are often incorrectly conflated. To work with LBGQ and TNB patients respectfully and competently, it is essential to be clear about these concepts and how they differ. Figure 12.1 represents the binary concept of male and female that excludes TNB individuals. Figure 12.2 illustrates a different conceptualization; instead of each individual fitting into one of two boxes, we can conceptualize gender and sexual orientation as containing four aspects.

Sex Assigned at Birth

Sex assigned at birth is a term that describes reproductive organs and presumed or confirmed chromosomal makeup. Individuals born with a penis, testicles, and XY chromosomes are assigned male at birth (AMAB). Individuals born with a vulva, uterus, ovaries and XX chromosomes are assigned female at birth (AFAB). Individuals born with reproductive anatomy that cannot be easily categorized as either male or female are assigned as intersex at birth. Sex assigned at birth does not determine sexual orientation and is not an indicator of gender identity. The distinction between sex assigned at birth, and gender identity is important clinically. It is necessary to be aware of a patient's anatomy to determine which screening tests are appropriate; for example, pap smears are recommended for individuals of appropriate age who have a cervix regardless of gender identity.

NOT TO BE MISSED

The term *cisgender* refers to someone whose gender identity matches their sex assigned at birth (i.e., a non-transgender individual).

Sexual Orientation

Good communication with patients requires being aware of the different aspects of sexual orientation.

Gender binary consisting of male and female as gender options

Figure 12.1 Binary concept of gender.

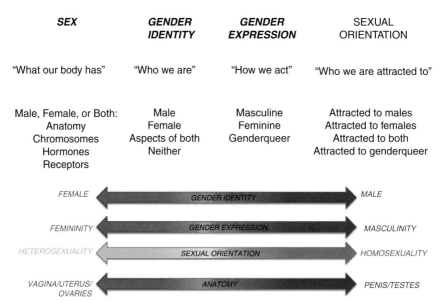

SEX	GENDER IDENTITY	GENDER EXPRESSION	SEXUAL ORIENTATION
"What our body has"	"Who we are"	"How we act"	"Who we are attracted to"
Male, Female, or Both: Anatomy Chromosomes Hormones Receptors	Male Female Aspects of both Neither	Masculine Feminine Genderqueer	Attracted to males Attracted to females Attracted to both Attracted to genderqueer

FEMALE ◄— GENDER IDENTITY —► MALE
FEMININITY ◄— GENDER EXPRESSION —► MASCULINITY
HETEROSEXUALITY ◄— SEXUAL ORIENTATION —► HOMOSEXUALITY
VAGINA/UTERUS/OVARIES ◄— ANATOMY —► PENIS/TESTES

Figure 12.2 Model illustrating four aspects of gender. (From Johnson B, Leibowitz S, Chavez A, Herbert SE. Risk versus resiliency: addressing depression in lesbian, gay, bisexual, and transgender youths. *Child Adolesc Psychiatr Clin N Am.* 2019;28[3]:509–521.)

Having good communication is necessary to making the patient feel comfortable and confident in the provider's care. If a provider communicates rigid, artificially simple concepts of sexuality, patients may not feel comfortable being open about their sexual behaviors. How an individual defines their sexuality can be different from that individual's sexual attraction and behavior. Research done in the late 1940s by Dr. Alfred Kinsey and colleagues showed that many individuals do not fit neatly into the categories of heterosexual or homosexual if sexual attraction is taken into account. Kinsey's survey of thousands of college students found that most were attracted to both males and females at least to some extent.[12,13]

It is important to remember that sexual orientation is not a singular experience; rather, it is composed of a number of different components including sexual attraction, identity, and behavior. Attraction can be further delineated into physical (i.e., sexual) attraction and emotional (i.e., nonsexual) attraction acknowledging that many individuals have committed, intimate relationships that do not involve sexual activity. The degree of alignment between these facets of sexual orientation varies, and in research they have been found to be poorly correlated.[14] In addition, rigid ideas of sexual orientation become problematic when sex assigned at birth and gender identity are understood as separate concepts that may not neatly align.

The fact that an individual's conception of their sexual identity may not match the reality of their behavior has important clinical significance, as does the fact that sexual identity and behavior can change throughout individuals' lives. For example, an individual may identify and present as heterosexual but may experience same-sex attraction and occasionally engage in same-sex sexual behavior. Or an individual who identifies as lesbian may currently have an AMAB partner or have had AMAB partners in the past. The majority of lesbians have had at least one AMAB partner in their lifetime, greater than 70% in some studies.[15,16] Similarly, more than 10% of females who identify as heterosexual have had an AFAB partner.[17] Information on sexual behavior is critical in determining sexual health risk factors; as such, merely knowing a patient's identity is not sufficient.

The most commonly used terms for sexual orientation are *lesbian, gay, bisexual, queer,* and *straight* or *heterosexual.* The term *lesbian* is typically reserved to describe those who identify as females, while *gay* is sometimes used as an umbrella term for all individuals who are not heterosexual. The lexicon of LGBQ and TNB identity is rich, diverse, creative, and culturally rooted; the terminology discussed in this chapter represents a small sampling of commonly used terms and is in no way exhaustive.

The term *queer* is a word that has been reclaimed by some LGBQ individuals. It has historically been used as a slur and continues to be used as hate speech today; for this reason, even positive use of the word continues to be experienced as harmful by many LGBQ individuals. Those who claim the term *queer* may do so for many reasons: as a political act, as an umbrella term, as a term that is entirely free from gendered connotations, or to express fluidity in one's sexual orientation.

Patients may or may not disclose their identification with the term *queer* in the context of a health care setting, even if they openly do so in other spheres of their lives. It is important to note that, although the term *queer* has an important role in LGBQ communities—and thus is incorporated throughout this chapter—its use by non-LGBQ individuals can be problematic given its history as hate speech. Therefore, health care providers should never use the term *queer* with patients unless expressly requested to do so and even then, should maintain caution when communicating with and about patients.

Additional terms for sexual orientation include *pansexual,* which describes an individual who is attracted to individuals of all gender identities, and *asexual,* which describes an individual who does not usually experience sexual attraction or engage in sexual behavior.

Most LGBQ individuals prefer not to use the term *homosexual,* although it is used in academic work. In speaking with patients, it would be best to avoid the term *homosexual* unless patients themselves use it to describe their sexual orientation.

There are some terms and acronyms used in medical and research settings that refer specifically to sexual behavior. In general, these terms are used to refer to sex assigned at birth rather than to gender identity. Table 12.1 provides a list of terminology.

Although helpful in clearly defining sexual behavior for individuals who are not transgender, there are no parallel terms for TNB individuals. Because good data are not available for TNB individuals, providers may need to extrapolate from the risk data and screening guidelines for cisgender patients when performing

TABLE 12.1   Binary and Cisnormative Sexual Behavior Terminology Used in Medical Research and in Screening Guidelines*

Term	Acronym	Definition
Lesbian or gay women	WSW	Women who have sex with women
Gay or gay men	MSM	Men who have sex with men
Bisexual	WSMW MSMW	Women who have sex with men and women Men who have sex with men and women
Heterosexual	WSM MSW	Women who have sex with men Men who have sex with women

*The terms *men* and *women* are used here to refer to male/female sex assigned at birth rather than to gender identity.

a sexual risk assessment. This can be done by focusing on anatomy instead of gender identity. For example, a transgender female patient with a penis who has sex with a cisgender male would be considered *MSM* (a man who has sex with men) for purposes of applying STI screening guidelines by the U.S. Centers for Disease Control and Prevention (CDC), even though the patient is not a male.

> **PATIENT-CENTERED CARE:** Because good data are not available for TNB individuals, providers may need to extrapolate from the risk data and screening guidelines for cisgender patients when performing a sexual risk assessment. This can be done by focusing on anatomy instead of gender identity.

For good reason, application of terms based on anatomy rather than gender identity may be experienced as disrespectful by TNB patients. In the aforementioned example, the transgender female patient who has sex with a cisgender male may find it offensive to be labeled as MSM because this directly conflicts with the patient's female gender identity. A transgender male patient who has sex with other transgender males might similarly be upset by being labeled as WSW (a woman who has sex with women). Individuals of all sexual orientations may also find it uncomfortable to be grouped into these broad categories that providers use as markers of risk,

rather than having their risk assessed in the context of their individual sexual behavior. As a result, these terms should be avoided or used with caution in direct patient communication.

Gender Identity

An individual's gender identity is their internal sense of who they are and how they think about their gender. Individuals with binary gender identities identify as either male or female. Those with non-binary gender identities do not identify as solely male or female or may identify as neither male nor female. As with sexual orientation, gender identity is multifaceted, and seeming discrepancies between identity and outward behavior or expression are common.

Terms describing gender identity are constantly changing and evolving, both in the medical world and in TNB communities. Clinicians must be familiar with terminology to communicate effectively with other providers as well as with their patients and to be flexible, changing the words they use with patients as terminology evolves. Table 12.2 provides a list of gender identity terminology. As with terminology related to sexual orientation, the terms used in this chapter represent a small sample of the rich language TNB communities have created. When communicating with patients, it is important to listen and use the terminology they prefer. Clinicians should never correct the terminology patients use to describe themselves, even if it seems incorrect or even pejorative. When communicating with other providers, it is wise to remember that there are wide ranges of knowledge about TNB identities, therefore it is important to be very clear about patients' gender identities as well what name and pronoun should be used.

> **CLINICAL SURVIVAL TIP** Terms describing gender identity are constantly changing and evolving, both in the medical world and in TNB communities. Clinicians must be familiar with terminology to communicate effectively with other providers as well as with their patients and to be flexible, changing the words they use with patients as terminology evolves.

The terms *transgender* or *trans* refer to someone whose gender identity is in some way different from their sex assigned at birth. These are often used as umbrella terms to describe a wide range of gender identities. *Non-binary, gender nonconforming, and gender-queer* are terms often used by individuals whose gender

TABLE 12.2   Gender Identity Terminology*

Term	Definition
AFAB	Assigned female at birth based on visual examination of external genitals and/or chromosomal status
AMAB	Assigned male at birth based on visual examination of external genitals and/or chromosomal status
Transgender Trans	An individual whose gender identity is different from the sex assigned at birth Often used as umbrella terms for both binary and non-binary gender identities
Transgender woman	A woman who was assigned male at birth
Transgender man	A man who was assigned female at birth
Non-binary Gender non-conforming Gender variant Genderqueer	An individual whose gender identity does not conform to a binary/dichotomous concept of gender May identify as both male and female, neither male nor female, or describe other identities that are not binary
Agender	An individual who does not identify with any gender designation
Cisgender	An individual whose gender is the same as their sex assigned at birth

*The terms in this table are not contingent on hormonal or surgical status. For example, a transgender woman does not need to undergo gender-affirming hormone therapy to have her female identity/womanhood validated.

identity is not solely male or female. Non-binary individuals may identify as both male and female, identify as neither male nor female, or describe other unique relationships to the concept of gender. *Gender fluid* is a term used to describe an individual whose gender identity shifts over time. *Agender* (without gender) is a term used to refer to individuals who do not experience themselves as gendered beings or do not identify with any gender designation. Throughout this chapter, the term *TNB* will be used to broadly encompass all non-cisgender gender identities.

The terms *cross-dresser, transvestite, drag king,* and *drag queen* all refer to an individual who dresses in ways that are different from what is considered normative for their sex assigned at birth as part of a gendered performance or for sexual pleasure. Being a cross-dresser or performing drag does not mean that an individual is TNB. The term *transvestite* is considered derogatory by many individuals and should not be used by clinicians.

Use of the term *transsexual* remains somewhat common in the medical community because of the *DSM's* prior use of the transsexualism diagnosis. Many TNB individuals find this term offensive because of its association with the idea of TNB identity being a mental illness.

Historically, there have been a number of terms used in medical communications and sometimes by transgender individuals to describe the trajectory of gender affirmation. These include male-to-female (MTF) and female-to-male (FTM). Although these terms may appear simple and concrete, they are medically inaccurate, lack the nuance that is required when discussing gender identity, and are often experienced as derogatory by TNB individuals (particularly non-binary individuals). These terms should be avoided along with other medically inaccurate and outdated terms such as *sex change surgery*. Some TNB individuals refer to undertaking medical interventions to better align their body and their gender expression as *transition*. Others prefer to refer to these interventions as *gender-affirming* or *gender-confirming* interventions. In this chapter, we recommend specific and medically accurate terminology coupled with the term *gender-affirming*. For example, taking testosterone may be referred to as *gender-affirming hormone therapy,* and hysterectomy may be referred to as *gender-affirming hysterectomy*.

Gender Expression

An individual's gender expression or gender presentation refers to how they present themselves in the world—how they communicate their gender. Gender is expressed through clothing, hairstyle, ways of talking, and other mannerisms. Gender expression is on a continuum with some individuals expressing themselves in what is interpreted as traditionally masculine or feminine ways and with others falling somewhere in between; this is true of cisgender individuals as well as TNB individuals. Terms for gender expression include *masculine, feminine,* and *androgynous.* The term *androgynous* is used to describe someone who appears neither masculine nor feminine. *Butch* is a term used to describe an extremely masculine gender expression, and *femme* describes an extremely feminine gender expression.

Gender expression is not an indicator of sexual orientation, and just as sexual behavior may not match sexual identity, perceived gender expression may or may not match gender identity. Additionally, TNB individuals may be more publicly expressive of their gender identity in some situations than in others. For example, they might be much more open about their gender identity with friends and family than they are at work or school. Because of pervasive homophobia and transphobia, safety concerns often inform personal decisions regarding gender expression.

The fact that gender expression and identity may appear discordant is clinically significant. Clinicians with less familiarity working with TNB patients may be hesitant to trust patients' self-report of their gender identity when it is in stark contrast with their gendered dress when they appear in clinic. Clinicians might mistakenly fear that a patient is "not ready" for hormone therapy if they are not already consistently presenting as their affirmed gender. However, there are many reasons that patients might wait until they have achieved significant appearance changes through gender-affirming hormone therapy before changing other aspects of their appearance. They might simply prefer to wait, which is valid in and of itself. They might feel protective of their internal self and not want to reveal this identity to others until their gender identity is more likely to be appropriately perceived. Or they might live or work in a setting in which they would be at risk of harassment or physical assault if their TNB status were detectable. Regardless of the reasons behind a patient's gender expression choices, the most important thing is for providers to trust the patient's self-reported gender identity. Because gender-affirming medication can be lifesaving in that it can prevent suicide, unnecessarily denying or delaying access to hormone therapy or surgical interventions could be a serious error on the part of the clinician.

> **PATIENT-CENTERED CARE:** Regardless of the reasons behind a patient's gender expression choices, the most important thing is for providers to trust the patient's self-reported gender identity.

ACCESS TO HEALTH CARE

Currently, many professional medical and nursing organizations encourage their members to provide comprehensive, culturally proficient care to LGBQ and TNB individuals. These include the American College of Nurse Midwives, American Academy of Nursing, American College of Obstetricians and Gynecologists, American Academy of Pediatrics, and American Public Health Association.[18] Despite significant gains, there still are important disparities in access to health care for LGBQ and TNB individuals.

Poverty and Lack of Insurance as Barriers to Access

Lack of health insurance is an important barrier to health care access for large numbers of LGBQ and TNB individuals. Same-sex couples may have problems with access to insurance because not all policies provide spousal coverage for same-sex partners.[5] Many insurance policies do not cover aspects of gender-affirming care, and some refuse to cover any care for patients identified as TNB. In 2015, the National Center for Transgender Equality conducted the U.S. Transgender Survey, a national survey exploring the lived experiences of over 27,000 TNB individuals living in the United States, its territories, and its overseas military bases. Twenty-five percent of respondents to the survey reported problems with insurance related to being TNB.[19]

Most Americans receive their health insurance through an employer.[20] This can be problematic for LGBQ and TNB individuals, who still face significant employment discrimination, including loss of employment when their sexual orientation is known.[21] In 2017, LBQT females had almost three times the unemployment rate of straight females, and 57% had been fired, not hired, or denied promotion because of their gender identity or expression.[23]

Ability to pay for health care can be another barrier to access even for LGBQ and TNB individuals who have insurance coverage. Needed health care is a lower priority than food or other necessities for individuals living in poverty.[22] LGBT females and TNB individuals are more likely to be poor than the general population. More than 36% of LBQ females live in poverty,[23] and they are more likely than the general population to forgo needed care because of cost.[5] In 2015, TNB adults were three times more likely to earn less than $10,000 per year than the general population, and 33% went without needed health care in the previous year because they could not afford it.[19]

Health Care Discrimination

LGBQ and TNB patients report alarming levels of mistreatment during health care encounters, often describing providers as being confused, upset, or accusatory when they reveal their gender identity or sexual orientation.[24] In a national survey on LGBQ and TNB health care, over 50% of LGBQ patients and 70% of TNB patients said that health care providers had been verbally or physically abusive, denied needed care, said that their sexual orientation or gender identity was the cause of their illness, or refused to touch them or used unnecessary precautions.[1] One TNB patient reported, "I was forced to have a pelvic exam by a doctor when I went in for a sore throat. The doctor invited others to look at me while he examined me and talked to them about my genitals."[25]

Health care systems and infrastructure are built around the needs of heterosexual and cisgender patients and thus are fraught with points of tension for LGBQ and TNB patients. For example, LGBQ and TNB patients rarely find themselves reflected in displayed artwork and patient education materials when receiving care; intake forms typically lack appropriate fields for relationship status and fail to collect critical information about gender identity, sexual orientation, and appropriate name and pronouns. Lacking standardized fields with which to track these important pieces of data, electronic medical records place patients, providers, and staff at a disadvantage and reduce the health care system's ability to systematically respond to health care disparities.[26] Additionally, TNB patients are frequently shamed and put in danger in public spaces such as waiting rooms when staff members reveal their TNB status by calling out their legal name. Safety issues also arise when health care facilities lack gender-neutral and/or single-stall patient restrooms.

Many LGBQ and TNB individuals avoid health care even when they are ill or know they need preventive care because of fear based on their own traumatic health care experiences as well as situations they have heard from others.[25]

HEALTH DISPARITIES

Because of LBQ and TNB invisibility, the data on health disparities are very limited. Sexual orientation and gender identity are not routinely documented during health care visits.[26] Without large data sets from electronic health records, it is not possible to accurately analyze the health risks of LGBT individuals.[26] In the research that does exist, categories such as *lesbian* and *bisexual* are not uniformly defined, so it is difficult to combine data from different studies. Studies that clarify the sex assigned at birth and gender identity of sexual partners are scarce; therefore it is not always clear, for example, if *male partners* refers to AMAB individuals or if this includes male-identified AFAB individuals. More will be learned about health disparities in the future when a larger quantity of more precise data becomes available and more research focuses on identifying and studying LGBQ and TNB health. In each of the disparities discussed here, the findings are limited and often inconclusive. However, clinicians can use the available evidence to inform clinical decision making.

Some LGBQ and TNB health disparities have been apparent, regardless of these difficulties with data collection. The HIV epidemic and the activism that followed helped bring awareness to the special health needs of gay males. Later, advocates within LGBQ and TNB communities as well as health care providers and researchers began focusing on the needs of previously neglected parts of the LGBT population. As a result, individuals other than cisgender gay males were found to have unique health concerns as well.

In 2011, the Institute of Medicine (IOM) published a research agenda on the health of LGBQ and TNB individuals, and national health surveys began to collect data specifically about the health status of LGBQ and TNB populations.[7] Some common health risks and diseases have been identified that disproportionately affect the LGBQ and TNB community. Overt discrimination as well as subtler forms of everyday insults have been shown to contribute to health disparities by their harmful effect on both mental and physical health.[28] For

LGBQ individuals, stressful prejudice events have been directly linked to deterioration in physical health,[29] and discrimination has been shown to lead to higher depression scores and lower levels of self-esteem and mastery.[30] LGBQ and TNB individuals who also belong to other stigmatized and marginalized groups, such as disabled and BIPOC (Black, Indigenous, and People of Color) LBGQ and TNB individuals, experience multiple unique sources of minority stress simultaneously.[31]

Mental Health

Like other stigmatized groups, LBQ and TNB individuals are more likely to have mental health concerns than the general population.[32-34] TNB individuals have much higher rates of serious psychological stress, suicidal thoughts, depression, and anxiety than their heterosexual and cisgender peers.[19,35] A very large proportion of TNB individuals have attempted suicide in their lives, with a rate of 40% compared with the 4.6% rate of the general U.S. population.[19]

One of the ways to identify mental health disparities in LBQ females is by categorizing them according to their sexual behavior. There is an increased incidence of mental health diagnoses among LBQ females, particularly depression, anxiety and posttraumatic stress disorder.[37] In 2013, only 0.5% of deaths were caused by suicide in heterosexual females, whereas the rate for LBQ females was 9%.[36]

With sexual identity as the variable, bisexual cisgender females experienced more psychological pain than lesbian and heterosexual cisgender females. In the 2013 National Health Information Survey, 11% of bisexual females had experienced what they described as serious psychological distress in the prior 30 days.[38]

> **! SAFETY ALERT**
>
> TNB individuals have much higher rates of serious psychological stress, suicidal thoughts, depression, and anxiety than their heterosexual and cisgender peers.

Alcohol, Tobacco and Other Substance Use
Alcohol

LBQ females are more likely than other females to binge drink or use alcohol excessively.[37-41] If they are college age, they also report more serious consequences from drinking such as nonconsensual sex and suicidal thoughts.[41] TNB individuals binge drink at only slightly higher rates than the rest of the U.S. population,[19] but in 2008, 26% said that they currently used or had used drugs and alcohol to help cope with discrimination.[25] Because of social and employment discrimination, TNB individuals are more likely than their peers to engage in the "underground economy," that is engaging in financial transactions that are not reported to the government and are not taxed or regulated. Often this involves selling drugs or trading sex for money or resources. This in turn has an impact on substance abuse behaviors. In 2015, rates of binge drinking among TNB individuals who were currently engaged in the underground economy were twice that of both the general U.S. population and TNB individuals not engaged in the underground economy.[34]

Tobacco

LBQ females smoke at a much higher rate than do heterosexual females, and they have an increased risk of smoking-related disease such as asthma.[39,41-43] LBQ youths have higher rates of smoking than other youths.[44] Additionally, LBQ females appear to be more receptive to tobacco advertising than heterosexual females.[46] Figure 12.3 shows that lesbian and bisexual females have higher rates of smoking than other females. When TNB individuals were first surveyed nationally, 30% reported being current smokers, significantly more than the 20.6% rate of the general population of U.S. adults. However, when transgender individuals were surveyed in 2015, only 20% were current smokers.

Other Substances

The use of prescription drugs in ways for which they were not prescribed as well as the use of illegal drugs and marijuana is more frequent in LBQ and TNB communities than in among cisgender individuals.[37,47] The rate of substance use for TNB individuals is 29% versus 10% for the U.S. population as a whole.[19] As with binge drinking, the rates for TNB individuals working in the underground economy—a reflection of stigmatization and marginalization—are even higher. Over two-thirds of TNB individuals who are employed in the underground economy reported using drugs illegally in the 30 days before they were surveyed in 2015.[19] Figure 12.4 shows how working in the underground economy is related to substance use in TNB individuals.

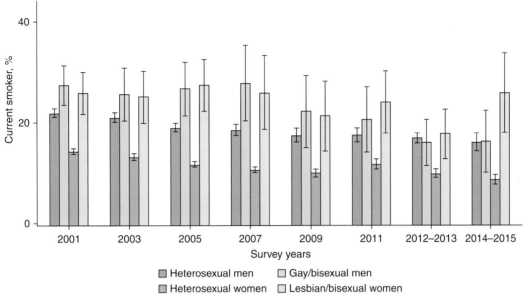

Figure 12.3 Percentage of current smokers by sexual orientation and gender over time. (Data from UCLA Center for Health Policy Research. *California Health Interview Survey, 2001–2015.* https://healthpolicy.ucla. edu/chis/Pages/default.aspx.)

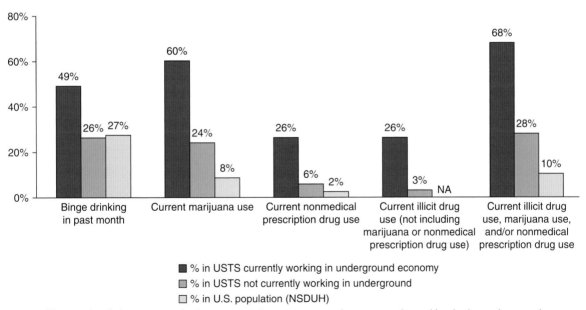

Figure 12.4 Substance use in the past month among respondents currently working in the underground economy. (From James SE, Herman JL, Rankin S, Keisling M, Mottet L, Anafi M. *The Report of the 2015 U.S. Transgender Survey.* Washington, DC: National Center for Transgender Equality; 2016. http://www. transequality.org/sites/default/files/docs/usts/USTS Full Report - FINAL 1.6.17.pdf.)

Cervical Cancer

LBQ females are less likely than heterosexual females to have pap smears as a screening test for cervical cancer.[49,50] One major reason for the disparity in screening of LBQ females is patients' and providers' erroneous belief that only heterosexual females get cervical cancer and that LBQ females do not need to be tested.[50,51] This belief is based on the fact that the human papillomavirus (HPV), which has been shown to be transmitted by heterosexual vaginal sex, causes virtually all cases of cervical cancer.[52] However, HPV is also passed by skin-to-skin contact and can be transmitted by digital intercourse or shared sex toys.[52] Additionally, because a high proportion of LBQ females have had sex with an AMAB individual at some time in their life, there is also the possibility of acquiring the virus by penile penetration.

Another contributing factor to lower pap smear screening rates in LBQ females of reproductive age is that they are less likely to access gynecological or contraceptive care than heterosexual females.[49] Primary care providers who emphasize pap smear testing can provide another avenue for LBQ female patients to have cervical cancer screening.

TNB individuals who have a uterus and a cervix, no matter what their gender identity, should have a pap smear on the recommended schedule. Sixty-six percent of adult females on the National Health Interview Survey reported having had a pap smear in the previous year, but in a different survey, only 27% of TNB individuals who had female on their original birth certificate had a pap smear in the same year.[19,53]

Multiple factors contribute to the lower rate of cervical cancer screening in the TNB population. Gynecologists and other reproductive health care providers may refuse to provide care to TNB patients; if these patients do succeed in being seen, they may receive insensitive care from providers who are untrained to meet their needs.[54-56] A pelvic examination can be uncomfortable for anyone; TNB individuals may feel even more discomfort with attention focused on genitals that do not match their gender identity, and they may fear mistreatment by the health care providers examining them. An additional difficulty that can cause avoidance of pap smears for TNB individuals who are receiving gender-affirming testosterone therapy is that low estrogen levels lead to atrophy of the vaginal epithelium, making speculum insertion painful and sample collection technically difficult. Transgender males, particularly those taking testosterone, have higher rates of unsatisfactory pap results than cisgender females.[58] Individuals who have unsatisfactory pap results are often lost to follow-up.[57] Figure 12.5 provides a poster used in an outreach effort to encourage routine cervical cancer screening for TNB individuals.

Finally, TNB individuals who have changed their gender marker on legal identity documents to male have had coverage denied by their insurance company for pap smears and other sexual and reproductive health care services.

> ### NOT TO BE MISSED
>
> TNB patients who have a uterus and a cervix, no matter what their gender identity, should have a pap smear on the recommended schedule.

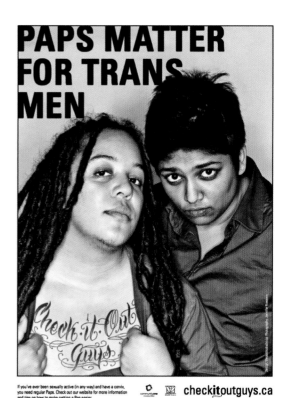

Figure 12.5 Poster encouraging Paps for trans males. (From Sherbourne Health. Pap Campaigns. Rainbow Health Ontario. https://www.rainbowhealthontario.ca/pap-campaigns/.)

Breast Cancer

Research suggests that LBQ females have more risk factors for breast cancer than heterosexual females.[59,60] These risk factors include higher age at first birth, never having had children, and a higher rate of alcohol use.[60] Data from the National Health Interview Survey and linked mortality files found that females in same-sex partnerships had over three times the risk of dying of breast cancer than other females.[60]

Lack of provider knowledge is a barrier to TNB individuals receiving screening according to the accepted guidelines. A 2015 survey of gynecologists revealed that almost 60% were unfamiliar with the breast cancer screening recommendations for transgender females.[62]

The incidence of breast cancer in transgender females is not higher (and is possibly lower) than that of cisgender females. However, there is evidence that breast cancer is diagnosed later and is more likely to be fatal in transgender females.[63]

Because cisgender females who take ethinyl estradiol (the form of estrogen in oral contraceptives) have a slightly increased incidence of breast cancer, there was concern that transgender females taking estrogen for feminization could also be at risk for breast cancer.[63] So far, the form of estrogen now used for feminization, 17-beta estradiol, does not appear to increase breast cancer risk for transgender females.[63,65,66]

Cardiovascular Health

As with other health disparities, there are limited data on the burden of cardiovascular disease among LBQ and TNB individuals because sexual orientation is not documented in health care visits and is often omitted from studies. Data on cardiac health in TNB individuals are particularly limited.

LBQ females have a higher incidence of important cardiac risk factors such as tobacco use, heavy alcohol consumption, and illicit drug use than heterosexual females.[41,67-69] However, these risk factors have not yet been shown to lead to higher incidence of cardiac disease.[67,68] The data on cardiac disease has mostly been self-reported from telephone interviews, which are not as reliable as data collected from medical records.[71] In the future, with more visibility of LBQ and TNB individuals, it is hoped there will be more reliable information on this important subject.

Large, retrospective studies of Dutch transgender females taking estrogen for feminizing hormone therapy have found as much as a 64% increased risk for cardiovascular mortality.[72,73] These studies showed a strong association between cardiovascular mortality and one form of estrogen, ethinyl estradiol, which might have accounted for the increase[72,73] Ethinyl estradiol, the same form of estrogen that is used in oral contraceptives, was previously used in high doses for feminization and is no longer recommended in accepted guidelines or prescribed for this indication in the United States.[74-76] Further research is needed to evaluate the cardiovascular implications and true risk level of current feminizing regimens using moderate doses of 17-beta estradiol.

Cisgender males who are athletes and take supraphysiological doses of testosterone have serious, adverse cardiovascular consequences.[77,78] However, no adverse effects have yet been shown for transgender males who take physiological doses of testosterone, and the limited research that is available is reassuring.[64,72,73,79]

Endocrine Function and Polycystic Ovarian Syndrome

Polycystic ovarian Syndrome (PCOS) is a group of symptoms in AFAB individuals that includes ovarian dysfunction and high androgen levels (see Chapter 17 for a discussion of diagnosis and management of PCOS). PCOS is linked to increased risk of metabolic syndrome, diabetes, cardiovascular disease, and infertility. There has been some evidence that this condition may be more prevalent in LBQ and TNB populations. However, research on risk and prevalence is complicated by differing diagnostic criteria and the lack of precise definitions for elements of the diagnostic criteria. To date, some studies have shown that LBQ females have a significantly higher incidence of PCOS,[80,81] and other larger studies have shown no significant difference.[81,82]

For TNB AFAB individuals, the possibility that masculinizing hormones might cause or contribute to PCOS is an important consideration. The research on this is inconclusive. In one study of 69 FTM participants taking testosterone, 58% had PCOS. In another study, histological changes compatible with PCOS were found in the ovaries of all 11 FTM participants who were taking testosterone. These findings are limited by the small sample sizes and the fact that because the participants were not evaluated before they began testosterone, it is unclear if a causal relationship is present.

Body Image and Composition

A number of studies have focused on the size and composition of the LBQ female's body. However, evidence demonstrates that the body mass index (BMI) is not a good indicator of risk of disease and future mortality.[70,85,86] Of greater importance than the size of one's body is the consequence of weight bias in health care. Many females with larger bodies delay care, particularly gynecological care, to avoid weight-based discrimination.[88] Weight bias on the part of health care providers thus increases the risk that chronic and acute medical conditions will go undetected early in the disease process, and contributes to a poorer prognosis by the time of diagnosis.

There is some limited research that indicates that TNB individuals may have a higher risk of disordered eating than the general population[89,90] and that TNB individuals may develop disordered eating because of a desire to conform to cultural gender ideals of muscularity or thinness.[91]

Sexually Transmitted Infections and Vaginitis

For LBQ and TNB individuals, a significant barrier to diagnosis and treatment of sexually transmitted infections (STIs) is providers' discomfort with and lack of skills in taking sexual histories or in even asking about sexual orientation or gender identity.[57,92,93] Because of the exclusion of LBQ and TNB identities from data and research, there is inadequate evidence available about prevalence or risk of STIs in these communities. The CDC periodically issues definitive guidelines on STI testing, but has only limited guidelines for TNB individuals and instructs providers to make screening decisions based on sexual behavior and anatomy.[94]

The high prevalence of HIV in TNB AMAB individuals, discussed in the following section, implies that this population is also at high risk for other STIs. There is very little information about STI risk for TNB AFAB individuals, but research indicates that significant risk is present;[95,96] in fact, the risk may be as high as that seen in their AMAB TNB counterparts.[97] Physiological changes to the vaginal epithelium with use of gender-affirming testosterone may have important implications for STI transmission risk; further research is needed to explore this.

The myth that LBQ females are very low risk for STIs is common, both among providers and within LBQ communities, and results in missed opportunities for necessary screening.[98] Although gay, bisexual, and queer AMAB individuals have been studied extensively, the risk for STIs in LBQ females is rarely examined.[99,100] Syphilis, hepatitis, and chlamydia have all been shown to be passed between AFAB individuals, and in one large population-based study, the incidence of chlamydia was significantly higher in LBQ females than in heterosexual females.[98,101]

Research has consistently shown that bacterial vaginosis (BV) is more common in LBQ females than in heterosexual females.[98] A study of African American females showed a higher rate of BV for bisexual females than for lesbian females.[102] Specific risk factors for BV among LBQ females have been identified including multiple female partners, shared sex toys, frequent oral-vulvovaginal sex, using lubricant, and having a partner with BV.[98,103] Although research is lacking on this issue, TNB AFAB individuals are likely predisposed to BV because of physiological changes to the vaginal epithelium associated with gender-affirming testosterone use.

Little is known about vaginitis in TNB AMAB individuals with surgically constructed vaginas. A 2008 study analyzed the microflora of 50 transgender females whose vaginas had been constructed from inverted penile skin.[104] The composition of organisms colonizing the vagina was similar to that of the skin, intestine, and the vaginas of AFAB individuals with BV. Although lactobacilli are common in the microflora of natal vaginas, only one study participant was found to have lactobacilli in her surgically constructed vagina. Elevated vaginal pH and foul vaginal odor were noted in most study participants.[104] In a later study of 63 transgender females in 2014, interestingly, the majority of research participants demonstrated comparable strains of lactobacilli to those seen in the vaginas of AFAB individuals.[105] The clinical significance of these data is uncertain as (1) no clear links have been made between vaginal symptoms and specific microflora, and (2) certain findings inherent to the surgically constructed vagina, such as elevated pH, can confuse the clinical diagnosis of vaginitis such as BV.[104] Vaginal irritation and bothersome vaginal discharge are common presenting complaints, but these symptoms may not be associated with a clinical diagnosis of STI or vaginitis (Chapter 5).

HIV and TNB Communities

The HIV epidemic has had a huge, well-documented effect on LGBQ and TNB communities because of the large number of gay men who died of AIDS in the 1980s and 1990s. The effect of HIV on TNB communities is only recently beginning to be measured. In 2015, a total of 1.4% of TNB respondents to the U.S. Transgender Survey stated they were HIV positive, almost five times the rate of the general population.[19] TNB AMAB individuals have been most deeply affected by HIV. Reviews of the research currently available have estimated that from 22% to 28% of transgender females in the United States are living with HIV; these numbers are probably falsely low because many transgender females have not been tested and do not know their HIV status.[106,107]

Various factors contribute to the high rate of HIV among TNB AMAB individuals, including a lack of legal employment opportunities because of job discrimination. Of TNB individuals surveyed in 2015, 16% of those who had ever been employed had lost a job because of their gender identity and expression.[19] Homelessness is also a common experience for TNB individuals, with 6% surveyed in 2015 having been denied a home or apartment in the previous year because of their gender identity.[19] Unemployment and homelessness can lead to participation in the underground economy, including sex work. Nineteen percent of U.S. Transgender Survey respondents reported that they had done any type of sex work in exchange for money, food, a place to sleep, drugs, or other goods.[19]

BIPOC transgender females bear the twin burdens of racial and gender discrimination, and are HIV positive at disproportionately high rates compared with their White peers (Figure 12.6).[19] Research on HIV among TNB AFAB individuals is scarce; significant additional research is needed to gain an understanding of prevalence and risk factors.

Applying Data in Clinical Practice

Understanding the data about health and health care disparities among LBQ and TNB populations enables providers to make better health care management decisions. Knowing about disparities in disease prevalence enables clinicians to screen appropriately. Knowing about disparities in access to care allows clinicians to be aware of important health care needs that may have been neglected and may need to be addressed in a current visit. Understanding barriers to care and historical trauma allows a provider to correctly interpret a patient's acting withdrawn or angry as an anticipatory response to past

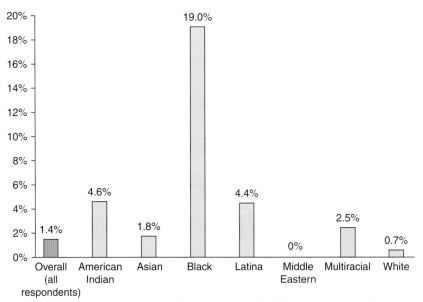

Figure 12.6 Race/ethnicity percentages of individuals living with HIV among transgender females. (From James SE, Herman JL, Rankin S, Keisling M, Mottet L, Anafi M. *The Report of the 2015 U.S. Transgender Survey.* Washington, DC: National Center for Transgender Equality; 2016. http://www.transequality.org/sites/default/files/docs/usts/USTS Full Report - FINAL 1.6.17.pdf.)

health care discrimination. This information also suggests approaches for reducing systemic barriers and improving health care for LBQ and TNB populations as a whole.

FOCUSED HISTORY AND PHYSICAL

Creating a Welcoming Environment

The clinical environment profoundly influences the provider's ability to take accurate, complete histories, particularly in the case of LBQ and TNB patients. If LBQ and TNB patients get the impression upon arriving that they are not safe because they fear that their privacy will not be respected, they will be assumed to be cisgender and heterosexual, or their care needs will not be understood, they will be less likely to be open and honest with the health care team. If the physical space of the clinical environment has visual cues that reflect an awareness of LGBQ and TNB individuals, patients will feel reassured. Examples are a poster showing a same-sex couple, a notice of a nondiscrimination policy that includes LGBTQ and TNB patients, a Healthcare Equality Index badge (Figure 12.7), LGBQ- and TNB-themed magazines, educational materials with messages directed to LGBQ and TNB patients, or a rainbow flag. The physical layout of the environment should also be taken into consideration. For example, restrooms are a difficult space for TNB patients. Patients may feel uncomfortable or unsafe using gendered, multistall bathrooms. They may have experienced harassment or assault in public bathrooms in the past. Additionally, patients may be fearful of asking directions to the restroom as this can result in being misgendered by a staff member who directs them to a restroom that does not match their gender identity or in which they do not feel safe. Gender-neutral single-stall bathrooms are the preferred option for all patients; any restroom that has just one toilet can be easily designated as all-gender with the simple addition of an appropriate sign or removal of gendered signs.

In addition to the physical environment, clinic systems and policies must be inclusive of LGBQ and TNB individuals. Intake forms that give limited options so the patient cannot fill them out honestly are problematic. All staff should be provided with appropriate training as each patient comes in contact with many different members of the health care team through the course of a visit. Frontline staff members in reception areas need a complex set of skills to avoid discriminating against LGB and TNB patients. They need to avoid assumptions about sexual orientation and gender identity. In addition, they need to find a way to avoid violating a patient's privacy while obtaining information, when many health care facilities require them to collect information in public spaces. As discussed earlier, individuals may present their gender differently in different settings. It could demean and endanger patients to have the name they use in the privacy of a health care encounter be heard in a public waiting room or to have their legal name called out publicly when their gender expression does not match their legal name. Staff training is crucial to avoid beginning a health care experience with discomfort or discrimination. Points of tension within the clinic system should be identified and strategies created to address them. Table 12.3 provides a list of excellent resources available for staff training.

Dealing With Homophobia and Transphobia Within the Health Care Team

Patient comfort and safety in the health care setting depends not only on the attitudes of clinicians but also on the attitudes of the entire health care team. Respect for LGBQ and TNB patients is still far from universal. It is inevitable that clinicians will encounter anti-LGBQ and anti-TNB comments and attitudes within the health care system, including within their own clinical environment. A clinician's response—either challenging these sentiments or offering complicity by ignoring

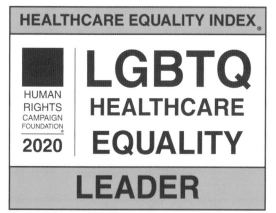

Figure 12.7 From HRC Foundation. (2020). Healthcare equality index 2020. HRC Digital Reports. Retrieved April 12, 2022, from https://reports.hrc.org/healthcare-equality-index-2020#hei-2020-leaders Copyright © 2020 Human Rights Campaign Foundation. All Rights Reserved. Reproduced with permission. Any further use without the express written consent of Human Rights Campaign Foundation is prohibited.

TABLE 12.3   Training on Best Practices for Working With LGBQ and TNB Patients

Name of Resource	Description	Where to Find It
Ready, Set, Go! Guidelines and Tips for Collecting Patient Data on Sexual Orientation and Gender Identity (SOGI)	Useful guide for systems and individuals at various levels of readiness	National LGBTQIA+ Health Education Center: https://www.lgbtqiahealtheducation.org/publication/ready-set-go-a-guide-for-collecting-data-on-sexual-orientation-and-gender-identity-2022-update/
Acknowledging Gender and Sex	Training for clinicians and frontline staff on two-step gender identity and sex differentiation	UCSF Center of Excellence for Transgender Health: https://prevention.ucsf.edu/transhealth/education/acknowledging-gender-sex
Transgender Healthcare Toolkit	Basic training modules for frontline and clinical staff including cultural information	Cedar River Clinics: http://www.cedarriverclinics.org/tran-stoolkit/
National LGBT Health Education Center online modules	A variety of online modules and recorded webinars for all levels of staff training	National LGBT Health Education Center: https://www.lgbtqiahealtheducation.org/
Affirmative Services for Transgender and Gender Diverse People—Best Practices for Frontline Staff	Very helpful guide for both providers and staff	National LGBT Health Education Center: https://www.lgbtqia-healtheducation.org/publication/affirmative-services-for-transgender-and-gender-diverse-people-best-practices-for-frontline-health-care-staff/
Taking Routine Histories of Sexual Health: A System-Wide Approach for Health Centers	Detailed guide on respectfully obtaining thorough sexual histories from LGBTQ patients. Note: contains some discrepancies with this chapter's approach to gender inclusivity.	National LGBT Health Education Center: http://www.lgbthealtheducation.org/wp-content/uploads/COM-827-sexual-history_toolkit_2015.pdf

them—helps set the tone for workplace culture. Each situation is different, but talking to the individuals involved privately is often a good idea rather than discussing the issue in front of patients or coworkers. If transphobic and homophobic comments and practices are endemic in a workplace, it can be helpful to talk with administrators who are able to change procedures and institute training.

In addition to reacting to problems as they come up, clinicians can be proactive by integrating positive sentiments about LGBQ and TNB individuals into their clinical environment. This can be accomplished by sharing interesting articles about LGBQ and TNB health with their peers, talking about a positive experience they recently had with a LGBQ or TNB patient, or presenting their own challenges (such as having misgendered a patient) to their peers for troubleshooting assistance. If a LGBQ or TNB patient reports feeling particularly validated or respected during a visit, this should be shared with the staff or providers involved. For example, during a visit a patient is smiling and states "When I got here, I asked the front desk person where the bathroom was and they told me where both the men's and women's rooms were so I could decide for myself where to go." That staff member should be approached in a timely matter so this positive feedback can be shared and they can be thanked for their excellent patient care.

Even providers who do not have control over the physical environment of their practices can demonstrate that the examination room is a safe place with placement

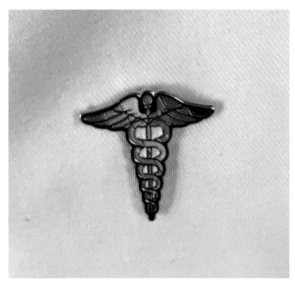

Figure 12.8 Rainbow caduceus pin. (Courtesy Kaleidoscope Health Alliance. LGBTQ ally pin. https://www.kaleidoscopehealth. org/product/lgbtq-ally-pin/.)

of LGBQ and TNB focused educational materials. They can wear a pin that indicates their support of LGBQ and TNB patients. See Figure 12.8 for an example.

History and Screening

Privacy, permission, and patient-centered communication are key elements of taking a good history and forming a therapeutic relationship with LBQ and TNB patients. It is often helpful to first discuss aspects of the history that are least likely to be linked to stigma and shame and, after establishing trust, to move to more sensitive subjects. The health and health care disparities discussed earlier guide the specific aspects of taking a history and determining appropriate screening for LGB and TNB patients.

Approach to History Taking

Providers are often unaware of the sexual and gender identities of their patients,[19] and many assume that their patients do not want to share this information.[108] However, the vast majority of patients report that they would choose to reveal their sexual orientation to their providers if asked and believe that knowledge of sexual orientation would help their providers know them better and ultimately provide better care.[108]

Sometimes health care providers avoid asking about gender identity or sexual orientation because they fear they will be seen as discriminatory.[109] Clinicians can

offer reassurance by offering assurance that they ask these questions of all patients, explaining the reason for their questions and explaining how those questions are relevant for a particular visit.

A sexual history should be included for any patient as necessary. However, LGBQ and TNB patients have reported painful, stigmatizing experiences such as coming to the emergency department for a broken hand and being "grilled about my sexuality for 10 minutes by the emergency department doctor."[57] If a lengthy sexual history is taken for an LGBQ or TNB patient when it would not be taken for a heterosexual or cisgender patient in the same situation, it is not appropriate. Additionally, providers should be mindful of the assumptions they may be making when forming questions for LGBQ or TNB patients, avoiding the pitfall of acting based on stereotypes.

Almost all LGBQ and TNB patients are aware of the homophobic or transphobic treatment they might expect to have when seeking care based both on their own previous experiences and those they have heard about. Out of self-protection, LGBQ and TNB patients may approach a health care encounter warily, picking up on subtle signals to determine if they can trust their providers. If providers make it obvious that they assume an LGBQ or TNB patient is heterosexual and cisgender, patients may not know if it is safe to correct them.

Because it is never possible to know a patient's sexual orientation or gender identity simply by their outward appearance or by their name, it is vitally important not to make assumptions about the gender identity or sexual orientation of any patient or their sexual partners. In many settings, some information about the patient's sexual orientation and gender identity is supplied by the medical record, but often this information is incomplete. For example, many records only offer options "male" and "female" for partners; this is not inclusive of patients who have TNB partners and can lead to confusion regarding risk factors and appropriate testing. A comprehensive question about sexual orientation gives options such as "not sure." A two-step method of asking about gender is recommended for registration forms (Box 12.1). A recommended registration question about sexual orientation is provided in Box 12.2.

Whatever amount of information is available in a medical record, respectfully asking about a patient's

---

BOX 12.1   Two-Step Approach to Obtaining Gender Identity and Sex Assigned At Birth

Do you think of yourself as:
- ☐ Male
- ☐ Female
- ☐ Female-to-male (FTM)/transgender male/trans man
- ☐ Male-to-female (MTF)/transgender female/trans woman
- ☐ Genderqueer, neither exclusively male nor female
- ☐ Additional gender category/(or other), please specify:

_____

- ☐ Something else

What sex were you assigned at birth on your original birth certificate? (Check one)
- ☐ Male
- ☐ Female
- ☐ Decline to answer

BOX 12.2   Sexual Orientation-Comprehensive Approach

Do you think of yourself as:
- ☐ Straight or heterosexual
- ☐ Lesbian, gay, or homosexual
- ☐ Bisexual
- ☐ Something else
- ☐ Do not know

---

sexual and gender identity can lead to a better understanding of how the patient defines their own identity. Each individual is different, and predefined categories may not fully express a particular individual's identity.[110] In addition, identities often change over time, particularly in times of exploration such as adolescence and young adulthood[112] or during gender affirmation.[112] A simple way to elicit information about changes in sexual behavior since the last sexual history is to ask, "Have there been any changes in your sexual activity that I should be aware of?" This opens the door for patients to disclose both changes in sexual attraction and sexual behavior.

To avoid making incorrect assumptions about sexual orientation or gender identity, providers should use gender-inclusive language. This is a new skill for many providers but can be easily learned with a short amount of practice. A good way to become comfortable with gender-inclusive language is to practice using it throughout entire patient encounters with all patients. It is particularly helpful to try this in visits that feel inherently gendered, such as contraceptive consults or prenatal visits. It will soon begin to feel natural and easy and often will be unnoticed by cisgender patients. Gender-inclusive language should be initially used with all patients in all circumstances; once rapport is established and the provider gets to know more about the patient, they can switch to language that is appropriate and affirming for that specific patient. This switch can be accomplished by "mirroring" the language the patient uses to describe themselves. The exception to this is language that might be perceived as discriminatory when used by a heterosexual or cisgender individual, as discussed earlier. Table 12.4 provides examples of gender-inclusive language.

> **CLINICAL SURVIVAL TIP** A good way to become comfortable with gender-inclusive language is to practice using it throughout entire patient encounters with all patients.

Talking about anatomy such as breasts and genitals may be difficult for TNB patients, who may have significant discomfort with these parts of their body. Avoiding specific anatomical terms such as *vagina* and *penis* until the patient has used them can provide the patient with the safety and comfort they need to talk openly with the clinician. It is also appropriate to directly solicit the patient's preferred terms and mirror these or to ask permission to use anatomical terms based on a clearly stated clinical rationale. For example, when assessing complaints of vulvar lesions, the provider could say: "I would like to use some very specific anatomical terms for different areas of your external genitals. This will help me figure out exactly what is going on and what the problem could be caused by. Would that be okay with you?"

Taking a careful history of any gender-affirming surgeries enables the provider to determine which organs are present in the patient's body. These organs should be screened appropriately, as discussed later in this chapter. If a patient has left the surgical history section of an intake form blank or you are otherwise unsure about

TABLE 12.4	Patient-Centered Language for Providers and Staff to Use With All Patients	
Category	Strategy	Examples
Patient's name	Upon meeting the patient, determine if they have a name they use that is not the name on their medical record. Determine the name they would like to use for health care encounters. Note this in the chart and use the appropriate name in all subsequent encounters.	Do not use the terms "Mr.", "Mrs.", or "Ms." You can say: "Many of my patients go by a name that is different from their legal name. Can you tell me what name you would like us to use for you in this clinic?"
Pronouns	Do not use gendered pronouns for patient either in documentation or in discussing patient until gender identity and correct pronouns have been discussed. Do not use gendered pronouns in referring to sexual partners or significant others until the patient has shared this information.	Do not say "he," "she," "him," or "her." Do say "they." Do mirror the language of the patient when referring to sexual partners.
Relationships	Do not use gendered descriptions of relationships	Do not say "boyfriend," "girlfriend," "husband," "wife," "son," "daughter," "mother," or "father" Do say "partner," "parent," and "child"
	Do not assume relationships of individuals who have come with the patient.	Do not say "Is this your mother, sister, brother, father, friend? Do introduce yourself and your role ("Hi, my name is _____. I am the nurse practitioner in clinic today.") If this does not prompt the patient to introduce their support person, you can say "Who is here with you today?" or "Tell me who's here with you for support today." If it is unclear who is the patient and who is the support person, ask both individuals to introduce themselves.

their current anatomy, it is appropriate to say "I have a few more questions to help me complete your full medical history. Have you ever had any gender-affirming surgery? Please tell me more about the surgeries you've had."

Cardiovascular Health. As discussed earlier, LBQ females, in comparison to heterosexual females, have a possible increased risk of heart disease. Evidence regarding the effects of testosterone and estrogen on heart health for TNB patients is reassuring, but not definitive. Therefore a history, appropriate screening, and treatment based on risk factors is particularly important for LBQ females and any TNB patients who are currently taking gender-affirming testosterone or estrogen. Risk factors include family or personal history of heart disease or thromboembolism, history of hypertension, diabetes, high LDL, low HDL, and clotting disorders as well as alcohol and tobacco use.

For TNB individuals taking gender-affirming hormone therapy, assessing cardiac risk to determine whether or not to prescribe statins or aspirin for prevention is complicated because risk assessment tools are gender specific.[113] The Center of Excellence for Transgender Health at the University of California San Francisco (UCSF) suggests that for those who begin hormone therapy later in life, it might be preferable to use the risk assessment tool for their sex assigned at birth. For those who began taking hormones as young adults or adolescents, the affirmed gender tool might be more appropriate. Age at which treatment was initiated and total duration of hormone exposure are key principles in determining the appropriateness of screening tools.[74] Given the lack of evidence about cardiovascular prevention practices in TNB patients, the decision to prescribe prophylactic aspirin or statins must be made based on careful consideration of the risks associated with these treatments.

Cancer Screening. All LBQ females and TNB individuals should receive routine cancer screening as a part of preventive care.

Cervical Cancer. As discussed earlier, LBQ females and TNB individuals with cervixes tend to have much lower cervical cancer screening rates when compared with the general population of cisgender females. When they present for care, there is a good chance that they may not be current on their pap smears. It is important to elicit the history of previous pap smears and any abnormal results, whether or not the reason for the visit is gynecological. Taking a history and making recommendations for pap screening should be undertaken with sensitivity to ensure that patients do not get the impression that their health care, including gender-affirming hormone therapy or contraception, will be "held hostage" until they are current on their pap screening. As always, a harm-reduction approach best facilitates rapport and patient engagement in care.

Getting a pap smear can be very challenging for TNB individuals with cervixes as well as some LBQ females, either because they have had negative experiences with genital examinations in the past with insensitive providers or because these examinations require sustained attention on genitals that may be incongruent with the patient's gender identity. TNB patients who are taking gender-affirming hormone therapy may have had painful examinations or unsatisfactory pap results caused by the effects of testosterone on the vaginal and cervical epithelium.[114] Providers should build a trusting relationship with the TNB patient before attempting to perform a speculum examination and pap smear. This can be accomplished by completing the first half of the visit with the patient fully clothed, in a non-examination room if this is available, or offering to postpone the pap smear to a separate appointment after the first meeting. The pap smear, like any test, is never done without the patient's consent, and gender-affirming hormone therapy should not be withheld from a patient who has not had a pap smear. The chances of success at obtaining consent for a pap smear are increased if the patient sets the pace. The pap smear can be delayed for as long as needed for the patient to be ready to have a speculum inserted.[74] More information on speculum and pelvic examinations for TNB patients is provided in the following section.

> **PATIENT-CENTERED CARE:** Providers should build a trusting relationship with the TNB patient before attempting to perform a speculum examination and pap smear. This can be accomplished by completing the first half of the visit with the patient fully clothed, in a non-examination room if this is available, or offering to postpone the pap smear to a separate appointment after the first meeting. The chances of success at obtaining consent for a pap smear are increased if the patient sets the pace. The pap smear can be delayed for as long as needed for the patient to be ready to have a speculum inserted.

Pap smears for LGB and TNB patients should follow the screening guidelines for cisgender female patients (see Chapter 5). As with cisgender patient, a TNB patient who has had a hysterectomy should have regular pap smears if the cervix is partially or fully intact. If the cervix has been removed, a pap smear is not needed unless the patient has a history of CIN2 or worse in the previous 20 years or has ever had cervical cancer.[115]

Breast Cancer. Screening for LGB female patients is important because they tend to be more likely to have certain risk factors than the general population, including nulliparity, smoking, and alcohol use, and they die of breast cancer at a higher rate.[60,61] LGB females have less frequent mammograms than heterosexual females,[115] so appropriate counseling and ordering of mammograms is of particular importance (Chapter 22).

According to the limited research that is available, TNB individuals who have used feminizing hormones probably have less risk for breast cancer than AFAB individuals and more risk for breast cancer than AMAB individuals.[74] The fact that feminizing hormone therapy leads to denser breast tissue than that seen in cisgender females and that TNB AMAB individuals tend to have their breast cancers diagnosed at later stages indicates the importance of screening.

TNB AFAB individuals who have not undergone gender-affirming chest surgery should have chest/breast cancer screening on the same schedule as cisgender females.[74] Chest surgery—often called *top surgery*—typically consists of a double mastectomy with reconstruction of chest tissue and nipple placement to create a traditionally masculine shape. Following chest surgery, the risk of cancer in the remaining tissue is not known. As there are no recommendations regarding routine chest wall palpation following chest surgery, the decision of whether or not to perform this screening should be based on shared decision making; however, any masses or new concerns should be promptly evaluated.[73] Mammography may not be possible after surgery because of scant tissue; when this is the case, ultrasonography or magnetic resonance imaging can be considered as alternative diagnostic tools. The provider can also do chest examinations and teach self-awareness of the remaining tissue to the patient as appropriate.

As with cisgender females, LGB and TNB patients may need earlier and possibly more frequent breast cancer screening if they have breast cancer risk factors.

> **! SAFETY ALERT**
>
> The risk of breast cancer after gender-affirming chest surgery is not currently known. Decisions about screening using palpation should be discussed and jointly decided by the provider and the patient. Any masses or concerns should be evaluated promptly.

Prostate Cancer. Screening according to the guidelines for AMAB individuals is the standard of care for all TNB patients with a prostate. The prostate is not generally removed during feminizing genital surgery. Prostate cancer is no more prevalent among TNB AMAB individuals with prostates than it is among cisgender men; in fact, it may be less common as estrogen therapy is one of the treatments for prostate cancer. Screening for TNB AMAB individuals is complicated by the fact that having low testosterone levels will have artificially lower prostate-specific antigen (PSA) levels, even in the presence of prostate cancer. The Center of Excellence for Transgender Health suggests setting the upper limit of normal for the PSA test at 0.1 ng/mL.[74] More information on prostate examination in TNB patients is provided later in this chapter.

Bone Health. In addition to the risk factors for osteoporosis in the general population (see Chapter 19), TNB patients may have some additional risks. There is limited evidence concerning the effect of gender-affirming hormone therapy, androgen blockade, and gonadectomy on bone mass; however, there are some strong indications that these treatments may increase the risk for osteoporosis in certain cases.

Feminizing Hormone Therapy. Research to date on the effect of feminizing hormones on bone mineral density (BMD) is conflicting, showing an increase, a decrease, or no change in BMD. This variation may be the result of differences in hormone therapy regimens and length of follow-up.[74] Following orchiectomy, most but not all patients continue to take estrogen. Those who do not are at increased risk for osteoporosis. It is recommended that TNB AMAB patients who have had no estrogen for 5 years after an orchiectomy begin screening for BMD.[74]

For those who have not undergone orchiectomy, androgen blockers play a role in osteoporosis risk. Cisgender males who are treated with androgen blockers for prostate cancer have decreased bone density and an increased risk of osteoporosis.[117] TNB AMAB patients who are using androgen blockers without taking estrogen or with estrogen doses that result in sub-physiological serum estradiol levels would be expected to have the same physiological response as cisgender males using androgen blockers, and it is recommended that they undergo BMD screening.[74]

> **NOT TO BE MISSED**
>
> TNB AMAB patients who are using androgen blockers without taking estrogen or with estrogen doses that result in sub-physiological serum estradiol levels would be expected to have the same physiological response as cisgender males using androgen blockers, and it is recommended that they undergo BMD screening.

Masculinizing Hormone Therapy. Taking testosterone increases bone mass, so TNB AFAB individuals who take testosterone have more bone mass than cisgender females.[118-121] Having an oophorectomy causes bone mass to decrease dramatically,[122] so TNB AFAB individuals who are not taking testosterone are advised to begin BMD screening within 5 years after an oophorectomy.[74]

Sexual History. Patients may be used to sharing details of their health at a medical visit, but they may not have ever been asked intimate details about their sexual practices. In addition to the reluctance shared with all patients, many LGB and TNB patients have come to fear questions about their sexuality, often asked out of voyeuristic curiosity.[24] Timing the sexual history after trust has been established and the patient has been given indications that the provider is respectful of all gender identities and sexual orientation can help patients feel comfortable disclosing their sexual history. Taking the time to get to know the patient as a whole person—including asking about their work, family life, and living situation—will increase trust and provide key preliminary information on sources of strength as well as possible risks. It is most appropriate to begin the sexual history with open-ended questions that will provide context on gender identity and sexual orientation and then ask specific follow-up questions as needed.

Permission. It is important to obtain permission for a sexual history and explain why the information is important. Each provider will find their own style and language. One possible introductory statement is to say "In order to give the best possible care, I ask all patients questions about their sexual history. Some of the questions are very personal. Is that okay?" Being asked for permission gives patients some control and may make them more comfortable to be open and honest with the provider. If the patient declines, this must be honored, however the provider can reopen the conversation later by explaining why a certain aspect of the sexual history is important and ask for some limited information.

Comfort. Provider comfort with discussing sexual health topics is an important influence on the LGB and TNB patient's comfort level. Patients have reported being met with blank stares, blushing, or confused looks on the part of providers when they openly answered questions about their sexuality.[57] In working with LGB and TNB patients, a provider might encounter a broader range of sexual expression than they have experienced or encountered with their cisgender heterosexual patients. Gaining knowledge of a wider range of sexual practices through reading, observing, and discussing cases with colleagues can increase knowledge, and as a result increase provider comfort. Comfort and knowledge enable a provider to ask appropriate follow-up questions and to help patients explore ways to make sex safer and more enjoyable.

Language. Some patients may be uncomfortable with traditional medical anatomical terms such as *penis* and *vagina*. Others may not be familiar with medical anatomical terms such as *vulva* or *scrotum*. Before using anatomical terms, the provider should ask which terms the patient prefers and confirm the patient's understanding during the discussion.

6 P's. Traditionally, the method of taking a comprehensive sexual history has been taught using the acronym of the "5 *P*'s,": *partners, practices, past* STIs, *prevention* of STIs, as well as *pregnancy* planning and prevention.[123] Some authors add another important component related to sexual enjoyment and function: the sixth "*P*," pleasure.[124]

Partners. Through previously filled-out forms or in-person history taking, the provider is already familiar with the patient's gender identity, sexual orientation, and anatomy. The clinician may need to ask additional questions beyond those on clinic forms if the forms only indicate if the patient has sex with "men, women, or both." The most salient clinical information needed relates to the anatomy of sexual partners, rather than their gender identities or sexual orientations. Therefore it is helpful to be specific by using questions such as "Do you partner with individuals who have penises, individuals who have vaginas, or both?" To facilitate respectful discussion, it is also important for clinicians to ensure that they are using the correct pronouns when discussing specific partners, regardless of that individual's anatomy.

In addition, questions about partners should include how many partners the patient has had in a specific timeframe in the past, such as 6 months or 1 year, and how many they currently have. Clinicians should also ask about partners' sexual risk factors such as other partners, history of STIs, injection drug use, and drug or alcohol use during sex.

The patient's relationship with partners is an important aspect of their sexual risk. Patients may have casual or anonymous partners, or they may be in a mutually monogamous relationship. Some patients may be in a primary couple relationship with one or both having relationships outside that couple, or they may be in a primary couple relationship with both partners having sex with a third person together. Patients may be polyamorous, having more than one committed, intimate relationship or sharing a committed, intimate relationship with more than one partner. Patients may not be familiar with the term *monogamous,* so the clinician could consider asking, "Do you and your partner only have sex with each other? Is there a possibility that your partner could have had sex with someone else during your relationship?"

Practices. The second *P,* practices, addresses how the patient has sex with partners. As noted earlier, it is most appropriate to start with open-ended questions and then ask additional clarifying questions as needed. Care should be taken to be clear and specific, as terms related to sexual activity can be vague and open to interpretation. It is helpful to be aware of common LGBQ and TNB community terms for sexual activity, keeping in mind that language does vary by region and culture and changes over time. Time-honored terms include *top, bottom, switch, cruising, rimming,* and *fisting.* If a patient states, "I bottom for anal sex," this typically means they are the receptive partner during anal intercourse. Patients who describe themselves as a "top" are typically the insertive partner. Patients who described themselves as a "switch" are sometimes the receptive partner and sometimes the insertive partner. Patients may top for one type of sexual activity and bottom for another. Providers can easily replace these terms with *give* and *receive;* for example, "Do you have anal sex? Do you give or receive penetration?" *Cruising* describes seeking anonymous partners in public spaces. *Rimming* describes oral-to-anal intercourse. *Fisting* describes the insertion of the entire hand and sometimes a portion of the wrist or arm into a partner's vagina or rectum.

It is critical that clinicians ask about all types of sexual activity and do not make assumptions about sexual behavior based on sexual orientation or gender identity. All patients should be asked if they take part in oral, vaginal, and anal sex. For each of these categories, the clinician should elicit information to determine if the patient is the receptive or insertive partner. For receptive intercourse, it is important to determine what is being used for penetration (i.e., penis, toys, fingers, hands). For each type of sex the patient engages in, it is important to know if they use safer-sex practices; when safer-sex practices are used inconsistently, the clinician should elicit information about how these decisions are made. Importantly, it cannot be assumed that all TNB

individuals have dysphoria in regard to their genitals; in fact, many TNB individuals and LBQ females with a more masculine gender expression very much enjoy using their genitals for sex.

Past Sexually Transmitted Infections. Because some patients feel shame and guilt about their past STIs, the clinician can help open the discussion by communicating a nonjudgmental attitude. The history should include specific infections, how the patient was treated, if partners were treated, if follow-up testing was performed if recommended, and if the patient is still in a relationship with a partner or partners who are likely sources of transmission.

Prevention of Sexually Transmitted Infections. Asking an open-ended question about what patients do to protect themselves from STIs is a good way to begin this discussion. The provider's goal is to understand prevention from the patient's point of view. If the patient uses safer-sex practices only in certain situations, the clinician should explore when and why. For example, patients may forego barrier methods with a primary partner—often referred to as being *fluid bonded*—but consistently use barrier methods with additional, non-primary sexual partners. Some patients will use barrier methods for anal or vaginal intercourse with non-primary partners but do not use barrier methods for oral intercourse. When discussing barrier methods, it is helpful to ask if the patient uses barriers "never, sometimes, or always" with each type of sexual intercourse they engage in. This information is very valuable and allows for exploration of how the patient perceives safety and risk. Some patients have misunderstandings about risks and prevention. This question often leads to education and counseling, which is covered later in this chapter.

Pregnancy Planning and Prevention. An initial question is to ask how the patient feels about the idea of becoming a parent or having more children, either now or in the future. Clarification of partners and practices will give the provider an indication if there is a possibility of pregnancy occurring in the patient's current situation. As discussed earlier, many LBQ females have sexual contact that could result in pregnancy. Many TNB individuals have sex that could result in a pregnancy even if they are taking gender-affirming medications that substantially affect spermatogenesis or the chance of ovulation. In a study of TNB AFAB individuals' experiences of pregnancy, pregnancy was experienced by 24% of participants who were not actively trying to conceive and had a history of gender-affirming testosterone therapy and by 44% of those who were not actively trying to conceive and had never taken testosterone.[125]

Some patients are very clear about their pregnancy intentions, whereas others are ambivalent or take the approach "If it happens, it happens." Every individual's relationship to the concept of when and how families are built is complex and culturally rooted; it is inappropriate to assume that pregnancies that occur when not actively trying to conceive are unplanned or unwelcome or that pregnancies that occur when actively trying to conceive are welcome. Education and counseling, discussed later in this chapter, should focus on contraception and preconception care as appropriate.

Pleasure. Sexual pleasure, desire, and function have an important role in individuals' lives, relationships, and motivation. Unless they are asked, patients may not feel comfortable bringing up concerns with discomfort during sex or their goals for sexual pleasure and function. Asking patients if they are satisfied with their level of desire and function or if they have any problems with pain during sex can help begin these conversations when they are ready to have them. Providers should be aware that specific sexual concerns can arise with gender-affirming hormone therapy, such as decreased lubrication and vaginal atrophy with testosterone use as well as erectile dysfunction with estrogen use. Hormone therapy may also alter libido and how orgasm is felt in the body. These may or may not be perceived as problematic by patients, depending on how they use their bodies for sex.

Communication and Etiquette

Relevance vs. Curiosity. When caring for any patient, health care providers must strike a balance between eliciting all information needed to provide excellent care and asking unnecessary questions. This is particularly true when there is cultural discordance between the provider and patient, such as a White provider caring for a BIPOC patient, or a heterosexual provider caring for an LBQ patient.

Both LBQ and TNB patients report being asked inappropriate questions by curious health care providers. It is never appropriate to ask personal questions that are irrelevant to the patient's care. A good rule of thumb is that if you would not ask a cisgender or heterosexual patient the same question in the same clinical scenario, then the question is not appropriate. For example,

a health care provider would never casually ask a cisgender patient, "How long have you been a woman?" or a heterosexual patient "How long have you been straight?" It follows that a health care provider should not ask, "When did you become transgender?" or "How long have you been gay?" It would not be appropriate to ask a patient being seen for a sprained ankle if they intend to have cosmetic breast surgery or to ask a TNB patient being treated for the same concern if they plan to have genital or breast surgery.

The corollary of this is that providers should never avoid necessary questions out of personal embarrassment. A good rule of thumb is that if you would ask a cisgender patient the same question in the same clinical scenario, you should respectfully ask the same question of a TNB patient. A common example of this is providers not taking sexual histories from LBQ and TNB patients because they feel nervous or embarrassed to do so.

It is important to note that clinicians often ask inappropriate questions such as those discussed earlier out of a genuine desire to learn and to connect with their patient. These desires are legitimate but must be addressed by different means. It is never the responsibility of a patient to educate the clinician, and questions that feel invasive or irrelevant facilitate distrust rather than rapport. In some cases, inappropriate curiosity can actually function as a denial of timely care.

Because of historical trauma within health care system, it is important to explicitly let LBQ and TNB patients know that sensitive questions are actually relevant to their health care by explaining the reason for the question. Additionally, patients from marginalized communities should never be treated as representatives of that group. For example, it is inappropriate to ask, "What does the lesbian community think about the new mayor?"

> **PATIENT-CENTERED CARE:** It is never appropriate to ask personal questions that are irrelevant to the patient's care. A good rule of thumb is that if you would not ask a cisgender or heterosexual patient the same question in the same clinical scenario, then the question is not appropriate.

Errors in Language. It is common for health care workers to accidentally *misgender* a patient (call them by the wrong pronoun or name) or to make an incorrect assumption about a relationship between the patient and one of their significant others, such as assuming a same-sex partner is a sibling. The best response is to apologize sincerely, make a clear statement that you will change your behavior in the future, and move on. The patient should not be expected to reassure the provider by having to respond to excessively emotional or multiple apologies. Additionally, health care consumers are aware of the scarce amount of time allotted to their visits; it is very frustrating to see that time is wasted as the provider processes the mistake inappropriately.

Knowledgeable Consumers. LBQ females, and even more so TNB individuals, frequently have to educate their providers about different aspects of sexual and TNB health. They therefore may enter a new provider-patient relationship with a significant amount of uncertainty about the provider's competence.

Many TNB patients are very knowledgeable about gender-affirming health care. They may have studied the same online evidence-based guidelines that are recommended in this chapter. In addition, they may be familiar with routine practices of different gender-affirming care providers. There are many Internet resources geared to the LGBQ community and the TNB community with information about legal issues, medical protocols and facilities, support groups, and online forums. Information about medical care is also obtained through communication with friends within the TNB community. Patients may present to care already having extensive experience with medication management as a result of obtaining gender-affirming medications online or through other informal means and managing their own care.

Online sources, including those led by the lay public, may contain accurate, helpful information about different approaches to transgender health care in different geographical areas. Because research is inadequate, current practice is constantly evolving as clinicians develop new surgical methods, medication regimes, or ways of managing hormone therapy for patients with medical conditions. A patient may learn about important new developments before the provider does.

Utilizing a shared decision-making approach, providers can help their patients evaluate the different sources of information they bring to the health care encounter. Providers can correct any misinterpretations that can arise when an individual does not have medical training. Together they can evaluate the evidence and weigh the different options for an individual management plan.

Formal medical and nursing training in gender-affirming care is inadequate, so providers must obtain most of their knowledge of the field through self-planned educational activities. Furthermore, the field is constantly evolving. Providers who have made efforts to learn about gender-affirming health care need not feel guilty or inadequate when confronted by a patient with an area in which they are not knowledgeable. The best approach is an honest, straightforward statement by the provider that they are not familiar with the subject and will find out more. The provider should make a plan to meet with the patient in a timely manner as soon as they have had time to research and/or talk with a more experienced colleague.

> **PATIENT-CENTERED CARE:** Utilizing a shared decision-making approach, providers can help their patients evaluate the different sources of information they bring to the health care encounter.

Focused Physical

Most aspects of the physical examination are covered elsewhere in this text because they are the same for LBQ and TNB patients as for the general population. This section will cover those aspects of the physical examination that are unique to LBQ and TNB patients.

Any physical examination can make LBQ and TNB patients feel particularly vulnerable. Many TNB patients have had traumatic experiences related to hostile responses to their bodies, and they can find physical examinations particularly difficult. The following strategies are a good standard of care for performing examinations on any patient, regardless of sexual orientation or gender identity, and are particularly important when working with LBQ and TNB patients.

Before being asked to undress or submit to an examination, the patient should be provided with specific and complete information about the recommended examination. The examination should not be undertaken without permission. Some patients may be comfortable having some essential parts of an examination but request to decline or postpone other portions. If the patient is comfortable with a limited examination, and this is handled with respect and dignity, the patient may be comfortable having a more extensive examination at a future visit.

Patients should be allowed to bring a support person into the room for the examination and to use any stress-reducing strategies they wish, such as listening to music on headphones. If support individuals are excluded by protocols for the purpose of public health, such as during the ongoing COVID-19 pandemic, institutionally acceptable exceptions may be possible. Another option is to virtually bring support individuals into the room via a video call. During the examination, the clinician should obtain permission before each step (or announce each next step), pause to allow time for the patient to voice concerns, and then inform the patient that the examination may be discontinued at any point if the patient wishes.

An oral benzodiazepine taken 20 to 60 minutes before a pelvic examination may be very helpful for some patients.[74] However, for patients with a history of trauma, anti-anxiety medication can cause dissociation.[126] This possibility should be discussed in advance with the patient to allow for informed consent and shared decision making. At a minimum, patients will need a driver for transportation to and from the visit as they will be unable to travel independently. It may be a good idea to arrange for one of the patient's support individuals to be present as a chaperone during the examination. It is also important to be aware, however, that for some TNB individuals, having a chaperone present may increase rather than decrease their distress. This may be because, for the patient, it is simply not tolerable to have more than one person viewing their genitals or to have anyone see them in the vulnerable position that allows their genitals to be examined.

Postsurgical Examinations

There are a wide variety of gender-affirmation surgeries, and the techniques and postsurgical presentations vary with each technique. Patients may present to a local provider for an examination when they are unable to follow up with their surgeon, which is often the case because many patients travel a long distance for surgery because of the dearth of experienced surgeons. The basic principles of wound healing will be valuable to the provider in this case, and additional information specific to gender-affirming surgical follow-up is available online. One good resource is the *Post-Surgical Care Guide* available in the Cedar River Clinic's Transgender Health Care Toolkit.[126] In addition, the surgeon can be contacted directly to advise on the normal postsurgical course, and

this should be done anytime providers are unsure if they understand what they are seeing.

> **CLINICAL SURVIVAL TIP** Patients may seek after-surgery care through a local provider rather than the surgeon because of distance of travel required. Knowing the basic principles of wound care and information specific to gender-affirming surgical follow-up is an invaluable skill. One good resource is the *Post-Surgical Care Guide* available in the Cedar River Clinic's Transgender Health Care Toolkit.

Breast/Chest Examination

Many TNB AFAB patients use the term *chest* for this examination, which should be done, as for cisgender females, only when indicated (see Chapter 21). Those who have not had gender-affirming chest surgery may use methods to flatten their chest tissue to create a flatter chest contour. They may have a compression shirt, a chest binder, a tightly fitting bra, or an ace bandage to remove for the examination. There may be rashes, skin breakdown, or infections from binding that is too tight or prolonged.

Patients who have had gender-affirming chest surgery typically have very little breast tissue, sometimes making mammography impossible. Without mammography as a screening method, examinations should be done based on risk factors and discussion of risks and benefits with the patient.

The Center of Excellence for Transgender Health recommends beginning breast cancer screening for individuals taking feminizing hormones at 50 years of age if they have taken hormones for at least 5 years.[74] It is not recommended to initiate routine screening before 5 years of hormone therapy, regardless of age. As with natal females, they may need earlier screening based on risk factors. As hormones cause new tissue growth, there will be breast changes, and a breast examination is indicated anytime a patient has concerns about possible masses or tenderness.

Vaginal Examination

The vaginal examination can be a source of significant anxiety for LBQ and TNB patients because of previous experiences with health care providers' inappropriate curiosity about or negative reactions to their genitals. Speculum insertion may be difficult for those who do not routinely experience vaginal penetration during sex, just as it is with heterosexual cisgender female patients. Dysphoria about having a vagina or fear that one's surgically constructed vagina will be approached with scorn or undue curiosity can also contribute to anxiety. Before beginning the vaginal examination, it is important to ensure that the patient knows the steps and that the clinician will discontinue the examination if the patient feels they need to stop before it is complete.

NOT TO BE MISSED

The vaginal examination can be a source of significant anxiety for LBQ and TNB patients because of previous experiences with health care providers' inappropriate curiosity about or negative reactions to their genitals.

TNB AFAB Patients. Patients who take gender-affirming testosterone will experience decreased vaginal lubrication and thinning of the vaginal epithelium, which can make speculum insertion painful. Physiologically this is similar to the way lowered estrogen levels affect speculum examinations for postmenopausal cisgender female patients. If the patient is willing to try it, a 2-week course of vaginal estrogen before the speculum examination can help thicken the vaginal epithelium and increase lubrication; this will in turn increase both patient comfort and likelihood of an adequate sample.[58] It is important to provider reassurance that this low-dose, local form of estrogen will not counteract the gender-affirming impact of testosterone.

> **CLINICAL SURVIVAL TIP** Patients taking gender-affirming testosterone have an increase in comfort and likelihood of an adequate sample if given a 2-week course of vaginal estrogen before the speculum examination.

The narrowest speculum that will allow visualization of the cervix should be used. A medium Pederson speculum works well for many patients. An extra-narrow Pederson speculum should also be available to use if needed, and if the vagina is short enough, a pediatric speculum should be used.

Using water-based lubricant or topical lidocaine on the outside of the speculum bills is very helpful and is not likely to interfere with pap smear collection. Putting

gentle downward pressure on the vaginal opening with a gloved finger and then gently pressing with the speculum against the introitus until the muscle relaxes is usually more comfortable for the patient than forcing the speculum past a tense introital muscle. Patients can also be offered the opportunity to insert the speculum themselves, with instructions from the clinician. For some patients, this will decrease tensing of the pelvic floor muscles and reduce feelings of vulnerability.

As noted earlier, TNB patients taking testosterone have a high rate of unsatisfactory pap smears. It is possible to decrease the likelihood of an insufficient sample by using more than one collection device and collecting several samples using a spatula, a broom, and a brush.[8] All three samples should be submitted together to increase the amount of cells collected.

TNB AMAB Patients. A surgically created vagina is most commonly formed by a penile skin inversion in which the tip of the penis forms the clitoris, the scrotum forms the vulva, and the skin of the penile shaft lines the vagina. The surgeon can also use intestinal tissue or skin grafts from other areas of the body. Because the lining of the vagina is not mucosal tissue, the microflora is different from the vagina of an AFAB individual. Vaginal irritation, vaginal odor, and unusual discharge are common complaints; these symptoms may be caused by buildup of sebum or other material in the vaginal vault or may be associated with vaginitis such as BV.

If penile tissue was used for the surgery, the epithelial cells do not self-lubricate, and any discharge is likely to be from sebaceous glands, dead skin, or retained semen or lubricant.[127] If there is any unusual odor or discharge, the clinician should check for lesions. A mild, blood-streaked yellowish discharge may be the result of granulation tissue from delayed healing following surgery. The vaginal examination should include checking for skin diseases that can be found on the penis such as skin cancer or psoriasis.

If intestinal tissue was used to form the vagina, there may be a normal discharge from digestive secretions, sometimes requiring the patient to wear a small pad. A greenish discharge may be the result of overgrowth of intestinal bacteria, which can be identified by a culture.[73]

The surgically created vagina is shallower and less elastic than the vagina of an AFAB individual (average depth is 15 cm[73]), so it is sometimes helpful to use a pediatric speculum or a clear plastic anoscope for the examination. The speculum should be inserted following the natural direction of the vagina, which is usually more posterior than the direction of the vagina in an AFAB individual. If the patient has not performed adequate dilation to keep the vagina patent, the vagina may have stenosed.

Prostate Examination

Prostate examinations for TNB AMAB patients should be done on the same schedule as for cisgender male patients. The examinations are usually begun at 50 years of age. As discussed earlier, the PSA level is altered by low testosterone levels. A sensitively performed prostate examination is an important method of screening for prostate cancer for TNB AMAB patients. If the patient has a surgically constructed vagina, the prostate examination is most comfortably done with fingers in the vagina, pressing against the anterior wall.

Summary

Ideally, a physical examination is a positive experience in which patients feel safe and trust that the clinician will treat them respectfully and competently screen for and investigate important health issues. The clinician can use the physical examination to build a therapeutic relationship by carefully ensuring consent throughout the process, listening and responding to patient concerns and questions, and describing at least some of the normal, healthy aspects noted during the examination.

TREATMENTS AND RECOMMENDATIONS

The bulk of care required by LBQ and TNB patients is routine primary care unrelated to sexual orientation or gender identity, and recommended treatments would be similar to those used in any other patient population. Accordingly, this section will focus on medical strategies for reducing the risk of HIV transmission (not unique to LBQ and TNB patients, but frequently indicated), and gender-affirming care.

Reducing HIV Acquisition in the Context of High-Risk Sexual Activities

Prevention of HIV infections through preexposure prophylaxis (PrEP) and postexposure prophylaxis (PEP) is particularly important in any population that is at high risk for HIV acquisition, including LBQ and TNB individuals who have MSM partners or engage in high-risk sexual activities. Barrier methods are the most important preventive measure against HIV infection. However,

using barrier methods is not practical or desirable for everyone. TNB patients with penises who are undergoing gender-affirming feminization may not be able to put a condom on a soft penis. Like cisgender female patients, TNB individuals who have little power in a coercive relationship may not be able to insist on barrier method use. This is particularly true for sex workers and individuals experiencing intimate partner violence. The two types of medications taken preventively by individuals who are not HIV positive are preexposure prophylaxis (PrEP) and non-occupational postexposure prophylaxis (nPEP).

PrEP is safe and effective to reduce the risk of HIV acquisition for patients at high risk. A single pill is taken daily. The CDC provides excellent detailed guidelines for prescribing PrEP.[130] As the name suggests, nPEP is medication administered after a concerning exposure. Use of nPEP for LBQ and TNB patients follows the same guidelines as for heterosexual and cisgender patients.[131] Any patient presenting for nPEP should be assessed as a potential candidate for PrEP in order to establish more effective protection on an ongoing basis. There are no contraindications to using PrEP or nPEP with gender-affirming hormone therapy.[74]

> **CLINICAL SURVIVAL TIP** The CDC provides a PDF guideline for providing PrEP that can be found at: www.cdc.gov/hiv/pdf/clinicians/materials/cdc-hiv-FlyerPrEPUpdateProvider508.pdf

Gender-Affirming Care

As discussed previously, many TNB individuals choose to take either masculinizing or feminizing medications. Primary care is the most appropriate setting in which to initiate and manage gender-affirming medical care because co-occurring medical problems can also be addressed in this setting.[131] The need for gender-affirming care is often what brings TNB patients to a primary care provider, perhaps after many years of health care avoidance because of fears of discrimination. Meeting immediate needs for gender affirmation can engage this underserved population in comprehensive primary care. Primary care physicians, nurse practitioners (including certified midwives and certified nurse midwives), and physician assistants are all recognized as qualified to manage masculinizing and feminizing hormone therapy.[132]

Building Provider Competence and Confidence

Providers may initially feel concerned about their competence to care for TNB patients, largely because the care needs of this population have historically been excluded from all formal medical and nursing education. However, this legacy of institutionalized transphobia does not excuse providers from an ethical obligation to provide care to all patients, regardless of gender identity. Providers may build their competence and confidence over time by seeking clinical experience, continuing education, and consultation with more experienced colleagues. As providers are in the process of acquiring the necessary knowledge, they can advance their skills and the services they offer over time.

All clinicians have an obligation to provide basic preventive and primary care for TNB patients using a patient-centered and TNB-positive approach. For example, as there is no difference between a sprained ankle in a cisgender patient and the same injury in a TNB patient, it would be unethical for a provider to refuse care or insist on referring the injured patient to a different provider. Preventive care services include basic pelvic and breast/chest care such as pap smears, prostate examinations, and mammography referrals, and these services should likewise never be denied or delayed on the basis of gender identity.

Managing gender-affirming hormone therapy and post-surgical care is squarely within the scope of all primary care providers but does require additional knowledge that clinicians must actively seek; clinical competence with this care will develop over time as with any other new skill. Providers may wish to attend several conferences or webinars before they begin to independently initiate and manage care in hormone-naïve patients. However, given the potential consequences of sudden loss of access to gender-affirming hormone therapy, particularly the risk of suicide, all providers can and should at a minimum provide bridging prescriptions for those who are already taking gender-affirming medications. A bridging prescription allows the patient time to find an experienced provider who is knowledgeable in managing their long-term care or for the provider to seek the needed support to take on the patient's care on a long-term basis.

> **PATIENT-CENTERED CARE:** The patient taking gender-affirming therapy is at risk for suicide when there is a sudden loss of access to these medications (from a variety of factors). At a minimum, providers should provide bridging prescriptions for these patients until they can establish care with a provider who is knowledgeable in managing this therapy.

Some patients seeking this support will have received a prior prescription from a licensed health care provider; others will have obtained their medications in other ways such as through friends or online. In either case, it is important that the medications be continued at the proper therapeutic doses so the patient can avoid gaps in care that cause significant emotional distress and can obtain the medications in the correct therapeutic dosages from an appropriately regulated pharmacy. The clinician should evaluate the patient's current treatment for safety and drug interactions and prescribe appropriate doses or medication as necessary.[75] Even those with no familiarity with gender-affirming care can easily do this by quickly checking one of the excellent care protocols discussed later in this chapter.

Every practice should maintain a referral list of hormone therapy providers for patients to access after they receive a bridging prescription.

Ultimately, all primary care providers should be comfortable initiating and managing gender-affirming hormone therapy. The following section provides an overview of this care and identifies resources for clinicians. Additional gender-affirming services that fall within the purview of primary care include clerical services and postoperative care. Clerical services include completing appropriate local and federal forms for a change of gender marker on legal documents, writing letters in support of gender-affirming surgery, and writing "travel letters" that aim to decrease harassment in settings such as TSA checkpoints.

Levels of Evidence

Until 2011, when the IOM outlined a research agenda for LGBQ and TNB health issues, most of the available research on gender-affirming care came from Europe.[134] Because the IOM report, medical researchers in the United States have done more research in this area. However, progress has been slow both in the United States and in Europe, and high quality, randomized controlled trials with adequate power have not been performed to determine either the efficacy or adverse effects of gender-affirming hormone therapy. Observational studies including cohort studies and case-control studies have been performed, but they lack sufficient sample sizes and follow-up times to yield conclusive results. Information about hormonal effects of the medications is available from studies done on cisgender individuals, but the applicability to TNB individuals is not known.

Fortunately, we have over 60 years of clinical experience with gender-affirming hormone treatments in the United States and over 70 years in Europe. Expert clinical opinion and available evidence have been compiled in several excellent sets of clinical guidelines. These are listed in Table 12.5.

Informed Consent

In 1979, the Harry Benjamin International Gender Dysphoria Association's *Standards of Care* was published.

This publication was the first compilation of current expert opinion on gender-affirming health care. The *Standards of Care* was expanded and edited over time and is now in its 7th edition, entitled *WPATH Standards of Care for the Health of Transsexual, Transgender, and Gender-Nonconforming Individuals.*[75] The *Standards of Care* helped legitimize gender-affirming care and afforded guidance for clinicians to begin providing it. The first edition of the *Standards of Care* reflected what was then the prevailing idea that there are two categories of TNB individuals.[135] One group could overcome their gender dysphoria and accept their birth gender through psychotherapy; these individuals were not considered "real" transsexuals, and it was thought that the risks of future regret or adverse physical effects did not justify treatments for this population.[135] The other category—the "real" transsexuals—were the only candidates approved for gender-affirming care. They exhibited what was believed to be a pathological condition termed

TABLE 12.5 Guidelines for Gender-Affirming Care		
Title	**Link**	**Notes**
Guidelines for the Primary and Gender-Affirming Care of Transgender and Gender Nonbinary People	https://transcare.ucsf.edu/guidelines	UCSF Center of Excellence for Transgender Health. The most comprehensive of the guidelines (updated periodically). Updated 2016.
Transgender Health Resources	https://fenwayhealth.org/wp-content/uploads/Medical-Care-of-Trans-and-Gender-Diverse-Adults-Spring-2021-1.pdf	Medical Care of Trans and Gender Diverse Adults. Issued by Fenway Health.
Feminizing and Masculinizing Hormone Therapy Protocols	http://www.cedarriverclinics.org/trans-toolkit/hormonetherapy/	Part of Cedar River Clinics' comprehensive Trans Health Care Toolkit. Updated 2021.
Endocrine Treatment of Gender-Dysphoric/Gender-Incongruent Persons: An Endocrine Society Clinical Practice Guideline	https://academic.oup.com/jcem/article/102/11/3869/4157558	Issued by the Endocrine Society. Published September 17, 2017. Link contains corrections in 2017 and 2018.
Protocols for the Provision of Hormone Therapy	http://callen-lorde.org/graphics/2018/05/Callen-Lorde-TGNC-Hormone-Therapy-Protocols-2018.pdf	Issued by Callen-Lorde Community Health Center. Updated 2018.
Standards of Care for the Health of Transsexual, Transgender, and Gender Nonconforming People	https://www.wpath.org/publications/soc	Issued by the World Professional Association for Transgender Health (WPATH). Available in different languages. Updated periodically. Volume 7, updated 2012. For updates, visit: https://www.wpath.org/soc8

gender identity disorder that could not be successfully treated with psychotherapy.[135] At the time, non-binary identities were not recognized as legitimate, and "real" transsexuals were expected to demonstrate binary male or female gender identities.[135]

Early editions of the *Standards of Care* required that before qualifying for gender-affirming medical care, a TNB individual must spend a certain amount of time completing a "real-life experience" of openly presenting as their affirmed gender in all aspects of life. This affirmed gender was expected to be binary, either male or female, and only once the "real-life experience" was completed could the patient obtain a letter from a therapist stating that they qualified for gender affirmation.[135] As TNB individuals and their social movements became more visible and the medical community began to recognize its obligation to treat TNB individuals as full human beings, problems with the old method of determining eligibility for gender-affirming care became evident. The "real-life experience" requirement subjected many TNB individuals to severe marginalization and abuse. Transgender females in particular were at high risk of harassment, assault, or murder when forced to wear women's clothing and use women's restrooms without the benefit of gender-affirming changes to secondary sex characteristics, regardless of where they lived.

Additionally, the lack of tolerance for gender diversity embodied by this approach forced all TNB individuals to present a homogenous representation of their gender identity. To qualify for treatment, TNB patients learned that they must provide a very specific narrative about their lives—one that conformed to the expectation of long-time identification as either male or female. It was expected that all TNB individuals felt they were born in the "wrong" body, had felt this way from early childhood, and desired a body in direct opposition to their sex assigned at birth, including a desire "to be rid of [their] own genitals."[137] Although this narrative was and continues to be true for some TNB individuals, it represents only one TNB experience. However, no other narrative could secure access to care, thus this became the medical and social definition of what it meant to be TNB. For the many TNB individuals who had a different experience with gender, this mandatory dishonesty interfered with the patient-provider relationship. The requirement for a therapist's letter placed undue burden on TNB individuals who had difficulty finding sympathetic TNB-positive therapists and usually had to take on the financial burden of paying for therapy.

Many in the medical community and the TNB community pointed out that this old model of determining eligibility denied TNB individuals the autonomy granted to others to make life-changing health care decisions, in contradiction to accepted medical standards of informed consent. This model drove some TNB individuals to obtain gender-affirming treatments from unregulated and potentially dangerous sources. Hormones could be obtained online or through other informal means and used without medical supervision, and those who could not travel to other countries for surgery sometimes turned to infusions of industrial-grade silicone and other fillers to create-affirming changes to body shape. The impact of this has been most pronounced for TNB AMAB individuals, who face a higher risk of thromboembolic events when unable to obtain the safest formulation of estradiol and experience medically and cosmetically catastrophic sequelae from silicone/filler "pumping."[129,138] Although these practices persist today because of financial barriers, safer options for care are becoming more and more accessible with changes to standards of care and the development of new approaches to service delivery.

In the early 1990s, some providers and health systems began to question the need for a therapist's evaluation before initiating gender-affirming care in patients without significant psychiatric comorbidities.[136] Eventually, many providers implemented what is known as the *informed consent model* for determining eligibility for gender-affirming medical treatments. Under this model, the same principle of informed consent is applied to gender-affirmation decisions as to any other health care decision: namely, patients are able to make informed choices after demonstrating understanding of the risks, benefits, and alternatives of treatment. For hormone therapy, discussion of risks and benefits should address all domains of life: physical, emotional, social, occupational, and financial. As with other health care decisions, before initiating treatment, clinicians should feel confident that the patient understands the information presented, can safely use any prescribed medications, and is competent to give consent. Therapy is encouraged in this model as it is helpful in navigating the process and impact of physical transition, but it is not required before initiation of hormone therapy. This model of care further acknowledges that TNB individuals are complex and nuanced individuals who may have significant co-occurring medical or mental health challenges. When this is the case, it is not a reason to deny treatment; rather, co-occurring conditions should be reasonably well controlled,[74] and referrals should be placed as appropriate. The informed consent model is now included as an option in the *WPATH Standards of Care*[75] as well as in respected clinical systems.[129,139,140]

Gender-Affirming Hormones

Gender-affirming medications are exogenous endocrine agents that act to reduce endogenous sex hormone levels or increase hormone levels to better align with their affirmed gender. Primary care providers are familiar with most of these medications, having prescribed them for other conditions such as benign prostatic hypertrophy, male pattern baldness, menopause management, contraception, and abnormal uterine bleeding.[74]

The goal of the treatment is to bring the patient's secondary sex characteristics into better congruence with their gender identity. TNB patients have a range of treatment goals. Some TNB patients wish to be consistently perceived as either male or female, while others desire a more androgynous or non-binary appearance. Although gender-affirming regimens can be personalized to meet individual goals, results vary and are unpredictable. It is important that patients understand that they may not achieve the level of masculinization, feminization, or androgyny that they desire or may experience undesired physical changes such as hair loss or erectile dysfunction. The efficacy of hormones is assessed, and dosages are adjusted as necessary throughout the treatment process by monitoring the patient's clinical response and satisfaction with outcomes.

It is important to note that the field of gender-affirming hormone therapy is rapidly evolving based on new research, clinical experience, and the needs of TNB patients. As such, it is important to remember that the following detailed clinical content is subject to change, and it is advisable to reference online protocols for changes as time passes from publication of this book.

Masculinizing Hormone Therapy

Masculinizing hormone therapy works by increasing testosterone levels in the body, in turn lowering estrogen. Increased testosterone levels produce changes to hair, skin, facial and body hair, muscle mass, fat distribution, genitals, menstruation, and voice. Table 12.6 provides a timeline of expected changes. It is also important for patients and clinicians to understand what testosterone will *not* change and that it is impossible to predict exactly how individuals will respond to therapy and which changes will endure if hormone therapy is discontinued. Testosterone will not cause changes to the bony skeleton in adults, increase height, or cause a significant reduction in chest size. It is also important to note that responses to hormone therapy (as responses to all medications) vary from patient to patient. Additionally, some changes such as facial and body hair growth are quite variable based on ethnicity and family history.

Fertility Considerations. Research exploring the long-term fertility impact of testosterone therapy is lacking. There is significant anecdotal evidence that some TNB individuals can and do achieve pregnancies after discontinuation of testosterone; however, we must assume there is also a possibility of permanent infertility. Given these uncertainties, it is important to both discuss fertility preservation options before initiation of testosterone and inform patients that testosterone is not a reliable form of contraception. Contraception is indicated for patients taking testosterone who have genital contact with sperm and do not want to be pregnant.

NOT TO BE MISSED

Long-term effects of testosterone on fertility are currently unknown, although limited evidence is reassuring. Counseling on fertility desires and options for family building should take place before initiation of testosterone therapy or at any time during the course of therapy as desired by the patient.

Dosage and Method of Administration. The most common method of administration of testosterone is intramuscular or subcutaneous administration. It is also available transdermally in patches, gels, and creams. Different providers have slightly different regimens, none of which have been proven to have superior efficacy. We have chosen to use the masculinizing regimen from the UCSF Center of Excellence for Transgender Health[74] (Table 12.7). All providers adjust dosages according to clinical response, which is determined at follow-up visits by the degree of masculinization, side effects, and blood tests for hormone levels.

TABLE 12.6	Timeline for Masculinizing Effects of Hormone Treatment		
Expected Changes	**Onset**	**Peak Effect**	**Likely Permanent?**

Skin changes
  Increased oiliness
  Increased acne
	1–6 months	1–2 years	No

Facial and body hair changes
  Facial hair growth
  Increased amount and thickness of
    hair on legs, arms, stomach, and
    chest
	6–12 months	4–5 years	Yes

Scalp hair changes
  Hair thinning
  Male pattern hair loss
	6–12 months	Ongoing	Yes

Muscle changes Increase in muscle size and strength	6–12 months	2–5 years	No

Fat redistribution
  Thinning of subcutaneous facial fat
  Body fat redistribution from hips,
    thighs, and buttocks to abdomen
	1–6 months	2–5 years	No

Vocal changes
  Thickening of vocal cords
  Deepening of voice
	6–12 months	1–2 years	Yes

Chest changes
  Decrease in tissue elasticity
  Less common: small decrease in
    volume of breast tissue
	Variable	Variable	No

Genital changes
  Clitoromegaly
  Vulvovaginal atrophy
	1–6 months	1–2 years	No

Amenorrhea
  Ovulation may cease; limited data are
    available
	1–6 months	Ongoing	No

Emotional changes
  Changes to emotional response
  Increased libido
	Variable	Variable	Unknown

Modified from Hembree WC, Cohen-Kettenis P, Gooren, L, et al. Endocrine treatment of gender-dysphoric/gender-incongruent persons: An endocrine society clinical practice guideline. *J Clin Endocrinol Metab*. 2017;102(11):3869–3903.

Monitoring and Laboratory Evaluation. Most providers establish a schedule of follow-up visits to monitor progress and laboratory values. Table 12.8 provides monitoring parameters by the Center of Excellence for Transgender Health.

Another excellent set of guidelines was created by Fenway Health and can also be utilized.[140] Whichever protocol is used, follow-up visits should be scheduled as needed to monitor co-occurring medical conditions or if the patient's history indicates they are at high risk for adverse effects.

Feminizing Hormone Therapy

For feminization, the most commonly used medication is estradiol, used with or without spironolactone. Estradiol increases the patient's estrogen levels and spironolactone blocks testosterone. Feminizing medications affect the skin, facial and body hair, muscles, fat distribution, breasts, genitals, and libido. Table 12.9 presents a timeline of expected changes. As with masculinizing therapy, it is important for patients and providers to understand what feminizing hormone therapy will *not*

Androgen	Initial: Low Dose[b]	Initial: Typical	Maximum: Typical[c]	Comment
Testosterone cypionate[3]	20 mg/week IM/SQ	50 mg/week IM/SQ	100 mg/week IM/SQ	For q 2 week dosing, double each dose
Testosterone enanthate	20 mg/week IM/SQ	50 mg/week IM/SQ	100 mg/week IM/SQ	
Testosterone topical gel 1%	12.5–25 mg q AM	50 mg q AM	100 mg q AM	May come in pump or packet form
Testosterone topical gel 1.62%[d]	20.25 mg q AM	40.5–60.75 mg q AM	103.25 mg q AM	
Testosterone patch	1–2 mg q PM	4 mg q PM	8 mg q PM	Patches come in 2-mg and 4-mg sizes. For lower doses, may cut patch
Testosterone cream[e]	10 mg	50 mg	100 mg	
Testosterone axillary gel 2%	30 mg q AM	60 mg q AM	90–120 mg q AM	Comes in pump only; one pump = 30 mg
Testosterone undecanoate[f]	N/A	750 mg IM, repeat in 4 weeks, then q 10 weeks ongoing	N/A	Requires participation in a manufacturer-monitored program[f]

TABLE 12.7   Masculinizing Hormone Therapy Regimen

[b]Initial: low dose recommended for genderqueer and non-binary dosing.

[c]Maximum dosing does not mean maximal effect. Furthermore, these dosage ranges do not necessarily represent a target or ideal dose. Dose increases should be based on patient response and/or monitored hormone levels. Some patients may require less than this amount, and others may require more.

[d]Doses of less than 20.25 mg with 1.62% gel or doses less than 30 mg with 2% axillary gel may be difficult because measuring one-half of a pump or packet can present a challenge. Patients requiring doses lower than 20.25 mg and whose insurance does not cover 1% gel may require prior authorization or an appeal.

[e]Testosterone creams are prepared by individual compounding pharmacies. Specific absorption and activity varies, and consultation with the individual compounding pharmacist is recommended.

[f]Testosterone undecanoate has been used extensively for transgender care outside of the U.S. for many years.[2,3] It has recently become available in the United States. Testosterone undecanoate has been associated with rare cases of pulmonary oil microembolism and anaphylaxis. As such, in the United States, the drug is available only through a restricted program called the AVEED Risk Evaluation and Mitigation Strategy (REMS) Program. All injections must be administered in an office or hospital setting by a trained and registered health care provider and monitored for 30 minutes afterward for adverse reactions.

[a]Available as standard U.S. Pharmacopeia (USP) as well as compounded products.

From UCSF Center of Excellence for Transgender Health; Deutsch MB, ed. *Guidelines for the Primary and Gender Affirming Care of Transgender and Gender Nonbinary People;* 2016. https://transcare.ucsf.edu/guidelines.

change, and that it is impossible to predict exactly how individuals will respond to therapy and which changes will endure if hormone therapy is discontinued. Feminizing hormone therapy does not cause changes to the bony skeleton in adults and will not decrease height, shoulder width, or hand/foot size. The voice will not be affected by feminizing medications, although many individuals are able to feminize their voices through voice training. Cartilage is not affected, so hormone therapy will not cause significant changes to the size or appearance of the "Adam's apple."

Fertility Considerations. Research exploring the long-term fertility impacts of feminizing hormone therapy is lacking. It is known that sperm production decreases and sperm abnormalities increase during hormone therapy, and permanent infertility is a possibility.[191] There is significant anecdotal evidence that TNB individuals can and do use their semen to achieve pregnancies after discontinuation of hormone therapy. However, sperm quality, which is affected by hormone therapy, is an important factor in fertility. For patients who might desire children in the future, the option with

TABLE 12.8	Laboratory Monitoring Guidelines for Masculinizing Hormone Regimens							
Therapy	Comments	Baseline	3 Months*	6 Months*	12 Months*	Yearly	PRN
Lipids	No evidence to support routine lipid monitoring at any time; use clinician discretion	Based on USPSTF guidelines					X
A_{1C} or fasting glucose	No evidence to support routine lipid monitoring at any time; use clinician discretion	Based on USPSTF guidelines					X
Estradiol							X
Total testosterone			X	X	X		X
Sex hormone–binding globulin (SHBG)†			X	X	X		X
Albumin†			X	X	X		X
Hemoglobin and hematocrit		X	X	X	X	X	X

*In first year of therapy only.
†Optional and may be helpful in complex cases (see text). Used to calculate bioavailable testosterone and to monitor bioavailable testosterone.
USPSTF, U.S. Preventive Services Task Force.
From UCSF Center of Excellence for Transgender Health; Deutsch MB, ed. *Guidelines for the Primary and Gender Affirming Care of Transgender and Gender Nonbinary People;* 2016. https://transcare.ucsf.edu/guidelines.

most likelihood of success is to use sperm banking before beginning hormone therapy. In addition, patients can also discontinue hormone therapy at any time to bank sperm, with the understanding that semen quality may be affected. Individual variations in sperm quality also affect fertility. Limited research has indicated that TNB AMAB individuals may tend to have impaired sperm quality relative to the general population, even before undertaking gender-affirming hormone therapy.[190] Given these uncertainties, it is important to both discuss fertility desire and family building options before initiation of therapy and inform patients that a reliable form of contraception is indicated if the patient does not want to cause a pregnancy in a AFAB sex partner.

NOT TO BE MISSED

Long-term effects of feminizing hormone therapy are currently unknown. Counseling on fertility desires and family-building options should take place before initiating this therapy or at any time during the course of therapy as desired by the patient.

Dosage and Method of Administration. The most common methods of administration of estrogen are a transdermal patch, tablets given orally or sublingually, and injections. As noted earlier, an androgen blocker may be used in addition to estradiol to counteract endogenous testosterone. The most commonly used androgen blocker is spironolactone. Finasteride can be

TABLE 12.9 Timeline for Feminizing Effects of Hormone Treatment

Expected Changes	Onset	Peak Effect	Likely Permanent?

Skin changes
  Softening of skin
  Decreased oiliness
  Decreased acne
	3–6 months	Unknown	No

Facial and body hair changes
  Slowing of growth of hair on face, legs, arms,
    stomach, and chest
  Possible thinning of facial and body hair
	6–12 months	3+ years	No

Scalp hair changes
  Possible slowing of scalp hair thinning and scalp
    hair loss
	Variable	Variable	No

Muscle changes Decreased muscle size and strength	3–6 months	1–2 years	No

Fat redistribution
  Increased facial subcutaneous fat
  Body fat redistribution from abdomen to hips,
    thighs, buttocks, and lower belly
	3–6 months	2–3 years	No

Breast changes
  Breast tenderness
  Slow increase in volume of breast tissue
  Final breast size typically smaller than in AFAB
    individuals, more tubular in shape
	3–6 months	2–3 years	Yes

Genital changes
  Decreased testicular size and volume
  Possible decrease in penile size
	3–6 months	2–3 years	No

Changes in sexual function
  Decreased/absent spontaneous erections
  Decreased ability to achieve and/or maintain
    desired erections
	1–3 months	3–6 months	No

Emotional changes
  Changes to emotional response
  Decreased libido
	Variable	Variable	Unknown

AFAB, Assigned female at birth.
Modified from Hembree WC, Cohen-Kettenis P, Gooren, L, et al. Endocrine treatment of gender-dysphoric/gender-incongruent persons: An endocrine society clinical practice guideline. *J Clin Endocrinol Metab.* 2017;102(11):3869–3903.

used for patients with male pattern baldness or if they are unable to take spironolactone. Androgen blockers are taken orally. If patients are taking angiotensin-converting enzyme (ACE) inhibitors or angiotensin II receptor blockers (ARBs), they should change to a different antihypertensive. If this is not possible, the patient should either discontinue the spironolactone or be started at a lower dose and carefully monitored. Table 12.10 provides the feminizing hormone regimen used by the Center of Excellence for Transgender Health. In all cases, doses are adjusted according to clinical response, which varies from patient to patient. Clinical response is monitored at follow-up visits.

It is important to note that some patients experience bothersome side effects with excessive androgen blockage, such as changes to mood, libido, sexual function, and energy; avoiding an androgen blocker or using a

TABLE 12.10   Feminizing Hormone Therapy Regimen

Hormone	Initial: low[b]	Initial	Maximum[c]	Comments
Estrogen				
Estradiol oral/sub-lingual	1 mg/day	2–4 mg/day	8 mg/day	If >2 mg, recommend divided bid dosing
Estradiol transdermal	50 mcg	100 mcg	100–400 mcg	Max single patch dose available is 100 mcg. Frequency of change is brand/product dependent. More than two patches at a time may be cumbersome for patients
Estradiol valerate IM	<20 mg IM q 2 weeks	20 mg IM q 2 weeks	40 mg IM q 2 weeks	May divide dose into weekly injections for cyclical symptoms
Estradiol cypionate IM	<2 mg IM q 2 weeks	2 mg IM q 2 weeks	5 mg IM q 2 weeks	May divide dose into weekly injections for cyclical symptoms
Progestogen				
Medroxyproges-terone acetate (Provera)	2.5 mg qhs		5–10 mg qhs	
Micronized proges-terone			100–200 mg qhs	
Androgen blocker				
Spironolactone	25 mg qd	50 mg bid	200 mg bid	
Finasteride	1 mg qd		5 mg qd	
Dutasteride			0.5 mg qd	

UCSF Center of Excellence for Transgender Health; Deutsch MB, ed. *Guidelines for the Primary and Gender Affirming Care of Transgender and Gender Nonbinary People;* 2016. https://transcare.ucsf.edu/guidelines.

very low dose of androgen blocker can be very helpful in addressing this concern. All individuals, including cisgender females, produce endogenous testosterone; therefore complete testosterone suppression is not a physiologically appropriate goal.

> **! SAFETY ALERT**
>
> Patients taking ACE inhibitors or ARBs should consider avoiding androgen blockers or changing to a different antihypertensive medication when started on androgen blockers.

Monitoring and Laboratory Evaluation. Most providers establish a schedule of follow-up visits to monitor progress and laboratory values. Table 12.11 presents monitoring parameters used at the Center of Excellence for Transgender Health. As discussed earlier, there are also excellent monitoring protocols from other gender specialty services such as Fenway Health.[140]

Whichever protocol is used, follow up visits should be scheduled as needed to monitor co-occurring medical conditions or if the patient's history indicates they are at high risk for adverse effects.

TABLE 12.11 Laboratory Monitoring Guidelines for Feminizing Hormone Regimens

Test	Comments	Baseline	3 Months*	6 Months*	12 Months*	Yearly	PRN
BUN/Cr/K+	Only if spiro used	X	X	X	X	X	X
Lipids	No evidence to support routine monitoring at any time; use clinician discretion	Based on USPSTF guidelines					X
A$_{1C}$ or glucose	No evidence to support routine monitoring at any time; use clinician discretion	Based on USPSTF guidelines					X
Estradiol			X	X			X
Total testosterone			X	X	X		X
Sex hormone–binding globulin (SHBG)†			X	X	X		X
Albumin†			X	X	X		X
Prolactin	Only if symptoms of prolactinoma						X

*In first year of therapy only.

†Used to calculate bioavailable testosterone: monitoring bioavailable testosterone is optional and may be helpful in complex cases (see text).

UCSF Center of Excellence for Transgender Health; Deutsch MB, ed. *Guidelines for the Primary and Gender Affirming Care of Transgender and Gender Nonbinary People;* 2016. https://transcare.ucsf.edu/guidelines.

Interpreting Laboratory Results

In addition to monitoring estradiol and testosterone levels, clinicians must interpret other laboratory tests ordered during their care for TNB patients. At this time, there are no established reference ranges for patients undergoing medical gender affirmation. Exogenous hormones and androgen blockers affect erythropoiesis, fat distribution, and muscle and bone mass, so the correct reference ranges for many tests are those of the affirmed gender.[192]

Patients who are well established on a feminizing regimen will have significantly lower levels of testosterone than they had before they began taking the medications, therefore muscle mass, bone mass, and erythropoiesis will be affected. Hemoglobin and hematocrit levels within the cisgender female range can be normal for a patient whose testosterone is well suppressed.[74]

Patients undergoing a masculinizing regimen can be expected to have higher muscle and bone mass than before they began taking the medication. Erythropoiesis will be enhanced. Masculinizing patients' hemoglobin and hematocrit are expected to increase as their testosterone levels increase to cisgender male levels and their estrogen production is suppressed.[74]

There are sex-based differences in the normal levels of cardiac troponin, a substance released when cardiomyocytes are damaged. The high-sensitivity cardiac troponin (hs-cTn) assay is commonly used to predict myocardial infarction. Sex-related differences in results are caused by differences in cardiac mass, which is probably not affected by gender-affirming hormones. Using the reference value of the sex assigned at birth is probably the most appropriate. To avoid missing an acute cardiac event, however, it is important to emphasize other findings such as electrocardiogram results, serial hs-cTn levels, and clinical history.[192]

Laboratories assume the sex of a patient from the designation on the insurance or laboratory requisition, and it is not always obvious which sex is referenced in a report. Clinicians should obtain and reference their laboratory's male and female ranges (which vary in different laboratories) to interpret a patient's results.

TABLE 12.12　Patients on Masculinizing Hormone Therapy

LOWER AND UPPER LIMITS OF NORMAL FOR SELECTED TESTS

Laboratory Test	Lower Limit of Normal	Upper Limit of Normal
Creatinine	Not defined	Male value
Hemoglobin/ hematocrit	Female value	Male value
Alkaline Phosphatase	Not defined	Male value

UCSF Center of Excellence for Transgender Health; Deutsch MB, ed. *Guidelines for the Primary and Gender Affirming Care of Transgender and Gender Nonbinary People;* 2016. https://transcare.ucsf.edu/guidelines.

TABLE 12.13　Patients on Feminizing Hormone Therapy

LOWER AND UPPER LIMITS OF NORMAL FOR SELECTED TESTS

Laboratory Test	Lower Limit of Normal	Upper Limit of Normal
Creatinine	Not defined	Male value
Hemoglobin/ hematocrit	Male value if amenorrheic. If menstruating regularly, consider using female lower limit of normal.	Male value
Alkaline phosphatase	Not defined	Male value

Center of Excellence for Transgender Health. *Primary Care Protocols for Transgender Patient Care.* 2nd ed. San Francisco, CA: University of California, San Francisco, Department of Family and Community Medicine; 2011. http://transhealth.ucsf.edu/trans?page=protocol-00-00.

> **CLINICAL SURVIVAL TIP** At this time, there are no established reference ranges for patients undergoing medical gender affirmation. Laboratories assume the gender of a patient from the designation on the insurance or laboratory requisition. Clinicians should obtain and reference their laboratory's natal male and female ranges to interpret a patient's results.

The Center of Excellence for Transgender Health has developed guidelines for normal ranges in some tests (Tables 12.12 and 12.13). In evaluating any laboratory result for a particular TNB patient, clinicians should consider how long the patient has been on gender-affirming medications, whether their endogenous hormones are well suppressed, and if they are having any symptoms.

Gender-Affirming Medications for HIV-Positive Patients

Being positive for HIV is not a contraindication to gender-affirming medical or surgical care. For HIV-positive patients, care should be co-managed with the provider managing their HIV care. Hormone regimens currently being prescribed have not been tested for interactions with medications used to treat HIV; however, there are no known interactions between HIV medications and testosterone, spironolactone, or other anti-androgens.[74] Up to 28% of transgender females in the United States are HIV positive, and some caution is warranted with feminizing hormone regimens.[107]

Taking an estrogen with either amprenavir (Agenerase) or unboosted fosamprenaivr (Lexiva) can decrease serum concentrations of amprenavir.[74] Therefore they should either not be co-administered with estradiol or only be administered with very close oversight by the patient's HIV health care provider.

There is a theoretical interaction between estrogens and protease inhibitors used for antiretroviral (ARV) therapy because there have been interactions between oral contraceptives and protease inhibitors.[74] When oral contraceptives are taken with some protease inhibitors, the HIV medication's efficacy is unchanged, but the patient may have a decrease or increase in blood levels of norethindrone, norgestimate, or ethinyl estradiol.[73] However, none of the hormones used in oral contraceptives are currently prescribed as feminizing hormones. If a feminizing patient on ARV medication experiences changes in the efficacy of the gender-affirming hormones or an increase in hormonal side effects, the estradiol dosage can be adjusted.[74] The patient's symptoms and estradiol blood levels can be monitored to assist in dosing changes, and the HIV health care provider should be consulted.

If patients living with HIV acquire opportunistic infections that are treated with trimethoprim-sulfamethoxazole, there can be a significant interaction between this medication and spironolactone.[74] Hospitalization and sudden death have been reported.[141,142] These two medications should not be taken together.

The effectiveness of treatments and recommendations will be greatly increased if they are accompanied by referrals, counseling, and education tailored to the patient's unique life situations. The following sections contain practical ideas for individualizing medical treatments to meet the needs of LBQ and TNB patients.

Cedar River Clinics provides a sample surgical referral letter in its Transgender Health Toolkit.[143,144]

> **PATIENT-CENTERED CARE:** The effectiveness of treatments and recommendations will be greatly increased if they are accompanied by referrals, counseling, and education tailored to the patient's unique life situations.

REFERRALS

Referrals are an important aspect of primary care for all patients, and every provider must have good referrals for specialty care. For LBQ and TNB patients, referrals should, as much as possible, be made to LBQ and TNB-knowledgeable and -welcoming providers. To decrease the likelihood that a patient will be turned away or given substandard care, it is best to learn about a provider's comfort and skill in working with LBQ and TNB patients before making a referral. Calling the provider and making a direct referral provides an opportunity to evaluate the provider and office staff to determine if the LBQ or TNB patient will feel comfortable. Asking LBQ and TNB patients about their experiences with local providers and cataloguing this information is a good method for developing a list of referrals. Table 12.14 provides other sources for compiling a comprehensive referral list.

Referrals for Gender-Affirming Surgery

For many individuals, surgery plays an important role in gender affirmation. Feminizing surgical options include breast augmentation, orchiectomy, vaginoplasty, tracheal shave (to reduce the prominence of the Adam's apple), and a number of facial surgeries. Masculinizing surgical options include chest reconstruction, hysterectomy with or without oophorectomy, metoidioplasty (release of the clitoral suspensory ligament to enlarge the appearance of the clitoris and approximate the position of a penis), and phalloplasty. Although some of these procedures are considered cosmetic when performed in cisgender individuals, they are medically indicated in the context of gender affirmation.

Many surgeons require a letter from the primary care provider validating the medical necessity of the surgery based on a diagnosis of gender dysphoria. The WPATH standards provide an excellent resource explaining the medical necessity of gender-affirming surgery, and

TABLE 12.14 Finding LGBQ- and TNB-Positive Providers

Resource	Explanation
GLMA Health Professionals Advancing LGBT Equality: *www.glma.org*	Go to "Find a Provider" for a list of U.S. providers who self-identify as LGBQ and TNB-positive. Not all areas and specialties are included, but it is possible to contact a provider and ask for help with referrals.
MyTransHealth: *http://mytranshealth.com/*	A location-based search tool that offers resources in four categories: medical, mental health, legal, and crisis care.
Human Rights Campaign's Healthcare Equality Index: *https://www.hrc.org/resources/healthcare-equality-index*	Evaluates health care facilities' policies and practices related to the equity and inclusion of their LGBTQ patients, visitors, and employees.
Centerlink Community of LGBT Centers: *www.lgbtcenters.org/Centers/find-a-center.aspx*	Directory of LGBT centers around the United States. LGBT centers often have valuable information about referrals.
Finding LGBTQ resources not listed above	Most communities have an LGBT resource of some kind that can lead you to referrals. Search: LGBT resources and the name of your community

PATIENT EDUCATION AND COUNSELING

A plan for care is never effective unless the clinician has an idea of the patient's life beyond the confines of the examination room. If clinicians can engage the patient in an open dialogue, they can develop the care plan with the patient and adapt it to the patient's unique needs. In this process, the clinician explores the patient's level of knowledge and understanding and provides clarification and information as necessary.

Exploring a patient's support system is relevant whenever their health care plan alters their life in any way, physically or emotionally. LBQ and TNB individuals have a wide variety of family and social support structures—some traditional and some nontraditional. It is helpful to acknowledge the strengths of a patient's support system as well as any limitations.

Gender Identity Disclosure

TNB individuals must make decisions about when, where, to whom, and how they will disclose their gender identity. There are many different factors that go into disclosure decisions, and many TNB individuals make different decisions as their lives change or based on the specific context in which they are making the disclosure decision. Sometimes the decision to not disclose is made to protect themselves from physical danger or from losing employment. In other cases, a TNB patient may decide not to disclose simply because it is exhausting to have to constantly explain or defend their gender identity when they would rather focus on all the other aspects of their life. Others may identify solely as male or female and may not identify as "transgender" at all; in this case, disclosure of one's sex assigned at birth may be seen as inappropriate or irrelevant, and it can be very painful. Limited social understanding of identities that do not confirm to the rigid gender binary can make disclosure particular fraught for non-binary individuals.

Non-Medical Methods of Gender Affirmation

Many strategies may be used by TNB individuals as an alternative to or in addition to medical and surgical treatments. Providers should be familiar with these strategies and promote efforts to ensure health and safety while managing gender dysphoria. This section will review common non-medical gender-affirming practices used by TNB individuals.

Voice

Aspects of voice that influence perceived gender are pitch, resonance, and intonation. Pitch is one of the aspects of voice that is most obviously interpreted as masculine or feminine. Masculinizing hormones enlarge the larynx and lower the pitch, but the amount of change varies. Feminizing hormones taken after puberty cannot affect the larynx size, and pitch is unchanged. There are surgeries to raise the pitch by reducing the size of the larynx, but results have been inconsistent.[74] Each individual has a pitch range in which they normally speak. The pitch floor (the lowest notes within an individual's natural range) is how listeners perceive gender. If desired, patients can learn to use range differently to change how their gender is perceived.[74] Resonance is primarily determined by the size of the sinus bones and is not affected by either masculinizing or feminizing hormones. However, training can change resonance to some extent. Intonation is the variation in pitch while speaking: for example, AFAB individuals tend to go higher at the end of a sentence, and AFAB voices are often breathier.[74]

Learning the skills to make vocal changes takes time and practice, and it is helpful to work with a qualified specialist such as language pathologist with training in TNB voice issues. Table 12.14 provides information on finding a referral. There are also videos and other online sources of information. It is important for TNB patients to know that their voice may continue to be perceived as that of their sex assigned at birth when on the phone or in other contexts in which additional gender cues such as physical appearance are not available to the listener.

Hair Removal

Body and facial hair can be a significant source of either gender dysphoria or gender euphoria in TNB individuals. Patients taking feminizing hormones may seek body and facial hair removal because the effect of feminizing hormones on hair is minimal. Some patients taking masculinizing hormones are uncomfortable with the degree of hair growth they experience and may seek hair removal. Additionally, non-binary individuals (both AFAB and AMAB) may find hair removal on some or all areas of their body to be gender-affirming. For some, facial or body hair can be removed effectively by a close shave. Topical hair removal products are typically not very effective on facial hair.

The two main methods of long-term or permanent hair removal used by TNB individuals are electrolysis and laser removal. Laser hair removal is quicker and less expensive than electrolysis but provides permanent reduction of hair rather than permanent removal and may require periodic repeat treatment after in intensive initial regimen is completed. In addition, laser hair removal does not work on all colors of hair. It concentrates a beam of light on a hair follicle. The pigment of dark hair absorbs the light, destroying the hair follicle. Laser treatments are less effective on red, blonde, or white hair.[74]

Electrolysis is a more permanent solution; although it does not remove all hair, it greatly reduces the volume. With electrolysis, a fine needle probes the hair follicle and destroys the root with an electric current. Both electrolysis and laser removal should be avoided in areas of the skin that are infected or have active dermatitis. Patients with pacemakers should consult their cardiologist before beginning treatment.[74] BIPOC individuals should work only with a technician who has experience performing hair removal on darker skin tones and has appropriate equipment to ensure patient safety.

When referring for electrolysis or laser hair removal, an experienced, TNB-supportive provider should be sought. See Table 12.14 for suggestions on finding providers. Some medical practices can bill insurance for laser or electrolysis, which can make a huge difference in the cost. If the practice does not provide local anesthesia, the primary care provider can prescribe a local anesthetic cream in advance of the appointment.

Tucking

To create a more feminine groin contour, some AMAB TNB individuals use their fingers to tuck their testicles up into the inguinal canals and push the penis and scrotal tissue back between the legs. Tape and/or snug-fitting underwear or a garment called a *gaff* are used to keep the genitals tucked in place. In general, tape should be avoided. If it is used, irritating tape such as duct tape should be avoided. Using medical tape and shaving the area before taping can help prevent skin irritation. For increased safety, the penis can be wrapped in a thin, soft cloth, and tape can be applied to this wrapping rather than directly to the skin. Prolonged tucking can cause mechanical damage, urinary problems, epididymo-orchitis, prostatitis, and scrotal pain. If scrotal pain does occur, it should be immediately investigated to rule out

other causes such as torsion, STIs, and inguinal hernia.[74] A primary care provider can consult with or refer to a specialist for chronic scrotal pain.

In counseling patients about safe tucking, it is important to be sensitive to the role that tucking plays in their lives. Some patients tuck 24 hours per day, even when sleeping, and changing this pattern could be very difficult for them if they have significant gender dysphoria. Gender-affirming genital surgeries may be a more appropriate option in this setting if the patient desires permanent removal of the gonads.

❗ SAFETY ALERT

Prolonged tucking can cause mechanical damage, urinary problems, epididymo-orchitis, prostatitis, and scrotal pain.

Packing

To create a more masculine groin contour, AFAB TNB individuals may use a variety of "packers," usually worn in the underwear or on a small packing strap that goes around the waist. Commercially available options include packers in the shape of a flaccid penis with testicles, "stand to pee" (STP) packers with a discrete urine funnel in the testicles and patent tube in the shaft of the penis through which urine can pass, and "pack and play" packers with a semi-firm shaft that allows for penetrative intercourse. Depending on the material, many packers must be stored in a bag of corn starch when not in use to preserve the integrity of the skin surface. More affordable packing options include socks or other soft fabrics.

Chest Binding

To create a more masculine, flatter chest profile, AFAB TNB individuals can safely compress breast tissue with sports bras, compression shirts, or special garments called *binders*. If an individual has very little breast tissue, athletic garments or compression shirts may be sufficient. Chest binders, specifically made for the purpose, can be very effective, even with quite large breasts.

Tape, elastic bandages, or binders that are too small can be very restricting and can interfere with breathing and cause pain in the shoulders, back, chest, and breasts.[144] Restriction of breathing can result in shortness of breath, dizziness, lightheadedness, or worsening of asthma or respiratory infections. Tape and elastic bandages should be avoided if possible as frequent, prolonged use may cause significant skin breakdown and serious skin infections.

Patients should be encouraged to use a well-fitting binder, although they can be very expensive. There are programs in which gently used binders are donated to those who cannot afford to purchase their own. Examples include the Big Brothers Binder Program (http://www.thetransitionalmale.com/BBUB.html) and the B4CK Binders for Confident Kids program for young individuals older than 13 years of age (https://b4ck.org/).

It is safest to wear a binder no more than 8 to 12 hours per day and to avoid wearing it when sleeping. A less restrictive binding method is preferable during exercise. The skin should be completely dry before placing the binder to avoid skin irritation.[145] If an otherwise well-fitting binder irritates certain areas of the skin, it can be altered.[146]

Breast Enhancement

Breast growth from feminizing hormones can take years to complete, and for many the amount of growth is minimal. An average amount of growth would bring a patient's breasts to the size of an A cup,[147] and many patients would like to enhance the appearance of their breast shape and size. Others prefer natural methods of breast enhancement without hormones. Bras can be filled with inserts made of silicone or foam that can be purchased in bra stores or online. Simply filling a bra with household items like socks is also a possibility. Silicone breast forms can stick comfortably to the chest and can be worn without a bra.

Silicone Injections

Injection of industrial-grade silicone or other fillers are sometimes used for feminizing facial and body contouring. Although the significant dangers have been publicized, some patients choose silicone injections because they are much less expensive than surgery and work much more quickly and often with more dramatic results than hormones.

Medical silicone injections are sometimes done by experienced practitioners in very small volumes of less than 0.1 cc for facial contouring.[74] However, non-medical silicone injections are done by unlicensed individuals using large volumes of silicone of up to several liters. Unlicensed individuals may use substances such as aircraft lubricant that are not medical-grade silicone and have not been developed for human use.[74] Also, the silicone or the injection equipment may not be sterile.

Patients who are considering non-medical silicone injections should be informed of the danger of local effects as well as the danger that silicone can migrate from the injection site to other areas causing disfiguration, infection, or emboli.[74] The most common complication is the formation of granulomas near the injection site, either inflammatory on non-inflammatory. The granulomas can also appear at distant sites as a result of silicone migration. Silicone emboli can cause pulmonary embolism, heart attack, stroke, or kidney damage. Infections can be local or systemic.

Patients who have had non-medical silicone injections should be educated that complications can occur not only immediately following the injection but also weeks or years later. TNB individuals may be reluctant to disclose their silicone injection history because they may fear being condemned or ridiculed for their decision to use fillers. However, it is important to report this history to avoid misdiagnosis and mistreatment of silicone injection–related complications. Building a relationship of mutual respect by demonstrating a non-judgmental attitude and harm-reduction approach will encourage patient disclosure.

For non-emergency treatment of complications, patients should be referred to a dermatologist or plastic surgeon with knowledge and experience with silicone injection sequelae. For emergency referrals such as a referral for a suspected pulmonary embolism, the new provider must be aware of the patient's history of silicone injections.

> **! SAFETY ALERT**
>
> Some patients seek injection with non–medical-grade silicone. Inflammation causing the formation of granulomatous tissue is the most common side effect, but silicone emboli can cause pulmonary embolism, heart attack, stroke, or kidney damage.

Reproductive Health Counseling

Education and counseling concerning contraception, preconception, donor insemination, and assisted reproductive technologies have aspects unique to LBQ and TNB patients. Providers can give LBQ and TNB patients useful information to assist them with the unique legal challenges they face in areas such as health care decision making and parenting.

Determining parenting and pregnancy intention for LBQ females and TNB individuals is an important and often neglected aspect of primary care that involves discussing an individual's hopes and plans for a future family. A good way to begin this conversation is to ask an open-ended question about a patient's thoughts on having children in the future. Although research on parenting desire in TNB individuals is limited, one qualitative research study found that participants want to be asked about this as part of their routine care; an emphasis was placed on asking this in a nonjudgmental manner and with the understanding that there are many routes to parenthood.[128]

Contraception

If an LBQ female patient or an AFAB TNB individual does not want children soon, a full, honest discussion of sexual partners and practices (as described earlier in the "Sexual History" section) will make it apparent if pregnancy prevention is indicated. Using a shared decision-making, patient-centered process, the patient and provider can discuss preferences about such factors as effectiveness, menstrual changes, side effects, how the method is used, and other considerations such as privacy.

Some patients feel that effectiveness is the most important characteristic of a method. For patients who are ambivalent about pregnancy or who say "If it happens, it happens," effectiveness is often not the most important consideration. Patients who use a less effective birth control method and can use abortion as a backup method may not place as high a value on effectiveness as those who do not have this option. Some patients do not want to use a method that requires touching their own genitals. There is no one method that should be recommended for any LBQ or TNB patient. In general, the best method is the one that the patient wants and will use, and the patient is more likely to be satisfied with a method that is chosen in a shared decision-making process.[148]

Although masculinizing gender-affirming hormones do decrease the change of pregnancy, it is best not to rely on them as contraceptives because their effectiveness has not been adequately studied, and unplanned pregnancies have been noted.[125] As with any other patient, TNB patients weigh the risks and benefits of their contraceptive options; some may choose to use hormone therapy alone as contraception with the understanding that efficacy is unknown. In the following sections, we will discuss information about contraception for TNB patients who are undergoing gender-affirming hormone therapy.

AMAB TNB patients who take feminizing hormones and have a penis and testicles may be able to create a pregnancy in an AFAB individual, either cisgender or TNB, who is fertile. Estrogen and spironolactone will almost certainly decrease the quantity and quality of sperm, but contraceptive effectiveness is unknown. Insertive condoms (commonly called *male condoms*) and receptive condoms (commonly called *female condoms*) both offer pregnancy and STD protection for individuals with a penis.

AFAB TNB patients may have receptive vaginal penetration by a penis as part of their sexual activity. If they have had a complete hysterectomy as a gender-affirming surgery, they have permanent contraception. If they are still fertile and do not want to be pregnant, contraception is indicated.

Individuals taking testosterone usually stop menstruating after 3 to 6 months,[125] but testosterone has not been studied as a contraceptive, and very limited research has been conducted to determine the effectiveness of testosterone at preventing ovulation or pregnancy.[193] However, pregnancy has occurred before resumption of menses in individuals who had previously taken testosterone.[125] Additionally, laboratory evidence in one small study showed spontaneous ovulation during gender-affirming testosterone use.[193] Both testosterone, which is probably the most frequently prescribed masculinizing hormone, and finasteride, which is sometimes prescribed to prevent baldness or as an anti-androgen, are classified as Pregnancy Category X, meaning there is strong evidence of fetal risk.[151,152] In the case of testosterone, limited data exist to support this categorization; however, it is the current standard of care to consider it as Category X, and is not appropriate to initiate or continue testosterone in the context of pregnancy. If a patient who is taking testosterone or finasteride could possibly become pregnant and does not want to use abortion as a backup, a highly effective method of birth control should be considered.

A goal for many AFAB TNB patients is to eliminate menstrual bleeding, and the effect of a contraceptive method on bleeding patterns may be an important consideration. The following methods tend to decrease or eliminate bleeding:

- Hormonal IUDs
- Contraceptive implants
- Contraceptive injections (Depo-Provera)
- Combined contraceptives (oral, patch, or ring) taken continuously without traditional spacing

If a patient takes testosterone, natural vaginal lubrication can be decreased, and lubricants are helpful with vaginal penetration. Receptive (female) or insertive (male) condoms come with their own lubrication, and either water-based or silicone-based lubricants can be added as needed. Oil-based lubricants break down the condom and make the condom ineffective and should not be used. Table 12.15 provides tools for patient-centered counseling that can be used with a shared decision-making approach and language that is inclusive of LBQ TNB individuals.

TABLE 12.15 Patient-Centered Contraceptive Counseling for TNB Patients	
Tool	**Explanation**
Birth Control Options Chart: *https://fpntc.org/ training-and-resources/ birth-control-method-options-chart*	All methods on a printable one-page chart, grouped according to common patient concerns
All About Birth Control Methods: *https://www. plannedparenthood. org/learn/birth-control*	Online explanation of each contraceptive method
Training Tools: Explaining Contraception: *https://rhntc.org/ sites/default/files/ resources/2017-10/ fpntc_explaining_ cc_2017.pdf*	Printable one-page explanation of each contraceptive method
Bedsider: *https://www. bedsider.org/*	Contraceptive information website with easy-to-understand pictographs regarding efficacy and risks, interactive material, and content for both AFAB individuals and AMAB individuals. May be particularly compelling for young people.

AFAB, Assigned female at birth; *AMAB,* assigned male at birth.

NOT TO BE MISSED

Testosterone and finasteride are categorized as Pregnancy Category X (strong evidence of fetal risk). If a patient who is taking testosterone or finasteride could possibly become pregnant, a highly effective method of birth control should be considered.

Options Counseling

LBQ and TNB patients need access to sensitive pregnancy options counseling (see Chapter 10). In receiving pregnancy-related care including abortion, prenatal care, and childbirth care, LBQ females and TNB AFAB individuals are particularly vulnerable to feeling isolated and to experiencing health care discrimination. Referrals to clinically and culturally responsive providers are particularly important. The resources in Table 12.14 are helpful for locating LBQ- and TNB-inclusive providers. In addition, large institutions that have gender specialty clinics can also be a good resource.

Preconception Counseling

Many LBQ and TNB patients want children. In a 2013 survey, 35% of LGBT respondents were parents. Of the participants younger than 60 years of age, 28% said they would like to have children someday, and 34% were not sure.[153] For LBQ and TNB individuals who want to have children, the route to parenthood can take many forms including pregnancy, adoption, fostering, surrogacy, gestational surrogacy, step parenting, and co-parenting with a close friend or partner.

All LBQ and TNB patients who want to have genetically related children in the next year, have contact with sperm, and are fertile should be offered preconception counseling. All of the usual aspects of preconception counseling such as treatment for chronic health conditions, avoiding teratogens, and taking folic acid should be covered[153] (Chapter 6).

Because fertility after initiation of gender-affirming hormone treatment has not been well researched, counseling and education are tailored to the patient's priorities and attitude toward risk. Financial considerations also come into play as some of the treatments to preserve fertility are quite expensive. Pregnancy is possible after hormone treatment is discontinued; however, there is no assurance that fertility will return.

Sperm Preservation. To increase the chance of having viable sperm available in the future, some patients choose to have their sperm frozen before beginning gender-affirming hormone therapy or to support delayed parenting regardless of hormone therapy intention. Discussion of this option should be offered as part of the informed consent process.[75] Cryobanks can be located online that offer home collection kits that can be used if it is not possible to find a local TNB-friendly cryobank. See Table 12.14 for suggestions on locating TNB-inclusive providers. This procedure is generally not covered by insurance.

Egg Banking. Egg banking can be done before beginning masculinizing hormone treatment or to support delayed parenting regardless of hormone therapy intention, and discussion of this options should be offered during the consent process before beginning a masculinizing hormone regimen.[75] The process for collecting eggs is an approximately 10-day course of hormonal stimulation followed by surgical egg retrieval.[155] This process is very expensive, often costing over $13,000 to $18,000,[156] and is not usually covered by insurance. Patients should also be informed that it involves a series of examinations and procedures that may heighten dysphoria, including transvaginal ultrasound and pelvic procedures.

Patients who are interested in egg banking, in vitro fertilization, or working with gestational carriers or surrogates should be referred to a reproductive medicine specialist. In 2015, the American Society of Reproductive Medicine's Ethics Committee published an opinion that TNB individuals have a right to these services, and many reproductive medicine specialists routinely care for LBQ and TNB patients. If providers are accustomed to treating LGBQ and TNB patients, it is usually reflected by the language on their websites. See Table 12.14 for other suggestions for finding providers.

Donor Insemination

If an LBQ or TNB patient has a uterus and ovaries and is fertile, insemination with donor sperm can be arranged. Insemination can be done either with or without a health care provider. Typically, insemination by a health care provider is done in the clinic setting, although it is sometimes offered in the home. Insemination without a health care provider is typically provided in the home. In addition to the options of intracervical insemination and vaginal insemination, which can be completed with or without a provider, health care providers can perform intrauterine insemination. If possible, patients who are planning insemination should consult an attorney who is familiar with the state's laws and policies around parental rights. In some cases, even if the child has a second, non-gestational parent whose name is on the birth certificate, it offers more security to the family if the non-gestational parent does a second parent or a step-parent adoption.[157]

Some patients choose an acquaintance, friend, or loved one as the sperm donor and arrange insemination privately; this is referred to as a *directed* (or *known*) donor. Directed sperm donation, particularly if insemination is completed at home without a health care provider, can provide a less medicalized, more personal way of becoming pregnant. It is also much less expensive than the option of using a sperm bank. However, legal issues can arise with use of directed donors because sometimes judges or state officials have deemed directed sperm donors to be fathers with parental rights and obligations.

The same insemination types and location options are available with a directed donor as with an anonymous donor, although fresh semen must be processed appropriately (referred to as being *washed*) by a health care provider before it can be used for intrauterine insemination. If they choose a clinical setting, patients will need to know if potential insemination health care providers have the materials needed to perform this procedure with fresh sperm and if any restrictions are placed on using fresh directed-donor sperm when there is no marital or sexual relationship between the donor and recipient. Before doing an insemination with directed-donor sperm, it is important for LBQ and TNB patients to discuss the donor's relationship with the child-to-be. Many have a written agreement to specify the donor's role, but courts have not always honored these agreements.

Legal Protections

Because the overall health of LBQ and TNB patients is affected by discrimination, a primary care provider's role of promoting wellness is enhanced with some basic knowledge of legal protections and resources for this population. Clinicians can provide information and referrals to assist patients in navigating areas such as legal recognition of families; medical decision making and visitation rights; and housing discrimination. Table 12.16 provides resources for legal issues.

TABLE 12.16 Resources for Help with Legal Issues	
Human Rights Commission Current information about LGBT legal rights and resources for many different aspects of housing Information about medical decision making and visitation rights	https://www.hrc.org/explore
Unmarried Equality Information about medical decision making and visitation rights	http://www.unmarried.org/health-care/hospital-rights/
Center for Lesbian Rights Current information about LGBTQ parenting issues Help with low-cost legal aid Some information in Spanish	https://www.nclrights.org/our-work/racial-economic-justice/legal-aid-legal-services/
Lambda Legal Information about rights related to employment, HIV, and gender as well as LGBTQ teens and young adult rights. Has an online Legal Help Desk	https://www.lambda-legal.org/know-your-rights

Health Care

Implementation of the Affordable Care Act (ACA) and the Supreme Court decisions in 2013 and 2015 that legalized same-sex marriage brought increased access to health care for LGBQ and TNB individuals in the United States. As a result, same-sex partners who were federal or state employees gained the same rights as other married couples for spousal insurance coverage. Additionally, specific prohibitions against insurance restrictions based on sexual orientation and gender identity were included in the ACA. As a result, at this writing, gender-affirming medical and surgical treatments are covered by Medicaid and other third-party payers.[5] Unfortunately, because of both Medicaid rules and the dearth of experienced surgeons, even this coverage does not guarantee that surgical care will be accessible.

Legal Parenting Issues

LBQ and TNB parents and their children are at high risk of experiencing anxiety and stress at the lack of recognition of their relationships and may face the threat of loss of custody. If an individual is not a legal parent, they may not be able to make decisions for their child such as giving permission for a field trip or a medical procedure. Marriage equality has helped legitimize LGBQ and TNB families, but marriage does not automatically confer legal parenthood unless the child is born to one of the partners after they are married.

The legal situation for parents is constantly shifting with new laws and new court and administrative decisions, and it varies from state to state. LBQ and TNB parents have widely divergent situations and levels of risk depending on their socioeconomic status, family support system, support of institutions such as schools with which the child interacts, personal preferences, and other factors. Primary care providers can help by learning more about their situations and giving support or referrals as needed.

ADOLESCENTS AND YOUNG ADULTS

Adolescence is a time of change for all young individuals as they develop physically, sexually, and emotionally, and LBQ and TNB youths have much in common with their peers (see Chapter 3 for a discussion of adolescent health). In addition, they have some unique health disparities including increased risk of homelessness, victimization, abuse, and STIs. These disparities make it crucial for providers to create a clinical environment in which young LBQ and TNB patients feel safe to talk openly and honestly. Providers must have skills in discussing sexual activity and gender identity as well as screening for personal safety. In addition, all primary care providers must be able to respond to common concerns about gender on the part of adolescents, young adults, and their parents. They should also be able to counsel TNB young adults and their families about appropriate puberty-delaying and gender-affirming medical care.

NOT TO BE MISSED

LBQ and TNB youths have some unique health disparities including increased risk of homelessness, victimization, abuse, and STIs.

Adolescent-Affirming Environment

Many of the methods discussed earlier in this chapter for creating a welcoming environment for all LBQ and TNB patients apply to adolescents and young adults. For LBQ and TNB patients, confidentiality is particularly important because homelessness or physical abuse will result for some youths if their parents learn of their LBQ or TNB status.[34,158] Adolescents may avoid needed health care if they fear that the information will be revealed to their parents.[158] At the beginning of a visit, it is important to inform an adolescent patient about limitations on confidentiality. One way to accomplish this would be to make a statement such as "I want you to know that everything here is confidential, meaning I will not talk to anyone else about what is happening unless you tell me that you are being hurt physically or sexually by someone or planning to hurt yourself."[159] (This statement should be modified to match the legal requirements of each jurisdiction.)

The entire health care team must work together to maintain confidentiality as serious breaches can occur at different points throughout a visit, particularly if a young patient is accompanied by a parent or guardian. Registration processes can be risky for preserving confidentiality (see Chapter 3 for a further discussion of confidentiality for adolescents).

There is an important distinction between privacy protection and the laws and regulations about consent for care. Although there are limits on minors' rights to receive medical care without parental consent, the rules about privacy allow adolescents more autonomy. Unless particular aspects of an adolescent patient's protected information must be revealed to protect the patient's health or to prevent the patient from harming someone else, neither parents/guardians nor any other authority should have access to an adolescent patient's protected health information without their express consent. For example, if an adolescent is suicidal and this fact must be reported, the patient's gender identity or sexual orientation should not be revealed without their permission.[161] Providers can assure the adolescent and young adult patient's confidentiality by providing privacy for consultation at some point during the visit, even when parents or guardians accompany them. A typical scenario would be to talk with the parent(s) and the patient together at the beginning of the visit, conduct a visit with only the patient, and then bring the parent(s) back to the conversation for the closing portion of the visit.

> ### NOT TO BE MISSED
>
> Unless particular aspects of an adolescent patient's protected information must be revealed to protect the patient's health or to prevent the patient from harming someone else, neither parents/guardians nor any other authority should have access to an adolescent patient's protected health information without their express consent.

If an adolescent or young adult has a name or pronouns that are different from those they were given at birth, they should be allowed to determine when those pronouns will be used. They may have different preferences for communication with other health care providers or with parents or schools. Documenting these preferences clearly in the medical record is critical to patient safety.

Discussing Sexual Orientation and Gender Identity

Many adolescents and young adults would like to talk with their providers about gender identity and sexual orientation, but this rarely happens.[162] Adolescents indicate that they would like to have the provider bring up the subject.[162,163] LBQ and TNB adolescents feel more able to be open about sexual orientation and gender identity if the provider demonstrates comfort asking about and discussing same-sex attractions and TNB gender identities.[162]

In the past, there were models describing a path for "coming out," or forming and publicly expressing a sexual identity. These models were created largely from the experiences of adult AMAB individuals in a time of great stigma without the cultural supports that exist in many contexts today.[161] During this time, full expression of sexual identity commonly occurred in full adulthood.[7] Little work has been done to document how expression of sexual identity progresses in current times, especially among AFAB and BIPOC individuals. Some youths may be ready to express their identity openly at an early age, and youths of any age may have important concerns about sexual orientation.

In encouraging an adolescent or young adult to discuss sexual orientation, in addition to asking about whether the patient is sexually active, it can be very helpful to ask about sexual attraction. Some young individuals may not yet be sexually active, or they may interpret a question about being sexually active as referring only to penis-vagina sex. Others may be just beginning to be aware of LBQ attractions.

Research about the process of gender identity formation is also limited, mostly based on clinical observations. Children often experiment with gender role behavior and expression including choosing playmates or styles of play that are atypical of their assigned sex or dressing or grooming themselves in ways that express gender variance. For some, these behaviors are precursors of an adolescent or adult TNB identity, and for others they are not. A few express a desire to be a gender other than their assigned gender, for example saying, "I wish I were a boy." A much stronger statement, thought to be strongly predictive of continuing gender discordance into adolescence, is for a child to state that rather than wishing to be a different gender, they *are* a gender other than their assigned gender, for example "I am a girl" or "I am not a boy."[164,165] There are indications that the strength of gender dysphoria in childhood correlates with the likelihood of dysphoria continuing into adolescence,[165,166] and gender dysphoria in adolescence is very strongly predictive of dysphoria continuing into adulthood.[167] One useful model for assessing the strength of gender variance is to evaluate the insistence, persistence, and consistency of a young patient's gender identity assertions.[168] It is important to remember that youths, like adults, may be non-binary. Some youths may say "I am not a girl or a boy" or make other statements that support a non-binary gender identity. These statements should be taken as seriously and with as much sensitivity as expressions of binary gender identities.

> **CLINICAL SURVIVAL TIP** One useful model for assessing the strength of gender variance is to evaluate the insistence, persistence, and consistency of a young patient's gender identity assertions, regardless of whether they are binary or non-binary.

The onset of puberty with the beginning development of secondary sex characteristics is a common time for becoming aware of a gender identity different from society's expectations. Interviews with TNB adults reveal that the ages from 10 to 13 years were particularly significant in determining their gender identity as they began to anticipate or acquire secondary sex characteristics, began to experience romantic and sexual

attractions, and experienced more gender segregation than had existed in childhood.[169] It is also common for young adults to express their TNB identity after they have completed puberty, and for many individuals, a TNB identity first becomes evident well into adulthood.

Each individual's process for establishing their gender identity is unique. Adolescents who experience their gender identity as different from societal expectations may have known about the discrepancy from an early age, or they may be just beginning to become aware of their gender identity. They may struggle with finding the words to express their new consciousness, or they may be able to fully articulate their identity. It is important to listen to patients, maintain respect, and work with them to explore their gender identity. For both young individuals and adults, it is important to remember that all aspects of identity formation in humans take place within the context of cognitive development, therefore changes may occur along the way.

Gender-related questions such as the name and pronouns to be used during patient interactions should be included on a registration form or prefaced by a statement indicating that the provider asks these questions of all patients. Not answering registration questions about gender identity or sexual orientation may indicate that a patient is not comfortable declaring their identity or orientation openly, but they may be willing to discuss this with a trusted provider. The provider could say, "I noticed you didn't fill out the part of the questionnaire about your gender (or sexual orientation). Is that something you would like to talk about?" The subject of gender identity or sexual orientation might come up at any point during the visit. If so, the provider can ask open-ended questions to explore the issue as much as the patient wishes. When taking a history, questions about pubertal changes could be followed by questions about how the patient feels about their body.

Screening for Personal Safety

Risk factors for LBQ and TNB youths make it important to evaluate whether they are safe. At school, they are vulnerable to physical, sexual, and verbal abuse from peers and sometimes from teachers.[19,170] At home, they have elevated rates of physical and sexual abuse.[19,170] The incidence of homelessness is high for these youths, either as a result of running away from an abusive situation or being kicked out of the home by their families.[19,171] Suicidal thoughts and attempts are more frequent in the LGBTQ adolescent population than in the general adolescent population.[34,172] Before asking questions about safety, it is important to inform the adolescent patient about limitations on confidentiality, as discussed earlier. In some cases, reporting abuse can endanger the adolescent. For example, an adolescent may need to evaluate whether a preliminary visit from a social worker to their home might seriously jeopardize their safety. One screening approach to determine danger of abuse and victimization is to ask directly if the patient feels safe at home and at school. In some situations, it can be more effective to ask open-ended questions about their experiences at home or at school.

In addition to a history of suicidal attempts or thoughts, there are some unique predictors of suicide in LBQ and TNB youths that, if present, warrant an in-depth suicide screening. LGBQ and TNB youths have a much higher rate of repeated suicide attempts within 1 year of a suicide attempt than do youths in general. Other important predictors of suicide in LGBQ and TNB youths are early age of same-sex attraction, lack of social support from parents, and having experienced hate-based harassment or assault because of their sexual orientation or gender identity.[173]

Patients may reveal abuse, victimization, or thoughts of suicide only after one or more visits, when they have formed a trusting relationship with a provider. A primary care provider may be the only person they have ever talked to about these issues. Within the limits of confidentiality, providers can and should be effective advocates for their LBQ and TNB patients with parents, within the legal and school systems, and with mental health providers.

> ### ❗ SAFETY ALERT
> Suicidal thoughts and attempts are more frequent in the LGBTQ adolescent population than in the general adolescent population.

The Role of Parents and Guardians

Parents' or guardians' support of LBQ or TNB youths is a key factor in their well-being. Often parents will come to primary care providers when a young individual's gender role behaviors concern them. Some parents may wish to support their children's sexual orientation or gender identity, and others may want advice on how to change them. In any case, providers can educate parents about normal exploration and development of gender identity and sexual orientation. The provider can lead parents to helpful resources such as literature, support groups, and mental health providers to help them learn more, cope with their own feelings, and better parent and advocate for their children. With the patient's permission, the provider can model correct name and pronoun usage when the parents or guardians are present. If the parents are supportive of their child's gender identity and sexual orientation, the provider can be a powerful co-advocate in dealing with the patient's needs in the school system and other settings.

Support Resources for LBQ and TNB Youths

LBQ and TNB youths may benefit greatly from working with a mental health professional to deal with depression, isolation, and anxiety that result from verbal, physical, or sexual victimization; suicidal ideation; or problems with peers or at school.[174,175] Many LBQ and TNB youths function very well and do not have serious psychological issues, particularly if they are supported by their families.[176,177] However, all LBQ and TNB youths can benefit from an affirmative therapeutic approach that helps them explore and express their identities, work through internal conflicts, and develop techniques to deal with a homophobic and transphobic world. Therapists can also help TNB youths make decisions about social transition and medical interventions.[74,161]

Parents and family members can also benefit from a supportive therapist to help them deal with their own process of coming to terms with the LBQ or TNB adolescent's identity as well as homophobia or transphobia directed at their loved one. Many parents of LGBTQ children experience a personal growth process including becoming more open-minded, developing closer family relationships, and becoming activists.[178]

There are varying approaches to psychological therapy for LGBTQ adolescents, some of which are damaging and should be avoided. Reparative therapies (sometimes referred to as *conversion therapies*) that focused on changing an adolescent or young adult's sexual orientation are widely regarded as both harmful and unsuccessful, and they have been disavowed by most major psychological associations.[179] These therapies may include use of aversive stimuli as well as psychological abuse. Similar therapies aimed at persuading TNB youths to change their gender identity are considered unethical because they have not been shown to be successful, and clinical observations show that they too are harmful.[75,164,180] Mental health providers who work with LBQ and TNB youths should utilize an affirmative approach, and if possible, they should have experience working with LBQ and TNB youths and their families. Even in remote areas, it is sometimes possible to access mental health services online (see Table 12.14).

In addition to support from mental health professionals, peer support is critical to the emotional and social well-being of LBQ and TNB youths. Many communities have general and/or youth-specific community centers serving LGBQ and TNB individuals. Many middle schools, high schools, and colleges also have Gay-Straight Alliances (GSAs), which can be a great source of support. GSAs are student-run clubs that offer a safe forum for discussing sexuality and gender identity issues, building community with fellow LGBQ and TNB youths, and organizing to improve conditions for LGBQ and TNB students on campus. For youths whose schools do not already have a GSA in place, the GSA Network (www.gsanetwork.org) provides students with the resources they need to start their own GSA and communicate with other GSAs throughout the country. If forming a GSA is not an option, clinicians and parents can help guide young LGBQ and TNB individuals toward safe and appropriate online peer support resources.

Social Gender Affirmation

Some youths, before entering adolescence, have already affirmed their gender in all aspects of their lives including with peers, at home, at school, and with extended family. Others may just be beginning to consider their options. A health care provider or a mental health professional can help TNB youths and their families consider when and how to make changes in their gender presentation as well as their name and pronouns. TNB youths must weigh considerations of safety as well as their readiness to handle transphobic responses from peers, family members, teachers, and school officials. As with adults, some will decide to be open about their gender in some environments and not in others.

Gender-Affirming Medical Care

Early adolescence is a crucial time for providers to identify TNB youths and assist them in getting the help they need. As discussed earlier, most individuals who identify as TNB in adolescence continue to do so into adulthood, and the onset of adolescence is a time when many youths

experience severe dysphoria. If they are initiated in time, fully reversible interventions can fully prevent the onset of secondary sexual characteristics, greatly reducing dysphoria and allowing the adolescent and/or the parents/guardians to explore and process issues surrounding gender identity. Another benefit of timely pubertal suppression is that if an adolescent goes on to become a TNB adult, they will not have had permanent changes that would have been irreversible without surgery. Later in adolescence, if the youth wants to continue with gender affirmation, hormones can be added to the pubertal suppression medications to allow the adolescent to go through puberty that is affirming to their gender. If a young patient decides to, they may stop pubertal suppression at any time and allow puberty with endogenous hormones to unfold.

Puberty Suppression. Puberty suppression is best initiated in Tanner stage 2, when youths develop long, downy pubic hair, AFAB individuals develop breast buds, and AMAB individuals' testicles begin to grow. Suppression can also be initiated in Tanner stage 3. If suppression is initiated in Tanner stage 3 or 4, it will be too late to block some permanent changes, but gender-affirming hormones can be used to assist in stopping further development of secondary sex characteristics and begin gender-affirming development. For all adolescents and particularly for TNB youths, it can be difficult to have a physical examination for interpretation of Tanner stages, but there are tools to help the adolescent accurately self-assess their own Tanner stage until enough trust can be established for the youth to allow an examination. There are questionnaires that a child or adolescent fills out in the office[181] as well as a pictorial version with written descriptions seen in Figure 2.11.[182]

Gonadotropin-Releasing Hormone (GnRH) Analogues. GnRH analogues have been used since the early 1980s to suppress precocious puberty.[183] A gender clinic in Amsterdam instituted a protocol for blocking puberty for TNB adolescents in 1998.[184]

Informed consent for adolescents and parents/guardians must include the fact that the patients who were the first to receive these treatments are not yet old enough to show long-term effects.[76] In addition, larger numbers of patients will need to be treated before it is possible to discover effects that only show up in small percentages of individuals. Effects of concern include bone development and height.[76] However, preliminary information indicates greatly improved psychological functioning[166] and no adverse physical effects.[184]

There are two medications most commonly used in the United States for puberty suppression. The first is leuprolide (Lupron Depot), which is given in intramuscular injections usually every 3 to 4 months.[74] The second is a histrelin implant, which is inserted under the skin in the inner arm and removed after 12 to 36 months.[74] Another implant can be inserted at the same time as the original one is removed.

When these medications are initiated, there is an immediate stimulation of gonadotropin secretion, which can lead to an upsurge in pubertal symptoms such as emotional lability; however, this response is usually brief and is usually followed by complete suppression.[185] About 6 to 8 weeks after initiation of blockers, the patient undergoes blood tests to determine if the hypothalamic pituitary axis has been suppressed.[74]

Ongoing care includes communication with the youth to ensure that they want to continue gender-affirming therapy. It is important that patients know they can stop treatment at any time and then will be able to continue puberty with endogenous hormones, usually within 6 months of discontinuation.[185] Other aspects of ongoing care include monitoring clinical effects and hormonal blood levels. At some point during puberty suppression, the TNB youth may be ready to add gender-affirming hormones to the GnRH analogues.[74] There are different protocols for the age of discontinuing GnRH analogues. In some settings, they are discontinued at 18 years of age if surgeries are planned. Some protocols continue the GnRH analogues into early adulthood, allowing the patient to take lower doses of gender-affirming hormones.[74]

Gender-Affirming Medications in Early Adolescence. There are some important aspects of informed consent for adolescents and their families before initiating gender-affirming hormones. If started before the ovaries or testes mature, undergoing gender-affirming hormone therapy means that the youth's bodies will never be able to create sperm or ova capable of reproduction.[74,187] Strategies currently being studied in children with cancer may hold promise for fertility preservation in the context of pubertal suppression as well as, for example, laboratory maturation of cryopreserved prepubertal ovarian and testicular tissue.[187] However, the viability and accessibility of these potential technologies is impossible to predict, and clinicians should be clear that permanent infertility is the most likely outcome. This means that the decision to forgo future biological offspring is made at an age before TNB youths may have a full sense of their own future desires for parenting. Another consideration for young AMAB individuals is that pubertal suppression before full development of the penile tissues can cause difficulties with future vaginoplasty. The most common vaginoplasty technique is penile inversion, and immature genitals may not provide sufficient tissue for this technique.[188,189] The impact of gender-affirming hormone therapy on sexual function and sexual pleasure in adulthood has not been adequately studied.

Given these unknowns regarding future fertility and sexual function as well as other adverse effects that may not yet be known, participation in this decision by parents/guardians involves weighing the psychological risks of not giving the medications versus the potential risks of giving them. Young patients must be involved in this decision-making process. One youth described a feeling about future unknown adverse effects of hormone therapy this way: "I know I may be shaving off some years of my life by taking testosterone, but when I considered the alternative of living my entire life miserable and depressed, it was an easy choice."[186] Another important aspect of informed consent is to ensure that the adolescent or young adult knows the limits of what the hormones can do and does not have unrealistic expectations.[74]

The Endocrine Society Guidelines state that gender-affirming hormones should not be initiated before 16 years of age, the age that was used in the initial studies at the gender clinic in Amsterdam.[76,166] Recently, specialty clinics and gender specialists have begun studying initiation around 14 years of age. An earlier start of hormones enables the adolescent to go through puberty at the same time as their peers rather than waiting until 16 years of age, which may have a significant impact on social interactions and social functioning. Another reason for starting hormones earlier is the possible effect on future bone development for adolescents who began puberty at a young age and might potentially go for 5 to 7 years without the hormones that initiate the pubertal growth spurt.[74]

Gender-Affirming Medications in Late Adolescence. In Tanner Stages 3 and 4, gender-affirming hormones can be combined with GnRH analogues. However, GnRH analogues may not be covered by insurance and are very expensive. The difference in efficacy of taking gender-affirming hormones with or without GnRH analogues is unknown.

Resources for Clinicians

The Center of Excellence for Transgender Health has an excellent and thorough set of guidelines for treating adolescents and young adults.[74] The Human Rights Campaign has an interactive map showing clinical care programs for gender-expansive children and adolescents.[190]

Summary

Providing health care to LBQ and TNB youths is an opportunity to support them at a very significant time in their development. By recognizing their challenges and health risks and by respecting and supporting each patient's unique process of self-discovery, providers can have a significant impact on the future lives of these patients.

CONCLUSION

LBQ and TNB individuals may face daunting challenges to leading healthy lives. Their access to health and the quality of their health care have been significantly affected by stigma and discrimination. However, LGBQ and TNB social movements have made LGBQ and TNB individuals more visible and have given birth to a strong LGBQ and TNB health movement that has done important research, created new care models, and developed practice guidelines. Progress in improving LGBQ and TNB health care has been accompanied by setbacks from forces that resist change, but social change to bring about full recognition of human rights takes time.

Until medical and nursing educational institutions can incorporate LGBQ and TNB health into all aspects of their curricula, providers will need to learn from more experienced clinicians and through self-study. As with all patients, an attitude of cultural humility is the key element in being able to provide good care.

As individual providers, we can provide culturally and clinically competent care in our own practices. We can also advocate for LGB and TNB populations within health care systems and within the larger society. In doing this, we have an opportunity to help advance an important worldwide movement for social justice and human rights.

KEY POINTS

- LGBQ and TNB individuals still experience health care discrimination.
- It is incumbent on all providers to minimize health care discrimination and disparities for this population.
- History of the treatment of LGBQ and TNB patients informs us why there is reticence and distrust in the health care system.
- Understanding the concepts of sex assigned at birth, sexual orientation, and gender identity is key to providing culturally competent care of LGBQ and TNB communities.
- Providing a safe and welcoming environment using inclusive language assists in providing a care experience that allows the patient to reveal sensitive information that informs their care.
- Some common health risks and diseases have been identified that disproportionately affect the LGBQ and TNB community.
- Examinations and health screening should be tailored to the reproductive organs that are present in the patient.
- There are many forms of gender-affirming therapies and techniques that are available, including medication and surgery.
- The long-term effects of hormone therapy on fertility are currently unknown.
- Adolescents and young adults among the LGBQ and TNB communities are at especially increased risk of threats to their safety.

REFERENCES

1. Lambda Legal. *When Health Care Isn't Caring: Lambda Legal's Survey on Discrimination against LGBT People and People Living with HIV*. New York: Author; 2010. www.lambdalegal.org/health-care-report.
2. Jones JM. *LGBT Identification Rises to 5.6% in Latest U.S. Estimate*; 2021. http://www.gallup.com/poll/201731/lgbt-identification-rises.aspx.
3. Williams Institute. (2021). *Well-Being of LBQ Women in the US*; 2021. https://williamsinstitute.law.ucla.edu/publications/lbq-women-in-us/.

4. Herman JL, Flores AR, O'Neill KK. *How Many Adults and Youth Identify as Transgender in the United States?*. Los Angeles, CA: The Williams Institute, UCLA School of Law; 2022. https://williamsinstitute.law.ucla.edu/publications/trans-adults-united-states/.

5. Kates J, Ranji U, Beamesderfer A, Salganicoff A, Dawson L. *Health and Access to Care and Coverage for Lesbian, Gay, Bisexual, and Transgender (LGBT) Individuals in the U.S*; 2018. https://www.kff.org/racial-equity-and-health-policy/issue-brief/health-and-access-to-care-and-coverage-for-lesbian-gay-bisexual-and-transgender-individuals-in-the-u-s/.

6. File T, Lee J-H. *Now Include SOGI, Child Tax Credit*. COVID Vaccination of Children; 2021. https://www.census.gov/library/stories/2021/08/household-pulse-survey-updates-sex-question-now-asks-sexual-orientation-and-gender-identity.html.

7. Institute of Medicine. *The Health of Lesbian, Gay, Bisexual, and Transgender People: Building a Foundation for Better Understanding*. Washington, DC: The National Academies Press; 2011.

8. American Psychiatric Association. Diagnostic and Statistical Manual of Mental Disorders. 3rd ed. Revised (DSM-III-R). *American Psychiatric Association*. 1987.

9. American Psychological Association, American Public Health Association. *Brief of Amici Curiae American Psychological Association and American Public Health Association in Supreme Court of United States*; 1986.

10. Beek TF, Cohen-Kettenis PT, Kreukels BPC. Gender incongruence/gender dysphoria and its classification history. *Int Rev Psychiatry*. 2016;28(1):5–12.

11. Rodríguez M. Gender incongruence is no longer a mental disorder. *J Mental Health Clin Psychol*. 2018;2:6–8.

12. Kinsey AC, Pomeroy WB, Martin CE, Gebhard PH. *Sexual Behavior in the Human Female*. Philadelphia: Saunders; 1953.

13. Kinsey AC, Pomeroy WR, Martin CE. Sexual Behavior in the Human Male. 1948. *Am J Public Health*. 1948;93(6):894–898.

14. Mendelsohn DM, Omoto AM, Tannenbaum K, Lamb CS. When sexual identity and sexual behaviors do not align: the prevalence of discordance and its physical and psychological health correlates. *Stigma Health*. 2022;7(1):70–79.

15. Muzny CA, Austin EL, Harbison HS, Hook EW. Sexual partnership characteristics of African American women who have sex with women; Impact on sexually transmitted infection risk. *Sex Transm Dis*. 2014;41(10):611–617.

16. Barefoot KN, Warren JC, Smalley KB. Women's health care: the experiences and behaviors of rural and urban lesbians in the USA. *Rural Remote Health*. 2017;2:1–16.

17. Nield J, Magnusson B, Brooks C, Chapman D, Lapane KL. Sexual discordance and sexual partnering among heterosexual women. *Arch Sex Behav*. 2015;44(4):885–894.

18. Gay and Lesbian Medical Association (GLMA). *Compendium of Health Profession Association LGBT Policy & Position Statements*; 2013. http://www.glma.org/_data/n_0001/resources/live/GLMA Compendium of Health Profession Association LGBT Policy and Position Statements.pdf.

19. James SE, Herman JL, Rankin S, et al. *The Report of the 2015 U.S. Transgender Survey* Washington, DC. ; 2016.

20. Long M, Rae M, Claxton G, Damico A. *Trends in Employer-Sponsored Insurance Offer and Coverage Rates 1999–2014*; 2016. http://kff.org/private-insurance/issue-brief/trends-in-employer-sponsored-insurance-offer-and-coverage-rates-1999-2014/.

21. Sears B, Mallory C. *Documented Evidence of Employment Discrimination & Its Effects on LGBT People*; 2011. https://williamsinstitute.law.ucla.edu/wp-content/uploads/Sears-Mallory-Discrimination-July-20111.pdf.

22. Feeding America. *Hunger in America 2014*; 2014. http://www.feedingamerica.org/hunger-in-america/our-research/hunger-in-america/.

23. Deleted in proofs.

24. Rounds KE, Burns B, McGrath EW. Perspectives on provider behaviors: a qualitative study of sexual and gender minorities regarding quality of care. *Contemp Nurse*. 2013;44(1):99–110.

25. Grant J.M., Mottet L.A., Tanis J., Herman J.L., Harrison J., Keisling M.. National Transgender Discrimination Survey Report on Health and Health Care; 2010:5

26. Callahan EJ, Hazarian S, Yarborough M, Sánchez JP. Eliminating LGBTIQQ health disparities: the associated roles of electronic health records and institutional culture. *Hastings Cent Rep*. 2014;44(suppl 4):S48–S52.

27. Cahill S, Singal R, Grasso C, et al. Do ask, do tell: high levels of acceptability by patients of routine collection of sexual orientation and gender identity data in four diverse American community health centers. *PLoS One*. 2014;9(9):e107104.

28. Paradies Y, Ben J, Denson N, et al. Racism as a determinant of health: a systematic review and meta-analysis. *PLoS One*. 2015;10(9):1–48.

29. Frost DM, Lehavot K, Meyer IH. Minority stress and physical health among sexual minority individuals. *J Behav Med*. 2013;38:1–8.

30. Khan M, Ilcisin M, Saxton K. Multifactorial discrimination as a fundamental cause of mental health inequities. *Int J Equity Health*. 2017;16(1):43.

31. Balsam KF, Molina Y, Beadnell B, Simoni J, Walters K. Measuring multiple minority stress: the LGBT People

of Color Microaggressions Scale. *Cultur Divers Ethnic Minor Psychol.* 2011;17(2):163–174.

32. Pascoe EA, Smart Richman L. Perceived discrimination and health: a meta-analytic review. *Psychol Bull.* 2009;135(4):531–554.

33. Cochran SD, Sullivan JG, Mays VM. Prevalence of mental disorders, psychological distress, and mental health services use among lesbian, gay, and bisexual adults in the United States. *J Consult Clin Psychol.* 2003;71(1):53–61.

34. James SE, Herman JL, Rankin S, Keisling M, Mottet L, Anafi M. *The Report of the 2015 U.S. Transgender Survey.* Washington, DC: National Center for Transgender Equality; 2016. *http://www.transequality.org/sites/default/files/docs/usts/USTS Full Report - FINAL 1.6.17.pdf.*

35. Budge SL, Adelson JL, Howard KAS. Anxiety and depression in transgender individuals: the roles of transition status, loss, social support, and coping. *J Consult Clin Psychol.* 2013;81(3):545–557.

36. Reisner SL, White JM, Mayer KH, Mimiaga MJ. Sexual risk behaviors and psychosocial health concerns of female-to-male transgender men screening for STDs at an urban community health center. *AIDS Care.* 2014;26:857–864.

37. Miranda K, Pace DA, Cintron R, et al. Sexually transmitted disease (STD) diagnoses and mental health disparities among women who have sex with women screened at an urban community center, Boston, Massachusetts, 2007. *Sex Transm Dis.* 2010;37(1):1358–1375.

38. Ward BW, Dahlhamer JM, Galinsky AM, Joestl SS. Sexual orientation and health among U.S. adults: National Health Interview Survey, 2013. *Natl Health Stat Rep.* 2014;(77):1–12.

39. Przedworski JM, McAlpine DD, Karaca-Mandic P, VanKim NA. Health and health risks among sexual minority women: an examination of 3 subgroups. *Am J Public Health.* 2014;104(6):1045–1047.

40. Blosnich JR, Farmer GW, Lee JGL, Silenzio VMB, Bowen DJ. Health inequalities among sexual minority adults: evidence from ten U.S. states, 2010. *Am J Prev Med.* 2014;46(4):337–349.

41. Kerr DL, Ding K, Chaya J. Substance use of lesbian, gay, bisexual and heterosexual college students. *Am J Health Behav.* 2014;38(6):951–962.

42. Farmer GW, Jabson JM, Bucholz KK, Bowen DJ. A population-based study of cardiovascular disease risk in sexual-minority women. *Am J Public Health.* 2013;103(10):1845–1850.

43. Simoni JM, Smith L, Oost KM, Lehavot K, Fredriksen-Goldsen K. Disparities in physical health conditions among lesbian and bisexual women: a systematic review of population-based studies. *J Homosex.* 2016;0(0):1–13.

44. Rosario M, Li F, Wypij D, et al. Disparities by sexual orientation in frequent engagement in cancer-related risk behaviors: a 12-year follow-up. *Am J Public Health.* 2016;106(4):698–706.

45. Deleted in proofs.

46. Blosnich J, Lee JGL, Horn K. A systematic review of the aetiology of tobacco disparities for sexual minorities. *Tob Control.* 2011;22:66–73.

47. Fallin A, Goodin A, Lee YO, Bennett K. Smoking characteristics among lesbian, gay, and bisexual adults. *Prev Med (Baltim).* 2015;74(2015):123–130.

48. Kerr D, Ding K, Burke A, Ott-Walter K. An alcohol, tobacco, and other drug use comparison of lesbian, bisexual, and heterosexual undergraduate women. *Subst Use Misuse.* 2015;50:340–349.

49. Agénor M, Krieger N, Austin SB, Haneuse S, Gottlieb BR. Sexual orientation disparities in Papanicolaou test use among US women: the role of sexual and reproductive health services. *Am J Public Health.* 2014;104(2):e68–e73.

50. Marrazzo JM, Koutsky LA, Kiviat NB, Kuypers JM, Stine K. Papanicolaou test screening and prevalence of genital human papillomavirus among women who have sex with women. *Am J Public Health.* 2001;91(6):947–952.

51. Charlton BM, Corliss HL, Missmer SA, et al. Influence of hormonal contraceptive use and health beliefs on sexual orientation disparities in papanicolaou test use. *Am J Public Health.* 2014;104(2):319–325.

52. Bosch FX, de Sanjosé S. The epidemiology of human papillomavirus infection and cervical cancer. *Dis Markers.* 2007;23(4):213–227.

53. Waterman L, Voss J. HPV, cervical cancer risks, and barriers to care for lesbian women. *Nurse Pract.* 2013;40(1):46–53.

54. U.S. Centers for Disease Control and Prevention. National Center for Health Statistics. *Pap Test Use.* https://www.cdc.gov/nchs/fastats/pap-tests.htm.

55. Bockting W, Robinson B, Benner A, Scheltema K. Patient satisfaction with transgender health services. *J Sex Marital Ther.* 2004;30(4):277–294.

56. Kosenko K, Rintamaki L, Raney S, Maness K. Transgender patient perceptions of stigma in health care contexts. *Med Care.* 2013;51(9):819–822.

57. Rounds KE, McGrath BB, Walsh E. Perspectives on provider behaviors: a qualitative study of sexual and gender minorities regarding quality of care. *Contemp Nurse.* 2013;44(1):99–110.

58. Peitzmeier SM, Reisner SL, Harigopal P, Potter J. Female-to-male patients have high prevalence of unsat-

isfactory paps compared to non-transgender females: implications for cervical cancer screening. *J Gen Intern Med.* 2014;29(5):778–784.

59. Case P, Austin SB, Hunter DJ, et al. Sexual orientation, health risk factors, and physical functioning in the Nurses' Health Study II. *J Women's Health.* 2004;13(9):1033–1047.

60. Dibble SL, Roberts SA, Nussey B. Comparing breast cancer risk between lesbians and their heterosexual sisters. *Women's Health Issues.* 2004;14(2):60–68.

61. Cochran SD, Mays VM. Risk of breast cancer mortality among women cohabiting with same sex partners: findings from the National Health Interview Survey, 1997–2003. *J Women's Health.* 2012;21(5):528–533.

62. Unger CA. Care of the transgender patient: a survey of gynecologists' current knowledge and practice. *J Women's Health (Larchmt).* 2015;24(2):114–119.

63. Brown GR, Jones KT. Incidence of breast cancer in a cohort of 5,135 transgender veterans. *Breast Cancer Res Treat.* 2014;149:191–198.

64. Swe NC, Ahmed S, Eid M, Poretsky L, Gianos E, Cusano NE. The effects of gender affirming hormone therapy on cardiovascular and skeletal health: a literature review. *Metabolism Open.* 2022;13:100173.

65. Rossouw JE, Anderson GL, Prentice RL, et al. Risks and benefits of estrogen plus progestin in healthy postmenopausal women: principal results From the Women's Health Initiative randomized controlled trial. *JAMA.* 2002;288(3):321–333.

66. Gooren LJ, van Trotsenburg MAA, Giltay EJ, van Diest PJ. Breast cancer development in transsexual subjects receiving cross-sex hormone treatment. *J Sex Med.* 2013;10:3129–3134.

67. Hatzenbuehler ML, McLaughlin KA, Slopen N. Sexual orientation disparities in cardiovascular biomarkers among young adults. *Am J Prev Med.* 2013;44(6):612–621.

68. Everett B, Mollborn S. Differences in hypertension by sexual orientation among U.S. young adults. *J Community Health.* 2013;38:588–596.

69. Caceres BA, Brody A, Luscombe RE, et al. A systematic review of cardiovascular disease in sexual minorities. *Am J Public Health.* 2017;107(4):13–22.

70. Roberson LL, Aneni EC, Maziak W, et al. Beyond BMI: The "metabolically healthy obese" phenotype & its association with clinical/subclinical cardiovascular disease and all-cause mortality—a systematic review. *BMC Public Health.* 2014;14:14.

71. Caceres BA, Brody A, Chyun D. Recommendations for cardiovascular disease research with lesbian, gay and bisexual adults. *J Clin Nurs.* 2016;25(23-24):3728–3742.

72. Asscheman H, Giltay EJ, Megens JAJ, De Ronde W, Van Trotsenburg MAA, Gooren LJG. A long-term follow-up study of mortality in transsexuals receiving treatment with cross-sex hormones. *Eur J Endocrinol.* 2011;164:635–642.

73. Gooren LJ, Wierckx K, Giltay EJ. Cardiovascular disease in transsexual persons treated with cross-sex hormones: Reversal of the traditional sex difference in cardiovascular disease pattern. *Eur J Endocrinol.* 2014;170(6):809–819.

74. UCSF Center of Excellence for Transgender Health. In: Deutsch MB, ed. *Guidelines for the Primary and Gender Affirming Care of Transgender and Gender Nonbinary People.* ; 2016. https://transcare.ucsf.edu/guidelines.

75. Coleman E, Bockting W, Botzer M, et al. Standards of care for the health of transsexual, transgender, and gender nonconforming people. *Int J Tansgenderism.* 2012;13(4):165–232.

76. Hembree WC, Cohen-Kettenis P, Gooren L, et al. Endocrine treatment of gender-dysphoric/gender-incongruent persons: an endocrine society clinical practice guideline. *J Clin Endocrinol Metab.* 2017;102(11):3869–3903.

77. Parssinen M, Seppala T. Steroid use and long-term health risks in former athletes. *Sport Med.* 2002;32(2):83–94.

78. Kanayama G, Hudson JI, Pope HG. Long-term psychiatric and medical consequences of anabolic-androgenic steroid abuse: A looming public health concern? *Drug Alcohol Depend.* 2008;98(1-2):1–12.

79. Wierckx K, Mueller S, Weyers S, et al. Long-term evaluation of cross-sex hormone treatment in transsexual persons. *J Sex Med.* 2012;9(10):2641–2651.

80. Baba T, Endo T, Honnma H, et al. Association between polycystic ovary syndrome and female-to-male transsexuality. *Hum Reprod.* 2007;22(4):1011–1016.

81. Robinson K, Galloway KY, Bewley S, Meads C. Lesbian and bisexual women's gynaecological conditions: a systematic review and exploratory meta-analysis. *BJOG.* 2017;124(3):381–392.

82. Smith HA, Markovic N, Matthews AK, et al. A comparison of polycystic ovary syndrome and related factors between lesbian and heterosexual women. *Women's Health Issues.* 2011;21(3):191–198.

83. Deputy NP, Boehmer U. Weight status and sexual orientation: differences by age and within racial and ethnic subgroups. *Am J Public Health.* 2014;104(1):103–109.

84. Eliason MJ, Ingraham N, Fogel SC, et al. A systematic review of the literature on weight in sexual minority women. *Women's Health Issues.* 2015;25(2):162–175.

85. Dias IBF, Panazzolo DG, Marques MF, et al. Relationships between emerging cardiovascular risk factors, z-BMI, waist circumference and body adiposity index (BAI) on adolescents. *Clin Endocrinol (Oxf).* 2013;79(5):667–674.

86. Bacon L, Aphramor L. Weight science: evaluating the evidence for a paradigm shift. *Nutr J.* 2011;10(9):1–13.

87. Flegal KM, Kit BK, Orpana H, Graubard BI. Association of all-cause mortality with overweight and obesity using standard body mass index categories: a systematic review and meta-analysis. *JAMA.* 2013;309(1):71–82.

88. Fikkan JL, Rothblum ED. Is fat a feminist issue? Exploring the gendered nature of weight bias. *Sex Roles.* 2012;66(9-10):575–592.

89. Ålgars M, Alanko K, Santtila P, Sandnabba NK. Disordered eating and gender identity disorder: a qualitative study. *Eat Disord.* 2012;20:300–311.

90. Vocks S, Stahn C, Loenser K, Legenbauer T. Eating and body image disturbances in male-to-female and female-to-male transsexuals. *Arch Sex Behav.* 2009;38(3):364–377.

91. Jones BA, Haycraft E, Murjan S, Arcelus J. Body dissatisfaction and disordered eating in trans people: a systematic review of the literature. *Int Rev Psychiatry.* 2016;28(1):81–94.

92. Sherman MD, Kauth MR, Shipherd JC, Street RL. Provider beliefs and practices about assessing sexual orientation in two veterans health affairs hospitals. *LGBT Health.* 2014;1(3):185–191.

93. Kano M, Silva-Banuelos AR, Sturm R, Willging CE. Stakeholders' recommendations to improve patient-centered "LGBTQ" primary care in rural and multicultural practices. *J Am Board Fam Med.* 2016;29(1):156–160.

94. Workowski KA, Bachman LH, Chan PA, et al. Sexually transmitted infections treatment guidelines, 2021. *MMWR Recomm Rep.* 2021;70(4):1–187.

95. Sevelius J. There's no pamphlet for the kind of sex I have": HIV-related risk factors and protective behaviors among transgender men who have sex with nontransgender men. *J Assoc Nurses AIDS Care.* 2009;20(5):398–410.

96. Feldman J, Romine RS, Bockting WO. HIV risk behaviors in the U.S. transgender population: Prevalence and predictors in a large internet sample. *J Homosex.* 2014;61:1558–1588.

97. Green N, Hoenigl M, Morris S, Little SJ. Risk Behavior and sexually transmitted infections among transgender women and men undergoing community-based screening for acute and early HIV infection in San Diego. *Medicine (Baltimore).* 2015;94(41):e1830.

98. Gorgos LM, Marrazzo JM. Sexually transmitted infections among women who have sex with women. *Clin Infect Dis.* 2011;53(suppl 3):S84–S91.

99. Logie CH, Lacombe-Duncan A, Weaver J, Navia D, Este D. A pilot study of a group-based HIV and STI prevention intervention for lesbian, bisexual, queer, and other women who have sex with women in Canada. *AIDS Patient Care STDS.* 2015;29(6):321–328.

100. Logie CH, Gibson MF. A mark that is no mark? Queer women and violence in HIV discourse. *Cult Health Sex.* 2013;15(1):29–43.

101. Singh D, Fine DN, Marrazzo JM. Chlamydia trachomatis infection among women reporting sexual activity with women screened in family planning clinics in the Pacific Northwest, 1997 to 2005. *Am J Public Health.* 2011;101(7):1284–1290.

102. Muzny CA, Sunesara IR, Austin EL, Mena LA, Schwebke JR. Bacterial vaginosis among African American women who have sex with women. *Sex Transm Dis.* 2013;40(9):751–755.

103. Marrazzo JM, Thomas KK, Agnew K, Ringwood K. Prevalence and risks for bacterial vaginosis in women who have sex with women. *Sex Transm Dis.* 2010;37(5):335–339.

104. Weyers S, Verstraelen H, Gerris J, et al. Microflora of the penile skin-lined neovagina of transsexual women. *BMC Microbiol.* 2009;9:102.

105. Petricevic L, Kaufmann U, Domig KJ, et al. Molecular detection of *Lactobacillus* species in the neovagina of male-to-female transsexual women. *Sci Rep.* 2014;4(3746):1–4.

106. Baral SD, Poteat T, Strömdahl S, Wirtz AL, Guadamuz TE, Beyrer C. Worldwide burden of HIV in transgender women: A systematic review and meta-analysis. *Lancet Infect Dis.* 2013;13(3):214–222.

107. Herbst JH, Jacobs ED, Finlayson TJ, McKleroy VS, Neumann MS, Crepaz N. Estimating HIV prevalence and risk behaviors of transgender persons in the United States: a systematic review. *AIDS Behav.* 2008;12(1):1–17.

108. Haider AH, Schneider EB, Kodadek LM, et al. Emergency department query for patient-centered approaches to sexual orientation and gender identity: the EQUALITY Study. *JAMA Intern Med.* 2017;177(6):819–828.

109. Beagan BL, Fredericks E, Goldberg L. Nurses' work with LGBTQ patients: "they're just like everybody else, so what's the difference". *Can J Nurs Res.* 2012;44(3):44–63.

110. Galupo MP, Mitchell RC, Davis KS. Sexual minority self-identification: multiple identities and complexity. *Psychol Sex Orientat Gend Divers.* 2015;2(4):355–364.

111. Savin-Williams RC, Joyner K, Rieger G. Prevalence and stability of self-reported sexual orientation identity during young adulthood. *Arch Sex Behav.* 2012;41(1):103–110.

112. Katz-Wise SL, Reisner SL, Hughto JW, Keo-Meier C. Differences in sexual orientation diversity and sexual fluidity in attractions among gender minority adults in Massachusetts. *J Sex Res.* 2016;53(1):74–84.

113. Goff DC, Lloyd-Jones DM, Bennett G, et al. 2013 ACC/AHA guideline on the assessment of cardiovascular risk: a report of the American College of Cardiology/American Heart Association Task Force on Practice Guidelines. *Circulation*. 2014;129(25 suppl 2):S49–S73.

114. Miller N, Bedard YC, Cooter NB, Shaul DL. Histological changes in the genital tract in transsexual women following androgen therapy. *Histopathology*. 1986;10:661–669.

115. American College of Obstetricians and Gynecologists (ACOG). *Practice Advisory*. Updated Cervical Cancer Screening Guidelines; 2021. https://www.acog.org/clinical/clinical-guidance/practice-advisory/articles/2021/04/updated-cervical-cancer-screening-guidelines.

116. Cochran SD, Mays VM, Bowen D, et al. Cancer-related risk indicators and preventive screening behaviors among lesbians and bisexual women. *Am J Public Health*. 2001;91(4):591–597.

117. Bienz M, Saad F. Androgen-deprivation therapy and bone loss in prostate cancer patients: A clinical review. *Bonekey Rep*. 2015;4:716.

118. Ruetsche AG, Kneubuehl R, Birkhaeuser MH, Lippuner K. Cortical and trabecular bone mineral density in transsexuals after long-term cross-sex hormonal treatment: A cross-sectional study. *Osteoporos Int*. 2005;16(7):791–798.

119. Mueller A, Haeberle L, Zollver H, et al. Effects of intramuscular testosterone undecanoate on body composition and bone mineral density in female-to-male transsexuals. *J Sex Med*. 2010;7(9):3190–3198.

120. Schlatterer K, Auer D, Yassouridis A, von Werder K, Stalla G. Transsexualism and osteoporosis. *Exp Clin Endocrinol Diabetes*. 1998;106(4):365–368.

121. Van Caenegem E, Wierckx K, Taes Y, et al. Bone mass, bone geometry, and body composition in female-to-male transsexual persons after long-term cross-sex hormonal therapy. *J Clin Endocrinol Metab*. 2012;97(7):2503–2511.

122. Garcia C, Lyon L, Conell C, Littell RD, Powell CB. Osteoporosis risk and management in *BRCA1* and *BRCA2* carriers who undergo risk-reducing salpingo-oophorectomy. *Gynecol Oncol*. 2015;138(3):723–726.

123. U.S. Centers for Disease Control and Prevention (CDC). Taking a Sexual History. https://www.cdc.gov/std/treatment/sexualhistory.pdf.

124. Streed Jr . KG. Medical history. In: Eckstrand K, Ehrenfeld JM, eds. *Lesbian, Gay, Bisexual, and Transgender Healthcare: A Clinical Guide to Preventive, Primary, and Specialist Care*. New York: Springer; 2016:74–76.

125. Light AD, Obedin-Maliver J, Sevelius JM, Kerns JL. Transgender men who experienced pregnancy after female-to-male gender transitioning. *Obstet Gynecol*. 2014;124(6):1120–1127.

126. Potter J, Peitzmeier SM, Bernstein I, et al. Cervical cancer screening for patients on the female-to-male spectrum: a narrative review and guide for clinicians. *J Gen Intern Med*. 2015;30(12):1857–1864.

127. Ellis SA, Gromko L. *Supporting Patients before and after Gender Affirming Surgery: A Brief Guide*. Cedar River Clinics; 2021. http://www.cedarriverclinics.org/transtoolkit/PDF/SurgicalCareGuide.pdf.

128. Ellis SA, Wojnar DM, Pettinato M. Conception, pregnancy, and birth experiences of male and gender variant gestational parents: It's how we could have a family. *J Midwifery Womens Health*. 2014;60(1):62–69.

129. UCSF Center of Excellence for Transgender Health. *Primary Care Protocols for Transgender Patient Care*. 2nd ed. San Francisco, CA: University of California, San Francisco, Department of Family and Community Medicine; 2011. http://transhealth.ucsf.edu/trans?page=protocol-00-00.

130. U.S. Centers for Disease Control and Prevention. US Public Health Service: Preexposure Prophylaxis for the Prevention of HIV Infection in the United States—2021 Update: A Clinical Practice Guideline. https://www.cdc.gov/hiv/pdf/risk/prep/cdc-hiv-prep-guidelines-2021.pdf.

131. Dominguez KL, Smith DK, Vasavi T, et al. *Updated guidelines for antiretroviral postexposure prophylaxis after sexual, injection drug use, or other nonoccupational exposure to HIV*; 2018. https://stacks.cdc.gov/view/cdc/38856.

132. Feldman J, Safer J. Hormone therapy in adults: suggested revisions to the sixth version of the Standards of Care. *Int J Transgenderism*. 2009;11:146–182.

133. Dahl M, Feldman JL, Goldberg JM, Jaberi A. Physical aspects of transgender endocrine therapy. *Int J Transgenderism*. 2008;9(3-4):111–134.

134. Institute of Medicine. *The Health of Lesbian, Gay, Bisexual, and Transgender People: Building a Foundation for Better Understanding*. Washington, DC: National Academies Press; 2011.

135. Nieder TO, Richter-Appelt H. Tertium non datur—either/or reactions to transsexualism amongst health care professionals: the situation past and present, and its relevance to the future. *Psychol Sex*. 2011;2(3):224–243.

136. Radix A. Medical transition for transgender individuals. In: Ekstrand KL, Ehrenfeld J, eds. *Lesbian, Gay, Bisexual, and Transgender Healthcare: A Clinical Guide to Preventive, Primary, and Specialist Care*. Switzerland: Springer International Publishing; 2016:351–361.

137. World Professional Association for Transgender Health. *Standards of Care for the Hormonal and Surgical Sex Reassignment of Gender Dysphoric Persons*. World Professional Association for Transgender Health; 1990.

138. Wilson E, Rapues J, Jin H, Raymend HF. The use and correlates of illicit silicone or "fillers" in a population-based sample of transwomen, San Francisco, 2013. *J Sex Med*. 2014;11(7):1717–1724.

139. Callen-Lorde Community Health Center. *Protocols for the Provision of Hormone Therapy*; 2015. New York https://issuu.com/callenlorde/docs/tg_protocols_2014_v.5.

140. Thompson J, Hopwood RA, deNormand S, Cavanaugh T. *Medical Care of Trans and Gender Diverse Adults*. Boston: Fenway Health; March 2021. https://fenway-health.org/wp-content/uploads/Medical-Care-of-Trans-and-Gender-Diverse-Adults-Spring-2021-1.pdf.

141. Antoniou T, Gomes T, Mamdani MM, et al. Trimethoprim-sulfamethoxazole induced hyperkalae-mia in elderly patients receiving spironolactone: nested case-control study. *BMJ*. 2011;343:d5228.

142. Antoniou T, Hollands S, Macdonald EM, Gomes T, Mamdani MM, Juurlink DN. Trimethoprim-sulfamethoxazole and risk of sudden death among patients taking spirono-lactone. *CMAJ*. 2015;187(4):E138–E143.

143. World Professional Association for Transgender Health. Position Statement on Medical Necessity of Treatment, Sex Reassignment, and Insurance Coverage in the U.S.A. https://www.wpath.org/newsroom/medical-necessity-statement.

144. Cedar River Clinics. Surgical referral letter. http://www.cedarriverclinics.org/transtoolkit/PDF/SurgicalReferral-Letter.pdf.

145. British Columbia Centre for Disease Control. *Smart Sex Resource*; 2015. https://smartsexresource.com/health-providers/blog/201505/addressing-chest-binding-transgender-and-gender-diverse-clients.

146. Erickson-Schroth L. *Trans Bodies, Trans Selves*. New York: Oxford University Press; 2014.

147. Ellis S, Sherley C, Gromko L. *Feminizing Hormone Therapy*; 2017. http://www.cedarriverclinics.org/transtoolkit/hormonetherapy/.

148. Dehlendorf C, Levy K, Kelley A, Grumbach K, Steinauer J. Women's preferences for contraceptive counseling and decision making. *Contraception*. 2013;88(2):250–256.

149. Luebbert H, Leo-Rosberg I, Hammerstein J. Effects of ethinyl estradiol on semen quality and various hormonal parameters in a eugonadal male. *Fertil Steril*. 1992;58(3):603–608.

150. Schneider F, Neuhaus N, Wistuba J, et al. Testicular functions and clinical characterization of patients with gender dysphoria (GD) undergoing sex reassignment surgery (SRS). *J Sex Med*. 2015;12(11):2190–2200.

151. National Library of Medicine. DailyMed: Depo-Testosterone-testosterone cypionate injection. Updated August 17, 2020. https://dailymed.nlm.nih.gov/dailymed/drugInfo.cfm?setid=cfbb53d4-b868-4a28-8436-f9112eb01c39&#!.

152. National Library of Medicine. Daily Med: Finasteride. https://dailymed.nlm.nih.gov/dailymed/drugInfo.cfm?setid=7d140366-2388-488e-bd86-67e6edf44345. Published 2015. Updated August 8, 2022.

153. Gates GJ. *LGBT Parenting in the United States*. Williams Institute, UCLA School of Law; 2013; February:1–6.

154. Raghuraman N, Tuuli MG. Preconception care as an opportunity to optimize pregnancy outcomes. *JAMA*. 2021;326:1.

155. Jones CA, Reiter L, Greenblatt E. Fertility preserva-tion in transgender patients. *Int J Transgenderism*. 2016;17(2):76–82.

156. Grifo J. Egg Freezing. *Lesson 7 of 8 The Costs of Egg Freezing*. https://www.fertilityiq.com/egg-freezing/the-costs-of-egg-freezing.

157. National Center for Lesbian Rights. *Legal Recognition of LGBT Families*; 2019. https://www.nclrights.org/wp-content/uploads/2013/07/Legal_Recognition_of_LGBT_Families.pdf.

158. Saewyc EEM, Skay CLC, Pettingell SSL, et al. Hazards of stigma: the sexual and physical abuse of gay, lesbian, and bisexual adolescents in the United States and Cana-da. *Child Welfare*. 2006;85(2):195–213.

159. Leichliter JS, Copen C, Dittus PJ. Confidentiality issues and use of sexually transmitted disease services among sexually experienced persons aged 15–25 years—United States, 2013–2015. *MMWR Morb Mortal Wkly Rep*. 2017;66(9):237–241.

160. Chopel A. *School Health Center Healthy Adolescent Relationship Program (SHARP)*. presented at the Preven-tion Peer Network Web Conference; November 20; 2014. http://www.cpedv.org/sites/main/files/file-attachments/ppn_schoolhealthcenters.pdf.

161. Makadon HJ, Mayer KH, Potter J, Goldhammer H. *Fenway Guide to Lesbian, Gay, Bisexual, and Transgen-der Health*. 2nd ed. Philadelphia: American College of Physicians; 2015.

162. Fuzzell L, Fedesco HN, Alexander SC, Fortenberry JD, Shields CG. I just think that doctors need to ask more questions": Sexual minority and majority adolescents' experiences talking about sexuality with healthcare providers. *Patient Educ Couns*. 2016;99(9):1467–1472.

163. Alexander SC, Fortenberry JD, Pollak KI, et al. Sexuality talk during adolescent health maintenance visits. *JAMA Pediatr*. 2014;168(2):163–169.

164. Ehrensaft D. From gender identity disorder to gender identity creativity: True gender self child therapy. *J Homosex*. 2012;59(3):337–356.

165. Steensma TD, McGuire JK, Kreukels BPC, Beekman AJ, Cohen-Kettenis PT. Factors associated with desistence and persistence of childhood gender dysphoria: A quantitative follow-up study. *J Am Acad Child Adolesc Psychiatry*. 2013;52(6):582–590.

166. De Vries ALC, Steensma TD, Doreleijers TAH, Cohen-Kettenis PT. Puberty suppression in adolescents with gender identity disorder: A prospective follow-up study. *J Sex Med*. 2011;8(8):2276–2283.

167. Steensma TD, Kreukels BP, de Vries AL, Cohen-Kettenis PT. Gender identity development in adolescence. *Horm Behav*. 2013;64(2):288–297.

168. Forcier MM, Haddad E. Health care for gender variant or gender non-conforming children. *R I Med J (2013)*. 2013;96(4):17–21.

169. Steensma TD, Biemond R, de Boer F, Cohen-Kettenis PT. Desisting and persisting gender dysphoria after childhood: a qualitative follow-up study. *Clin Child Psychol Psychiatry*. 2011;16(4):499–516.

170. Friedman MS, Marshal MP, Guadamuz TE, et al. A meta-analysis of disparities in childhood sexual abuse, parental physical abuse, and peer victimization among sexual minority and sexual nonminority individuals. *Am J Public Health*. 2011;101(8):1481–1494.

171. Corliss HL, Goodenow CS, Nichols L, Bryn Austin S. High burden of homelessness among sexual-minority adolescents: Findings from a representative massachusetts high school sample. *Am J Public Health*. 2011;101(9):1683–1689.

172. Robinson JP, Espelage DL. Bullying explains only part of LGBTQ-heterosexual risk disparities: Implications for policy and practice. *Educ Res*. 2012;41(8):309–319.

173. Mustanski B, Liu RT. A longitudinal study of predictors of suicide attempts among lesbian, gay, bisexual, and transgender youth. *Arch Sex Behav*. 2013;42(3):437–448.

174. Reisner SL, Vetters R, Leclerc M, et al. Mental health of transgender youth in care at an adolescent urban community health center: A matched retrospective cohort study. *J Adolesc Health*. 2015;56(3):274–279.

175. D'Augelli AR, Grossman AH, Starks MT. Childhood gender atypicality, victimization, and PTSD among lesbian, gay, and bisexual youth. *J Interpers Violence*. 2006;21(11):1462–1482.

176. Travers R, Bauer G, Pyne J, Bradley K, Gale L, Papadimitriou M. *Impacts of strong parental support for trans youth: a report prepared for Children's Aid Society of Toronto and Delisle Youth Services*; 2012. http://transpulseproject.ca/wp-content/uploads/2012/10/Impacts-of-Strong-Parental-Support-for-Trans-Youth-vFINAL.pdf.

177. Olson KR, Durwood L, DeMeules M, McLaughlin KA. Mental health of transgender children who are supported in their identities. *Pediatrics*. 2016;137(3). e20153223–e20153223.

178. Gonzalez KA, Rostosky SS, Odom RD, Riggle EDB. The positive aspects of being the parent of an LGBTQ child. *Fam Process*. 2013;52(2):325–337.

179. Drescher J, Schwartz A, Casoy F, et al. The growing regulation of conversion therapy. *J Med Regul*. 2016;102(2):7–12.

180. Olson J, Forbes C, Belzer M. Management of the transgender adolescent. *Arch Pediatr Adolesc Med*. 2011;165(2):171–176.

181. Carskadon MA, Acebo C. A self-adminstered rating scale for pubertal development. *J Adolesc Health*. 1993;14(3):190–195.

182. Rasmussen AR, Wohlfahrt-Veje C, Tefre de Renzy-Martin K, et al. Validity of self-assessment of pubertal maturation. *Pediatrics*. 2015;135(1):86–93.

183. Lewis KA, Eugster EA. Experience with the once-yearly histrelin (GnRHa) subcutaneous implant in the treatment of central precocious puberty. *Drug Des Devel Ther*. 2009;(3):1–5.

184. Cohen-Kettenis PT, Schagen SEE, Steensma TD, De Vries ALC, Delemarre-Van De Waal HA. Puberty suppression in a gender-dysphoric adolescent: A 22-year follow-up. *Arch Sex Behav*. 2011;40(4):843–847.

185. Olson J. In: Bodies Trans, Selves Trans, eds. *Medical intervention for trans children*. New York: Oxford University Press; 2014:442–443.

186. Ehrensaft D. One pill makes you boy, one pill makes you girl. *Int J Appl Psychoanal Stud*. 2009;6(1):12–24.

187. Johnson EK, Finlayson C. Health preservation of fertility potential for gender and sex diverse individuals. *Transgender Health*. 2016;1(1):41–44.

188. de Vries ALC, Cohen-Kettenis PT. Clinical management of gender dysphoria in children and adolescents: The Dutch approach. *J Homosex*. 2012;59(3):301–320.

189. Khatchadourian K, Amed S, Metzger DL. Clinical management of youth with gender dysphoria in Vancouver. *J Pediatr*. 2014;164(4):906–911.

190. Human Rights Campaign. Interactive Map: Clinical Care Programs for Gender-Expansive Children and Adolescents. https://www.hrc.org/resources/interactive-map-clinical-care-programs-for-gender-nonconforming-childr.

191. Rodriguez-Wallberg KA, Häljestig J, Arver S, Johansson ALV, Lundberg FE. Sperm quality in transgender women before or after gender affirming hormone therapy—A prospective cohort study. *Andrology*. 2021;9(6):1773–1780.

192. Cheung AS, Lim HY, Cook T, et al. Approach to interpreting common laboratory pathology tests in transgender individuals. *J Clin Endocrinol Metab*. 2021;106(3):893–901.

193. Taub RL, Ellis SA, Neal-Perry G, Magaret AS, Prager SW, Micks EA. The effect of testosterone on ovulatory function in transmasculine individuals. *Am J Obstet Gynecol*. 2020;223(2):229. e1–229.e8.

13

Menopause in the Primary Care Setting

Diana Drake

OBJECTIVES

- Describe the menopause transition encounter in primary care.
- Develop a plan of care for assessment, management, and health promotion of female patients during the menopause transition.

- Utilize and incorporate current national evidence-based guidelines into menopausal care interventions.
- Describe interprofessional collaboration in menopause care.

INTRODUCTION TO MENOPAUSE IN PRIMARY CARE

Demographics

The menopause transition is a normal physiological event that affects females by the fifth decade of life or earlier. In the United States, it is estimated that 6000 females are currently reaching menopause age daily and are also living longer lives.[1] In the Western world, the average female life expectancy is just over 81 years. Most females will live one-third or more of their lives after menopause, and the number of postmenopausal females is expected to increase to 1.1 billion worldwide by 2025.[1] The combination of an increasing postmenopausal female demographic combined with an increased female lifespan represents a significant shift for health care delivery. Caring for female patients in midlife transition is an essential emerging health care skill set for the advanced practice registered nurse (APRN) primary care provider. It is an opportunity to care for the patient's gender-specific life transition symptoms and at the same time provide a broad primary care perspective of aging and wellness for the patient (Fig. 13.1).

Midlife Health Context

The menopause transition is a sentinel event in the patient's life and offers a unique opportunity for discussions between the patient and the primary health care provider. Although some females will navigate the menopause transition without any bothersome symptoms, others will regularly seek health care services. It is an important time for implementing behavioral changes to ensure healthy aging.[1] Women's health care at midlife is a whole systems experience that is far broader than treating menopausal symptoms alone. It is a key time to evaluate a wide variety of primary midlife health issues, initiate age-related health screenings, and encourage healthy lifestyle practices.

Midlife health risks for females change partially because of decreasing hormones and partially because of the increased risk of illnesses associated with aging such as osteoporosis, cardiovascular disease, obesity, and diabetes.[2] Lifestyle counseling in midlife should include tobacco cessation; alcohol and drug safety; diet and exercise; injury prevention and bone health; breast health; prevention of sexual transmitted infections (STIs) and pregnancy; eye and dental health; abuse assessment; and medication and supplement management.[1]

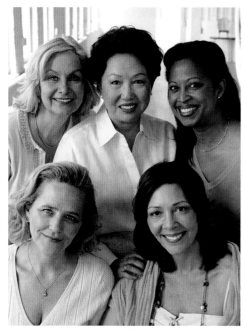

Figure 13.1 The ethnic variety of the older female population. (From iStockPhoto.com/72420378.)

In a large study on preventive services in the 40 to 64 years age group, it was found that the percentage of adults who are up to date with standard recommendations for clinical preventive services remains alarmingly low, particularly among adults 50 to 64 years of age; fewer than 1 in 4 adults in this age group received core preventive care. It is estimated that by the time adults in the United States reach the sixth decade, 70% will have been diagnosed with one or more chronic health conditions, and nearly one-half will have two or more conditions.[3]

NOT TO BE MISSED

A midlife female patient's quality of life (QoL) is not limited to menopausal symptoms alone. QoL involves a global sense of well-being that is inclusive of physical, mental, and emotional domains and can be reflective of the patient's culture, beliefs, and expectations. Assessment of a patient's QoL is a valuable therapeutic tool. The Utian Quality of Life Scale is one tool used in to assess QoL in the menopausal patient.[4]

MENOPAUSE DEFINED

Description

Menopause occurs in response to normal physiological changes of aging in the hypothalamic-pituitary-ovarian axis and results in the decline of ovarian follicular estrogen production. It is recognized retrospectively by the cessation of menstrual bleeding for a continuous 12-month period from the final menstrual period (FMP; sometimes referred to as the *last normal menstrual period* [LNMP]). The permanent end of menstruation also signals the end of the childbearing cycle. The average age of menopause in the United States is 52 years, but it can vary widely from 41 to 58 years. Because of the relative wide age range for natural menopause, chronological age alone is a poor indicator for the beginning or end of the menopausal transition.[5] Other factors that can influence the age of menopause include genetic determinants, smoking, and body size. Smokers typically experience menopause earlier than nonsmokers.[2] Undernourished females and vegetarians may experience an earlier menopause, and those with greater adipose tissue can potentially have a later menopause as body fat stores can convert to estrogen.[6]

Females who experience menopause between 40 and 45 years of age are considered to have *early menopause;* this occurs in approximately 5% of the population.[1] *Premature menopause* is defined as menopause occurring before 40 years of age. About 1 in 100 females will experience premature menopause for unknown reasons.[1] Premature menopause may also be induced by either bilateral oophorectomy or iatrogenic ablation of ovarian function by chemotherapy or pelvic radiation. The term *primary ovarian insufficiency* (POI) is the preferred term for premature menopause as the condition may be transient as a result of ovarian dysfunction related to temporary treatments or conditions.[1] Although the etiology of POI is often idiopathic, it may be caused by genetic abnormalities, metabolic disturbances, pelvic surgery, radiation therapy, chemotherapy, or immune disorders.[1]

❗ SAFETY ALERT

Females who have induced or premature menopause are at a greater risk for developing cardiovascular disease, osteoporosis, and cognitive impairment with aging.[1]

Stages of the Menopause Transition

Perimenopause is a term used to define the highly symptomatic period leading to the menopause transition and continuing through the 12 months of amenorrhea. It is characterized by irregular menstrual cycles that fluctuate in duration, interval, and amount of bleeding and/or other menopause type symptoms.

NOT TO BE MISSED

A diagnosis of perimenopause is a clinical diagnosis of exclusion, and it requires an awareness of the disease processes that could cause similar symptoms such as hypothyroidism, hyperprolactinemia, pregnancy, polycystic ovarian syndrome and other causes of abnormal uterine bleeding (AUB).[1]

A key issue in caring for female patients in the perimenopausal phase is that ovulation is still possible until there has been 12 months of continuous amenorrhea.

NOT TO BE MISSED

During the perimenopausal period, up to 75% of pregnancies in females older than 40 years of age are unintended.[5]

Symptom management must be combined with contraceptive management. Treating symptoms with hormone therapy (HT) alone is not adequate to prevent unintended pregnancy. Age is a significant predictor of non-use of contraception. Studies show that 24% of 40- to 44-year-old females report not using contraception; 48% of pregnancies among females older than 40 years of age are unintended; and 46% of these pregnancies end in abortion. Contraception should be continued until natural sterility is reached: amenorrhea for 2 years if younger than 50 years of age; amenorrhea for 1 year if older than 50 years of age based on fertility statistics; and a general approach for all females 55 years of age.[7] Table 13.1 provides a summary of menopause transition terminology.

Common Menopause Transition Symptoms

The individual experience of the menopause transition varies widely and is likely to be affected by multiple factors including the overall health of the patient before the menopause transition. The most common reported symptoms in the menopause transition are hot flashes, irregular bleeding, and vaginal dryness.[1] Other commonly reported symptoms are disturbed sleep and fatigue, dyspareunia, low libido, hair thinning and/or loss, cognitive and memory issues, weight gain, and increased depression and anxiety. The menopause encounter visit provides an opportunity for the clinician to assess multiple midlife health concerns that may or may not be associated with the menopause transition. Depression and fatigue may be a secondary result of sleep disturbance related to nightly hot flashes, or they can be preexisting conditions that worsened in the menopause transition.

Hot Flashes

Hot flashes, hot flushes, and *night sweats* all describe the same phenomenon and are medically defined as *vasomotor symptoms* (VMS; Fig. 13.2). Generally, hot flashes last from 1 to 5 minutes and can create heat, flushing, sweating, and frequently cause chills to occur afterwards. The exact mechanism behind hot flashes is not completely understood. Females with hot flashes appear

TABLE 13.1 Summary of Menopause Transition Terminology[21, 22, 23]		
Menopause Terminology	Average Age/Range	Description
Premature ovarian insufficiency (POI)	<40	Cessation of menses because of ovarian failure as a result of genetic or autoimmune disorders.
Premature menopause	<40	Cessation of menses as a result of genetics, autoimmune disease, medical procedures or treatments.
Early menopause	<45	Can be the same cause as premature menopause with the only difference being age of onset.
Perimenopause	4 to 8 years before the final menses	Varied duration prior to and 12 months past the last menstrual period. The period of the greatest symptoms due to erratic hormones.
Menopause	52/40 to 58	The cessation of menses.
Postmenopause	Start varies, lasts through end of life.	The time after the last menses, consists of early and late stages.

to have a thermoregulatory zone that is narrow, thus small increases in core body temperature can trigger hot flashes.[8] The thermoregulatory zone is the range in which the skin temperatures adjust to maintain a constant core temperature in a resting person. The onset of VMS can be the hallmark of starting the menopause transition, and hot flashes are the second most frequently reported symptom in perimenopause.

NOT TO BE MISSED

Health care education and medical treatment can assist in managing hot flashes, but there isn't a "cure" for the menopausal transition of the aging process, the treatment is based on providing symptoms relief.[1]

CLINICAL SURVIVAL TIP Up to 75% of perimenopausal females experience hot flashes, and the degree of severity varies greatly per individual. It is estimated that 25% of the females experiencing hot flashes in the menopause transition experience have symptoms that are sufficient to seek health care services.[1] Unless bothersome to the patient, hot flashes do not require medical intervention, and they will eventually subside on their own.

Perimenopausal Menstrual Changes

Menstrual changes can herald the onset of the menopause transition, and approximately 90% of females experience 4 to 8 years of menstrual changes before menopause.[1] The irregular bleeding is attributed to a decreased frequency in ovulation and erratic levels of ovarian hormones. Anovulation resulting in irregularly

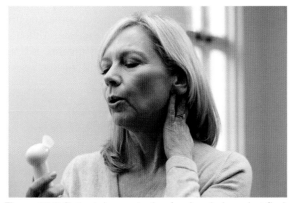

Figure 13.2 Patient demonstrating fanning during a hot flash. (From iStockPhoto/Highwaystarz-Photography.)

timed menses in the perimenopausal phase is not uncommon. For this reason, slight changes in the menses pattern are to be expected and are a normal change leading to menopause. Other issues, such as uterine polyps, fibroids, and adenomyosis, can also be the cause of abnormal bleeding, and pathology should be ruled out.[9] A consideration with symptoms of abnormal bleeding during the menopause transition years is the possibility of endometrial cancer, which characteristically manifests as irregular bleeding. Endometrial cancer is the most common gynecological malignancy in North America, and the risk of endometrial hyperplasia increases with age.[1] By 40 to 49 years of age, the risk for endometrial cancer is 36.5 cases in 100,000 females.[6]

! SAFETY ALERT

The American College of Obstetricians and Gynecologists (ACOG) recommends endometrial biopsy (EMB) in any female older than 45 years of age who has symptoms of abnormal bleeding, unless the patient is pregnant or there is a clear reason to avoid biopsy.[10]

In the postmenopausal woman, AUB is defined as uterine bleeding 12 months or more after regular menses have stopped. Approximately 20% of postmenopausal bleeding is associated with hyperplasia of the uterine lining.[1] Abnormal uterine bleeding accounts for more than 70% of all gynecological consults in the perimenopausal years.[10]

During the perimenopause transition, laboratory evaluation for AUB based on the clinical situation may include testing for complete blood count, pregnancy, coagulation, sexually transmitted infections (STIs), liver function, thyroid, prolactin, follicle-stimulating hormone, estradiol, progesterone, testosterone, and dehydroepiandrosterone sulfate. Procedures may include office endometrial biopsy (EMB), transvaginal ultrasonography, saline infusion sonohysterography, office hysteroscopy, and dilation and curettage (Table 13.2).

Depending on the services available in the primary care setting, referrals to women's health specialists may be warranted. Family nurse practitioners (FNPs) trained in EMB can perform the procedure at the time of the menopause clinical encounter, or it can be referred to a women's health nurse practitioner (WHNP) (Fig. 13.3). Further evaluation for diagnostic imaging and procedures should also be referred to an obstetrics and gynecology clinical setting.

TABLE 13.2   Summary Evaluation of Abnormal Uterine Bleeding[10]

Uterine Evaluation Methods	Procedure Description
Endometrial biopsy	Inexpensive, office-based procedure with sensitivity ranging from 60% to 97% in diagnosing endometrial cancer.
Transvaginal ultrasonography	Vaginal probe used to measure the thickness of the uterine lining and evaluate the uterine and adnexal anatomy. If the endometrial lining is 4 mm or less, endometrial sampling is not required unless bleeding persists.
Hysteroscopy	Endoscope is inserted through the cervix to visualize the uterine cavity. The uterus is distended with fluid or carbon dioxide to view focal lesions, polyps, and fibroids.
Dilation and curettage	The cervix is dilated, and the uterine lining and/or contents of the uterus are removed by curettage.

*Further information on abnormal uterine bleeding can be found in Chapter 17.

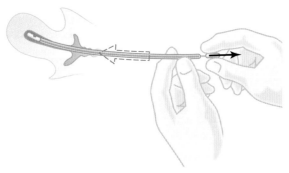

Figure 13.3 A pipelle used to obtain endometrial tissue sampling. (From Hacker NF, Gambone JC, Hobel CJ. *Hacker & Moore's Essentials of Obstetrics and Gynecology.* Elsevier; 2016.)

In the symptomatic perimenopausal patient, there are several options for symptom management that also provide birth control.

> **CLINICAL SURVIVAL TIP** Combined oral contraceptives have the benefit of restoring a regular menses cycle, decreasing dysmenorrhea and heavy bleeding, and improving acne that may flare up in the menopause transition. They also have the added benefit of suppressing VMS.

Intrauterine contraception offers another highly effective birth control option and can result in very light cyclical bleeding or amenorrhea over time. The progestin-only birth control pill is an option for cigarette smokers over 35 years of age and is considered for patients with hypertension, a history of venous thromboembolism, or any issue in which estrogen is contraindicated. The subdermal implant and injectable progestin are also options to regulate bleeding and provide birth control.

> **! SAFETY ALERT**
>
> According to the U.S. Medical Eligibility Criteria (US MEC) for Contraceptive Use guidelines from the U.S. Centers for Disease Control and Prevention, no contraceptive methods are contraindicated on the basis of age alone.[1]

Genitourinary Syndrome of Menopause

The decrease in estrogen can create a collection of symptoms effecting the external genitalia, urethra, bladder, and vagina. It is estimated that 10% to 40% of menopausal females will experience one or more symptoms of genitourinary syndrome of menopause (GSM).[8] Vaginal dryness, burning, irritation, and the sexual symptoms of lack of lubrication are common menopause symptoms. Dyspareunia, loss of labial adipose tissue, and impaired sexual function can occur secondary to these changes. Vaginal walls may become thin, dry, pale, and smooth, and pain during vaginal penetration is often the presenting symptom. Urinary symptoms of urgency, dysuria, and urinary tract infections (UTIs) may also increase. Although not all females will experience these symptoms, it is an important component of the clinician menopause assessment.

> **PATIENT-CENTERED CARE:** GSM can negatively affect the female patient's overall quality of life, particularly regarding sexual health and intimate relationships. Comprehensive and holistic assessment techniques can encourage the patient to discuss GSM issues to help decide on the available options for treatment.

MENOPAUSE HEALTH CARE ENCOUNTER

A patient's health care visit for menopause symptoms may coincide with the annual well-woman examination. Recommendations for well-woman examinations, age-related laboratory tests, and preventive screenings in the 40- to 64-year-old age group are well defined by the ACOG.[11] A healthy menopause transition is based on maintaining overall midlife good health and healthy lifestyle practices. To better understand the patient's narrative in the initial menopause health care encounter, the clinician must utilize a holistic assessment technique that is patient centered and comprehensive while reviewing overall health and lifestyle expectations for the visit. If the patient is being seen for a menopause concern and has had a recent normal well-woman examination, the encounter may be focused solely on menopause symptoms and midlife concerns. A thorough history and focused examination can guide the clinician and patient in making management decisions.

> **CLINICAL SURVIVAL TIP** The goal of the encounter is to provide relief from common menopausal symptoms, rule out other disorders, and at the same time work with the patient to prevent osteoporosis, heart disease, cancer risks, and other age-related disease.

History

The history includes the following:

Personal History Questionnaire-9 (PHQ9), Becks Depression Inventory,[12] and Generalized Anxiety Disorder-7 (GAD 7)[13]

Rationale: The PHQ-9 and GAD-7 are frequently used mental health assessment surveys with scored results that indicate the level or category of depression and anxiety. An estimated 1 in 10 U.S. adults report depression, and an estimated 1 in 7 report stress/anxiety. The risk of depression and anxiety increases at midlife as a result of hormonal fluctuations and potential midlife stressors.[5]

Breast cancer screening

Rationale: Mammogram screening guidelines vary based on age and risk factors. Resources for screening guidelines include the American Cancer Society, ACOG, and U.S. Preventive Services Task Force.

Colorectal screening

Rationale: Colonoscopy is the preferred screening recommended by 50 years of age; it may be recommended at an earlier age if there are personal or family risk factors.[11]

Diabetes screening

Rationale: Diabetes screening is recommended at 45 years of age; if it is normal, repeat at a minimum of 3-year intervals.[11]

Pap screening

Rationale: Discontinue screening at 65 years of age if there is adequate negative prior screening. Adequate negative screening includes three consecutive negative pap tests *or* two consecutive negative co-tests (HPV negative) *or* two consecutive negative high-risk HPV (hrHPV) tests in the preceding 10 years.[14]

> **NOT TO BE MISSED**
>
> Pap screening can cease if the patient has had a hysterectomy with removal of the cervix and does not have a history of high-grade precancerous cervical lesion or cancer.[14]

Lipid assessment

Rationale: Screening is recommended every 5 years beginning at 45 years of age; it may occur sooner if the patient has a positive family history, positive personal history, or other risk factors.[11]

STI screening

Rationale: The risk of STIs continues throughout the lifespan.[11]

Lifestyle and health habits

Rationale: Other areas to assess the impact on health and disease prevention include nutrition, physical activity, stress, substance use, caffeine, prescription drugs, herbal treatment and supplements, and recreational drug use.[2]

> **NOT TO BE MISSED**
>
> Greater than one-third of U.S. adults used complementary health approaches that include but are not limited to herbs, acupuncture, supplements, relaxation techniques, and massage.[15] Midlife females are the highest users of complementary therapies, and the menopause transition often heralds the increased use of over-the-counter supplements and integrative therapies for self-treatment and symptom relief.

Physical Examination

The physical examination includes the following:

Vital signs including body mass index (BMI), blood pressure, and pulse

Rationale: More than one-third of the U.S. population is considered obese (35.7%), and 25.8 million children and adults in the United States have diabetes. During the menopause transition, females can gain an average of approximately 5 lb.[1]

Thyroid

Rationale: Thyroid disorders are common in females and increase with age; thyroid disorder symptoms can mimic common menopause symptoms.[1]

Heart and lungs

Rationale: Cardiovascular disease is the leading cause of death for females worldwide. Asthma is more prevalent in females; age-related decreased lung volumes and pulmonary symptoms become more prevalent. Some specific cardiovascular and/or pulmonary conditions are a contraindication to estrogen therapy (ET).[5]

NOT TO BE MISSED

If patient is asymptomatic for GSM, abnormal uterine bleeding, or other pelvic concerns, the evidence to do a pelvic examination is limited and contradictory.[5]

Pelvic Examination

The pelvic examination includes the following:

External genitalia assessment for infection, pain, lesions, atrophy/thinning with loss of adipose tissue.

Rationale: At least 1 in 3 females will experience GSM. The mucus membranes of vulvar and vaginal tissue may become thin with a resulting loss of elasticity (Fig. 13.4). This condition is described as *atrophy.* Loss of lubrication can also occur, making infections more likely and sexual activity more painful. Decreasing estrogen may cause the urethra to shorten, which increases the risk of UTIs. Urinary incontinence also increases the risk of UTIs.[5]

Urethral os: Assess changes related to decreasing estrogen.

Rationale: Assess for signs of irritation, bleeding, atrophy, and urethrocele

Pelvic floor integrity: Assess for tone, cystocele, rectocele, uterine prolapse, and urinary leakage with coughing

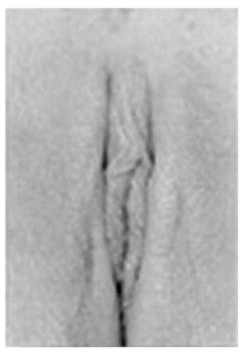

Figure 13.4 Vulva demonstrating postmenopausal labial fat loss, redness, and dryness. (From Mazloomdoost D, Crisp CC, Westermann LB, et al. Survey of male perceptions regarding the vulva. *Am J Obstet Gynecol.* 2015;213(5):731.e1–731.e9.)

Rationale: Pelvic floor prolapse is more common with aging and can interfere with normal urinary, bowel, and sexual functioning.[1]

Vaginal speculum examination for visual inspection

Rationale: Assess for signs of infection, vaginal lesions, bleeding, irritation, or atrophy.

Cervical visual inspection

Rationale: Assess for common changes related to decreased estrogen; shortened cervix pale in color; os may be stenotic. Endocervical polyps may be present and can be a cause of abnormal bleeding.

Uterus: Palpation assessment

Rationale: Manually assess for tenderness, size, shape, mobility, and contour. A decrease in uterine size is normal with aging. Uterine fibroids are associated with abnormal bleeding.

Adnexa: Palpation assessment

Rationale: Manually assess for masses, tenderness, and mobility. Ovaries decrease in size with aging and become less palpable. Perform a manual and visual rectal inspection.

Rationale: Assess for irritation, hemorrhoids, bleeding, and rectocele.

Bone density scan

Rationale: If 65 years of age or older or with a history of fracture, risk factors of osteoporosis, or body weight less than 127 lb.[9]

> **CLINICAL SURVIVAL TIP** The use of hormone testing to determine menopause status is not routinely indicated. VMS are generally the best predictor of the menopause transition. Follicle-stimulating hormone (FSH) may be indicated if symptoms are atypical or occur at an early age.[1]

SYMPTOM MANAGEMENT INTERVENTIONS

Intervention selection includes counseling about options for treatment of menopause-related symptoms and encouraging the patient to have an active role in decision making. Understanding that the menopause transition is a phase in the patient's life, a natural event, and not a disease is a helpful place to begin the discussion. The clinician can utilize open-ended questions and reflective statements to partner with the patient in jointly selecting the best options. Studies have shown that female patients respond well to language that is free from heterosexual assumptions and that disclosing sexual orientation increases communication satisfaction, making it more likely that they will continue to seek medical help.[1]

> **PATIENT-CENTERED CARE:** Effective counseling encompasses viewing the menopause transition from the perspective of the patient's culture, beliefs, sexual orientation, gender identification, and other individual influences. Providers can describe all of the necessary information for the patient in an unbiased, factual, and comprehensive manner that explains the benefits and risks of any therapeutic options in lay terms.

It is important to elicit and include patient preferences in any recommendations and to understand the patient's comprehension and capacity to participate in treatment choices. The clinician must be well aware of the benefits and the common side effects of the non-hormonal and hormonal medications within the context of the most current evidence-based practice guidelines.

Nonpharmacological Interventions

Clinicians have the responsibility to be well informed about the emerging research in menopause treatment options and the level of evidence for the wide array of options currently available to midlife female patients.

> **⚠ SAFETY ALERT**
>
> Evidence-based (EB) recommendations increase patient safety and treatment effectiveness through application of effective and appropriate therapies. Following EB recommendations eliminates the underuse of effective therapies and the use of inappropriate or ineffective therapies.

A narrative review conducted by Biglia et al. presented an update on non-hormonal treatments for VMS.[16] Some of the frequently advised lifestyle recommendations were not found to have any impact on VMS. Cooling techniques such as dressing in layers, drinking ice water, using a fan, and lowering room temperature are not supported by clinical evidence, and relaxation techniques show insufficient evidence in reduction of VMS in healthy perimenopausal and postmenopausal females. The following nonpharmacological lifestyle-related treatments were found to be effective in reducing VMS:

- Cognitive behavioral therapy
- Weight loss
- Yoga and exercise
- Acupuncture

Non-hormonal Therapy Interventions

Non-hormonal medications were also reviewed, and a low-dose paroxetine salt (7.5 mg daily) is the only non-hormonal medication approved by the U.S. Food and Drug Administration (FDA) for management of VMS.[16] However, other selective serotonin reuptake inhibitors (SSRIs) and serotonin-norepinephrine reuptake inhibitors (SNRIs) were found to be effective. Gabapentinoids and clonidine show evidence of efficacy but have been less well studied. S-equol derivatives of soy isoflavones may also be beneficial, however more studies are needed. When considering the use of an SSRI or SNRI for VMS, the clinician should utilize an individualized approach based on the patient's medical history, personal preferences, and the risk-benefit to the patient.[1] Table 13.3

summarizes the non-hormonal medication options with recommended dosage and potential side effects.

Over-the-counter supplements such as purified pollen extract (PPE) and black cohosh are being used by females to relieve hot flashes. PPE has been shown to reduce hot flashes versus placebo by 65%; however, although black cohosh has been used by both Native American and European females for centuries, randomized controlled trials have not shown any statistically significant difference in the frequency or severity of hot flashes.[16]

In the treatment of GSM, non-hormonal options can serve as initial therapy for vaginal dryness and irritation. Lubricants are available without a prescription and provide temporary measures to relieve vaginal dryness related to pain during intercourse. They can be used on both partners before and during sex and are immediate-acting. Vaginal moisturizers provide longer-term relief of vaginal dryness and are shown to increase comfort. These products are FDA approved under the heading of cosmetics.[16]

Hormone Therapy Interventions

HT is approved by the FDA for five indications: bothersome VMS; prevention of bone loss; hypoestrogenism caused by hypogonadism; POI; and GSM.[17] When considering HT, it is important to evaluate the patient's complete medical history and symptoms, identify any individual risks for HT, and engage in a discussion on evidence-based risks and benefits. The HT prescription is guided by patient symptoms, expectations, preferences, and any other health concerns. The contraindications to HT are listed in the Safety Alert box.

! SAFETY ALERT

Contraindications to Hormone Therapy

- Abnormal uterine bleeding (accounts for more than 70% of all gynecological consults in the perimenopausal years)[10]
- History of breast cancer
- High-risk endometrial cancer
- Active or history of deep vein thrombosis or pulmonary embolism
- Active or history of arterial thromboembolic disease (stroke, transient ischemic attack, myocardial infarction)
- Liver dysfunction or disease
- Known or suspected pregnancy

NOT TO BE MISSED

An estimated 50% to 80% of midlife U.S. females use non-hormonal, nonprescription therapies to treat VMS.[16]

TABLE 13.3   Non-hormonal Medications for Vasomotor Symptoms[16]

Non-hormonal Therapies	Dosage	Side Effects
Paroxetine (Paxil, Brisdelle)*	7.5 mg/day (FDA-approved dose) 10–25 mg/day	Asthenia, sweating, nausea (20-mg dose), somnolence, anorgasmia, decreased libido, blurred vision
Venlafaxine (Effexor)*	37.5–150 mg/day; up-titrate when starting therapy	Nausea, vomiting, dry mouth, decreased appetite, constipation
Desvenlafaxine (Pristiq)*	100–150 mg/day	Nausea, dizziness and headache only in first week of treatment
Citalopram (Celexa)*	10–20 mg/day	Nausea, diarrhea, vomiting, increased sweating, increased appetite, weight changes, anorgasmia
Escitalopram (Lexapro)*	10–20 mg/day	Somnolence, dizziness, insomnia, heartburn, constipation, decreased sex drive, anorgasmia
Oxybutynin (Ditropan)	5–15 mg/day	Dizziness, somnolence, blurred vision, dry mouth, diarrhea, constipation
Gabapentin (Neurontin, Gralise)	Initial dose 900–2,400 mg/day	Somnolence, dizziness, ataxia, fatigue, weight gain, possible suicidal ideation
Pregabalin (Lyrica)	150–300 mg/day	Somnolence, dizziness, ataxia, constipation, edema, breast swelling, blurred vision, memory problems, weight gain, possible suicidal ideation

*First-line option for hot flashes.
†Second-line option for hot flashes.

Bioidentical Hormones

Bioidentical hormones are hormones that are chemically identical to those made in the human body. The chemical structure of the hormone, not its source, determines if a hormone is bioidentical. There are FDA-approved bioidentical forms of estrogen and progesterone that are widely available. These include 17 beta estradiol and micronized progesterone. Bioidentical hormones have not been found to be safer or more effective than non-bioidentical hormones.[1]

NOT TO BE MISSED

Bioidentical hormones have not been found to be safer or more effective than non-bioidentical hormones.[1]

Estrogen Therapy

ET is available for systemic use in oral and transdermal forms (Fig. 13.5). For specific treatment of GSM, estrogen is available in creams, rings, and suppository tablets (Table 13.4). Systemic ET alone is only recommended for female patients who have had a hysterectomy and do not need uterine protection with progestogens to prevent uterine cancer. Estrogen-progestogen therapy (EPT) is required when treating a patient with a uterus. Estrogen for symptom relief should be combined with a progestogen to protect the endometrium.

⚠ SAFETY ALERT

Systemic ET alone is only recommended for female patients who have had a hysterectomy and do not need uterine protection with progestogens to prevent uterine cancer. EPT is required when treating a woman with a uterus. Estrogen for symptom relief should be combined with a progestogen to protect the endometrium.[1]

Systemic ET is associated with risks, such as an increased risk of stroke, blood clots, and possibly breast cancer if used long term. ET should be used at the lowest effective dose consistent with the patient's treatment goals. EPT is associated with side effects similar to ET and should be used at the lowest effective dose consistent with treatment goals. The risk of breast cancer appears to be higher with EPT, especially when used long term (more than 5 years). Low-dose vaginal ET is effective for GSM. Treating GSM locally with vaginal estrogen is preferred because of its safety profile.[5] ET effectively alleviates atrophic vaginal symptoms related to menopause. Local therapy is advised for the treatment of female patients with only vaginal symptoms. All low-dose systemic estrogen formulations are FDA approved for the treatment of atrophic vaginitis.

The list of hormone products on the market is extensive. A full list of approved products can be found on the North American Menopause Society (NAMS)

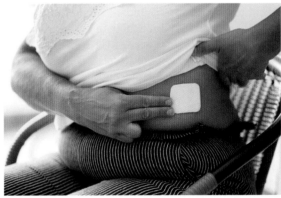

Figure 13.5 Patient wearing a hormone replacement patch. (From iStockPhoto.com/AndreyPopov.)

TABLE 13.4 Hormone Therapy Options[1,8]			
Hormone Options	**Estrogen Therapy (ET)**	**Progestin Therapy (PT)**	**Combined Therapy Estrogen/ Progestin Therapy (EPT)**
Systemic effect	Oral	Oral	Oral
Systemic effect	Transdermal patch Gel Spray Cream	Cream: Evidence for endometrial protection is limited	Transdermal patch
Localized treatment	Vaginal ring Suppository Cream	Progesterone intrauterine device (IUD). Not FDA approved for endometrial protection with ET use	

website: www.menopause.org. A brief summary is provided in Table 13.4.

HT regimens are classified as follows: (1) continuous-cycle, sequential daily estrogen with 12 to 14 days per month of progesterone; (2) continuous-cycle, long-cycle daily estrogen and progesterone for 12 to 14 days every 2 to 6 months; and (3) continuous combined daily estrogen and daily progesterone.[1] There are pros and cons to the types of regimens prescribed and the routes of administration. Clinical decision making in HT prescribing is multifactorial and based on risk factors, patient preference and symptoms, surgical history, and other issues addressed throughout this chapter.

When considering the type of HT to use, the symptom management goal is to decrease VMS and GSM symptoms, help regulate perimenopausal bleeding, and provide contraception if indicated.

Patient counseling and follow-up encounters can establish a consistent pattern of safe use and the maximum benefit to patients. In general, VMS may begin to decrease 2 to 6 weeks after initiating HT, but the full effect is not reached until 8 to 12 weeks.[1] A return visit is recommended 1 to 2 months after beginning consistent HT therapy.[2] The clinician should assess adequate symptom management and whether the patient has found the route of administration a satisfactory method.

The following recommendations of the NAMS[1] and the ACOG[8] provide a summary of key HT prescribing criteria:

- There is good data supporting the initiation of HT around the time of menopause to treat menopause-related symptoms. The absolute risk of HT is low between the 50 and 59 years of age. The benefits outweigh the risks for most healthy, symptomatic females younger than 60 years of age or within 10 years of the final menstrual period. For females who initiate HT more than 10 years from menopause onset or are 60 years of age or older, the benefits appear less favorable than for earlier HT use because of the greater absolute risk of CHD, stroke, VTE, and dementia.[17]
- HT is recommended as the first-line therapy for female patients with VMS of menopause without contraindications.
- The HT formulation, timing, and route of administration are important. The lowest effective dose needed for symptom relief should be used, and individualization of therapy should be based on the patient's health history and risk factors.
- If the patient has a uterus, systemic HT must include a progestin to decrease the risk of endometrial hyperplasia.
- If progesterone is not needed, ET alone has a better risk-to-benefit ratio than combined estrogen-progesterone therapy.
- Systemic HT and low-dose vaginal ET are very effective treatments for moderate to severe symptoms of vulvar and vaginal atrophy (vaginal dryness, dyspareunia, and atrophic vaginitis).

TABLE 13.5   Hormone Therapy Side Effects and Management[24]

Side Effects	Management
Breast tenderness (sometimes enlargement)	Stop current therapy. Start hormone therapy at a lower estrogen dose, slowly titrate dose up. Switch to transdermal delivery that gives constant levels of hormones. Switch progestin component to either norethindrone or oral micronized progesterone. Augment with methyltestosterone.
Hot flashes or night sweats	Increase estrogen dose to twice original for 4 to 6 months, then titrate dose down to patch. Add testosterone.
Breakthrough bleeding	Decrease estradiol to the next lowest dose. Increase oral micronized progesterone to 200mg or 400mg on days 14-28. 400mg may cause morning tiredness. If younger than 35, perform endometrial biopsy Switch to progesterone IUD. Switch to either cyclical combined or continuous sequential cycling.
Cognitive issues (memory loss, less sharp)	Ensure 7 to 8 hours of sleep regularly. Increase estradiol in small increments every month.
Vaginal dryness	Augment current treatment with ½ applicator of estrogen vaginal cream 2 to 3 nights a week. Augment current treatment with Estring vaginal ring every 3 months.
Mood changes	On combined oral contraceptives-switch to low-dose contraceptive. On cyclical combined therapy-switch to low-dose patch on the progestin cycle, through the menstrual cycle. Switch progesterone to oral micronized progesterone 100-200mg at bedtime on progestin cycle. Increase exercise. Take Vit B6 50-100mg every day. Decrease sodium and sugar intake.

- Low-dose vaginal estrogen is also recommended as the first-line treatment for female patients with isolated GSM. For patients with premature menopause, HT can be prescribed until reaching the median age of menopause.
- An increased risk of breast cancer was seen with 3 to 5 years of estrogen-progestogen therapy in the Women's Health Initiative, whereas no increased risk of breast cancer was seen with 7 years of ET use, allowing for more flexibility in duration of ET use in female patients without a uterus.
- Both transdermal ET and low-dose oral ET have been associated with a lower risk of venous thromboembolism and stroke compared with standard-dose oral ET in observational studies, but evidence from randomized, controlled trials is lacking. Systemic HT and low-dose vaginal ET are very effective treatments for the moderate to severe symptoms of GSM.

The guidelines for when HT should be discontinued have evolved over time. According to current ACOG guidelines, discontinuation of HT may be associated with recurrent VMS in approximately 50% of females, regardless of age and duration of use.[8]

NOT TO BE MISSED

There is consensus that HT does not need to stop routinely at 60 or 65 years of age. Treatment should be individualized, and the risks and benefits should be evaluated regularly.[17]

NOT TO BE MISSED

Currently there is insufficient evidence to recommend one method of HT discontinuation (abrupt or tapering) over the other to prevent recurrent symptoms.

When to Discontinue Hormone Therapy

The decision to continue HT should be individualized and based on the patient's symptoms and the risk-to-benefit ratio, regardless of age. Because some females 65 years of age and older may continue to need systemic HT for the management of VMS, the ACOG recommends against routine discontinuation of systemic estrogen at 65 years of age. As with younger female patients, the use of HT and ET should be individualized based on each patient's risk-to-benefit ratio and clinical presentation.

Intervention Summary

Interprofessional Care of the Midlife Female Patient

In addition to the role of the primary care nurse practitioner, comprehensive menopause management may include a team of health care professionals. The team may include referrals to a women's health nurse practitioner, psychologist, pharmacist, nutritionist, and physician to help provide the patient with the best care. It has been shown that health care providers who work within an interprofessional practice model increase the practice of safe, high-quality, accessible, patient-centered care desired by patients and providers alike.[18] The family nurse practitioner can work to establish community resources and referrals for the menopausal and midlife female patient that will ultimately provide more evidence-based options for treatment. Community resources can include low-cost and accessible programs for weight management, exercise, stress reduction, integrative therapies, and support groups. Well-being and healthy aging are dependent on healthy communities with a strong integration of medical systems and community resources. Females go through the menopause transition within the context of their lived experiences, therefore connectivity to work, family, and community are essential components of their health.

Population Considerations

Ethnicity. Keeping a perspective on population health outcomes alongside individual care can help the primary care provider achieve a health system goal of improved health and health equity across the lifespan.[19] To date, there is a paucity of research on ethnicity and the menopause experience. The data collected has primarily been focused on middle class, educated White females.[1] In one study, Caucasian females were found to be concerned about aging and loss of youthful appearance, while African American females were more welcoming of menopause as a normal event.[1] In general, females with higher incomes and education reported better overall health, fewer symptoms, and a better quality of life than low-income menopausal females

attending primary care clinics. Hot flash frequency may vary per ethnic group; one large study found that Black females reported VMS most frequently (45.6%), followed by Hispanic (35.4%), White (31.2%), Chinese (20.5%), and Japanese females (17.6%).[20]

Obstacles to Health Care. Health care access and affordability with aging is an issue for both genders. Females at midlife may experience more obstacles in this age group that can include decreased mobility, lack of insurance, decreased income level, transportation difficulties, and cultural norms.

> **PATIENT-CENTERED CARE:** Studies indicate that lesbian females seek health care services less frequently than heterosexual females and feel a lack of open communication with health care providers. Instilling trust through unbiased communication regarding sexual orientation in language that is free from heterosexual assumptions can establish a therapeutic relationship.[1]

Mental Health. Counseling a female patient at midlife on healthy aging includes encompassing the biophysical changes of the menopause transition, health risks, and options to reduce those risks. Risk factors, morbidity, and mortality patterns combined with access to health care can vary widely in different populations. Females in midlife have multiple roles and responsibilities that may include a spouse and partner, employee and employer, parent and caregiver, friend, and community citizen. The experience of midlife can be influenced by current health status, cultural and familial beliefs on aging, education, income, and ethnicity. Counseling patients during the menopause transition involves patient-centered care that is specific to individual priorities and utilizes evidence-based guidelines.

> **PATIENT-CENTERED CARE:** Females who can identify a comprehensive health plan for the promotion of their physical, emotional, and social health will be more able create a template for success as they age.

CONCLUSION

Menopause is a natural transition in a female's life and marks a key landmark at midlife. It is the end of the reproductive years and a natural part of the aging process. Every female transitions through perimenopause to menopause in a unique way. If symptomatic and seeking care, it is the patient's decision on which therapies to use based on individual risk factors and available options. Although many females will make the transition without incident or the desire to seek medical care, many will also experience VMS and GSM.

> **PATIENT-CENTERED CARE:** For the primary care provider, improving the patient's quality of life through symptom management is the focus of treatment. A combination of healthy lifestyle modifications with hormonal and/or non-hormonal therapies can decrease symptoms and improve the patient's quality of life.

As more and more females enter the menopause transition years, clinicians are in a prime position to offer counseling and screening for other age-related disease risks. The menopause encounter provides an opportunity to address additional midlife health issues that may encompass weight management, cardiovascular disease, diabetes, cancer, osteoporosis, thyroid disorders, smoking cessation, sleep, depression, and stress management. The clinician can partner with patients to develop self-management strategies for healthy aging and encourage the potential for personal growth and positive change during the menopause transition years.

KEY POINTS

- The menopause transition is a normal physiological event that affects females by the fifth decade of life or earlier. It is a key time to evaluate a wide variety of primary midlife health issues, initiate age-related health screenings, and encourage healthy lifestyle practices.
- The average age of menopause in the United States is 52 years of age, but it can vary widely from 41 to 58 years of age. Because of the relative wide age range for natural menopause, chronological age alone is a poor indicator for the beginning or end of the menopausal transition.
- A diagnosis of perimenopause is a clinical diagnosis of exclusion, and it requires an awareness of the disease processes that could cause similar symptoms such as hypothyroidism, hyperprolactinemia, pregnancy, polycystic ovarian syndrome, and other causes of abnormal uterine bleeding.
- During the perimenopausal period, up to 75% of pregnancies in females older than 40 years of age are unintended. Symptom management must be combined with contraceptive management.
- The individual experience of the menopause transition varies widely and is likely to be affected by multiple factors including the overall health of the patient before the menopause transition.
- The most common reported symptoms in the menopause transition are hot flashes, irregular bleeding, and vaginal dryness.

- Non-hormonal, nonpharmacological, and a variety of hormone therapies are available for symptom management of the menopause transition.
- Health care education and medical treatment can assist in managing hot flashes, but there is no "cure" for the menopause transition or aging. Treatment is based on symptom relief.[1]
- Systemic ET alone is only recommended for females who have had a hysterectomy and do not need any uterine protection with progestogens to prevent uterine cancer.
- EPT is required when treating a patient with a uterus.
- Treating GSM locally with vaginal estrogen is preferred because of its safety profile.[5]
- The decision to continue HT should be individualized and based on the patient's symptoms and the risk-to-benefit ratio, regardless of age.
- Every female transitions through perimenopause to menopause in a unique way. If symptomatic and seeking care, it is the patient's decision on which therapies to use based on individual risk factors and available options.
- Female patients who can identify a comprehensive health plan for promotion of their physical, emotional, and social health will be more able create a template for success as they age.

REFERENCES

1. North American Menopause Society. *Menopause Practice: A Clinician's Guide.* 5th ed. Mayfield Heights, Ohio: NAMS; 2014.

2. Alexander IM, Atkin KP, Andrist LC. Menopause. In: Schuiling KD, Likis FE, eds. *Women's Gynecologic Health.* 3rd ed. Burlington, MA: Jones & Bartlett; 2017:261–302.

3. U.S. Centers for Disease Control and Prevention, American Association of Retired Persons, American Medical Association. *Promoting Preventive Services for Adults 50–64: Community and Clinical Partnerships.* Atlanta, GA: National Association of Chronic Disease Directors; 2009.

4. Utian W, Janata J, Kingsberg S, Schluchter M, Hamilton J. The Utian Quality of Life (UQOL) Scale: development and validation of an instrument to quantify quality of life through and beyond menopause. *Menopause.* 2002;9(6):402–410.

5. Shifren J, Gass M. North American Menopause Society Recommendations for Clinical Care of Midlife Women. *Menopause.* 2014;21(10):1038–1062.

6. Fritz M, Speroff L. *Clinical Gynecologic Endocrinology and Infertility.* 8th ed. Wolters Kluwer Lippincott; 2011.

7. Black. A. (2019). Contraception during the menopause transition: Choices and challenges. [PDF]. https://www.menopause.org/docs/default-source/speaker-slides/black-2019.pdf.

8. American College of Obstetricians and Gynecologists. Management of Menopausal Symptoms: January 2014. *Practice Bulletin Number.* 2014;141.

9. Lebovic D, Gordon J, Taylor R. *Reproductive Endocrinology and Infertility.* 2nd ed. Arlington VA: Scrubhill Press; 2014.

10. American College of Obstetricians and Gynecologists. *Diagnosis of Abnormal Uterine Bleeding in Reproductive Age Women: July 2012.* Practice Bulletin Number 2014: 128.

11. Women's Preventive Services Initiative. *Recommendations for Well-Woman Care—a Well-Woman Chart.* Washington, DC: ACOG Foundation; 2018. https://www.womenspreventivehealth.org/wellwomanchart/.

12. Kroenke K, Spitzer R, Williams J. The PHQ-9 validity of a brief depression severity measure. *J General Internal Med.* 2001;16(9):606–613.

13. Spitzer R, Kroenke K, Williams J. A Brief measure for assessing generalized anxiety disorder. *J General Internal Med.* 2006;66(10):1092–1097.

14. American College of Obstetricians and Gynecologists. ACOG Practice Advisory. *Updated Cervical Cancer Screening Guidelines;* 2021. https://www.acog.org/clinical/clinical-guidance/practice-advisory/articles/2021/04/updated-cervical-cancer-screening-guidelines.

15. Clarke TC, Barnes PM, Black LI, Stussman BJ, Nahin RL. *Use of Yoga, Meditation, and Chiropractors Among U.S. Adults Aged 18 and Over. Nchs Data Brief, No. 325.* Hyattsville, MD: National Center for Health Statistics; 2018.

16. David, P. S., Smith, T. L. Nordhues, H. C., & Kling, J. M. (2022). A clinical review on Paroxetine and emerging therapies to treat vasomotor symptoms. doi: 10.2147/IJWH.S282396.

17. The NAMS 2017 Hormone Therapy Position Statement Advisory Panel. The 2017 hormone therapy position statement of The North American Menopause Society. *Menopause.* 2017;24(7):728–753.

18. Interprofessional Education Collaborative. *Core Competencies for Interprofessional Collaborative Practice: 2016 Update.* Washington, DC: Interprofessional Education Collaborative; 2016.

19. Hawkins JW, Roberto-Nichols DM, Stanley-Haney JL. *Guidelines for Nurse Practitioners in Gynecologic Settings.* 11th ed. New York: Springer Publishing Company; 2016.

20. Gold E, Sternfield B, Kelsey JL, et al. Relation of demographic and lifestyle factors to symptoms in a multiracial/ethnic population of women 40–55 years of age. *Am J Epidemiol.* 2000;152(5):463–473.

21. U.S. Department of Health & Human Services. Early or premature menopause. (n.d.). *Office on Women's Health.* https://www.womenshealth.gov/menopause/early-or-premature-menopause.

22. Pinkerton, J. V. (2021). Menopause. *Merck Manual Professional Version.* https://www.merckmanuals.com/professional/gynecology-and-obstetrics/menopause/menopause.

23. The North American Menopause Society. (n.d.). Menopause 101: A primer for the perimenopausal. https://www.menopause.org/for-women/menopauseflashes/menopause-symptoms-and-treatments/menopause-101-a-primer-for-the-perimenopausal.

24. Sherif. K. (2013). *Hormone therapy: Monitoring effects and side effects.* In: Hormone Therapy. Springer. https://doi.org/10.1007/978-1-4614-6268-2_10.

14

Mental-Behavioral Health Screening and Treatment for Women

Laura Thiem

OBJECTIVES

- Identify psychiatric diagnoses commonly found in females.
- Identify screening tools available to screen for common psychiatric disorders in primary care.
- Develop a pharmacotherapeutic plan of care using appropriate interventions based on diagnoses and current evidence.
- Provide patient education related to the plan of care.

INTRODUCTION

Female patients with mental health symptoms frequently present to the primary care setting for initial evaluation. Physical and mental health are intrinsically tied, and the advanced practice provider cannot separate one from the other in patient interaction. Failure to recognize mental health symptoms in the primary care setting can be detrimental to a patient's overall well-being.

Epidemiological data reveals that 40% of Americans who completed suicide visited their primary care provider within 24 hours before completion of the suicide.[1] The question of whether the patients were assessed for depression, anxiety, or suicide risk during their primary care visit was unknown.[1] The primary care provider plays a critical role in the early identification and treatment of depression.[2] Patients may experience delays of longer than one week to be seen by a behavioral health provider because of a national lack of access to mental health services.[3]

During the Coronavirus (COVID-19) pandemic, depression and anxiety increased, especially in females and adolescents.[4] The greatest number of patients with depression and anxiety were in the 15- to 20-year-old demographic.[4] An additional 53.2 million individuals were diagnosed with major depression caused by the pandemic over the baseline of previous years. Anxiety

disorders increased by 76.2 million over baseline.[4] Mental health services, already strained before the pandemic, were further limited by lockdowns and quarantines. Many providers shifted to telehealth to provide services that may have been covered by insurers, allowing them to continue to provide care to patients.[5]

The National Institute of Mental Health (NIMH) funded the Sequenced Treatment Alternatives to Relieve Depression (STAR*D) study to determine the patient response to various treatments of major depression.[6] Patients are likely to achieve remission from depressive symptoms within the first two steps of the STAR*D algorithm.[6] Primary care providers reported time constraints; conflicting priorities; inadequate preparation for screening, diagnosis, and treatment of mental health disorders; and avoidance of mental health topics as reasons for low rates of mental health diagnosis in practice.[7]

Patients with depression can be three times more likely to be nonadherent to a treatment plan for other illnesses as noted in a meta-analysis performed by DiMatteo et al.[8] In another meta-analysis, Grenard et al.[9] identified that patients with a diagnosis of depression were 1.76 times more likely not to take prescription medications as directed for comorbid chronic illnesses. Adams and Folds[10] recognized a correlation between self-efficacy and adherence in diabetes care and depression. As depressive symptoms increased, self-efficacy and

275

adherence to the recommended treatment decreased. In females with comorbid depression and type 2 diabetes, the risk of mortality is 2.5 times higher than females who have either disease process alone.[11,12]

The physiology of females differs from their male counterparts, therefore knowledge is required to navigate the complexities of mental health diagnosis and treatment. Mental illness is often a combination of genetic predisposition, environmental effects, or biochemical imbalances.[13] The effects of hormones (primarily estrogen) during puberty, menstruation, the perinatal period, the postpartum period, and menopause affect the neurotransmitters responsible for cognition and memory.[14,15] Genetic predisposition can also contribute to mental health disorders.[15] The effects of stress from the home, work, and social environments contribute to difficulties maintaining mental wellness. Females were excluded from medical and behavioral health research studies until 1991.[16] The primary care Advance Practice Registered Nurse (APRN) must have an understanding of these intricacies to screen, diagnose, and provide treatment for female patients with mental health symptoms.

The Anatomy and Physiology of the Brain and Mental Health

The basic conduction of the brain includes the neurons and synapses (Fig. 14.1). Physiologically, electrical impulse transmission occurs as chemical communication through the action of the neurotransmitters including dopamine, serotonin, acetylcholine, norepinephrine, glutamate, and GABA. Additional neuromodulators, transmitters, and hormones affecting brain chemistry include histamine, estrogen, testosterone, and progesterone. The neurotransmitters exist in the synaptic areas and move to the neuron neuroreceptors during electrical transmission.[15]

The chemical activity and electrical transmission vary. Some transmission is linear in which the pre-synaptic neuron signals to the post-synaptic neuron. Some transmission is retrograde in which the post-synaptic neuron signals back to the pre-synaptic neuron. Another form of transmission does not require synaptic activity; transmission arises from volume-dependent transfusion.[15] A cascading effect is created by the simpler neurotransmissions as the neurotransmitters combine or fit with other proteins at the cellular level. Eventually, the cascade can result in alterations in genetic code expressions. This alteration is thought to be the basis of many psychiatric disease processes. Subsequently, treatment is directed at the neurotransmitters and neuroreceptors early in the cascade.[15]

Within the brain, many different areas are responsible for cognition, executive function, mood, anxiety, craving, satiety, and memories. The prefrontal cortex is responsible for concentration, executive function, attention, mood, and self-esteem. Another area responsible for mood is the amygdala, which also controls memory, emotion, feelings of reward, guilt, and self-esteem. The hypothalamus directs the necessities for survival including food and rest. The nucleus accumbens affects pleasure, energy, and fatigue.[15]

The reward pathway of the dopaminergic/cortical/limbic systems is activated in substance use and gambling. Reward conditioning and memory of the pleasure obtained from the substance occur in the limbic region including the amygdala and hippocampus. Alteration of the reward system contributes to craving and the neglect of normal needs including food, sleep, and self-care in pursuit of the substance or activity.[15,17]

Presently the technology is not available to measure the neurotransmitters directly. Positron emission topography (PET) scanning has been used to identify brain activities, primarily circulation, and glucose metabolism in response to medications and other interventions. The use of PET scanning for psychiatric consideration remains investigational.[17]

Pharmacogenomics is testing of the individual's genetic response to various medications or substances. The results offer the prescriber additional information regarding an individual's body processes and medication metabolism. The prescriber can use genomic testing in patients who have unexpected or poor responses to medications. Pharmacogenomics reduce the trial-and-error approach to prescribing for most disease processes in addition to psychiatric uses.[17]

The Prevalence of Diagnoses

The Global Burden of Disease Study 2013 identified that approximately 25% of patients with chronic illness have comorbid psychiatric/mental health illnesses.[18] The impact is exemplified with two calculations: Years Lived with Disability (YDL) and Disability-Adjusted Life Years (DALY). YDL are calculated by multiplying the prevalence of a disorder

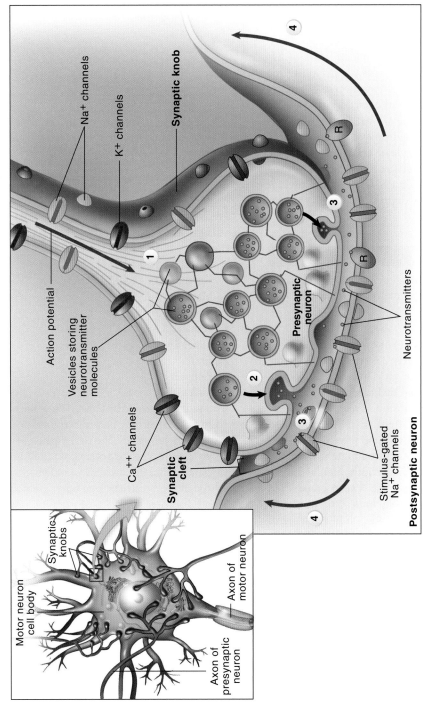

Figure 14.1 Neuronal transmission and the synaptic cleft. Details illustrate the synaptic knob of a pre-synaptic neuron, the plasma membrane of a postsynaptic neuron, and a synaptic cleft. (1) Action potential arrives at the synaptic knob. (2) Rapid exocytosis of neurotransmitter molecules from vesicles in the knob occurs. (3) The neurotransmitter diffuses into the synaptic cleft and binds to the receptor molecules (R) in the plasma membrane of the postsynaptic neuron. The postsynaptic receptors directly or indirectly trigger the opening of stimulus-gated ion channels, initiating a local potential in the postsynaptic neuron. (4) The local potential may move toward the axon, where an action potential may begin. (From Patton KT. *Anatomy and Physiology*. 10th ed. St. Louis, Mosby; 2019.)

by the short- or long-term loss of health associated with the disability (disability weight). Using this formula, the Global Burden of Disease Study 2019 reported that psychiatric disorders are second to musculoskeletal disorders US YDL at 11%.[19] DALY are calculated by adding the number of years of life lost to the number of years lived with disability for a certain disease or disorder. Psychiatric disorders were second to musculoskeletal disorders at 8%. This is an improvement from the Global Burden of Disease 2013 study in which neuropsychiatric disorders combined were reported to lead US DALY at 18.6% with mental health disorders at 13.6%, while neurological disorders were only 5.1%. Of all of the mental health diagnoses observed, depressive disorders led at approximately 2.5%.[19]

NOT TO BE MISSED

Approximately 25% of patients with chronic illness have comorbid psychiatric/mental health illnesses.

According to the National Survey on Drug Use and Health, in 2019 approximately 25% of the U.S. female population responded that they had a diagnosable mental health condition that included mood, anxiety, eating, impulse control, substance use, and adjustment disorders.[20] Autism, attention-deficit disorder, schizophrenia, substance use, and psychotic disorders were excluded. In 2019, approximately 7% of the U.S. female population had a serious mental illness that was so debilitating that they were considered disabled.[20] The assessments include U.S. noninstitutionalized civilian residents older than 18 years of age with a permanent residence. Members of the military, homeless individuals, transient individuals, and institutionalized patients were not represented in the survey. Additionally, the response rate was approximately 65%. The potential exists that individuals with mental illness may be underrepresented.

The lifetime prevalence of anxiety disorders in the U.S. population is approximately 31% of the U.S. population.[21] Of those persons diagnosed with anxiety, 22.8% suffered serious impairment, and 33.7% had moderate impairment.[21] The approximate lifetime prevalence for specific disorders not delineated by sex in the United States can be found in Box 14.1.

BOX 14.1   Lifetime Prevalence for Specific Disorders in the United States[22]

- Agoraphobia: 1.3%
- Generalized anxiety disorder: 5.7%
- Obsessive compulsive disorder: 2.3%
- Panic disorder: 4.7%
- Posttraumatic stress disorder (PTSD): 6.8%
- Social phobia: 12.2%
- Specific phobia: 12.5%
- Attention deficit disorder: 8.7%
- Persistent depressive disorder (dysthymic disorder): 2.5%
- Bipolar disorder: 4.4%

Females have a higher prevalence of eating disorder diagnosis. In 2012, Kessler et al. reported the following[22]:

- Anorexia nervosa
  - Females 1%
  - Males 0.3%
- Binge eating disorder
  - Females 3.5%
  - Males 2%
- Bulimia
  - Females 0.5%
  - Males 0.1%

In a study performed by Dove, 87% of the females surveyed indicate that they had uncertainty or displeasure with their appearance.[23] The participants also reported low body esteem (feeling good about their body). Study participants indicated that they would put their health at risk through food restriction or other methods.

Mood disorders affect 9% of the adult population in the United States.[22] Over their lifetime, females are 50% more likely to be diagnosed with a mood disorder than males.[22] In the 2019 National Survey on Drug Use and Health, 9.6% of females reported having a major depressive episode in the past year.[20.]

The Substance Abuse and Mental Health Services Administration (SAMHSA) revealed that nearly 18% of females in the United States reported use of an illegal drug, marijuana, or misused prescription medication in the previous year.[24] Specifically, over 3% of females admitted to misusing prescription drugs according to the same study. According to the U.S. Centers for Disease Control and Prevention (CDC), a female patient presents to the emergency department every 3 minutes for prescription pain medication overdose. Death from prescription pain medication overdose in females has increased by 400% since 1999. In the same time frame, the overdose rate for males only increased 265%.[25]

Substance use in the perinatal period puts the mother and fetus at risk. The mother is at increased peril of hypertensive crisis, seizure, or death from sudden withdrawal or use during pregnancy.[26] The infant may experience neonatal abstinence syndrome (NAS) after delivery because of the mother's substance use during pregnancy. NAS may result in low birth weight, respiratory problems, and prolonged hospitalization.[27] Infants with NAS increased 300% between 2000 and 2013.[27]

In 2020, 11% of females in the United States were current cigarette smokers.[29] The CDC reports that 1.8% of females in the United States use smokeless tobacco products.[28] Smoking remains the leading cause of preventable morbidity and mortality in the United States.[29]

Although malingering is not considered a psychiatric disease process with pathophysiology, the APRN provider is likely to encounter malingering in practice. Malingering is a deliberate attempt to accomplish an external incentive by exaggerated symptoms of physical or mental disease. External incentives may include remuneration; avoidance of military service, jury duty, or employment activities; or acquisition of prescription medications. Nearly one-half of Social Security disability examinations are attributable to feigned illness.[30]

History and Subjective Data

Collecting a complete history is critical to identification and diagnosis of mental health disorders in female patients. Initial assessment of the patient's health literacy offers the clinician the opportunity to alter the interaction to meet the literacy needs of the patient.[31] A mnemonic such as OLDCARTS can be used to explore *o*nset, *l*ocation, *d*uration, *a*ggravating factors, *r*elieving factors, *t*iming, and *s*everity. This mnemonic can help identify key information to assist with diagnosis and identify past medical diagnoses that may have a higher incidence of comorbid mental health conditions, such as cardiovascular disease, diabetes mellitus, chronic pain, or a history of myocardial infarction or stroke.[32]

The clinician should inquire if the patient has a personal or family history of mental health diagnosis. Mental disorders have a genetic predisposition, and this information may be helpful in the diagnosis process.[13]

The use of broad general screening questions can guide the clinician toward the need for additional evaluation. Patient-centered care permits patients to guide their care and select which questions they will answer. Assure patients that these questions are asked of every patient, and give them the opportunity to decline.[32] Culture affects the patient's experience and interaction with the clinician. Requesting clarification or explanation of terms or traditions with which the clinician is unfamiliar can improve the relationship and communication between the patient and clinician. If the clinician is not fluent in the patient's language, an appropriate interpreter must be provided and utilized.[31]

> **PATIENT-CENTERED CARE:** Use general screening questions, and allow patients to guide their care by selecting the questions they will answer. Terms or traditions of a culture that the clinician is unfamiliar with should be clarified to facilitate a positive relationship and enhance communication. Always use an interpreter when a language barrier exists.

The clinician should inquire about a history of trauma. Females who have experienced or witnessed trauma, violence, or abuse are likely to have anxiety, depression, eating disorders, sleep disorders, or substance use.[33-35] Medical settings can be difficult for patients with a history of trauma because of personal questions, removal of clothing, invasive procedures, vulnerable body positions, physical touch, gender of the clinician, and perceived power differential between the patient and clinician.[36] Awareness of the patient's trauma experience can help the clinician avoid retraumatizing the patient inadvertently and guide to potential comorbid disorders and treatment.[35]

> **CLINICAL SURVIVAL TIP** Providing effective care and improving patient engagement and treatment adherence for patients affected by trauma requires the clinician to use a trauma-informed care approach. To learn more about implementing trauma-informed care into practice, visit www.samhsa.gov/sites/default/files/programs_campaigns/childrens_mental_health/atc-whitepaper-040616.pdf.

Obtain information about military service. Veterans have an increased risk of mental health disorders including depression, posttraumatic stress disorder

(PTSD), and substance use compared with civilians.[37] Patients with military service may also have a higher risk of interpersonal violence, sexual assault, or abuse than civilians.[38]

Adolescent female patients frequently present to the primary care practice with somatic complaints rather than seeking care for mood or anxiety.[39] Adolescents in the United States who are 13 to 18 years of age have an estimated 49.5% lifetime prevalence of mental health disorder of any type.[40] Of the adolescents diagnosed with anxiety, only one-third of children and adolescents were being treated within the previous year.[41] Adolescents have a 25% lifetime prevalence of anxiety and 14% lifetime prevalence of mood disorder.[41] Diagnosed mental illness in adolescents remains undertreated. Preston et al.[42] identified that only one-half of the patients were receiving treatment for a diagnosed mental health disorder.

Older adult patients may present with somatic complaints of fatigue and pain instead of mood or anxiety symptoms.[43] The prevalence of mental health diagnoses in older adults is significant. In 2015, Reynolds et al. reported that 11% of older adults experienced anxiety, 6% suffered with mood disorders, and nearly 4% had substance use disorders in the previous year.[44] Females were more likely to be diagnosed with depression and anxiety.[44]

For patients with known psychiatric disorders, a review of the symptoms assists the primary care APRN to collaborate with the psychiatric provider. The patient can be screened for efficacy or adverse effects of medications and treatment including akathisia (motor restlessness), tardive dyskinesia (abnormal, involuntary muscle movement), or neuroleptic malignant syndrome. New or changing symptoms can be discovered requiring urgent evaluation to rule out additional disease processes.

Depression

The U.S. Preventive Services Task Force (USPSTF) recommends screening adults for depression.[45] The Personal Health Questionnaire-2 (PHQ-2) is a two-question screening tool.[46] The patient is asked to select one of the following to quantify their symptoms:
- Not at all = 0
- Several days = 1
- More than half the days = 2
- Nearly every day = 3

The screening questions are as follows:

In the past 2 weeks, have you been bothered by any of the following problems:
- Little interest or pleasure in doing things
- Feeling down, depressed, or hopeless

With a potential score ranging between 0 and 6, a score of 3 or higher indicates the need for additional screening. Varieties of screening instruments are available and may exist in an electronic health record. The clinician can select a tool based on preference, ease of use, or availability with the knowledge that the available tools range between 80% and 90% sensitivity and 70% and 85% specificity.[32]

Manic Symptoms

Additional inquiry during the history can reveal symptoms of mania, one aspect of bipolar disorder. The mnemonic DIG FAST identifies the principal symptoms of mania. These symptoms include *d*istractibility, *i*ndiscretion, *g*randiosity, *f*light of ideas, *a*ctivity increase, *s*leep deficit, and *t*alkativeness.[47] *Indiscretion* is further defined as excessive involvement in pleasurable activities such as sex, spending, or gambling. Sleep deficit presents as a decreased need for sleep.[47]

Female patients with bipolar disorder are more likely to present for an episode of depression. Males are more likely to present for care with an episode of mania. Screening for manic symptomology assists the clinician in identification of bipolar disorder. Bipolar mania may be activated if an antidepressant medication has been prescribed to a patient with unrecognized bipolar disorder.[15]

Grief

Inquire about recent losses. Commonly grief is associated with bereavement (loss of a loved one), but grief encompasses any significant loss. These losses can include employment, financial stability, health, physical function, pets, or items of significance. The clinician should determine the length of time since the loss, the impact of the loss on daily function, and coping mechanisms the patient is using. Symptoms of grief are similar to symptoms of depression and anxiety. The patient may not make the correlation between the symptoms and the loss. *Anticipatory grief* may begin before a loss occurs, as in terminal illness or injury. *Complicated grief* occurs when symptoms continue over an extended period or are interfering with daily needs and activities.[48]

Anxiety

The clinician can screen for anxiety by inquiring about the patient having anxiety or panic attacks. The question "Do you have anxiety or panic attacks?" helps the clinician discern between anxiety and panic. Questioning if the patient has had to limit activities as a result of anxiety helps determine the level of impairment and if the patient may have agoraphobia.[47] Screening tools for anxiety include the Generalized Anxiety Disorder (GAD-7) scale. This scale is a seven-question review of anxiety symptoms.[49] An assessment tool is also available at https://adaa.org/sites/default/files/GAD-7_Anxiety-updated_0.pdf.

Eating Disorders

Examining the patient's perception of weight can assist the clinician in uncovering an eating disorder. If the question, "Have you ever felt that you are overweight?" is answered with a definitive "No," an eating disorder is unlikely. If the answer is affirmative, additional questions about dieting, restrictive eating, laxative use, or purging are indicated.[47]

Substance Use/Medication Misuse

Because of the prevalence of substance use/medication abuse, patients should be assessed for use of illegal substances, alcohol intake, marijuana use, tobacco use, misuse of their own prescription medication, and use of prescription medication prescribed to others. The clinician should offer reassurance that these questions are asked of all patients. The use of open-ended questions versus a "yes/no" question may elicit more information. An example of an open-ended question such as, "Tell me about how much alcohol you've taken in this week" invites the patient to share as well as quantify the intake for the clinician. Similar questions can be used for all substances. Alternatively, formal screening tools such as the CAGE Questionnaire, AUDIT, BMAST, TWEAK, and RAPS with variable sensitivity and specificity can be used[50] (Box 14.2).

The Substance Use Brief Screen (SUBS) questionnaire is a four-item tool developed to screen for use of all substances in the primary care setting. The sensitivity and specificity for identifying unhealthy substance use were 97.8% and 95.7%, respectively. A limitation of the tool is that it was developed to be delivered using a computer or electronic device versus paper and pencil.[51]

BOX 14.2 CAGE Substance Abuse Screening Tool

Directions: Ask your patients these four questions, and use the scoring method described below to determine if substance abuse exists and needs to be addressed.

CAGE Questions
1. Have you ever felt you should cut down on your drinking?
2. Have people annoyed you by criticizing your drinking?
3. Have you ever felt bad or guilty about your drinking?
4. Have you ever had a drink first thing in the morning to steady your nerves or to get rid of a hangover (eye-opener)?

Case Questions Adapted to Include Drug Use (CAGE-AID)
1. Have you ever felt you ought to cut down on your drinking or drug use?
2. Have people annoyed you by criticizing your drinking or drug use?
3. Have you ever felt bad or guilty about your drinking or drug use?
4. Have you ever had a drink or used drugs first thing in the morning to steady your nerves or to get rid of a hangover (eye-opener)?

Brown RL, Leonard T, Saunders LA. Papasouliotis O. The prevalence and detection of substance use disorder among inpatients ages 18 to 49: An opportunity for prevention. *Preventive Medicine.* 1998;27:101–110.

Thoughts of Suicide, Self-Harm, or Threat to Others

Investigation into thoughts of self-harm, suicide, or homicide is needed for the patient who presents with mental health symptoms or makes indirect statements such as, "Life isn't worthwhile." The clinician should ask, "Have you had thoughts of hurting yourself or someone else?" as a direct question. If the answer is affirmative, the clinician must assess for a plan and whether the patient has the means to attempt or complete the plan; evaluate the lethality of the plan; and assess the resources the patient may have available to provide safety and support. Patients who have previous suicide attempts, substance use, impulsivity, or anxiety are at increased risk for death from suicide and may require emergency department evaluation or hospitalization.[52]

Psychosis

Psychotic symptoms such as bizarre thoughts, responding to hallucinations, or delusions may be evident during the interview. Patients with psychosis may appear guarded, paranoid, or suspicious. Psychosis may be a symptom of depression, bipolar disorder, substance use, schizophrenia, or neurocognitive disorders (dementia).[47] Psychotic thought processes warrant hospitalization or an immediate consult with a psychiatric provider such as a psychiatrist or psychiatric mental health nurse practitioner.

The clinician may inquire about voices the patient hears that others do not hear or things the patient sees that no one else sees. Hallucinations may also include sensations on the body that others cannot see, such as reporting insects on or in the skin. Delusions are a strongly held belief that is disproved by evidence, yet the patient cannot be dissuaded. For example, the patient may believe that the U.S. president has invited them to lunch at the White House today and has sent a private plane to the patient's home to transport the patient. It is important to carefully assess the evidence that supports or refutes the claim. The clinician can include additional historians for corroboration if available with patient permission.[17]

Cognitive Deficits

A brief assessment of cognition can be performed during the history. The clinician should ask the patient to state the date and current location. The patient is then instructed to repeat three words such as *trust, blue,* and *pencil.* Then the clinician advises the patient that they will be asked to recall these words after a few more questions. The patient is asked to provide information about a prominent public figure from the past, such as a president. The clinician then requests that the patient repeat the three words. Additional cognitive testing is indicated if the patient cannot correctly identify the date or place, recall at least two of the three words, or provide historical information.[47]

Malingering

Malingering, an exaggerated or feigned illness, may be indicated by any of the following examples. The symptoms reported by the patient seem exaggerated and do not correlate with the physical presentation. Additionally, the patient may report involvement in legal proceedings seeking compensation for injury or illness. The patient may also be uncooperative or impatient with the interview, examination, or treatment plan. If the patient has a diagnosis of antisocial personality disorder, malingering may be likely. Although these criteria may indicate malingering, the criteria may also be applicable to many other mental health disorders.[53] A consultation with a behavioral health provider who can perform additional testing should be arranged.

Adolescent Tools

Many of the tools available for adults have not been validated for used with adolescents. The clinician may want to utilize alternative tools to screen for depression, anxiety, attention-deficit disorder, or social difficulties. The PHQ-2 and PHQ-9 have a revision appropriate for use with adolescents. Other tools include the HEEADSSS Psychosocial Interview for Adolescents, the Pediatric Symptom Checklist 17 or 35 questions, Strengths and Difficulties Questionnaire, Kutcher Adolescent Depression Scale, Kutcher Generalized Social Anxiety Scale, CRAFFT, and SAD-Persons. As with the adult tools, the sensitivity and specificity vary with the tool.[54] The CRAFFT questionnaire is available at https://crafft.org/.

Review of Systems

The review of systems provides the opportunity to review past and current symptoms or disease processes. Using a systematic approach, the clinician can inquire about symptoms that may assist in the diagnostic process. Body systems to be reviewed include the general state of health, integumentary, head/ears/nose/throat, respiratory, cardiovascular, gastrointestinal, urogenital, musculoskeletal, neurological, and endocrine. Symptoms presented in the review of systems may also indicate other disorders that will need to be investigated.[49]

Physical Examination

The physical examination permits the clinician to investigate symptoms discovered in the reason for visit, history, and review of systems. Examining areas of concern to the patient and those of importance to the clinician will assist with diagnostic reasoning.[49] The use of physical examination helps the clinician test the hypothesis of probable diagnosis for coherence, adequacy, parsimony, diagnostic probability, and elimination of competing hypotheses.[32]

Metrics

Measurement of temperature, blood pressure, respirations, pulse oximetry, height, weight, and body mass index (BMI) should be performed with each visit. These recorded measures can validate other physical findings or patient symptoms and can indicate comorbid disorders. The record of vital signs offers the clinician the opportunity to observe changes occurring with medications or interventions.[49]

General Appearance

Observe gait and muscle movement. Inability to sit without fidgeting may be an indicator of anxiety, substance use, or akathisia. Slowed movements may occur with depression or neurocognitive disorders. Unusual posturing may be a symptom of schizophrenia.[49]

Evaluate body posture and position. Slumped posture may indicate depression or organic brain disease. Guarded, rigid posture, tightly folded arms, or tense muscles may indicate anxiety, thyroid disease, or past trauma.[35,49]

Note the patient's grooming and clothing. Neglect of grooming may indicate depression, mania, or organic brain syndrome. Odd clothing combinations, excessive cosmetics, or clothing inappropriate to season and setting may be indicative of mania or schizophrenia.[49] Clothing that fully covers all extremities may be an attempt to cover injection sites in the patient who injects substances.

Behavior

Note the patient's level of consciousness. The expected findings are that the patient is alert and aware of the setting and environment and responds to questions or stimuli within a reasonable time frame. Drowsiness, falling asleep, or inability to follow a conversation may indicate brain disease, medication effects, or substance use.[17,49]

Observe the patient's facial expressions and affect. Eye contact is expected to be comfortable for the patient and clinician. Avoidance of eye contact can be culturally appropriate. A full range of facial expression appropriate to setting and questions is anticipated. Lack of facial expression can occur in depression, parkinsonism, trauma history, or advanced neurocognitive disorders.[36,49] A minimal or fixed facial expression can be attempted to mimic psychiatric disorders in malingering.[55]

Speech should be conversational, clear, and even-paced. Difficulty selecting words or incorrectly selecting words may be an indication of aphasia or apraxia. Struggles with pronunciation, enunciation, or verbalization can indicate a neurological disorder or problems with the pharynx. Slow speech may be present in depression, trauma history, or parkinsonism.[36,49] Rapid, pressured speech can be a sign of mania, stimulant use, or distress from trauma history.[36,49]

Mood

Mood is evaluated by direct questioning as well as observation. Use of the PHQ-2 and DIG FAST or similar tools offer the clinician consistent screening methods. As noted earlier, surveillance of the patient's affect, body position, and speech may also contribute to the assessment of mood.[49] Altered mood is significant to mood disorders as well as a symptom of other diseases or side effects of medications.

Cognition

Expected findings include the patient being able to identify the date and location/setting. The patient should be able to recall three or four unrelated words after 5 minutes. The ability to follow a sequence of commands is also anticipated as a normal finding. Remote memory is intact if the patient can describe historical persons. Caution must be used to determine that the historical figure is appropriate to the patient's age and culture.[49] Alterations in cognition can be symptomatic of delirium, neurocognitive disorders, or substance use disorders.[49] Impaired cognition may also be a symptom of trauma history.[36]

Thought Processes and Content

The patient's thoughts and communication should be logical, coherent, and relevant to the setting, interview, and examination.[49] Content that is not pertinent, consistent, or coherent may indicate delirium, delusions, or neurocognitive disorders. A deliberate cessation of stream of thought, called *thought blocking,* may indicate psychosis or schizophrenia.[36,49] In addition to thought blocking, patients with abnormal thought processes may display any of the following:

- *Neologism:* Creation of a new word, possibly from a phrase. The meaning of the word is unique to the patient and may not be understood by the clinician.
- *Confabulation:* Creation of information to replace missing details. It can be difficult to identify without external corroboration and is frequently seen in dementia.
- *Circumlocution:* The use of more words than necessary.
- *Loose associations:* A change in topic without recognition that the topic is not related. It is frequently seen in psychosis and schizophrenia.
- *Flight of ideas:* A rapid transition from one topic to another. The topics may be related. It may be seen in mania, schizophrenia, or substance use disorders.

- *Word salad:* A collection of unrelated words lacking grammar or logical thought. It may be seen in neurocognitive disorders, delirium, or schizophrenia.
- *Preservation:* A repeated statement of response, although some of the content may change.
- *Echolalia:* Mimicking of a word or statement. It may be seen in neurocognitive disorders, delirium, and schizophrenia.
- *Clanging:* Rhyming of unrelated words. It is seen in neurocognitive disorders, delirium, and schizophrenia.[49]

Abnormal thought content can include the following:

- *Compulsion:* An unwanted feeling that an act must be performed to prevent or relieve discomfort or to prevent disaster.
- *Obsession:* Intrusive thoughts that are uncomfortable. The patient cannot remove the thoughts through logic.
- *Phobia:* An irrational fear that is strong, persistent, and drives the patient to avoid a stimuli or situation.
- *Delusion:* A strongly held belief that is disproved by evidence, yet the patient cannot be dissuaded from the belief.[49]

Patients presenting for malingering may not be able to replicate the subtleties of abnormal thought processes, especially during an extended, detailed interview and examination.[55] The clinician should record examples of the abnormal thought processes or content verbatim in the medical record.

Patients with personality disorders may present with a pattern of behavior that is different from the cultural standard. The traits persist over time and are apparent with impairment in two of these four areas: cognition, affect, interpersonal function, and impulse control. The onset of personality disorder is usually in adolescence or early adulthood.

Perceptions

Abnormal perceptions can include illusions and hallucinations. Illusions are a misinterpretation of environmental stimuli. Hallucinations include hearing, seeing, or feeling effects that are not verifiable by others. These altered perceptions can indicate neurocognitive disorders, schizophrenia, or substance use or withdrawal.[49]

Neurological Examination

A brief assessment of the cranial nerves, deep tendon reflexes, sensation, muscle strength, and movement offer the provider needed information to support or refute diagnostic hypotheses. The neurological examination provides a baseline for future treatment. Adverse effects of medications may affect the neurological system.[49] Deficits or abnormal findings may be further evaluated with the National Institutes of Health (NIH) Stroke Scale.[56]

Symptom-Specific Physical Examination

Depending on the presenting symptoms and information revealed in the review of systems, additional examination may be indicated. Additional examinations should be limited to the areas of concern. The clinician should explain the necessity yet offer the patient the opportunity to refuse any aspect of the examination.[32,34,49] Examples of additional examinations include the following:

- Cardiac examination for report of palpitations or syncope
- Thyroid examination for anxiety, panic, or palpitations
- Respiratory examination for shortness of breath, anxiety, or panic
- Integumentary examination for abnormal sensations or lesions
- Abdominal examination for nausea or abdominal pain
- Genitourinary examination for pelvic pain or dyspareunia[49]

Examination of additional systems can also identify comorbid disorders or adverse effects of medications.[49]

Pharmacological Interventions

This section will briefly review the diagnoses and hypothetical pathophysiology of each disorder with evidence-based treatments targeted to remission of disease and symptomology. Direct evidence supporting the various hypotheses is not available. The selection of a treatment plan should be individualized based on comorbidities, patient preference, socioeconomic factors, and available resources. In patient-centered care, when the patient selects treatment goals, adherence to the plan is more likely.[32]

Mood Disorders: Depression and Bipolar Disorder

The monoamine neurotransmitter system hypothesis implicates three neurotransmitters in mood disorders. These include dopamine, norepinephrine, and serotonin, also known as the *happy chemical*. When the system is balanced, the mood is euthymic. Alterations in the interactions of these three neurotransmitters are hypothesized to contribute to depression, mania, and dysthymia. The monoamine receptor hypothesis implicates malfunctions of the receptors for the three neurotransmitters. Building on the monoamine neurotransmitter depletion theory, the receptor hypothesis suggests that other postsynaptic neurotransmitters attempt to compensate. Genetic predisposition to mood disorders may lie in the type of serotonin transporters inherited from the patient's ancestors. One type is expressed as resiliency, while the other is expressed as vulnerability to stressors resulting in depressive symptoms.[15]

Medications used to treat mood disorders alter the neurotransmitters, the receptors, or the cascade of neurotransmitter effects. See Box 14.3 for the medication classes discussed here.

In the treatment of depression, the STAR*D trial resulted in an algorithm for use in medication selection.[16] In the algorithm after evaluating for suicidality, comorbidities, substance use, childbearing potential, and potential effects of age treatment is initiated with a selective serotonin reuptake inhibitor (SSRI). The patient is also referred to a mental health provider for therapy. If the patient has not had a complete remission of symptoms with dosage titration and reevaluation at 14 to 16 weeks, the prescriber and patient may elect to change medications to a different SSRI, a norepinephrine-dopamine reuptake inhibitor (NDRI), or a serotonin-norepinephrine reuptake inhibitor (SNRI). Another option is to augment the original SSRI with an NDRI or serotonin partial agonist/reuptake inhibitor (SPARI). Referral to a psychiatric provider is indicated if the patient has a poor response or lack of remission with the first two steps of the algorithm.[57]

NOT TO BE MISSED

Complete remission should occur within 14 to 16 weeks with dosage titration. If it does not, a change in medications or addition of an NDRI or SPARI to the original SSRI can be tried.

CLINICAL SURVIVAL TIP The reader is advised to use current resources as newer agents are introduced, additional research is performed, and side-effect profiles are augmented and reviewed. Additional sources of information include pharmaceutical manufacturers' prescribing information and U.S. Food and Drug Administration (FDA) advisories.

Selective Serotonin Reuptake Inhibitors. The SSRI class is often the first-line agent in the treatment of depression. These medications have similar effects of blocking the transport of unbound serotonin in the synapse into the pre-synaptic neuron, preventing signal transmission from the pre-synaptic neuron. As the transport is blocked, serotonin availability increases for binding with the post-synaptic neuron.[15] The SSRIs with indications for depression include citalopram (Celexa), escitalopram (Lexapro), fluoxetine (Prozac), paroxetine (Paxil), and sertraline (Zoloft).

The SSRIs are inhibitors of the cytochrome P450 (CYP450) pathway, resulting in many interactions with other medications.[15] The prescriber should perform drug reconciliation and monitor for potential drug-drug interactions to reduce the risk of serotonin syndrome. Serotonin syndrome occurs when the brain has excess serotonin resulting from too high of an initial medication dose, increasing the medication dose rapidly, the body's genetic inability to regulate serotonin, or interactions with other prescription medications, over-the-counter medications, or supplements. Initial symptoms include diaphoresis, nausea, and diarrhea. The symptoms can progress to confusion, autonomic and musculoskeletal system disorders, and death. Supportive care is required while the medication is

---

BOX 14.3   Medication Classes Used to Treat Mood Disorders*

- Selective serotonin reuptake inhibitors (SSRIs)
- Serotonin partial agonist/reuptake inhibitors (SPARIs)
- Serotonin-norepinephrine reuptake inhibitors (SNRIs)
- Norepinephrine-dopamine reuptake inhibitor (NDRI): bupropion
- Serotonin antagonist/reuptake inhibitors (SARIs)
- Nonselective norepinephrine-serotonin reuptake inhibitors (NNSRIs)
- Monoamine oxidase inhibitors (MAOIs)
- Mood-stabilizing agents
- Atypical antipsychotic agents

*The intended effects, side effects, and black box warnings will be discussed with each class.

adjusted or withdrawn. The patient may require hospitalization for monitoring and support during agitation and withdrawal.[15]

Withdrawal symptoms can occur if the patient has been taking the SSRI medication consistently for more than 5 weeks. Withdrawal symptoms include irritability, anxiety, altered balance, nightmares, difficulty concentrating, gastrointestinal upset, electric shock sensations, or fatigue. Gradual reduction is recommended over the course of a few weeks.[58,59]

! SAFETY ALERT

In 2004, the FDA issued a black box warning regarding increased risk of suicidality in children and adolescents who were prescribed antidepressant medications or received dosage adjustments. This warning was issued to alert patients and families to monitor for suicidal ideation after starting medication and was published after an increase in suicidal deaths related to initiation of antidepressant medication. The warning was revised in 2007 to include young adults up to 23 years of age. Unintended consequences included fewer children, adolescents, and young adults being diagnosed and treated for depression.[60]

Serotonin Partial Agonist/Reuptake Inhibitors. The SPARIs have partial agonist activity for serotonin 5-HT1. The agents are hypothesized to increase serotonin by several different paths.[15,61] Newer agents include vilazodone (Viibryd) and vortioxetine (Trintellix). The risk profile and warnings for these medications are similar to those in the SSRI class.[62]

Serotonin-Norepinephrine Reuptake Inhibitors. The SNRIs block the reuptake of two neurotransmitters: norepinephrine and serotonin. Blockage of the reuptake increases the availability of both norepinephrine and serotonin in the brain.[15] The medications approved for use in depression include desvenlafaxine (Pristiq), duloxetine (Cymbalta, Drizalma Sprinkle), levomilnacipran (Fetzima), and venlafaxine (Effexor XR, Venbysi XR).[62] The side-effect profiles are similar to the SSRI class but also have added side effects of hypertension and insomnia. The norepinephrine effect increases the lethality of these medications. Careful consideration must be given to use in patients with a history of hypertension, sleep disorders, or suicidal ideation or risk.[15]

Norepinephrine-Dopamine Reuptake Inhibitor

Bupropion. Bupropion is thought to inhibit the neuronal reuptake of norepinephrine and dopamine, subsequently increasing the availability of these two neurotransmitters. Bupropion is the only NDRI available and comes in immediate-release, slow-release (SR), and extended release (XL) formulations. Side effects include tremor, nervousness, dry mouth, and sweating.[15] The medication may interfere with sleep, so the slow-release form should be administered several hours before bedtime, and the extended-release form should be taken only in the daytime. Bupropion may worsen anxiety. The medication is contraindicated in patients with a history of seizures or hepatic dysfunction.[17,62]

Serotonin Antagonist/Reuptake Inhibitors. SARIs block serotonin reuptake as well as the postsynaptic serotonin subtype 5-HT2.[17] The two available SARIs are nefazodone and trazodone. Side effects include sedation, hypotension, and anticholinergic effects. Nefazodone has an FDA-issued black box warning for hepatotoxicity.[62] Because of the side-effect profile, neither drug is considered a first choice for the treatment of depression.[17]

Nonselective Norepinephrine-Serotonin Reuptake Inhibitors. NNSRIs are also known as *tricyclic antidepressants*. This class is no longer considered as a first choice because of the extensive side-effect profile. NNSRIs inhibit the reuptake of norepinephrine and serotonin in the presynaptic areas. Serotonergic, alpha-adrenergic, histaminic, and muscarinic receptors are also blocked. The result is an increase in norepinephrine and serotonin availability to connect to the post-synaptic receptors with the intent of improving mood and sleep.[17] The medications included in the NNSRI class of medication include amitriptyline, amoxapine, clomipramine (Anafranil), desipramine (Norpramin), doxepin, imipramine (Tofranil), mirtazapine (Remeron, Remeron SolTab), nortriptyline (Pamelor), protriptyline), and trimipramine.[62] Side effects include dry mouth, constipation, blurred vision, delirium, and urinary retention.[17]

! SAFETY ALERT

NNSRI overdose can occur with a small quantity of medication. The potential for death is a result of cardiac arrhythmias, hypotension, sedation, or seizures. Avoid prescribing the NNSRI class to patients with suicidal ideation or risk.[17] These medications should also be avoided in patients with a history of arrhythmias, seizures, or prostatic hypertrophy and in older adults because of an increased risk of adverse events.[62-64]

Monoamine Oxidase Inhibitors. Monoamine oxidase inhibitors (MAOIs) act by binding and deactivating the body enzyme monoamine oxidase. Monoamine oxidase degrades the three monoamine neurotransmitters: dopamine, norepinephrine, and serotonin. By removing monoamine oxidase, the monoamine neurotransmitters increase. Strict dietary restrictions are applied when the patient is prescribed an MAOI. Monoamine oxidase is used by the body to detoxify tyramine, another amine. Without monoamine oxidase to regulate tyramine, sudden and severe tachycardia and hypertension can occur and can be life-threatening. Additional side effects include hypotension, insomnia, edema, weight gain, and sexual dysfunction.[17] Symptoms of overdose include agitation, hyperthermia, hypertension, tachycardia, tachypnea, dilated pupils, and hyperactive reflexes.[17] The MAOI class should only be prescribed by a psychiatrist, psychiatric mental health nurse practitioner, or psychiatric mental health clinical nurse specialist.

The primary care provider may encounter patients who are currently prescribed MAOI medications. The MAOIs include isocarboxazid (Marplan), phenelzine (Nardil), Selegiline transdermal (Emsam transdermal), and tranylcypromine (Parnate). Knowledge of tyramine-containing foods such as aged meats, cheese, or foods that are fermented including wine, beer, sauerkraut, and soy sauce is essential in caring for these patients. The primary care provider should be aware of the symptoms of hypertensive crisis and assist the patient in seeking emergency evaluation or hospitalization.[17]

Mood-Stabilizing Agents

Lithium. Lithium has been used for mood stabilization and suicide risk reduction for many years. Side effects include gastrointestinal effects, weight gain, tremor, sedation, altered cognition, and incoordination. Long-term effects include development of thyroid disorders and renal failure.[17] The medication has a narrow therapeutic index requiring frequent laboratory testing for serum lithium levels and renal function.[17] The relatively low expense of the medication is offset with the expense of laboratory testing.

Anticonvulsants. The anticonvulsant class of medications has been used to reduce mania and stabilize mood. The hypotheses of action vary for the different agents. Common anticonvulsant medications used to treat bipolar disorder include carbamazepine, lamotrigine (Lamictal), and valproic acid (Depakote).[62] Side effects of carbamazepine include bone marrow suppression and sedation.[14] Frequent laboratory monitoring of complete blood counts offsets the relative low expense of the medication. Lamotrigine is well tolerated except for the potential for rash and life-threatening Stevens-Johnson syndrome.[17] The side-effect profile of valproic acid includes hair loss, weight gain, and sedation. Valproic acid may also contribute to liver and pancreatic failure as well and menstrual irregularities, polycystic ovarian syndrome, and insulin resistance in females.[17] All three of these medications are contraindicated in pregnancy and reduce the efficacy of oral contraceptives. Consideration must be given to the risk of pregnancy in the female patient of childbearing age.[57]

Second-Generation/Atypical Antipsychotic Agents. Atypical antipsychotic agents have also been used to stabilize mood and/or as adjunct medications in the treatment of depression. The mechanism of action is not known. Studies indicate improved efficacy of atypical antipsychotic agents in the remission of bipolar symptoms over mood-stabilizing medications.[15,16] The atypical or second-generation antipsychotics include aripiprazole (Abilify, Aristada), asenapine (Saphris), brexpiprazole (Rexulti), cariprazine (Vraylar), clozapine (Clozaril, Fazaclo, Versacloz), iloperidone (Fanapt), lumateperone (Caplyta), lurasidone (Latuda), olanzapine (Zyprexa), paliperidone (Invega), quetiapine (Seroquel), risperidone (Perseris, Risperdal), and ziprasidone (Geodon).[62] Many of these medications have varying delivery methods including 12-hour and 24-hour oral preparations or a long-acting injectable preparation. Knowledge of these formulations may assist the clinician with increasing patient satisfaction and compliance.

> **❗ SAFETY ALERT**
>
> All medications in this class have a black box warning regarding increased mortality with use in older adults.

The side effects are specific to each medication. Aripiprazole side effects include nausea, headache, insomnia, tremor, agitation, and akathisia.[57] Asenapine has somnolence and akathisia as side effects.[57] Common side effects for brexpiprazole include weight gain, akathisia, somnolence, restlessness, and tremor.[65] Cariprazine is reported to cause akathisia, insomnia, nausea, constipation, weight gain, and tachycardia.[66] Clozaril has special requirements for prescribing because of black box warnings addressing agranulocytosis, seizures, myocarditis, and other cardiovascular and respiratory adverse events. Other side effects include changes in heart rhythm or blood pressure, gastrointestinal symptoms, hypokinesia/akathisia, and somnolence.[67] Serious side effects of Iloperidone are cardiac arrhythmias, changes in blood counts, severe dysphagia, and hyperprolactinemia.[68] Lumateperone side effects include changes in white blood cell counts or liver function tests, tardive dyskinesia, somnolence, and dry mouth.[69] Lurasidone side effects include somnolence, akathisia, gastrointestinal symptoms, weight gain, and agitation.[70] Olanzapine is often sedating, so evening administration is preferred. Additional side effects include increased appetite and weight gain.[57] Paliperidone side effects include extrapyramidal symptoms (EPS), tachycardia, dyspepsia, weight gain, and somnolence.[71] Risperidone may cause the side effects of hypotension, bradykinesia, akathisia, and agitation. Gradual dosage titration reduces the risk of these side effects.[57] Quetiapine is reported to cause dizziness, weight gain, orthostatic hypotension, and somnolence. At the lower doses, it is sedating; as the dose is increased, the sedation decreases.[57,71] The side effects of ziprasidone include drowsiness, gastrointestinal complaints, and dizziness.[57]

Pimavanserin (Nuplazid) is also classified as an atypical antipsychotic, however this medication is only indicated for psychosis and hallucinations associated with Parkinson's disease. Side effects can include peripheral edema and confusion.[72]

The atypical antipsychotic medications have many potential drug-drug interactions. Medication reconciliation is advised. Consider obtaining a baseline electrocardiogram with each of these medications. Additional considerations include alterations of insulin sensitivity, altered lipid profiles, and prolactinemia. The primary care provider may care for patients taking these medications and may be responsible for monitoring for adverse reactions.[56,62,70]

Anxiety/Panic

The treatment of anxiety and panic disorders utilizes many of the same medications used for mood disorders. There are no large studies of anxiety; several randomized controlled trials indicate efficacy of SSRIs and SNRIs in the treatment of anxiety and panic. The treatment algorithm for anxiety includes screening for specific anxiety disorders and then screening for medical, psychiatric, and substance use comorbidities. With this information, the clinician can select an SSRI or SNRI with an appropriate indication and refer the patient to a mental health provider for counseling. If the patient does not achieve remission or responds poorly, referral to a psychiatric provider is indicated.[6] Please refer to the information provided in the "Mood Disorders: Depression and Bipolar Disorder" section earlier in this chapter as many of the medications also have an indication for anxiety disorders.

Selective Serotonin Reuptake Inhibitors. Fluvoxamine is a medication with an indication for anxiety and obsessive-compulsive disorder but does not have an indication for mood disorder.[62]

Serotonin-Norepinephrine Reuptake Inhibitors. All of the SNRIs listed in the "Mood Disorders: Depression and Bipolar Disorder" section except desvenlafaxine (Pristiq) and levomilnacipran (Fetzima) have indications for anxiety disorders.[62]

Buspirone. Buspirone is a GABA agonist that acts on the 5-HT1A receptor as a partial agonist with an indication for the treatment of anxiety. It has a slow onset and requires dosing two to three times per day. The medication has a low side-effect profile but does have a substance-drug interaction with alcohol.[15]

Benzodiazepines/GABA-ergics. Benzodiazepines act on the chloride ion channel of the GABA-A receptors. This action results in an increase of GABA-A neurotransmission, which, in turn, slows the reactivity of the brain to stimuli.[15] The medications have approved indications to relieve anxiety, provide anterograde amnesia, act as anticonvulsants, provide muscle relaxation, and provide sedation. Short-acting agents include oxazepam, and triazolam (Halcion). Intermediate-acting agents include alprazolam (Xanax), estazolam, lorazepam (Ativan), and temazepam (Restoril). Long-acting agents include chlordiazepoxide, clorazepate (Tranxene), diazepam (Valium), flurazepam, and quazepam (Doral).[15]

The side effects of the benzodiazepine class include dependence, withdrawal symptoms, risk of overdose, and death. The medications can cause respiratory depression and impaired cognitive and motor function. If used for an extended period, the medications must be tapered to reduce the risk of seizures. Hospitalization may be required to monitor and stabilize the patient during reduction and withdrawal.[15]

> **⚠ SAFETY ALERT**
>
> Each of the benzodiazepine medications have a black box warning addressing potential misuse, addiction, abuse, and death from withdrawal or concomitant opioid use.

Antihistamines. The action of antihistamines is antagonism of the histamine 1 receptor site. Many of the antihistamines are not selective to the histamine 1 receptor site and also have effects on the antimuscarinic receptors. The additional antimuscarinic effects are likely responsible for the common side effects including blurred vision, constipation, dry mouth, and sedation.[15] Hydroxyzine has an approved indication for anxiety.[62]

First-Generation Antipsychotics. The first-generation antipsychotic medications are strong dopamine (D_2) antagonists. The medications act in the mesolimbic dopamine pathway.[15] Prochlorperazine has an approved indication for the treatment of anxiety. Common side effects include abnormal muscle movements, neutropenia, sedation, dry mouth, constipation, and urinary retention.[62]

Eating Disorders

Fluoxetine, an SSRI, has an indication for bulimia nervosa, with the most favorable response at 60 mg. The medication is started at 20 mg and increased over several days to the 60-mg dose.[17] No medications have approved use in binge eating disorder. Medications have not proved to be effective in anorexia nervosa.[17]

Substance Use/Medication Misuse

Currently 10 classes of substances are considered in the substance use diagnoses in the *Diagnostic and Statistical Manual of Mental Disorders,* 5th edition *(DSM5).*[53] The substance categories include alcohol, tobacco, cannabis, stimulants, opioids, caffeine, hallucinogens, inhalants, sedatives/hypnotics/anxiolytics, and unknown. Medications used to treat substance use disorders are intended to replace the substance with a less lethal substance; replace the substance while new habits or rewards are created; produce aversion to the substance; or support the patient during withdrawal.[15] The primary care APRN may prescribe these medications or encounter the medications in the care of patients with comorbidities and substance use disorders. This section will focus on the specific substances and corresponding medications used in treatment.

Alcohol. Medications used to create an aversion or interrupt the reward of alcohol in the brain include acamprosate, disulfiram, and naltrexone (ReVia, Vivitrol). Side effects of acamprosate include depression and suicidality, nausea, dizziness, and gastrointestinal complaints. Adverse effects of disulfiram include severe nausea and vomiting with alcohol use, psychosis, hepatotoxicity, neuropathy, and optic neuritis. A common complaint with disulfiram use is a metallic taste. Naltrexone has serious side effects including suicidality, depression, and hepatotoxicity. The patient should be screened or tested for opioid use before initiation of the medication. Common side effects include insomnia, gastrointestinal complaints, headache, myalgia, and loss of appetite.[62]

The benzodiazepine class of medication may be used in support of alcohol withdrawal in the inpatient setting to reduce the risk of seizure activity. Diazepam (Valium) has an approved use for treatment of alcohol withdrawal.[62]

Tobacco

Nicotine Replacement. Nicotine replacement permits the gradual reduction of nicotine content to zero over time. The current forms of nicotine replacement include gum, inhaler, lozenges, mini-lozenges, nasal spray, and transdermal patches. The gum, lozenges, and transdermal patches are available over the counter. The Nicotrol inhaler and Nicotrol nasal spray require a prescription.[75] Side effects include nausea, vomiting, and headache if the products are used incorrectly or in conjunction with tobacco products. Local irritation of the skin can occur with the transdermal patches. Irritation of the mucous membranes of the mouth may happen with the gum and lozenges. Nasal and ocular symptoms may occur with the nasal spray. Cough, dyspepsia, and irritation of the mouth and throat occur with the inhaled form.[75] None of the current nicotine replacement products have an approved indication for smokeless tobacco cessation.

Bupropion. The mechanism of action for bupropion in smoking cessation is not known. A combination of bupropion and the transdermal nicotine patch is reported to be more successful than the patch alone. The use of bupropion in smoking cessation should be evaluated periodically. If the patient has not made a significant reduction in smoking by the seventh week, bupropion should be discontinued.[75]

Nicotinic Receptor Partial Agonists. Varenicline (Chantix) decreases nicotine binding to the nicotine receptors. This action reduces dopaminergic pleasure and reward for smoking. Side effects include nausea, insomnia, headaches, and nightmares. Suicidal ideation and action; altered behavior; depressed mood; and agitation have occurred in some patients. The medication should be used with caution in patients with a known psychiatric diagnosis.[75]

Cannabis. Currently, there are no medications approved for use in cannabis use disorder.[76] Research is ongoing, with a focus on medications that improve the common complaints of impaired sleep and cognitive function. Screening for comorbidities and subsequent treatment is indicated.[77]

Stimulants. There are no medications approved for current use in stimulant use disorders.[78] Research continues, with a focus on medications that affect the dopamine and norepinephrine neurotransmitters. Screening for comorbid disorders is warranted.[77]

Opioids. Opioid receptor antagonists are used in combination with therapy or counseling to reduce the risk of relapse in opioid use disorder. The medications naltrexone (ReVia, Vivitrol) and buprenorphine (Probuphine) or the buprenorphine/naltrexone (Suboxone) combination medication bind to the opioid receptors without activating the receptors. This reduces the reward and craving effects of the opioid substances. Naloxone is used to reverse opioid overdose. Side effects include severe opioid withdrawal, seizures, cardiac arrest, gastrointestinal complaints, and shortness of breath. Methadone is substituted for abused substances including heroin in approved detoxification programs. Side effects include hypotension, respiratory depression, cardiac arrhythmias, and bradycardia. Overdose or concurrent intake of opioid agonists can result in cardiac arrest, respiratory arrest, and death.[17]

Caffeine, Hallucinogens, and Inhalants. No medications are approved for use in the treatment of substance use disorders involving caffeine, hallucinogens, or inhalants.

Sedatives/Hypnotics/Anxiolytics. No medications are approved for use in the treatment of sedative, hypnotic, or anxiolytic withdrawal. The preferred method of cessation is a gradual reduction over an extended period.[17]

Grief

There is limited evidence regarding the use of pharmacotherapeutics in the treatment of grief. Complicated grief has recently been recognized with diagnostic criteria. Patients with complicated or prolonged grief should be screened for other disorders. A trial of an SSRI in conjunction with therapy or counseling may be beneficial.[79] No SSRIs have an approved use in the treatment of grief.

Psychosis/Schizophrenia

Immediate intervention is indicated for acute psychosis. Acute schizophrenia may present as severe agitation. Psychosis may also be the result of a manic episode or substance use. Hospitalization may be required to stabilize and monitor the patient.[17] After the patient is stabilized and psychotic symptoms are in remission, the patient may continue on long-term therapy. The medications used for maintenance require monitoring and screening for adverse effects.[17]

First-Generation Antipsychotics. The first-generation antipsychotics include chlorpromazine, fluphenazine, haloperidol, loxapine molindone, perphenazine, prochlorperazine, thioridazine, thiothixene, and trifluoperazine. Common side effects include hypotension, sedation, and anticholinergic effects. At higher doses or potency, the patient will commonly experience EPS, which include akathisia, dyskinesia, dystonia, and pseudoparkinsonism. EPS are treated by changing agents or administering anticholinergic medications (discussed later in this section).[17]

Second-Generation/Atypical Antipsychotic Agents. In addition to the agents discussed earlier in the "Mood Disorders: Depression and Bipolar Disorder" section, clozapine (Clozaril, FazaClo, Versacloz), iloperidone (Fanapt), and paliperidone (Invega) have an indication for schizophrenia and psychosis. Clozapine is restricted for use in patients who have responded poorly to other medications. Registry is required for pharmacies, prescribers, and patients. Clozapine has a high risk of neutropenia and requires frequent blood counts to monitor for this adverse effect.[17]

Antihistamines. Diphenhydramine (Benadryl) has an indication for reversal of the dystonic side effects of antipsychotic medications.[62] Common side effects include drowsiness and dry mouth.

Acetylcholine/Histamine Receptor Antagonists. Commonly known as *anti-parkinson medications*, this class of medication includes benztropine, carbidopa/levodopa (Sinemet), and trihexyphenidyl. The medications are used to reduce or eliminate the EPS caused by the antipsychotic medications. Common side effects include dry mouth, constipation, blurred vision, and memory loss.[15] Bromocriptine is used as an intervention for neuroleptic malignant syndrome.[15]

Nonpharmacological Interventions

Electroconvulsive therapy (ECT) is used in patients who have poor response to or have failed pharmacotherapies. The mechanism of action with the induction of seizures is downregulation of the post-synaptic beta-adrenergic receptors. ECT is indicated for major depressive disorder, mania, and acute exacerbation of schizophrenia. Regulations and availability vary by state.[15]

Brain stimulation to purposefully alter neuronal firing through the use of magnetic fields or electrical current is also used. These modalities include ECT, transcranial magnetic stimulation, transcranial direct current stimulation, and cranial electrical stimulation. The prolonged effects intend to improve synaptic efficiency and modulate cortical excitability and connectivity. The efficacy varies, with ECT remaining the gold standard. Regulations and availability depend on the state.[15]

Various modalities of counseling and therapy offer significant support in specific mental health disorders. Cognitive behavioral therapy is recommended for mood disorders, anxiety, and schizophrenia. Eye movement desensitization and reprocessing (EMDR) therapy has shown improvement in PTSD symptoms (Fig. 14.2). Family and marital therapies can improve interpersonal communication in the family unit or marital couple. Personality disorders may require dialectical behavioral therapy or psychotherapy.[15]

The APRN provider must have comprehensive knowledge of counseling professionals to ensure appropriate referral and collaboration. Psychologists are prepared at the doctoral level to provide psychological evaluation and diagnosis using a variety of validated tools. Psychological evaluation may include intelligence, personality traits, cognition, vocation, and neuropsychological function.[80] Psychologists provide counseling services using a variety of therapy formats depending on the diagnosis and the patient's needs. Currently in four states in the United States, psychologists have the authority to prescribe psychotropic medications after completing additional training.[81]

Counseling services are also provided by other types of professionals. These professions include social workers, licensed professional counselors, mental health counselors, nurse psychotherapists, psychiatric–mental health clinical nurse specialists, marital/family therapists, and pastoral counselors. Most of these professions are prepared with education at the master's degree level or higher.[82]

If the primary care APRN determines that the patient requires prescription management beyond their own knowledge and comfort, the patient may be referred to a psychiatric provider. Some circumstances requiring psychiatric referral include poor patient response to medication, suicidal ideation, severe medication adverse effects, or complex presentations of mental health disorders.[5] Psychiatric providers with specialized training in prescribing for mental or behavioral health include psychiatric–mental health nurse practitioners (PMHNPs), psychiatric mental health clinical nurse specialists (PMHCNSs),[83] and psychiatrists.[82] A psychiatrist is a physician who specializes in psychiatric conditions. Psychiatric providers may not provide counseling services.[82]

Patient Education

Patient education is provided both verbally and written in a language and format that the patient can understand. Provide information regarding the disease process and expected outcomes. Patient education includes taking each prescription medication consistently as prescribed. Identify and discuss any usual symptoms that need to be reported to the prescriber promptly. Provide direction on the methods to contact the provider or nursing staff with questions and concerns. Request that the patient not discontinue the medication abruptly without contacting the provider. The patient must be instructed to seek emergency care for symptoms of dystonia, serotonin syndrome, or

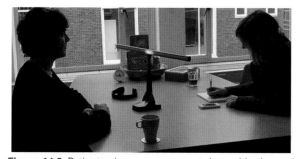

Figure 14.2 Patient using eye movement desensitization and reprocessing (EMDR) in a provider's office. (From Wireless emdr kit (SET). EMDR Kit. (2022, February 16). Retrieved April 5, 2022, from www.emdrkit.com.)

neuroleptic malignant syndrome including sweating, nausea, diarrhea, confusion, dizziness, muscle aches, or unusual muscle movements.[15]

Assist the patient in the identification of routine screenings indicated per age and risk factors. Discuss the plan of care and planned future visits. Incorporate the patient's expectations of future care in the plan of care.

KEY POINTS

- The USPSTF recommends that all adults be screened for depression.
- Females are more likely to be diagnosed with a mental health disorder than males.
- The pathophysiology of mental health disorders in females is different from that in males and is compounded by estrogen production through the life cycle.
- A thorough history and physical examination is important in ruling out medical conditions as causative factors when assessing mental health.
- Multiple medications can be used by primary care providers to treat mental health disorders. MAOIs should be prescribed by mental health professionals only.
- Substance use/medication misuse disorders may be treated by primary care providers, understanding that cannabis, stimulants, caffeine, inhalants, hypnotics, hallucinogens, anxiolytics, and sedatives have no pharmacological treatment.[78]
- Care must be taken when prescribing medications for mental health disorders. Patients require close follow-up with screening for suicidal/homicidal ideation, psychosis, and adverse side effects.
- Counseling is a valuable adjunct to pharmacological management of mental health disorders.

REFERENCES

1. Muxworthy H, Bowllan N. Barriers to practice and impact on care: an analysis of the psychiatric mental health nurse practitioner role. *J N Y State Nurses Assoc.* 2011;42(1-2):8–14.
2. Huynh NN, McIntyre RS. What are the implications of the STAR*D trial for primary care? A review and synthesis. *Prim Care Companion J Clin Psychiatry.* 2008;10(2):91–96.
3. National Council for Behavioral Health. *New Study Reveals Lack of Access as Root Cause for Mental Health Crisis in America.* https://www.thenationalcouncil.org/press-releases/new-study-reveals-lack-of-access-as-root-cause-for-mental-health-crisis-in-america/.
4. COVID-19 Mental Disorders Collaborators. Global prevalence and burden of depressive and anxiety disorders in 204 countries and territories in 2020 due to the COVID-19 pandemic. *Lancet.* 2021;398(10312):1700–1712.
5. Koonin LM, Hoots B, Tsang CA, et al. Trends in the use of telehealth during the emergence of the COVID-19 pandemic—United States, January–March 2020. *MMWR Morb Mortal Wkly Rep.* 2020;69(43):1595–1599.
6. Weber M, Estes K. Anxiety and depression. In: Woo TM, Robinson MV, eds. *Pharmacotherapeutics for Advanced Practice Nurse Prescribers.* 4th ed. Philadelphia: F.A. Davis; 2016:897–912.
7. Ramsawh HJ, Chavira DA, Stein MB. Burden of anxiety disorders in pediatric medical settings: prevalence, phenomenology, and a research agenda. *Arch Pediatr Adolesc Med.* 2010;164(10):965–972.
8. DiMatteo MR, Lepper HS, Croghan TW. Depression is a risk factor for non-compliance with medical treatment: meta-analysis of the effects of anxiety and depression on patient adherence. *Ann Intern Med.* 2000;160(14):2101–2107.
9. Grenard JL, Munjas BA, Adams JL, et al. Depression and medication adherence in the treatment of chronic diseases in the United States: a meta-analysis. *J Gen Intern Med.* 2011;26(10):1175–1182.
10. Adams J, Folds L. Depression, self-efficacy, and adherence in patients with type 2 diabetes. *J Nurse Pract.* 2014;10(9):646–652.
11. Egede LE, Nietert PJ, Zheng D. Depression and all-cause and coronary heart disease mortality among adults with and without diabetes. *Diabetes Care.* 2005;28(6):1339–1345.
12. Pan A, Lucas M, Sun Q, et al. Increased mortality risk in women with depression and diabetes mellitus. *Arch Gen Psychiatry.* 2011;68(1):42–50.
13. Emory University School of Medicine, Department of Human Genetics, Division of Medical Genetics. *Family History of Mental Illness.* Atlanta: Emory University; 2008. https://genetics.emory.edu/documents/resources/Emory_Human_Genetics_Family_History_Mental_Illness.PDF.
14. Craig MC, Murphy DG. Estrogen: effects on normal brain function and neuropsychiatric disorders. *Climacteric.* 2007;10(suppl 2):97–104.

15. Stahl SM. *Stahl's Essential Psychopharmacology: Neuroscientific Basis and Practical Application*. 4th ed. Cambridge, UK: Cambridge University Press; 2013.

16. National Institute of Mental Health (NIMH). *Sequenced Treatment Alternatives To Relieve Depression (STAR*D) Study*. https://www.nimh.nih.gov/funding/clinical-research/practical/stard/index.shtml.

17. Sadock BJ, Sadock VA, Ruiz P. *Kaplan & Sadock's Synopsis of Psychiatry: Behavioral Science/Clinical Psychiatry*. 11th ed. Philadelphia: Wolters Kluwer; 2015.

18. Global Burden of Disease Study 2013 Collaborators. Global, regional, and national incidence, prevalence, and years lived with disability for 301 acute and chronic diseases and injuries in 188 countries, 1990–2013: a systematic analysis for the Global Burden of Disease Study 2013. *Lancet*. 2013;386(9995):743–800.

19. Institute for Health Metrics and Evaluation. *Global Burden of Disease Study 2019 (GBD 2019) Data Resources*. Seattle: University of Washington; 2019. https://vizhub.healthdata.org/gbd-results/.

20. National Institute of Mental Health. *Mental Illness*. https://www.nimh.nih.gov/health/statistics/mental-illness.

21. National Institute of Mental Health. *Any Anxiety Disorder*. https://www.nimh.nih.gov/health/statistics/prevalence/any-anxiety-disorder-among-adults.shtml.

22. Kessler RC, Phetukova M, Sampson NA, Zaslavsky AM, Wittchen H-U. Twelve-month and lifetime prevalence and lifetime morbid risk of anxiety and mood disorders in the United States. *Int J Methods Psychiatr Res*. 2012;21(3):169–184.

23. Dove. *The Dove Global Beauty and Confidence Report*. London, UK: Edelmen Intelligence; 2016.

24. Substance Abuse and Mental Health Services Administration. *2020 NSDUH Detailed Tables*; 2021. https://www.samhsa.gov/data/report/2020-nsduh-detailed-tables.

25. U.S. Centers for Disease Control and Prevention. *Vital Signs: Prescription Painkiller Overdoses: A Growing Epidemic, Especially Among Women*; 2013. Atlanta; www.cdc.gov/vitalsigns/prescriptionpainkilleroverdoses/index.html.

26. U.S. Centers for Disease Control and Prevention. Incidence of neonatal abstinence syndrome—28 States, 1999–2013. *Morbid Mortal Wkly Rep*. 65(31):799–802. https://www.cdc.gov/tobacco/data_statistics/fact_sheets/smokeless/use_us/index.htm

27. U.S. Centers for Disease Control and Prevention. Cigarette smoking among adults—United States, 2005–2015. *Morbid Mortal Wkly Rep*. 2016;65(44):1205–1211.

28. U.S. Centers for Disease Control and Prevention. *Smokeless Tobacco Product Use in the United States*. Atlanta.

https://store.samhsa.gov/sites/default/files/d7/priv/sma14-4816_litreview.pdf.

29. Centers for Disease Control and Prevention (2022). *Smoking and tobacco use: Fast facts and facts sheet*. https://www.cdc.gov/tobacco/data_statistics/fact_sheets/fast_facts/index.htm.

30. Chafetz M, Underhill J. Estimated costs of malingered disability. *Arch Clin Neuropsychol*. 2013;28(7):633–639.

31. U.S. Department of Health and Human Services, Office of Disease Prevention and Health Promotion. (2010). *National Action Plan to Improve Health Literacy*. Washington, DC: Author. https://health.gov/sites/default/files/2019-09/Health_Literacy_Action_Plan.pdf.

32. Dains JE, Baumann LC, Scheibel P. *Advanced Health Assessment and Clinical Diagnosis in Primary Care*. 6th ed. St. Louis: Elsevier; 2019.

33. Epstein R, Street R. The values and value of patient-centered care. *Ann Fam Med*. 2011;9(2):100–103.

34. Center for Substance Abuse Treatment. Treatment improvement protocol (TIP) Series, No. 57: Trauma-Informed Care: A Sociocultural Perspective. *Trauma-Informed Care in Behavioral Health Services*. Rockville (MD): Substance Abuse and Mental Health Services Administration; 2014. https://www.ncbi.nlm.nih.gov/books/NBK207195/.

35. McHugo GJ, Kammerer N, Jackson EW, Markoff LS, Gatz M, Larson MJ, Mazelis R, Hennigan K. Women, Co-occurring Disorders, and Violence Study: evaluation design and study population. *J Subst Abuse Treat*. 2005;28(2):91–107.

36. Substance Abuse and Mental Health Services Administration. National Center for Trauma-Informed Care & Alternatives to Seclusion and Restraint. *Promoting Alternatives to the Use of Seclusion and Restraint*. Rockville, MD. https://www.samhsa.gov/sites/default/files/topics/trauma_and_violence/seclusion-restraints-1.pdf.

37. Substance Abuse and Mental Health Services Administration. Health Resources & Services Administration Center for Integrated Care. *Trauma-Informed Care in Behavioral Health Services*; 2012. https://store.samhsa.gov/sites/default/files/d7/priv/sma14-4816_litreview.pdf.

38. Government Accountability Office. *VA Mental Health: Number of Veterans Receiving Care, Barriers Faced, and Efforts to Increase Access*. Washington, DC; 2012. http://www.gao.gov/new.items/d1212.pdf.

39. Kimerling R, Gima K, Smith MW, Street A, Frain S. The Veterans Health Administration and military sexual trauma. *Am J Public Health*. 2012;97(12):2160–2166.

40. Ginsburg GS, Riddle MA, Davies M. Somatic symptoms in children and adolescents with anxiety disorders. *J Am Acad Child Adolesc Psychiatry*. 2006;45(10):1179–1187.

41. National Institute of Mental Health. *Mental Illness*. https://www.nimh.nih.gov/health/statistics/mental-illness.

42. Preston JD, O'Neal JH, Talaga MC. *Child and Adolescent Clinical Psychopharmacology Made Simple*. 2nd ed. Oakland, CA: New Harbinger Publications; 2010.

43. Drayer RA, Mulsant BH, Lenze EJ, et al. Somatic symptoms of depression in elderly patients with medical comorbidities. *Int J Geriatr Psychiatry*. 2005;20(10):973–982.

44. Reynolds K, Pietrzak RH, El-Gabalawy R, Mackenzie CS, Sareen J. Prevalence of psychiatric disorders in U.S. older adults: findings from a nationally representative survey. *World Psychiatry*. 2015;14(1):74–81.

45. U.S. Preventive Services Task Force. *Depression in Adults: Screening*; 2016. https://www.uspreventiveservicestaskforce.org/Page/Document/RecommendationStatementFinal/depression-in-adults-screening1.

46. Center for Quality Assessment and Improvement in Mental Health. Patient Health Questionnaire (PHQ-2); 2008. http://www.cqaimh.org/pdf/tool_phq2.pdf.

47. Carlat DJ. The psychiatric review of symptoms: A screening tool for family physicians. *Am Fam Physician*. 1998;58(7):1617–1624.

48. University of Wisconsin Integrative Medicine. *Pearls for Clinicians: Coping with Grief*; 2013. http://www.fammed.wisc.edu/files/webfm-uploads/documents/outreach/im/module_grief_clinician.pdf.

49. Jarvis C. *Physical Examination and Health Assessment*. 7th ed. St. Louis: Elsevier; 2016.

50. Cherpitel CJ. Brief screening instruments for alcoholism. *Alcohol Health Res World*. 1997;21(4):348–351.

51. McNeely J, Strauss SM, Saitz R, et al. A brief patient self-administered substance use screening tool for primary care: Two-site validation study of the Substance Use Brief Screen (SUBS). *American J Med*. 2015;128(7):e9–e19.

52. Office of the Surgeon General (US); National Action Alliance for Suicide Prevention (US). *2012 National Strategy for Suicide Prevention: Goals and Objectives for Action: A Report of the U.S. Surgeon General and of the National Action Alliance for Suicide Prevention*. Washington (DC): US Department of Health & Human Services (US); 2012. https://www.ncbi.nlm.nih.gov/pubmed/23136686.

53. American Psychological Association. *Diagnostic and Statistical Manual of Mental Disorders*. 5th ed. Arlington, VA; 2013.

54. American Academy of Pediatrics. *Guidelines for Adolescent Depression in Primary Care (GLAD-PC): Part 1. Practice Preparation, Identification, Assessment, and Initial Management*; 2018. https://pediatrics.aappublications.org/content/141/3/e20174081.

55. LeBourgeois III HW. Malingering: key points in assessment. *Psychiatric Times*. 2007;24(5):21. http://www.psychiatrictimes.com/forensic-psychiatry/malingering-key-points-assessment.

56. National Institutes of Health. *NIH Stroke Scale*. https://www.stroke.nih.gov/documents/NIH_Stroke_Scale_508C.pdf.

57. Woo TM. Drugs affecting the central nervous system. In: Woo TM, Robinson MV, eds. *Robinson Pharmacotherapeutics for Advanced Practice Nurse Prescribers*. 4th ed. Philadelphia: F.A. Davis; 2016:225–294.

58. U.S. Food and Drug Administration. *Information by Drug Class: Antidepressant Use in Children, Adolescents, and Adults*. MD: Silver Spring; 2007. https://www.fda.gov/drugs/drug-safety-and-availability/information-drug-class.

59. Thibault R. Selective serotonin reuptake inhibitor antidepressant treatment discontinuation syndrome: A review of the clinical evidence and the possible mechanisms involved. *Front Pharmacol*. 2013;4:1–10.

60. Busch SH, Barry CJ. Pediatric antidepressant use after the black-box warning. *Health Aff*. 2009;28(3):724–733.

61. U.S. Food and Drug Administration. *Trintellix Medication Guide*. MD: Silver Spring; 2017. http://general.takedapharm.com/content/file.aspx?applicationcode=396066C6-E50F-4113-ABAD-54FE9525BF7E&filetypecode=TRINTELLIXPI&cacheRandomizer=4b358a5b-d9a9-43ea-b981-b35fd8a97c56.

62. Stahl SM. *Stahl's Essential Pharmacology: Prescriber's Guide*. 7th ed. Cambridge, UK: Cambridge University Press; 2020.

63. Agency for Healthcare Quality and Research. *American Geriatrics Society 2015 Updated Beers Criteria for Potentially Inappropriate Medication Use in Older Adults*; 2015. Rockville, MD https://psnet.ahrq.gov/issue/american-geriatrics-society-2019-updated-ags-beers-criteria-potentially-inappropriate.

64. Khouzam HR. Depression in the elderly: How to treat. *Consultant*. 2012;52(4). http://www.consultant360.com/article/depression-elderly-how-treat.

65. U.S. Food and Drug Administration. *Rexulti Medication Guide*. MD: Silver Spring; 2015a. https://www.accessdata.fda.gov/drugsatfda_docs/label/2015/205422Orig1Orig2s000lbl.pdf.

66. U.S. Food and Drug Administration. *Vraylar Medication Guide*. MD: Silver Spring; 2015b. https://www.accessdata.fda.gov/drugsatfda_docs/label/2017/204370s001lbl.pdf.

67. Novartis. *Clozaril*. https://www.accessdata.fda.gov/drugsatfda_docs/label/2010/019758s062lbl.pdf.

68. Vanda Pharmaceuticals, Inc. *Fanapt*; 2009. https://www.accessdata.fda.gov/drugsatfda_docs/label/2009/022192lbl.pdf.

69. Sunovion Pharmaceuticals Canada Inc. *Product Monograph*. Latuda; 2020. https://www.sunovion.ca/monographs/latuda.pdf.

70. U.S. Food and Drug Administration. *Caplyta*; 2019. https://www.accessdata.fda.gov/drugsatfda_docs/nda/2019/209500Orig1s000lbl.pdf.

71. Ortho-McNeil-Janssen Pharmaceuticals, Inc. *Invega*; 2010. https://www.accessdata.fda.gov/drugsatfda_docs/label/2010/021999s018lbl.pdf.

72. AstraZeneca Canada Inc. *Product monograph including patient medication information*. Seroquel; 2021. https://www.astrazeneca.ca/content/dam/az-ca/downloads/productinformation/seroquel-product-monograph-en.pdf.

73. Üçok A, Gaebel W. Side effects of atypical antipsychotics: An overview. *World Psychiatry*. 2008;7(1):58–62.

74. Acadia Pharmaceuticals, Inc. *Nuplazid*; 2016. https://www.accessdata.fda.gov/drugsatfda_docs/label/2016/207318lbl.pdf.

75. Miller BJ. Smoking cessation. In: Woo TM, Robinson MV, eds. *Robinson Pharmacotherapeutics for Advanced Practice Nurse Prescribers*. 4th ed. Philadelphia: F.A. Davis; 2016:1205–1215.

76. National Institute on Drug Abuse. *Available Treatments for Marijuana Use Disorders*. https://www.drugabuse.gov/publications/research-reports/marijuana/available-treatments-marijuana-use-disorders.

77. National Institute on Drug Abuse. *Substance Use in Women*. https://www.drugabuse.gov/publications/research-reports/substance-use-in-women.

78. Haile CN, Kosten TR. Pharmacotherapy for stimulant-related disorders. *Curr Psychiatry Rep*. 2013;15(11):415.

79. Simon NM. Treating complicated grief. *JAMA*. 2013;310(4):416–423.

80. American Psychological Association. What do practicing psychologists do? https://www.apa.org/topics/psychotherapy/about-psychologists.

81. American Psychological Association Practice Organization. *About Prescribing Psychologists*. https://www.apaservices.org/practice/advocacy/authority/prescribing-psychologists?_ga=2.96557727.1413408084.1636216847-1087168104.1636216847.

82. Mental Health America. *Types of Mental Health Professionals*. https://www.mhanational.org/types-mental-health-professionals.

83. American Psychiatric Nurses Association. *About Psychiatric–Mental Health Nursing*. https://www.apna.org/i4a/pages/index.cfm?pageid=3292#1.

15

Vaginitis, Sexually Transmitted Infections, and Human Immunodeficiency Virus

Debra Ilchak, Sarah B. Freeman, and Kimberly Gray

OBJECTIVES

- Understand the epidemiology and pathogenesis of selected vaginal infections and sexually transmitted infections (STIs).
- Develop focused assessments that include a history and physical examination tailored toward selected vaginal infections and STIs.

- Formulate a plan of care for selected vaginal infections and STIs that includes diagnosis and management that is based on the most current U.S. Centers for Disease Control and Prevention (CDC) Sexually Transmitted Disease Treatment Guidelines.
- Implement strategies for the prevention of vaginitis and STIs.

INTRODUCTION

STI and vaginitis are frequently encountered problems in women's health. Vaginitis is one of the most common causes of a women's health visit to the office. These conditions can lead to a decrease in quality of life as well as possible long-term complications and should be diagnosed and treated immediately. Education should always include not only treatment but strategies to promote prevention of the disorders. This chapter is divided into two sections. The first section will deal with vaginitis, and the second section will provide treatment plans for STIs. All treatment plans are based on the latest guidelines provided by the CDC.

VAGINITIS

Vaginitis is a general term used for any inflammation or infection of the vagina. It is the most common infection in reproductive-age females, with a prevalence of 29% nationally.[1] Vaginal discharge accounts for more than 10 million office visits per year.[2] Although there

are many organisms that can cause vaginitis, changes in the normal vaginal flora is a major contributing factor. The three most common causes of vaginitis are bacterial vaginosis (BV), vulvovaginal candidiasis (VVC), and trichomoniasis, accounting for 75% to 95% of all vaginal infections.[1] Despite its prevalence, 85% of females remain undiagnosed or attempt self-treatment only.[1] Many females will also experience vulvar symptoms. Because of the magnitude of the problem, it is important for clinicians that provide care to female patients to know the causes, workup, and management of these problems.

Pathophysiology

The pathology associated with vaginitis is complex and deals with the fragile environment of the vaginal canal. Vaginal health is related to maintaining the balance of the microorganisms of the vagina. BV, VVC, and trichomoniasis are categorized as vaginitis/vaginosis syndromes. The two most common vaginal infections, BV and VVC, represent overgrowth of organisms that are

TABLE 15.1   Causative Organism for Vaginitis[2,3]

Vaginitis	Causative Organism	Comments
BV	*Gardnerella vaginalis* *Mycoplasma hominis* *Mobiluncus* species *Prevotella* species *Atopobium vaginae* *Bacteroides* species	BV is caused by an overgrowth of the bacteria normally found in the vagina.
VVC	*Candida albicans* (most common) *Candida glabrata* *Candida tropicalis*	VVC is caused by an overgrowth of a yeast organism normally found in the vagina.
Tricho- moniasis	*Trichomonas vaginalis*	This is a sexually transmitted disease.

BV, Bacterial vaginosis; *VVC,* vulvovaginal candidiasis.

normally found in the vagina (Table 15.1).[2,3] Risk factors for development of vaginitis include the following:

- Age
- Hormonal balance
- Sexual activity
- Immunological status
- Underlying chronic disease

Critical to maintaining the proper vaginal environment is the maintenance of a vaginal pH between 3.8 and 4.5. Normal physiological vaginal secretions are made up of substances from the vulvar, sebaceous, sweat, Bartholin, and Skene glands; exfoliated cells from the vagina; and both cervical mucus and secretions from the endometrial cavity and fallopian tubes. These substances are rich in glycogen, which forms the substrate for Doderlein lactobacilli. These lactobacilli convert the glycogen to lactic acid, thus creating the acidic vagina.

Many things can change the acidity of the vagina and predispose a female to the development of vaginitis. Some of the more common substances that are found in the vagina that negatively affect the pH are sperm and blood. Vaginal ecology can also be affected by hormonal changes at different phases of the menstrual cycle or during pregnancy, STIs, douching or use of feminine hygiene products, foreign bodies present in the vagina, contraceptive choice, and other factors. This disruption of the normal ecosystem increases the likelihood of

vaginitis by providing favorable conditions for bacteria and yeast found in the vagina to overgrow.[3,4]

Vaginitis affects females at any age from all ethnic backgrounds. Of the three most common causes, reproductive-age females are at the greatest risk. Although sexual activity is not necessary for the development of both BV and VVC, sexually active females are at increased risk.[3,5]

A change in vaginal discharge is one of the reported symptoms of vaginitis. The amount and quality of the discharge changes with the menstrual cycle. Discharge is greatest at midcycle as the cervical mucus increases around the time of ovulation. Although normal, some patients may perceive this as abnormal, so education as to the nature and character is an important component of care. Stress has also been known to cause an increase in discharge as a result of increased cell turnover. Patients usually do not have symptoms with a physiological discharge, but symptoms of irritation, pruritus, and odor may be present if it is pathological. An abnormal discharge adheres to the vaginal walls. The discharge can vary in appearance and be thick to watery or frothy, and it can range in color from white to yellow, gray, or green.[3]

NOT TO BE MISSED

An imbalance in the vaginal ecosystem is an important factor in the development of vaginitis. Assessment of pH provides a snapshot of the vaginal environment.

Prognosis

Although vaginitis is thought to be a mild disease, it can affect quality of life. Although the medications are effective in treatment, recurrence can be high as a result of changes in the vaginal ecosystem. If recurrent, vaginitis can lead to chronic irritation and psychosocial and emotional stress. Both trichomoniasis and BV are associated with an increased risk for adverse outcomes during pregnancy. Complications of BV include an increased risk of STIs, such as human immunodeficiency virus (HIV), human papillomavirus (HPV), herpes simplex virus 2 (HSV-2), trichomoniasis, chlamydia, and gonorrhea, as well as wound infection after gynecological surgery. Chronic vaginal infection can increase susceptibility to HIV transmission.[6]

CLINICAL SURVIVAL TIP Although vaginal infections are considered a mild disease, serious long-term complications are possible if not treated.

Assessment

A history and physical examination are important to the diagnosis of a vaginal infection. Exploration of risk factors provides a foundation for the differential diagnoses as some are more prevalent in certain diseases (Table 15.2). The history includes assessment of risk factors, prior history of similar conditions, and current symptoms such as the following:

- Previous symptoms that were similar
- Contraceptive method
- Last menstrual period (LMP)
- Abnormal bleeding
- Douching
- Use of feminine hygiene products
- Antibiotic use
- General medical history
- Systemic symptoms
  - Abdominal pain
  - Fever
  - Chills
  - Nausea and vomiting

NOT TO BE MISSED

The etiology of vaginal discharge should not be based only on worsening symptoms.

The history also includes assessment of common symptoms associated with vaginal infection. Ask about itching, odor, and discharge (Table 15.3). Discharge should be investigated in relationship to the following:

- Quantity
- Color
- Consistency
- Odor

NOT TO BE MISSED

Although the presenting symptoms of all three major vaginal infections are similar, it is important to know which symptoms are most closely related to which of the major disorders (see Table 15.3).

The focus of the physical examination for a patient presenting with vaginal discharge is a complete pelvic examination. The external genitalia and vagina are inspected, and any erythema is noted. If itching is present, the external genitalia may be excoriated because of the patient's scratching. If excoriations or fissures are noted, check the skin on the under thigh for rash or redness. While visualizing the vagina, the amount, color, and odor of the discharge should be noted. Note the upper vaginal wall and cervix for the presence of petechiae. These lesions are seen with trichomoniasis.

While the speculum is in place, collect any specimens needed to assist with the diagnosis. A cotton swab can be used to collect vaginal fluid for microscopic examination. Once the specimen is collected, it can be placed in a tube with saline to preserve the organism while completing the examination. A pH is performed at this time. The specimen for the pH should be collected from the lateral vaginal wall. Place the discharge on the pH paper, and note the color. Vaginal soreness may be noted on bimanual examination, but there is usually no cervical motion tenderness or pain

TABLE 15.2	Risk Associated With Specific Vaginal Infections[6,11]	
Bacterial Vaginosis	**Vulvovaginal Candidiasis**	**Trichomoniasis**
New sexual partner	Pregnancy	History of incarceration
More than one sexual partner	Diabetes (uncontrolled)	Two or more sexual partners during the
Multiple male sexual partners	Certain medications	previous year
Female partner	Oral contraceptives	Having less than a high school education
Douching	Antibiotics	Living below the national poverty level
Nonuse of condoms	Steroids	Nonuse of condoms
HSV-2 seropositivity	Weakened immune system	
	HIV	

HSV-2, herpes simplex virus 2; *HIV*, human immunodeficiency virus.

TABLE 15.3 Differential Diagnoses of Vaginal Infections[1,3,4,6]

Parameters	Normal	Bacterial Vaginosis	Vulvovaginal Candidiasis	Trichomoniasis
Symptoms	Usually nothing May report increased discharge	Odor Discharge-homogenous thin, milky white	Pruritus Dyspareunia Thick discharge (usually white) Fissures and vulvar rash	Odor Discharge maybe gray to yellow-green Post-coital spotting Dyspareunia Dysuria
Signs	Discharge-white or transparent, thin to thick, non-malodorous	Discharge adheres to the vaginal wall Vaginal walls not inflamed	Vaginal and vulvar erythema and edema Discharge may adhere to vaginal wall	Vulvovaginal erythema Cervical and vaginal petechiae
Vaginal pH	3.8 to 4.5	>4.5	4.0 to 4.5	>4.5
Wet prep Saline 10% KOH	PMN:EC ratio <1 Dominant flora: rods Squames-+++ Negative	PMN:EC ratio <1 Dominant flora: loss of rods with increased cocco-bacilli Clue cells: 1 in 5 epithelial cells Negative	PMN:EC ratio <1 Dominant flora: rods Squames-+++ Pseudohyphae: 40% of patients with non-albicans Candida-budding yeast WBCs Pseudohyphae: 70% of patients	PMN++++ Dominant flora: mixed Motile trichmonads: 60% of patients Negative
Amine test	Negative	Positive	Negative	Often positive

PMN, Polymorphonuclear leukocyte; *EC,* vaginal epithelial cells; *KOH,* potassium hydroxide; *WBCs,* white blood cells.

on deep palpation. If these exist, further evaluation for pelvic inflammatory disease (PID) is warranted.[1,3,6-8]

CLINICAL SURVIVAL TIP: Diagnosing Vaginitis/Vaginosis[9]
- A lack of itching makes the diagnosis of VVC unlikely.
- A lack of odor makes the diagnosis of BV unlikely.
- Inflammatory signs are most common in VVC.
- Presence of a fishy odor is most common with BV.

Microscopic Examination

NOT TO BE MISSED

Wet prep remains the hallmark for diagnosing vaginal infection.

The history and physical examination alone is not enough to make a positive diagnosis of vaginal infections. Clinical evaluation of vaginal secretions is used to diagnose vaginal infection. A microscopic evaluation of vaginal secretions (wet prep/wet mount) collected from either the posterior vaginal fornix or the lateral vaginal wall is the most appropriate test to perform. It has the advantage of being an office-based test, and the patient can obtain the results and receive treatment at the same visit. Table 15.4 is the procedure for performing a wet prep.[3,6,8,9] Although the wet prep is the test of choice to use when diagnosing a vaginal infection, there are other tests available. Normal findings under the microscope are found in Figure 15.1.

CLINICAL SURVIVAL TIP The ability to diagnose a vaginal infection with a wet prep is directly dependent on the quality of the slide, so it is important to be properly trained in this technique.

If a microscope is not available, the nucleic acid amplification test (NAAT) can be used. These tests are not the first-line choice because they do not provide immediate feedback and add to the cost of care. Tests can be performed on either a vaginal specimen or urine

TABLE 15.4   Wet Prep Examinations[3,6,8]

Indication	Use for Patients Presenting With Signs and Symptoms of Vaginal Infection
Contraindication or less than ideal conditions	Menstrual blood can obscure the finding, so not an ideal time to perform Douched within the past 24 hours Use of vaginal medication with the past 2–3 days Tampon use within the past 24 hours because it can affect amount of discharge and pH
Materials	Spatula or sterile swab 0.9% saline 10% KOH Glass or plastic test tube (for indirect method) Glass microscopic slide Glass coverslip Microscope-compound Dropper (indirect method)
Collection of discharge	Use the spatula or applicator to obtain a sample from the vaginal wall. The discharge that pools in the speculum can also be used. Use either the direct or indirect method to prepare the discharge.

Preparation of discharge
  Direct method
  Indirect method
	After obtaining the discharge, apply a small portion directly to a clean slide. Add a drop of saline, mix to suspend the discharge, and cover the suspension.
	Repeat with KOH.
	One or two slides may be used.
	Place the swab in a test tube that contains 1.0 mL of saline.
	Mix the swab with the saline gently.
	Use the swab or a dropper to place a drop of discharge on a clean slide.
	Cover with a coverslip.
	Prepare a KOH slide by adding a drop of KOH to the mixture, and repeat the procedure for making the slide.
	Note: Do not allow specimen to dry out.
	KOH must react with the sample for 30–60 seconds before viewing.

Examination	Examine under both low power (10×) and high power (40×).
	Examine the entire slide by moving until you have seen the four quadrants of the slide.
	Once the KOH is added, examine for a fishy odor.
	Observe for:
	  Round or oval budding cells around 3–10 per field (yeast)
	  Vaginal epithelial cells covered with small coccobacilli (clue cells)
	  Flagellated organism recognized by the rapid movement (trichomonas)
	  Spherical cells with single or multiple nuclei (white blood cells)
	  From 10–30 per field

KOH, Potassium hydroxide.

specimen. If a urine test is performed, it is best to use the first-void urine, so patients should bring the specimen to the visit. The Affirm DNA test can detect both trichomonas (80%) and BV (94%). If unable to diagnosis BV with wet prep or there is recurrent BV, the Affirm may provide further information to guide the plan of care.

Gram staining to detect BV is both sensitive (89% to 97%) and specific (79% to 85%). It requires special stains for making the slides and adds additional time to the visit. The results are available before the end of the patient visit, so it does not delay treatment. With resistant or recurrent yeast, Gram stain as well as culture with either Nickerson media or Sabouraud agar can be performed. If a non-albicans infection is suspected, culture can be used to identify the specific causative yeast organism.[3]

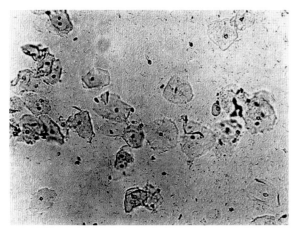

Figure 15.1 Normal findings of a wet prep under the microscope. (From Gupta S, Kumar B. *Sexually Transmitted Infections.* Elsevier; 2012.)

Treatment for the major types of vaginal infections are based on the history, physical examination, and laboratory findings. Figure 15.2 provides an algorithm for the workup and management of vaginal discharge.

BACTERIAL VAGINOSIS

Epidemiology

BV is caused by an alteration in the normal vaginal flora. Although it is the most common cause of vaginitis in sexually active reproductive-age females in the United States, the incidence is underestimated because many females to do not seek treatment, and it is not a reportable disease.[10] Higher rates of BV have been found in females of color, lower socioeconomic status, and lower educational levels.[11] BV is associated with a number of both gynecological and obstetrical complications including the following:[6,10,12]

- Increased risk of PID
- Preterm delivery
- Postpartum endometritis
- Recurrence of BV
- Increased transmission of some STIs
  - HIV
  - Gonorrhea
  - Chlamydia
  - HSV-2

Pathogenesis

The etiology of BV is unknown, but it occurs when there is a disturbance in the normal vaginal environment. Lactobacillus, the normal predominant vaginal flora,

maintains the normal acidic vaginal pH and creates a hostile environment for other bacteria, but these flora are diminished or absent in BV, resulting in an alkaline environment and overgrowth of organisms.[6] This can lead to replacement of the lactobacilli with high concentrations of *Gardnerella vaginalis* and other various anaerobic bacteria.[12] The bacteria adhere to the vaginal epithelium and result in a non-inflammatory response that leads to the symptoms seen with BV. The non-inflammatory response is used for the designation of vaginosis instead of the use of the term *vaginitis*.[12]

BV is a sexually associated condition.[13] In heterosexual females and women who have sex with women (WSW), the role of sexual contact in the transmission of the anaerobic bacteria may affect the development of BV. Intercourse is also known to have an impact on the vaginal environment and may predispose to the destruction of lactobacilli, thus starting the pathological response that leads to BV.[9] Table 15.2 provides examples of risk factors for developing BV.

Screening

Routine screening for BV in asymptomatic non-pregnant females is not recommended. Additionally, the evidence is insufficient to recommend screening for BV in asymptomatic pregnant females at risk for preterm delivery because it does not reduce the risk of preterm birth.[10,13]

Focused History and Physical Examination

BV is asymptomatic in an estimated 50% to 75% of females.[10] The vaginal symptoms may be acute or chronic and recurring.[6] Symptoms are found in Table 15.3.

On physical examination, a thin, off-white or milky, homogenous, and malodorous discharge that adheres to the vaginal walls may be seen (Fig. 15.3).[6,10] The discharge does not cause vulvar swelling, and there are no signs of vaginal or cervical inflammation.[10]

> **CLINICAL SURVIVAL TIP** Lack of inflammation is a hallmark sign of BV.

Diagnosis

Amsel's diagnostic criteria can be used to diagnose BV based on clinical signs (Box 15.1). Performed with the use of a wet prep, it is used most commonly in the office.[13] Figure 15.4 provides a look at the criteria as seen under a microscope. Vaginal Gram stain is the gold standard

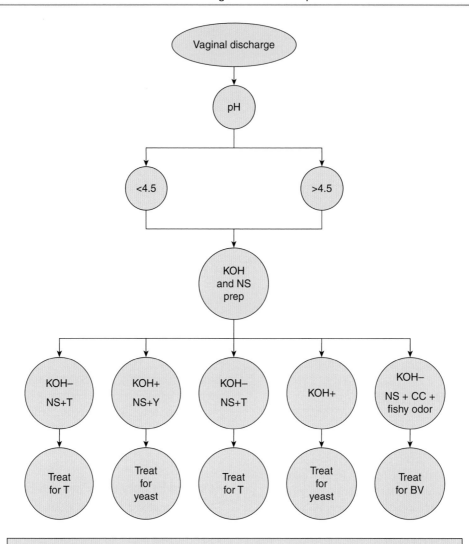

Figure 15.2 Algorithm for the evaluation of vaginal discharge. (Modified from Goje O. *Overview of Vaginitis*. Merck Manual; 2021. http://www.merckmanuals.com/professional/gynecology-and-obstetrics/vaginitis,-cervicitis,-and-pelvic-inflammatory-disease-pid/overview-of-vaginitis; U.S. Centers for Disease Control and Prevention. Sexually transmitted infections treatment guidelines, 2021. *MMWR Morbid Mortal Wkly Rep.* 2021;70[4]:1–187; Frobenius W, Bogdan C. Diagnostic value of vaginal discharge, wet mount and vaginal pH: An update on the basics of gynecologic infectiology. *Geburshilfe und Freuenheilkunde.* 2015;75[4]:355–366; Paladine HL, Desai UA. Vaginitis: diagnosis and treatment. *Am Fam Physician.* 2018;97[5]:321–329.)

for diagnosing BV because it can be used to quantify the amount of lactobacilli. Additional diagnostic tests include polymerase chain reaction (PCR) assays, DNA hybridization probe test, and indirect testing for enzymatic activity associated with the organisms causing BV.[6,13]

NOT TO BE MISSED

Because *Gardnerella vaginalis* is common to the vagina and found in asymptomatic females, vaginal culture is not useful in diagnosing BV.

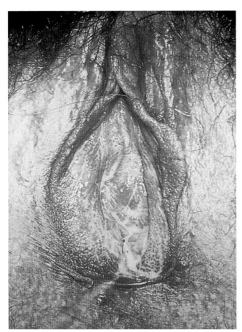

Figure 15.3 Classic gray-white thin discharge seen in bacterial vaginosis. (From Andrews G. *Women's Sexual Health*. New York: Elsevier; 2005.)

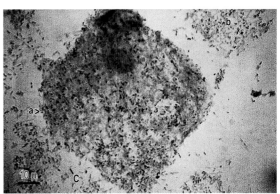

Figure 15.4 Wet prep under the microscope demonstrating clue cells in bacterial vaginosis. Note the epithelial squamous cells with multiple bacteria adherent to their surface *(a>)*, clue cells *(b)*, normal epithelial cells *(C)*, and bacteria. (From Symonds IM, Arulkumaran S. *Essential Obstetrics and Gynaecology*. Elsevier; 2020.)

BOX 15.1   Amsel's Diagnostic Criteria for Bacterial Vaginosis[13]

Must have at least three of the following findings:
- Vaginal pH >4.5
- Presence of >20% per high-power field of "clue cells" on wet mount examination
- Positive amine or "whiff" test
- Homogeneous, non-viscous, milky-white discharge adherent to the vaginal walls

---

BOX 15.2   U.S. Centers for Disease Control and Prevention Recommendations for Management of Bacterial Vaginosis[6]

Recommended Regimens
- Metronidazole 500 mg orally twice a day for 7 days
  OR
- Metronidazole gel 0.75% one full applicator (5 g), intravaginally, once a day for 5 days*
  OR
- Clindamycin cream 2%, one full applicator (5 g) intravaginally at bedtime for 7 days

Alternative Regimens
- Tinidazole 2 g orally once daily for 2 days
  OR
- Tinidazole 1 g orally once daily for 5 days
  OR
- Secnidazole 2 g orally once
  OR
- Clindamycin 300 mg orally twice daily for 7 days
  OR
- Clindamycin ovules 100 mg intravaginally once at bedtime for 3 days

* Recommended regimen in pregnancy.
From Centers for Disease Control and Prevention (CDC). (2021). Sexually transmitted infections treatment guidelines, 2021. *MMWR, Morbidity Mortality Weekly Report, 70*(4).

Management

For female patients with symptoms, treatment is recommended for symptom relief and to potentially decrease risk for acquiring other STIs. See Box 15.2 for the CDC-recommended guidelines for management of BV. Education is crucial to the successful use of any drug. Previous warnings of disulfiram-like reactions with alcohol and metronidazole have not been borne out by clinical studies, therefore avoidance of alcohol during treatment with metronidazole or tinidazole is no longer required.[6,10] Alternative regimens to metronidazole or tinidazole include clindamycin (oral or ovules), astodrimer 1% gel, and secnidazole.[6,10] Latex condoms and diaphragms should not be used for 5 days after use of clindamycin cream and ovules because they might be weakened by this oil-based medication.

> **PATIENT-CENTERED CARE:** The treatment regimen for BV is the same in females with HIV infection, but the rates of recurrence are higher.

Nonpharmacological

There are limited data on nonpharmacological treatment for BV. Most treatments involve recommendations that help maintain the vaginal environment, such as avoiding douching. Females who douche regularly encounter more health problems than those who do not douche. Many studies have shown a statistically significant reduction in BV recurrence with the use of probiotics, but there is no agreement on the type of probiotic, duration, and route of administration. Additional quality research is needed.[14]

> **PATIENT-CENTERED CARE:** Treatment of BV is recommended for symptomatic pregnant patients. They can be treated with the oral or vaginal regimens recommended for non-pregnant patients.

Education and Counseling

Patients diagnosed with BV should be tested for HIV and other STIs because of the increased chance of transmission.[6] Treatment of sex partners is not recommended because it has not been shown to decrease recurrence. Females should abstain from sexual intercourse or use condoms during treatment as this may help reduce recurrence. If symptoms resolve, follow-up is not necessary. If symptoms persist or recur, patients should return for evaluation. In patients with persistent or recurrent BV, the evidence is limited on optimal management strategies. It is recommended to retreat with the same regimen after the first occurrence. Metronidazole gel 0.75% can be used intravaginally twice weekly for 4 to 6 months, or monthly oral metronidazole 2 g with fluconazole 150 mg can be prescribed for patients with multiple reccurrences.[6]

TRICHOMONIASIS

Epidemiology

Trichomoniasis, commonly known as *trich,* is the most prevalent non-viral, curable STI in the United States and is caused by the protozoan parasite *Trichomonas vaginalis.* Although not a required reportable condition in the United States, it is estimated to affect 3.7 million individuals. In reproductive-age females in the United States, the estimated prevalence of infection is 2.1%.[6,15]

Trichomoniasis is associated with adverse gynecological and obstetrical health outcomes such as the following:[6]
- Increased risk of acquiring HIV
- Increased risk of cervical cancer
- Preterm birth
- Premature rupture of membranes
- Low birth weight infant

It should be considered as a possible diagnosis for any patients presenting with the cardinal signs of vaginitis.

> **NOT TO BE MISSED**
>
> Clinical manifestations of trichomoniasis in females can range from an asymptomatic carrier state to an acute, severe inflammatory disease.

Pathogenesis

T. vaginalis is the only known protozoan parasite to infect the genital tract. The single-celled protozoa have four flagella responsible for the jerky motility of the organism seen under a microscope.[16] Trichomoniasis may be transmitted during penile-vaginal sex as well as vaginal to vaginal contact. Undetected infections can persist for months or years in the genital tract.[17] Nonsexual transmission has not been proven.[16] The exact incubation period is not known. Studies suggest an incubation period between 4 to 28 days in about 50% of patients.[16] Co-occurrence of *T. vaginalis* and BV pathogens occurs commonly, with a co-infection rate of 60% to 80%.[16]

Screening

Routine screening for asymptomatic trichomoniasis is not recommended for pregnant or non-pregnant females. Screening should be considered in areas such as STI clinics and correctional facilities and in asymptomatic females at high risk. At-risk populations include females with multiple sex partners, history of STIs, sex workers, and those with substance use disorders.[6]

Routine screening is recommended at least annually in non-pregnant, asymptomatic females with HIV because of the association of PID and trichomoniasis.

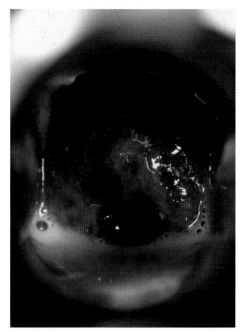

Figure 15.5 Frothy vaginal discharge of trichomoniasis with a strawberry cervix (ecchymotic petechiae). (From Lewis D. Trichomoniasis. *Medicine*. 2014;42[7]:369–371. https://doi.org/10.1016/j.mpmed.2014.04.004.)

Screening for pregnant patients should occur if there is a high index of suspicion for infection.[6]

Focused History and Physical Examination

Trichomoniasis is often asymptomatic; patients may report vaginal discharge that is yellow-green and malodorous, vulvar irritation, itching, dysuria, pain with intercourse, and abdominal pain. The external genitalia may exhibit signs of erythema, excoriations, or edema.[18] During the speculum examination, the vaginal discharge may be frothy, profuse, yellow to green, and malodorous, and the cervix and vaginal walls may have ecchymotic petechiae (Fig. 15.5). The vaginal pH will be greater than 4.5 (Box 15.3).[6,16]

> **CLINICAL SURVIVAL TIP** The clinical signs and symptoms of trichomoniasis are not sufficiently sensitive or specific to allow a positive diagnosis.

Diagnosis

Patients who present with a complaint of vaginal symptoms should be evaluated for vaginal infections

> ### BOX 15.3   U.S. Centers for Disease Control and Prevention Recommended Treatment for Trichomoniasis
>
> * Recommended Regimen: Metronidazole 500 mg orally twice daily for 7 days
> * Alternative Regimen and Recommended Regimen for Women: Tinidazole 2 g orally in a single dose

From U.S. Centers for Disease Control and Prevention. Sexually transmitted infections treatment guidelines, 2021. *MMWR Morbid Mortal Wkly Rep.* 2021;70(4):1–187

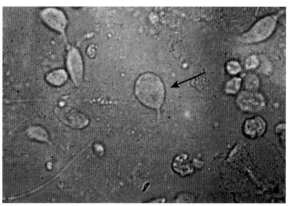

Figure 15.6 Wet prep under microscope demonstrating trichomonads with flagella. Arrow points to trichomonad. (From Hacker NF, Gambone JC, Hobel CJ. *Hacker & Moore's Essentials of Obstetrics and Gynecology.* Elsevier; 2016.)

including testing for *T. vaginalis*. The diagnosis of *T. vaginalis* is based on laboratory testing as follows:[6,16]

* Motile trichomonads on wet mount
* Positive culture
* Positive NAAT
* Positive rapid antigen or nucleic acid probe test [6,16]

The use of NAATs is highly recommended for testing for *T. vaginalis* in females because their high sensitivity and specificity increases the likelihood of detection of the disease.[6] Microscopic examination of vaginal discharge is a convenient, low-cost test and is often the first step used to diagnose trichomoniasis. Diagnosis can be made by visualization of mobile trichomonads on a saline wet prep (Fig. 15.6). However, the sensitivity of the wet mount is low at 48% to 68%.[6] The slide with the vaginal specimen should be viewed immediately as the motility of the trichomonads is reduced when cold or the specimen dries.[6,17] If the wet prep is non-diagnostic and no mobile organisms are seen, a NAAT should be performed.[16] An abundant amount of white blood cells may be seen on the slide as a result of inflammation, and a positive "whiff" test or an amine odor may be present when potassium hydroxide (KOH) is added to the vaginal specimen.[17] If trichomoniasis is diagnosed, consider testing for other STIs.[18]

Management

> **NOT TO BE MISSED**
>
> Treatment is indicated for both symptomatic and asymptomatic females.

Pharmacological

The only classes of antimicrobial medications effective against *T. vaginalis* infections are nitroimidazoles. It is no longer necessary to warn patients against alcohol consumption while taking this class of medications.[6,10] Because there are no other effective drugs to treat trichomoniasis other than the nitroimidazoles, it is suggested that patients with an allergy to metronidazole or tinidazole be referred for desensitization.[6]

> **PATIENT-CENTERED CARE:** For HIV-positive females, the CDC recommends that metronidazole 500 mg twice a day for 7 days be prescribed rather than single-dose therapy.

> **CLINICAL SURVIVAL TIP** Nitroimidazole drugs given in both a single dose and longer results in a 90% cure rate for trichomoniasis.

Nonpharmacological

There are no nonpharmacological treatments that can be used to treat and cure this disease. The patient should be counseled on preventive therapy such as condom use and limiting the number of partners.

> **PATIENT-CENTERED CARE:** For refractory trichomoniasis, increase the dose and duration of both metronidazole and tinidazole when retreated.

Education and Counseling

All sex partners should be referred for presumptive therapy and treated concurrently to prevent transmission and reinfection. Expedited partner therapy (EPT), the practice of treating the sex partners of patients with an STI without a medical evaluation, can be used in states where it is legal. EPT is usually provided through patient-delivered partner therapy (PDPT). Further research is needed to determine the true value of this strategy in the treatment of trichomoniasis.[19] Females should abstain from sex until they and their sex partners have completed treatment and any symptoms have resolved. Retesting within 3 months is recommended in female patients, even if the patient's partner completed treatment because of the high rate of reinfection. Consistent and correct condom use during penile-vaginal sex is effective in preventing trichomoniasis.[6]

VULVOVAGINAL CANDIDIASIS

Epidemiology

VVC, a disease characterized by the symptoms of vulvar and vaginal inflammation, is the second most common of the vaginal infections, accounting for about one-third of vaginal symptoms. The exact prevalence of VVC is difficult to determine because not all cases are confirmed with an examination. Many females experiencing symptoms will self-treat and not seek medical advice unless the symptoms do not disappear. Because some clinicians do not confirm the diagnosis, but treat on symptoms, as many as 50% of unconfirmed VVC diagnoses may be wrong.[20] The highest rate of occurrence is found among reproductive-age females.

The CDC estimates that 75% of females will have at least one episode of VVC, and 40% to 45% will have two or more occurrences.[6] Recurrent VVC or resistant VVC is the most frequent complication. VVC is classified as uncomplicated or complicated based on the following:

- Clinical presentation
- Microbiology
- Host condition
- Response to treatment[6]

  Table 15.5 defines the classifications for VVC.

Pathogenesis

Candida albicans is the mostly likely causative agent for VVC, accounting for 80% to 92% of infections.[21] The other 8% to 20% are caused almost exclusively by *Candida glabrata*.

The emergence of other *Candida* species may be caused by widespread use of over-the-counter drugs as

TABLE 15.5	**Classification of Vulvovaginal Candidiasis[6]**
Uncomplicated	Infrequent occurrence
	Mild to moderate infection
	Most likely causative agent: *Candida albicans*
	Nonimmunocompromised
Complicated	Recurrent
	Three or more episodes in less than 1 year
	Severe
	Edema
	Excoriation/fissure formation
	Most likely causative agent: non-albicans
	Preexistence of
	Diabetes
	Debilitation
	Immunosuppression such as human immunodeficiency virus
	Immunosuppressive therapy such as corticosteroids

well as the use of frequent short courses of antifungal drugs. Candida organisms are found normally in both the gastrointestinal and vaginal tract. The development of symptomatic disease is dependent on an overgrowth that penetrates the superficial epithelial cells and becomes symptomatic.

Host factors seem to play an important role in the development of symptomatic disease. Conditions such as increased estrogen levels (pregnancy or postmenopausal estrogen therapy), uncontrolled diabetes, genetic variations, immunosuppressive disorders, as well as the use of antimicrobials alter the host environment and can lead to an active overgrowth of the organism.[6,21]

Recurrent vulvovaginal candidiasis (RVVC) is defined as four or more episodes in a 12-month period.[21] Recurrent disease is thought to be caused by relapse from a persistent vaginal reservoir of organisms. It is usually a reinfection with the identical strain of susceptible *C. albicans*. Rarely, infection is caused by a different *Candida* species[22]. RVVC has been associated with a decrease in the vivo concentration of mannose-binding lectin (MBL) and increased concentration of interleukin-4 (Il-4). There is a direct interaction of MBL with *C.*

albicans. It is an important component of the ability to resist candidiasis, so any impairment of the interaction appears to predispose females to recurrent vulvovaginal Candida infection. Female patients in whom the MBL is decreased will have a strong response to the presence of Candida organisms in amounts that usually do not cause a response. The function of Il-4 is to block the anti-Candida response; therefore when the IL-4 levels are elevated, an inhibition of the local defense mechanisms helps protect from infection with the Candida organism.[22]

Screening

There are no recommendations for routine screening for VVC in either pregnant or non-pregnant females. All females should be screened and treated if symptoms are present.

Focused History and Physical Examination

The history should focus on the identification of symptoms (see Table 15.3). The most common presenting symptom is that of intense itching, which may be accompanied by vulvar and vaginal pain. Ask about pain as it relates to the following:

- Intercourse, especially on entrance into the vagina
- Burning pain with urination associated with the vulva
- Vaginal soreness

The patient may or may not perceive the presence of a discharge. If present, the discharge is described as thick,

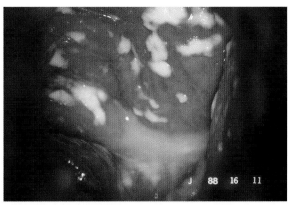

Figure 15.7 Classic "cottage-cheese" discharge seen in vulvovaginal candidiasis. (From Bailey WR, Tille PM. *Bailey & Scott's Diagnostic Microbiology.* Elsevier; 2017.)

white, "cottage cheese" or curdlike discharge (Fig. 15.7). The discharge usually has no offensive odor.

On physical examination, make note of signs of increased erythema of both the vagina and the vulva, vulvar and/or vaginal edema, fissures, and excoriations. The degree of vulvar and vaginal symptoms will determine whether the infection is uncomplicated or complicated. White, "cheesy" discharge may be present. The discharge is non-offensive. Foul-smelling or purulent discharge suggests bacterial infection (see Box 15.1). Although this is the typical appearance of the discharge, it can also appear as thin and loose, watery, or homogeneous and can be indistinguishable from other types of vaginitis. [21]

Satellite lesions on the upper thigh or lower abdomen may be present. If the patient is obese, examine the folds of the skin for lesions as both the vaginal area and the skin may require treatment. The cervix usually appears normal.[21]

The presentation of chronic and recurrent VVC may include the aforementioned symptoms as well as marked edema and lichenification of the vulva. Lichenification causes poorly defined margins, which can lead to difficulty in diagnosing. The vulva and vagina may take on a grayish color as a result of changes in epithelial cells caused by the effect of the Candida organisms. Patients usually report severe itching that may keep them up at night as well as burning, irritation, and increased pain. Patients with severe or chronic VVC should be checked for the presence of diabetes and immunosuppression.[23]

Diagnosis

A positive diagnosis can be made with use of the following:
- Wet prep with saline and 10% KOH demonstrates budding yeast, hyphae, and pseudohyphae (Fig. 15.8).
- Cultures[6]

> **CLINICAL SURVIVAL TIP** The use of KOH assists in the diagnosis by destroying the cellular elements and facilitates the recognition of budding yeast, pseudohyphae, and hyphae.

The presence of budding yeast only may indicate an infection with *C. glabrata* as opposed to *C. albicans*. *C. glabrata* grows as small, elliptical, budding, unicellular yeasts. They rarely form a chain.[24] Wet prep

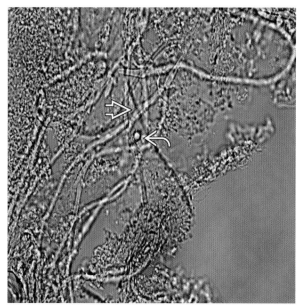

Figure 15.8 Wet prep with saline and 10% potassium hydroxide (KOH) demonstrates budding yeast, hyphae, and pseudohyphae. (From *Diagnostic Pathology: Gynecological, Second Edition,* 2019, Elsevier.)

alone is not sufficient for a type-specific diagnosis.[21] Wet prep is the first line of diagnosis and should be performed on all patients with a vaginal infection. If the results are positive, the patient should be treated.[6] If the patient has a negative wet prep and signs and symptoms of VVC, a culture for Candida should be considered.

Culture of asymptomatic patients is not recommended as 10% to 20% of females will test positive for Candida. If no symptoms are present, treatment is not needed. Because culture is more sensitive and specific, it remains the gold standard for diagnosing VVC.[6] Culture should be performed for female patients with persistent or recurrent symptoms because many of these patients have a non-*albicans* infection resistant to azoles.

Management

Pharmacological

> **NOT TO BE MISSED**
>
> Oral and vaginal azoles are equally effective in the treatment of uncomplicated VVC.

Antifungal drugs or azoles are used to treat uncomplicated VVC. Short-course formulations ranging from 1 to 3 days are effective, and short-course treatment is well-accepted by patients. Treatment with azoles results in both symptom relief and an 80% to 90% cure rate in patients who finish therapy. See Table 15.6 for the CDC-recommended treatment for uncomplicated VVC.[6]

NOT TO BE MISSED

Creams and suppositories are oil based and can weaken both latex condoms and diaphragms.

Treatment for complicated VVC may need to be extended over a longer period. If the condition is severe, there is usually a lower clinical response rate, so a 7- to 14-day topical azole is needed. If treating with oral fluconazole, two sequential doses of 150 mg given 72 hours apart is recommended.[6]

PATIENT-CENTERED CARE: Consider longer therapy (7 to 14 days) in patients on immunosuppressive therapy.

With RVVC, the short duration of the treatment course may not be effective in treating *C. albicans*. Consider the use of a longer duration of therapy, such as a topical azole for 7 to 14 days or fluconazole 100, 150, or 200 mg every third day to attempt to achieve remission in mycological activity.[6] Maintenance therapy can be used to help prevent recurrence. Oral fluconazole is first-line therapy for maintenance. It can be given weekly for up to 6 weeks. Although suppression therapy is effective, 30% to 50% of patients experience recurrence once therapy is discontinued. You may want to refer patients with RVVC to a specialist.[6]

PATIENT-CENTERED CARE: The rate of vaginal Candida is higher among HIV-positive patients, but the treatment remains the same; however, female patients with HIV may benefit from suppressive therapy.

Non-albicans is often difficult to treat because of the lack of effective antifungal preparations available for treatment. CDC recommendations are to treat for 7 to 14 days with a non-fluconazole azole.[6] When treating a glabrata infection, moderate success (70%) has been achieved with

TABLE 15.6 **Treatment for Uncomplicated Vulvovaginal Candidiasis**	
Over-the-Counter Intravaginal Agents	**Prescription Intravaginal Agents**
Butoconazole 2% cream 5 g intravaginally for 3 days OR	Butoconazole 2% cream (single dose bioadhesive product), 5 g intravaginally for 1 day OR
Clotrimazole 1% cream 5 g intravaginally for 7–14 days OR	Nystatin 100,000-unit vaginal tablet, one tablet for 14 days OR
Clotrimazole 2% cream 5 g intravaginally for 3 days OR	Terconazole 0.4% cream 5 g intravaginally for 7 days OR
Miconazole 2% cream 5 g intravaginally for 7 days OR	Terconazole 0.8% cream 5 g intravaginally for 3 days OR
Miconazole 4% cream 5 g intravaginally for 3 days OR	Terconazole 80 mg vaginal suppository, one suppository for 3 days
Miconazole 100 mg vaginal suppository, one suppository for 7 days OR	
Miconazole 200 mg vaginal suppository, one suppository for 3 days OR	
Miconazole 1200-mg vaginal suppository, one suppository for 1 day OR	
Tioconazole 6.5% ointment 5 g intravaginally in a single application	
	Oral Agents
	Fluconazole 150-mg oral tablet, one tablet in a single dose

Modified from U.S. Centers for Disease Control and Prevention. Sexually transmitted infections treatment guidelines, 2021. *MMWR Morbid Mortal Wkly Rep.* 2021;70(4):1–187.

intravaginal boric acid (600 mg capsule once daily for 3 weeks).[6] *Candida krusei* is generally resistant to fluconazole but is extremely susceptible to topical azole creams and suppositories such as clotrimazole, miconazole, and terconazole. Treatment should be for 7 to 14 days. *C. krusei* also responds to oral itraconazole (200 mg twice daily for 7 to 14 days) or ketoconazole (400 mg daily for 7 to 14 days). These oral agents have varying toxicities including hepatotoxicity, so topical treatment is recommended for first-line therapy.[22]

> ### ⚠ SAFETY ALERT
>
> Boric acid capsules can be fatal if swallowed.

> **PATIENT-CENTERED CARE:** VVC occurs frequently in pregnancy and should be treated with topical azoles for 7 days. Oral agents are not used in pregnancy.

Nonpharmacological

Data are lacking for a positive recommendation in most nonpharmacological treatments. Table 15.7 discusses the most frequent of these remedies along with available studies. Product safety can be an issue because of the lack of regulation. Discuss side effects, and counsel patients to discontinue the product and return for a visit if side effects develop.

Education and Counseling

Counseling includes proper use of the prescribed medication. Completing the course of therapy can be useful in preventing recurrence. VVC is not considered a sexually transmitted disease (STD), so unless the partner is showing signs of infection, no treatment is needed.[6] If a male partner is experiencing signs of balanitis, treatment with a topical azole is warranted. Follow-up is not needed unless the symptoms persist or return.

Prevention strategies are useful for the patient and may help prevent return. Antibiotic therapy can increase the risk of VVC, so it is helpful to use an azole at the start and end of antibiotic therapy in female patients who are susceptible to symptomatic yeast infections. Fluconazole 150 mg can be used to help prevent post-antibiotic VVC. [21] If the patient is diabetic, maintaining good glycemic control can help prevent VVC. Although there is no strong evidence, avoiding douching and irritants such as strong soaps or bubble baths may help protect the integrity of the vagina and help prevent vaginitis.

SEXUALLY TRANSMITTED INFECTIONS

STIs are the most common and preventable causes of morbidity in health care today. STDs are the diseases that are sequelae to STIs. Depending on the type of infection, untreated disease can result in PID, infertility, ectopic pregnancy, and chronic pelvic pain. Ten to twenty percent of STIs result in long-term problems.[25] STIs are also associated with high maternal morbidity and adverse fetal outcomes in pregnancy, therefore all pregnant patients must be screened for STIs at their first prenatal visit.[25]

Finally, STIs may increase the likelihood of HIV transmission.[6] Primary prevention of STIs must be one of the highest priorities in clinical practice. This section discusses assessment, diagnosis, treatment, and prevention of common STIs encountered in primary care.

Pathology and Epidemiology

STIs are a group of diseases that are caused by infection with bacteria, virus, or parasites. Some are exclusively transmitted sexually, and some are predominately transmitted this way. Contributing to the pathological process seen with STIs is the problem of the way in which it is transmitted. The social stigma associated with sexual transmission can complicate the ability of the clinician to effectively diagnose and treat the disease.[26]

The rate of STIs is currently on the rise.[27] Many diseases such as HSV and HPV are not reportable, so the increase we see is only part of the larger problem we face.

Some populations experience increased risk of contracting STIs. Gay and bisexual males face a combination of social, epidemiologic, and individual risk factors that increase the likelihood of developing STIs. An increased prevalence of infection within their sexual networks increases the likelihood of acquiring an STI. The burden of barriers to receiving STI services, such as lack of access to quality health care, homophobia, or stigma also contribute to increased risk. Young people between 15 and 24 years of age acquire approximately one-half of the estimated 26 million new STIs diagnosed each year.[27] These trends highlight the need for risk assessment, screening, and promotion of prevention.

> ### NOT TO BE MISSED
>
> STI screening must be a standard part of health care, especially in pregnant patients. Integrate STI prevention and treatment into prenatal care and other routine visits.

TABLE 15.7	Nonpharmacological Treatment for Vulvovaginal Candidiasis		
Treatment	**Use**	**What We Know**	**Reference(s)**
Boric acid	600 mg intravaginally for 2 weeks	Has been shown to work with *C. glabrata* infection and with proven azole resistance Can be toxic in large amounts	26–28
Gentian violet	Apply to affected areas of the vulva and vagina daily for 10 to 14 days	Used before azole therapy was available Useful as a vulvar antipruritic Can be useful for refractory cases of vulvovaginal candidiasis Used with azole resistance	29
Probiotic	Can be used orally Vaginal suppositories Plain Greek yogurt (intravaginally)	No evidence that vaginal flora are deficient in lactobacilli that must be replaced in females with recurrent vulvovaginal candidiasis Data not contradictory in regard to lactobacilli recurrent infection Evidence not strong enough to support a recommendation May be more useful with bacterial vaginosis Most common recommendation is further research	30–32
Tea tree oil	Vaginal suppositories	No randomized clinical trials No human data Never take orally because of toxicity	33
Apple cider vinegar	Add ½ cup to a lukewarm bath, and soak for 20 minutes	No data Patient reports of some improvement of itching Supposed to help eliminate *Candida* organisms from the skin.	No data
Garlic	Increase garlic intake in food to try for 40 mg a day of allicin (a garlic clove contains 3–5 mg per clove Insert a garlic clove in the vagina daily	No human data on oral garlic No data Vaginal burning has been reported	34
Oregano essential oil	3 to 5 drops with a carrier oil; apply to the vulva area Inhale with a diffuser	Found to have an antifungal effect in mice No human data Do not take essential oil by mouth	35
Vitamin C	Take daily to boost the immune system Use as a suppository at times of active growth	Vitamin C is an immune system booster Used intravaginally, it can cause burning; use with care	No data

Prognosis

Prognosis varies according to the disease present. Overall, for the bacterial infections, there are antibiotics that are effective in eradicating the disease. Prognosis depends on screening, early recognition, and proper treatment for both the patient and partner to prevent the long-term sequelae associated with the diseases. If left untreated, the bacterial infections can lead to long-term reproductive problems. The viral diseases are not curable, so early diagnosis and treatment is aimed at reducing the burden of the disease symptoms. Because of the nature of transmission, both partners must receive adequate treatment before intercourse can be resumed, or one partner will reinfect the other. The CDC recommends that clinicians have a plan for the treatment or referral of partners of patients with STIs to help reduce the rate of reinfection.[6]

Assessment
Focused History and Physical Examination

Risk assessment through routine sexual histories is critical to identify at-risk individuals. Risk factors for STIs can include behavioral and demographic factors as well as biological markers. Because of the personal nature of the questions, it is critical that the data be collected in a nonjudgmental way that shows respect for the patient being interviewed. Behavioral factors associated with a high risk of STIs include the following:

- Multiple sex partners
- A sex partner with multiple concurrent sex partners
- Sex with partners recently treated for an STI
- Inconsistent condom use
- Trading sex for money or drugs
- Sexual contact (oral, anal, penile, or vaginal) with sex workers
- Alcohol and drug use

NOT TO BE MISSED

Accurate risk assessment, along with education and counseling of at-risk individuals, is one of the only ways to avoid STIs and reduce the occurrence of these diseases.

The Five *P*'s framework for taking a sexual history (Table 15.8)[6] provides a systematic way of addressing the behavioral risk and offers questions that can be used to guide the interview. This tool can be used to provide a beginning for the counseling that is so important for patients. As risks are identified, counseling and preventive strategies can be discussed.

Demographic factors are important to identifying at-risk individuals. There are several high-risk groups that require specific considerations for STI screening and counseling. Some demographic groups identified as having a higher prevalence of STIs include the following:

- Young age (15 to 24 years of age)
- Men who have sex with men (MSM)
- History of a prior STI
- Unmarried status
- Lower socioeconomic status or a high school education or less
- Admission to a correctional facility or juvenile detention center
- Illicit drug use

Sexually active adolescents are considered to be at increased risk for STIs. The Youth Risk Behavior

TABLE 15.8   The Five *P*'s of Sexual History

Five Ps	Questions
Partner	Do you have sex with males, females, or both? Is your current partner(s) a male, female, or both? In the past 2 months, how many partners have you had sex with? In the past 12 months, how many partners have you had sex with? Is it possible that any of your sex partners in the past 12 months had sex with someone during the same period they were having sex with you?
Prevention of pregnancy	Are you trying to get pregnant? If not, what are you using to prevent it?
Protection	What do you do to protect yourself against human immunodeficiency virus (HIV) and sexually transmitted infections (STIs)?
Practice	To help you understand your risk of contracting STIs, I need to know the kind of sex you practiced over the past 12 months. What are your sexual practices, and do you understand the risk of these practices? *To be specific, ask*: Vaginal sex, Anal sex, Oral sex. Do you use condoms? If never: Why? If sometimes: In what situations?
Past history	Do you have a history of either STIs or HIV? Do any of your partners have a history of either STIs or HIV?
Other usual questions	Have you or any of your partners ever injected intravenous drugs? Have you or any of your partners exchanged money or drugs for sex? Is there anything else about your sexual practices that you think I should know?

Modified from U.S. Centers for Disease Control and Prevention. Sexually transmitted infections treatment guidelines, 2021. *MMWR Morbid Mortal Wkly Rep.* 2021;70(4):1–187.

Surveillance System (YRBSS) monitors six categories of health behaviors in this age group:[28]
- Behaviors that contribute to unintentional injuries and violence
- Tobacco use
- Alcohol and other drug use
- Sexual behaviors related to unintended pregnancy and STIs
- Unhealthy dietary behaviors
- Physical inactivity

Data for 2019 showed that 27.4% of high school students had a history of sexual intercourse, and 26.9% reported four or more lifetime sexual partners. The proportion of sexually active students reporting condom use decreased from 57% to 54.3% between 2015 and 2019 after having increased from 46% in 1991.[28]

MSM are also at increased risk of contracting an STI. The higher prevalence of these infections in the MSM community increases the likelihood of transmission.[6] Sexual risk assessment with a careful sexual history and counseling on risk reduction should be performed at all visits for MSM patients.[29,30] MSM who also have sex with females place the females at the same increased risk.

NOT TO BE MISSED

For transgender individuals, the risk of STIs depends on the current anatomy and sexual behavior. STI risk assessment as well as screening and counseling should be tailored to the patient's anatomy and risk behavior.

Pregnant patients, although not more likely to develop an STI, should be screened and counseled regarding STIs. Transmission during pregnancy can be both intrauterine and perinatal. There is the potential for high morbidity among pregnant patients with STIs and poor fetal outcomes with maternal infection. The CDC recommends that a risk assessment be performed on pregnant patients at the first prenatal visit, followed by appropriate screening.[6] Follow-up screening is based on the risk identified at the first screening.

Other than sexual history and risk assessment, the history should also include questions related to possible symptoms. Two of the major ways that STIs present is with signs and symptoms of discharge or with lesions; general questions related to these areas can be useful. It is also important to remember that not all STIs are symptomatic, and the absence of a presenting symptom does not mean absence of disease. This lack of symptoms is one of the reasons that screening is so important. The gynecological history is important when looking for symptoms of STIs. Be sure to ask about the following:
- Vaginal discharge or odor
- Dysuria, frequency, or urgency
- Itching or irritation
  - Vulvar
  - Anal
  - Pubic area
  - Perineum
- Abnormal vaginal bleeding
- Genital sores/ulcers/lesions, bumps/warts, masses, or rashes
  - Painful
  - Recurrent
- Dyspareunia
- Rectal/perianal symptoms
  - Pain
  - Discharge
  - Bleeding
  - Itching
  - Sores
  - Masses

Extend the history to other systems depending on the probable diagnosis as the genital tract is not the only system that is at risk for sexually transmitted organisms. Other systems to consider are as follows:
- Oral/pharyngeal symptoms
- Lymph node swelling or tenderness
- Non-genital skin rashes
- Abdominal complaints
  - Nausea
  - Vomiting
  - Constipation
  - Diarrhea
- Systemic or constitutional symptoms
  - Acute arthritic symptoms
  - Neurological symptoms

A focused physical examination for STI evaluation is concentrated mainly in two areas, the pelvic examination and a generalized inspection of the skin and hair. Other areas will depend on the clinician's differential diagnoses and the body areas that have been exposed. Examinations to consider are as follows:
- Inspection of the mouth and throat

- Lesions
- Redness
- Swelling
- Inspection of the trunk, forearms, and palms
  - Signs of rash lesions
- Inspection of external genital, pubic, and perianal areas
  - Bleeding
  - Discharge
  - Irritation
  - Lesions
  - Rash
- Palpation of the inguinal nodes
  - Swelling
  - Tenderness
- Inspection of the urinary meatus
  - Redness
  - Swelling
  - Discharge
  - Mucoid
  - Mucopurulent
  - Purulent

To complete the examination, perform a pelvic examination including the following:

- Palpate the Skene glands
  - Tenderness
  - Swelling
- Palpate the Bartholin glands
  - Tenderness
  - Swelling
- Assess vaginal discharge
  - Amount
  - Consistency
  - Color
  - Odor
  - pH
- Assess for any abdominal pain
- Inspect the cervix and vaginal wall
  - Redness
  - Swelling
  - Lesions
  - Discharge
- Bimanual examination
  - Cervical motion tenderness
  - Adnexal masses and tenderness
  - Uterine enlargement and tenderness
  - Abnormalities on palpation

Determine if other examination is needed based on the patient's specific needs.

> **CLINICAL SURVIVAL TIP** When performing a risk assessment, it is also important for clinicians to ask patients about symptoms consistent with common STIs, including urethral discharge, dysuria, ulcers, or anorectal symptoms.

Screening

The CDC estimates that nearly 68 million STIs occurred in 2018 in the United States, and almost one-half occurred in a younger population (15 to 24 years of age).[27] Two of the CDC's five strategies for the prevention and control of STIs are related to screening. Identification of asymptomatic individuals and effective diagnosis, treatment, counseling, and follow-up are major strategies recommended by the CDC. The U.S. Preventive Services Task Force (USPSTF) has issued clinical recommendation statements on screening for STIs, similar to those from the CDC. Table 15.9 reports the current recommendations of these two organizations.[6,31] Screening recommendations with strong evidence are the same among the major organizations that publish screening guidelines. Testing is recommended more frequently for patients who engage in risky behaviors and those who present with STI symptoms. Without routine screening, it would be impossible to eradicate STIs because of the number that appear to be asymptomatic.

When the patient requests an STI evaluation, it is likely prompted by either a known exposure or an unexpected risky behavior. Discerning the rationale for the requested testing can facilitate effective, patient-centered counseling. Routine screening includes the following:

- Gonorrhea (at genital and, if exposed, at rectal and pharyngeal sites)
- Chlamydia (at genital and, if exposed, at rectal sites)
- Syphilis
- HIV

Consider HBV and HCV testing if the patient has not been screened within the past year, especially if there was a possible exposure from a new or unknown partner. Offering routine screening can be useful in trying to control the spread of STIs. There are a number of STIs that are reportable to the CDC. It is the clinician's responsibility to report these diseases, usually to the local health department. Reportable diseases are as follows:

- Chlamydia
- Gonorrhea

TABLE 15.9 Sexually Transmitted Infection Screening for Female Patients[6,31]			
Population	Recommendation	Frequency	Additional Recommendations and Comments
<25 years	Chlamydia Gonorrhea HIV	Once a year Once a year At least once	Screen based on risk for syphilis, trichomoniasis, HBV, and HCV
<25 years	HIV	At least once	Screen based on risk for syphilis, trichomoniasis, HBV, HCV, chlamydia, and gonorrhea
HIV infected	Chlamydia Gonorrhea Syphilis HBV HCV	Once a year Once a year Once a year First visit First visit	
Pregnant	Chlamydia Gonorrhea Syphilis HBV HCV	Test of all on the first visit	If at increased risk, repeat in the third trimester If at risk for HCV, screen at the first prenatal visit Also screen pregnant HIV-positive patients for trichomoniasis at the first visit
WSW			Dependent on risk factors and if the patient had contact with a male since the last visit.
Transgender			Dependent on risk factors
Incarcerated	Chlamydia Gonorrhea Syphilis	<35 years of age <35 years of age On admission	It has been shown that individuals entering a correctional institution have a higher incidence of chlamydia and gonorrhea if 35 years of age or younger This should be performed based on the prevalence seen in the local area
Other women	HCV	Once	Individuals born between 1945 and 1946

HBV, Hepatitis B virus; *HCV,* hepatitis C virus; *WSW,* women who have sex with women. Adapted from U.S. Centers for Disease Control and Prevention. (2021). Sexually transmitted infections treatment guidelines, 2021. *MMWR Morbid Mortal Wkly Rep, 70(4),* 1–187 and Meyers, D., Wolff, T., Gregory, K., Marion, L., et al. (2008). USPSTF recommendation for STI screening. *Am Fam Phys., 15(77),* 819–824.

- Acute HBV
- Acute HCV
- HIV
- Syphilis

If the patient tests positive for gonorrhea, chlamydia, syphilis, or trichomoniasis, sex partners should be notified as they must be treated before sexual activity can resume, thus preventing reinfection. In most clinical situations, the patient is responsible for providing the notification. If your practice does not provide partner treatment, the patient should be given a list of options where her partner can receive treatment. Rescreening is dependent on resolution of symptoms, success of getting partners treated, and further risky behavior. Setting a schedule for rescreening should be tailored to personal risk as some patients may require more frequent screening.

Prevention

Prevention is key to control of the problems related to STIs. First in the realm of prevention is the preexposure vaccination. Vaccines are available for the prevention of several STIs. These include hepatitis A virus (HAV), hepatitis B virus (HBV), and HPV. Although HAV is not exclusively sexually transmitted, recommendations for vaccination for females is important. The CDC's Advisory Committee on Immunization Practices (ACIP) develops recommendations and guidelines that serve as the vaccine schedule in the United States.

Reduction in risky behavior is important to the prevention of STIs. One of the most reliable methods of preventing STIs is to avoid exposure. Abstinence from oral, vaginal, and anal sex will decrease risk. Skin-to-skin transmissions may lead to diseases that present as genital ulcers or lesions. One of the second-best prevention methods is to be in a mutually monogamous relationship with a partner known to be STI free. When discussing a monogamous relationship, be sure that you and the patient are defining the term alike. Many females practice serial monogamy as they have only one partner at a time. Follow-up a response that the patient is in a monogamous relationship with a question about how long the patient has been in that relationship and how many lifetime sexual partners the patient has had. This becomes an important question as the most likely transmission of infections is at the beginning of a new relationship.

NOT TO BE MISSED

Reducing the number of sexual partners reduces the risk of STIs.

Discussion of individual risk is important to control and reduce the identified risk. Counseling includes assessing the patient's knowledge and misconceptions regarding STIs and the circumstances affecting the patient's behavior.

The next step should include an assessment of the patient's readiness for change. Then a goal for behavioral change can be set, and a concrete first step to take toward this goal can be negotiated. Counseling also includes providing realistic steps toward obtaining the goal. Concrete behavior to lower risk, such as condom use, should be suggested and discussed with the patient. Abstinence should always be offered as an option for patients.

CLINICAL SURVIVAL TIP Risk-reduction counseling should be directed toward patient-centered change.

Condom use is one of the most important means of preventing STIs. Overall, the current evidence supports the efficacy of condoms in preventing most STIs. However, there may be some difference based on the type of STI that the patient is exposed to. Condoms have been shown to be effective in the prevention of HIV.[32] Condoms have also been shown to be highly effective against chlamydia, gonorrhea, and trichomoniasis. By limiting the transmissions of these STIs, there may also be a reduction in the risk for the development of PID.[33,34] In addition, the use of condoms has been shown to reduce

the risk of HPV- and HPV-related diseases, genital herpes, HBV, syphilis, and chancroid when the site of potential exposure is covered.[6]

Latex condoms are the most common type of condoms used in the United States. They are tested for strength and, when used correctly, are excellent at helping to prevent STIs. According to research, the rate of condom breakage is approximately 2 per 100.[35] The problem with condom failure is more likely to be from either nonuse or improper use.[36] It is important to use condoms within their expiration date. Expired condoms have a higher failure rate, as the latex weakens after 5 years.[6]

For patients with a latex allergy, there is the option to use either condoms made with polyurethane or natural membrane. When looking at effectiveness of the polyurethane condom, it has been shown to be comparable to the latex condoms in the prevention of STIs.[33] They are also more resistant and can be used with oil-based lubricants. Polyurethane condoms may be more expensive and are not as widely available. Although a few other synthetic condoms are available, they have not been studied, so their efficacy is not known.

The use of natural membrane condoms does not provide the same level of protection. These condoms made from the cecum of lambs are more porous, and although effective at keeping sperm out, they can allow the passage of some viruses. Studies have shown that HBV, HSV, and HIV can cross the barrier, so they are less effective in the prevention of these diseases. Natural membrane condoms are not recommended for use in the prevention of STIs.[8]

NOT TO BE MISSED

Teaching a female patient how to use a condom helps ensure that her partner is using it correctly.

Consistent and correct use is one of the most effective preventive measures used today. Assessment of condom use is generally by self-report, which may be unreliable. Incorrect use of condoms that would reduce their efficacy is rarely evaluated, and frequency of condom use is usually recorded as a static measure, when it may change over time. Each of these factors would underestimate the efficacy of appropriate condom use. There are several important messages that must be included in the education for proper use. Although many seem like common sense, it is better to give the information than send the patient out without the means to be successful. Many female patients are embarrassed to ask for information they feel they should already know, so the inability to use correctly continues. Even in patients that are using condoms, it may increase their use if they receive the information. The following information is important to the success of condom use:

- Use a new condom with each act of intercourse. If you have oral, anal, and vaginal intercourse during the same encounter, a new condom must be used each time.
- Be careful when handling condoms. Anything sharp can damage it. This includes fingernails, teeth, and any other sharp object.
- Use water-based lubricants with latex condoms. Oil causes the latex to break down, and failure is more likely.
- With synthetic condoms, either water-based or oil-based condoms can be used.
- Be sure to have adequate lubrication when having vaginal or anal sex. Use a water-based lubricant if needed. Without adequate lubrication, the condom can be damaged, and failures occur.[6]
- You may also need to instruct the patient on how to place a condom on the penis.
  - Put the condom on when the penis is erect but before it touches the partner's mouth, vagina, or rectum.
  - Direct genital contact can transmit some diseases. The liquid that comes out of the penis before orgasm can contain sexually transmittable virus.
  - If uncircumcised, push the foreskin back before putting on the condom. This lets the foreskin move without breaking the condom.
  - Squeeze the air out of the tip of the condom to leave room for semen, and unroll the rest of the condom down the penis.
  - Do not "double bag" (use two condoms). Friction between the condoms increases the chance of breakage.
  - After orgasm, hold the base of the condom, and pull out before the penis gets soft.
  - Remove the penis from the vagina before the erection is completely lost. Hold onto the base of the condom while removing the penis, and remove the condom well away from the vaginal area.[37]

Condoms should be stored away from extreme heat, cold, or friction. This includes both a wallet and a car glove compartment. All of these can lead to a weakening of the condom and increase the likelihood of failure. Check the expiration date. Do not use outdated condoms. Expired condoms are more likely to fail.

Female condoms provide a female-controlled mechanism for STI protection. Although use of the female condom provides some protection against STIs, the data are limited, and there is a need for further study.[38] Male and female condoms should not be used together, as they can stick to each other and lead to failure as a result of tearing. The female condom can be placed up to 8 hours before intercourse.[39] Again, providing instructions on use is important if the patient is to succeed in maximizing prevention.

- Put the condom in place before genital contact with the penis.
- For use in the vagina, insert the narrow end of the condom that contains the ring in the vagina as far back as it will go. This is performed by holding the inner ring between the thumb and middle finger and pushing it into the vagina.
- The larger end covers part of the vulva and may protect from some skin-to-skin contact transmission.
- When intercourse begins, guide the penis into the vagina to make sure it does not enter the vagina under the condom.
- After intercourse, remove the condom before standing up. Twist the large end to keep the semen inside. Gently pull the condom out, and throw it away.[40]

The female condom has been used with penis and anal intercourse, but there are no data on its effectiveness in preventing STIs.[41] If used for anal intercourse, the condom is placed on the penis and inserted into the anus with penetration.

Partner services refer to strategies like clinical evaluation of the partner, counseling, and treatment. Although not a preventive strategy, it can help reduce the risk of reinfection. The clinician can provide EPT for the partner of a patient being treated for chlamydia and gonorrhea if allowed by state law. This service allows the clinician to provide the patient with the medication that she can then give to the partner. Providing the actual medicine with instructions is the CDC-preferred method of EPT because many partners will not have the prescription filled. Up-to-date information on states that allow this can be found at https://www.cdc.gov/std/ept/legal/default.htm. Data from three U.S. clinical trials of men who have sex with women (MSW) reported that more partners received treatment, and two of the studies showed a statistically significant decline in the reinfection rate. The third study showed not only a decline in the reinfection rate but also a lower risk of persistent infection. There are no data to support the use of EPT in the treatment of syphilis.[6]

> ### NOT TO BE MISSED
>
> Reporting STIs allows for the collection of statistics that show incidence of the disease. This helps researchers identify disease trends and track disease outbreaks and can help control future outbreaks.

Reporting Criteria for Sexually Transmitted Infections

Some STIs are required by law to be reported. This is done because of the need to assess the morbidity trends, allocate resources, and assist local health authorities with both partner notification and treatment. Syphilis, gonorrhea, chlamydia, chancroid, HIV infection, and acquired immunodeficiency syndrome (AIDS) are reportable in all 50 states. Monitoring the incidence of these diseases allows us to identify areas where the disease is most prevalent. It helps identify disparities and allocate resources more appropriately to help improve public health.

The reporting of other STIs differs by state, and the clinician should check with the state health department to see what is required in that state. Because states may vary as to who is responsible for reporting (the clinician, laboratory, or both), clinicians again must check with the state health department if unsure of their responsibility. Reported information is confidential, and the provider is protected by a state statute or regulation in most jurisdictions.[6]

OTHER SEXUALLY TRANSMITTED INFECTIONS

Many diseases are partially or completely transmitted sexually. This chapter will discuss the most common diseases likely to be seen by the clinician in primary care. A complete list with the recommended treatment can be found in the most current CDC guidelines for treating STIs. STIs can be divided into two groups: (1) those characterized by infections of the urethra and/or the cervix and (2) diseases that cause lesions. Although these categories are not mutually exclusive, they provide a symptomatic place to begin the evaluation.

Diseases That Cause Urethral and Cervical Problems

Urethritis is characterized by inflammation of the urethra. General symptoms include the following:
- Dysuria
- Urethral itching
- Discharge (mucoid, mucopurulent, or purulent)

Cervicitis is characterized by mucopurulent or purulent discharge that is visible in the cervical canal as well increased friability of the cervix. It is important to remember that cervicitis can be asymptomatic in many patients, but if the signs are present, the patient should be worked up and properly treated. The most common causes of both urethritis and cervicitis in females are gonorrhea and chlamydia. Figure 15.9 provides an algorithm for the workup of a patient suspected of having gonorrhea and/or chlamydia.

Gonorrhea
Epidemiology
Gonorrhea, caused by *Neisseria gonorrhoeae,* is the second most commonly reported notifiable disease in the United States with approximately 820,000 new infections each year.[6] In 2019, the highest rates of gonorrhea in females were among those 15 to 24 years of age, and the rate of infection in Black females was 8.6 times the rate in White females.[27] In 2014, there were 350,062 reported cases of gonorrhea (a rate of 110.7 per 100,000). This is an increase of 15.1% over 2013 and poses a public health threat.[27]

Untreated gonorrhea can cause PID in females. PID can cause serious complications such as tubal scarring, infertility, ectopic pregnancy, and chronic pelvic pain. An infection of the Bartholin glands or Skene glands can be another complication of gonorrhea in female patients. Disseminated gonococcal infection (DGI) is rare but more common in females. DGI is a systemic gonococcal infection that causes petechial or pustular skin lesions, septic arthritis, tenosynovitis, and polyarthralgia.[6]

Pathogenesis
N. gonorrhoeae is an aerobic, oxidase-positive, gram-negative, diplococcus microorganism that attaches to

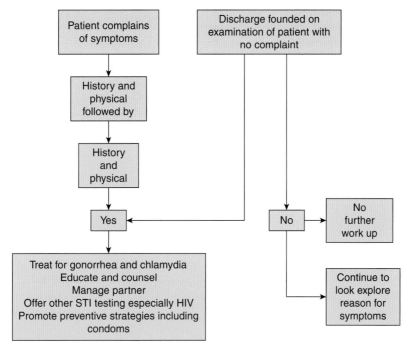

Figure 15.9 Algorithm for the workup for complaints related to urethral/cervical discharge. (Modified from Workowski KA, Bachmann LH, Chan PA, et al. *Sexually Transmitted Infections Treatment Guidelines, 2021. MMWR Recomm Rep.* 2021;70[4]:1–187.)

epithelial cells and infects the mucous membranes of the cervix, uterus, fallopian tubes, urethra, mouth, throat, eyes, and rectum.[12] Antibiotic resistance poses an urgent public health threat in addressing rising gonorrhea rates.[43] Transmission of gonorrhea occurs through sexual contact with the vagina, penis, mouth, or anus of an infected partner. Gonorrhea in neonates can result from perinatal exposure to an infected cervix and result in ocular infections.[6] Nonsexual transmission is rare.[12]

Screening
Sexually active females younger than 25 years of age and older females who are at increased risk for infection should be screened annually for gonorrhea.[44] See Table 15.9 for complete screening recommendations. Screening for gonorrhea should be performed at the first prenatal visit and again during the third trimester for pregnant patients younger than 25 years of age or in older female patients if at increased risk.[6]

Focused History and Physical Examination
Gonorrhea is asymptomatic in at least 50% of females. Symptoms differ according to the site of infection.

Table 15.10 is a list of the different presentations for gonorrhea.[6,27] If symptoms do occur, most develop within 10 days of exposure. The sexual history should assess if the patient has had any recent travel with sexual contacts outside of the United States.[6] Figure 15.10 provides an example of the presentations seen with gonorrhea, but it is important to remember that the physical examination may also be negative.

> **CLINICAL SURVIVAL TIP** Gonorrhea cannot be reliably distinguished from syndromes caused by other pathogens on the basis of signs and symptoms alone. Testing is required.

Diagnosis
NAAT and culture can be used to test for *N. gonorrhoeae*. The sensitivity of NAAT for urogenital and non-urogenital detection of *N. gonorrhoeae* is superior to culture and can be collected via endocervical swabs, vaginal swabs, and urine. Although NAAT is more generally sensitive than culture, the sensitivity of the

TABLE 15.10	**Symptoms of Gonorrhea Infection**[6,42]	

Urethritis	May be asymptomatic	Dysuria
		Pruritis
		Peri-urethral discharge
		    Mucoid
		    Mucopurulent
		    Purulent
		May involve the Skene and Bartholin glands

Cervicitis	May be asymptomatic
	Incubation period up to 10 days
		Symptoms range from mild to severe
		Dysuria
		Vaginal discharge
		Cervical discharge
		    Mucopurulent
		    Purulent
		Increased redness of the cervix
		Bleeding when the cervix is touched
		    From examination
		    From sexual contact

Pelvic inflammatory disease	Occurs in 10%–20% of females	Lower abdominal pain
		Pain usually bilateral
		Dyspareunia
		Marked tenderness over the
		    Adnexa
		    Cervix
		    Abdomen

Anorectal	May appear erythematous if examined with a proctoscope More frequent in MSM	Anal itching Discharge (cloudy in appearance) Soreness Bleeding Painful bowel movements
Pharyngeal infection	Usually asymptomatic	Sore throat
Disseminated gonorrhea infection (DGI)	Also called *arthritis-dermatitis syndrome* Reflects bacteremia	Fever Migratory pain or joint swelling Skin lesions (pustules)

Septic arthritis	More localized than DGI
	Arthritis with effusion
		Pain
		Usually involves large joints
		Acute onset
		    Fever
		    Severe joint pain
		    Limited joint movement
		    Overlying skin is warm to touch

Fitz-Hugh-Curtis syndrome	More common in females May also be caused by chlamydia Mimics hepatic disease	Right upper-quadrant abdominal pain Fever Nausea Vomiting

Modified from U.S. Centers for Disease Control and Prevention. (2021). *National Overview—Sexually Transmitted Disease Surveillance, 2019.* https://www.cdc.gov/STI/statistics/2019/overview.htm#:~:text=In%202019%2C%20 129%2C813%20 cases%20of,11.2%25%20during%20 2018%E2%80%932019; U.S. Centers for Disease Control and Prevention. (2021). *National Overview—Sexually Transmitted Disease Surveillance, 2019.* https://www.cdc.gov/STI/statistics/2019/overview.htm#:~:text=In%20 2019%2C%20 129%2C813%20cases%20of,11.2%25%20during%20 2018%E2%80%932019.

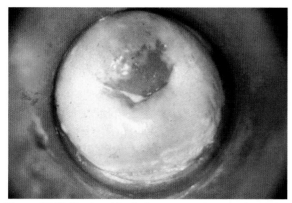

Figure 15.10 Cervix with discharge seen in gonorrhea infection. (From U.S. Centers for Disease Control and Prevention. *STD Clinical Slides;* 2020. https://www.cdc.gov/std/training/clinicalslides/default.htm.)

> ## BOX 15.4 Treatment Regimens: Uncomplicated Gonococcal Infections of the Cervix, Urethra, Rectum, and Pharynx
>
> ### Recommended Regimen
> - Ceftriaxone 500 mg IM in a single dose (for those weighing <150 kg)
> - Ceftriaxone 1 g IM in a single dose (for those weighing ≥150 kg)
>   If Chlamydia infection has not been ruled out, doxycycline 100 mg orally twice daily for 7 days
>
> ### Alternative Regimen
> - Gentamicin 240 mg IM in a single dose
>   *PLUS*
> - Cefixime 800 mg orally in a single dose
>   *OR*
> - Azithromycin 2 g orally in a single dose
>   If chlamydia has not been ruled out, doxycycline 100 mg orally twice daily for 7 days

From U.S. Centers for Disease Control and Prevention. Sexually transmitted infections treatment guidelines, 2021. *MMWR Morbid Mortal Wkly Rep.* 2021;70(4):1–187.

> **CLINICAL SURVIVAL TIP** Because of emerging resistance, there is a limited choice of effective antibiotics. It is important to follow treatment guidelines to avoid further resistance and to optimize treatment results.

individual NAAT varies by NAAT and specimen type. Proper specimen collection technique varies by test and affects the accuracy. Suspected non-genital infection requires a culture of the affected area. Culture provides the added advantage of testing for antibiotic sensitivity if the patient is allergic to the recommended treatment. With a persistent infection, a resistant organism should be considered, and a culture is recommended.[6]

Management

Pharmacological. Treatment for gonorrhea has been affected by antimicrobial resistance and has led to cephalosporin as the only remaining class of antimicrobial recommended for treatment of *N. gonorrhoeae* in the United States. Dual therapy using two antimicrobials with different mechanisms of action is recommended to improve treatment effectiveness and potentially slow the resistance to cephalosporins. In addition, patients who are infected with *N. gonorrhoeae* are often co-infected with *Chlamydia trachomatis*, therefore inclusion of doxycycline in the dual therapy provides treatment for chlamydia. See Box 15.4 for the recommended treatment for uncomplicated gonorrhea of the urogenital tract and rectum. If the alternative treatment is used, a test of cure should be performed in 2 weeks as this treatment is less effective. Patients allergic to cephalosporins should be treated with azithromycin 2 g orally as a single dose. A test of cure in 2 weeks is recommended as this treatment is less effective for treatment of more complicated cases. There are no nonpharmacological options for the management of gonorrhea.

Education and Counseling

All recent sex partners should be referred for evaluation and presumptive dual therapy to prevent transmission and reinfection. EPT using the alternative regimen can be used in states where permissible by law. This treatment option should be limited to females with gonorrhea who report that a partner(s) is unavailable or unlikely to receive prompt evaluation and treatment.[19] Females diagnosed with gonorrhea should be tested for other STIs, including chlamydia, syphilis, and HIV. Females should abstain from sex for 7 days after they and their partner(s) have completed treatment and any symptoms have resolved. Retesting for gonorrhea in females, even if their partner completed treatment, is recommended 3 months following initial treatment because of a high rate of reinfection. Consistent and correct use of condoms during penile-vaginal sex and a mouth-to-genital barrier during oral-genital sex can prevent gonorrhea.[6]

Chlamydia

Epidemiology

Chlamydia, caused by *C. trachomatis,* is the most common reportable infectious bacterial disease in the United States, with over 1.8 million cases reported in 2019.[6,27] The actual number of annual infections is anticipated to be significantly higher than reported because many cases go undetected. In 2019, the highest rates of chlamydia were among females 15 to 24 years of age, and the rate of infection in Black females was 4.5 times the rate in White females. [27] Chlamydia infections, like gonorrhea, have been increasing. Since 2018, the rate has increased 2.8%. There were approximately 1.4 million reported cases of chlamydia in 2014 for a rate of 456.1 cases per 100,000 individuals.[27]

Untreated chlamydia can cause PID in females. PID can cause serious complications such as fallopian tube scarring, infertility, ectopic pregnancy, and chronic pelvic pain.[6] Chlamydia is the leading cause of tubal factor infertility. Females with an asymptomatic infection are also at risk for subsequent infertility.[12]

Pathogenesis

C. trachomatis is an obligate, gram-negative, intracellular bacterium that can only reproduce within host cells. Columnar epithelial cells at mucosal sites serve as a host for *C. trachomatis* resulting in urogenital, rectal, oropharyngeal, and conjunctival infections.[12]

NOT TO BE MISSED

C. trachomatis causes trachoma or an STI; maternal transmission can cause neonatal conjunctivitis and/or pneumonia.

Transmission of chlamydia occurs through sexual contact with the vagina, penis, mouth, or anus of an infected partner. Vertical transmission from a mother to an infant occurs when the newborn passes through an infected genital tract during delivery. Exposure during delivery can result in ophthalmia neonatorum (conjunctivitis) or neonatal pneumonia.[6]

PATIENT-CENTERED CARE: Consider chlamydia infection with neonates if they present with conjunctivitis within 30 days or pneumonia within 3 months of delivery.

C. trachomatis has a slow replication cycle and a poorly defined incubation period. The incubation period is estimated to be 7 to 21 days in females who develop symptoms. Chronic infections may last months or even longer than 1 year if undetected, therefore routine screening is important because even asymptomatic infection can lead to damage that causes fertility problems.[12]

NOT TO BE MISSED

Chlamydia is considered to be a leading preventable cause of PID and female infertility worldwide.

Screening

Annual chlamydia screening is recommended for sexually active female patients younger than 25 years of age and older female patients who are at increased risk for infection.[44] Screening is also recommended at the first prenatal visit and again during the third trimester for pregnant patients younger than 25 years of age or in older female patients if at increased risk. Widespread prenatal screening and treatment of pregnant patients has resulted in less frequent neonatal complications from chlamydia.[6]

Focused History and Physical Examination

Chlamydia is asymptomatic in an estimated 70% of females. It is considered a "silent" infection because of the absence of symptoms and abnormal physical examination findings. Female patients with a urogenital infection may present with cervicitis or urethritis. Symptoms may include vaginal discharge, intermenstrual or postcoital bleeding, urinary frequency, dysuria, or abdominal or pelvic pain. Mucopurulent or purulent cervical discharge (Fig. 15.11), easily induced cervical bleeding, cervical motion tenderness, or uterine or adnexal tenderness may be present on examination as well as pyuria (presence of sterile pus) in the urine.[6]

Diagnosis

NAATs and cultures can be used to test for *C. trachomatis.* The sensitivity of NAATs for urogenital and non-urogenital detection of chlamydia is superior to culture and can be collected via vaginal swabs, endocervical swabs, and first-void urine. In females, vaginal swabs can be collected by either the patient or clinician and are the optimal specimen to screen. NAATs can be used with liquid-based cytology specimens collected for Pap

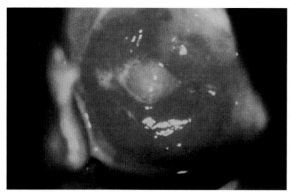

Figure 15.11 Mucopurulent cervical discharge seen in chlamydial infections. (Courtesy of C. Celum, MD, MHP, and W. Stamm, MD, Seattle, WA.)

BOX 15.5   Recommended Regimens for the Treatment of Chlamydia

Doxycycline 100 mg orally twice a day for 7 days

Alternative Regimens
- Azithromycin 1 g orally in a single dose
  OR
- Levofloxacin 500 mg orally once daily for 7 days

Treatment in Pregnancy
- Azithromycin 1 g orally in a single dose
  OR
- Amoxicillin 500 mg orally 3 times daily for 7 days

From U.S. Centers for Disease Control and Prevention. Sexually transmitted infections treatment guidelines, 2021. *MMWR Morbid Mortal Wkly Rep.* 2021;70(4):1–187.

---

smears, but the sensitivity for chlamydia is lower than the vaginal and endocervical swabs.[6]

Management

Pharmacological. Treatment should be provided as soon as possible after diagnosis, as delays can increase the risk of PID and other complications. Azithromycin is safe for use during pregnancy. Doxycycline is category D and is contraindicated for use during pregnancy. See Box 15.5 for recommended treatment for chlamydia. There are no effective nonpharmacological treatments. Retesting for chlamydia in female patients, even if their partner completed treatment, is recommended 3 months following initial treatment because of a high rate of reinfection. A test of cure 3 to 4 weeks after completion of therapy to assess for therapeutic failure is not recommended unless the patient is pregnant, has persistent symptoms, did not complete the medication as prescribed, or suspects reexposure or reinfection.[6]

Education and Counseling

All sex partners within the past 60 days or the most recent partner if greater than 60 days should be referred for evaluation and presumptive treatment to prevent transmission and reinfection.[6] EPT can be used in states where permissible by law and should be limited to heterosexual females with chlamydia who report that a partner(s) is unavailable or unlikely to receive prompt evaluation and treatment.[4] EPT should include written instructions and education for the partner.[6] Female patients diagnosed with chlamydia should be tested for other STIs, including gonorrhea, syphilis, and HIV. To avoid reinfection, females should abstain from sex for 7 days after they and their partner(s) have completed treatment and any symptoms have resolved.[6] Advocate for the correct use of condoms during penile-vaginal sex and a mouth-to-genital barrier during oral-genital sex.

Sexually Transmitted Infections That Present As Ulcers

Ulcerative STIs penetrate the skin of the external genitalia, colonize the subcutaneous tissue, and produce tissue damage. This damage can lead to ulceration in both skin tissue and mucosal tissue. Usually either skin abrasion or microtrauma is present, leading to the penetration of normal skin. With the disruption of the mucosal barrier, there is an increased risk of HIV transmission. Three common STIs characterized by genital ulcers are chancroid, HSV, and syphilis. Table 15.11 demonstrates a comparison of these three STIs.

Of these, HSV is most likely to be the cause; however, conditions may vary by geographic area as well as population studied. Assessment for a genital ulcer should include a history and physical examination, but these alone are not usually enough to make a positive diagnosis. Assessment should also include the following (Fig. 15.12):
- Culture or NAAT for *Haemophilus ducreyi* (chancroid)
- Serology or dark-field examination for syphilis
- Culture or NAAT (HSV)

Biopsy is usually reserved for patients who do not respond to treatment. Because early and aggressive treatment is necessary for control of these diseases, the CDC recommends that both syphilis and the initial outbreak

TABLE 15.11	Comparison of Sexually Transmitted Infections That Cause Genital Ulcers				
Disease	**Organism**	**Ulcer Appearance**	**Incubation**	**Painful**	**Adenopathy**
Herpes simplex virus	Herpes simplex Types 1 and 2	Multiple small groups, erythematous vesicles and shallow ulcers	2–7 days	Yes	Reactive nodes
Syphilis	*Treponema pallidum*	Indurated, smooth, firm borders, clean base, usually singular, may clear spontaneously	7–90 days	No	Firm, rubbery discrete nodes, tender
Chancroid	*Haemophilus ducreyi*	Sharply circumscribed, irregular borders, may see exudate at base	3–10 days	Yes; marked pain	Painful, usually unilateral, involves mainly the inguinal nodes, may rupture and drain

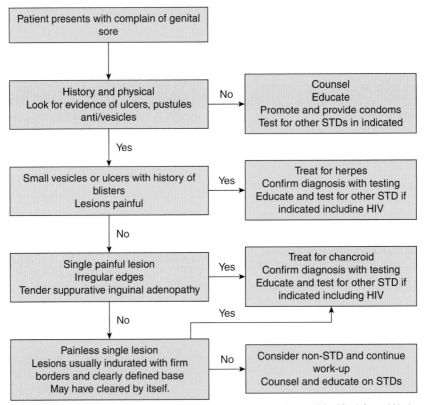

Figure 15.12 Algorithm for assessment and treatment of genital ulcers. (Modified from Workowski KA, Bachmann LH, Chan PA, et al. Sexually Transmitted Infections Treatment Guidelines, 2021. *MMWR Recomm Rep.* 2021;70[4]:1–187.)

of HSV be treated presumptively while awaiting test results. Treatment is based on history and physical findings, and testing is performed to confirm the diagnosis. Figure 15.12 provides a comparison of the three diseases to be discussed here.

Chancroid

Epidemiology

Reported cases of chancroid in the United States declined steadily between 1987 and 2001. In 2019, there were no reported cases of chancroid in the United States.[27] The true incidence of chancroid is unclear as many facilities do not test for the causative organism. *H. ducreyi* is difficult to isolate in the laboratory.[6] Males have a higher rate of chancroid than females, and uncircumcised males are more likely to develop the disease. The disease is greater in minorities and is associated with low socioeconomic status, poor hygiene, prostitution among sex workers, and drug use. Although rare in the United States, it is still a problem in some countries, so travel history is important when genital ulcers are present. Chancroid may still occur in parts of Africa and the Caribbean.[6] It is easily treated with antibiotics. Left untreated, the genital lesion usually resolves within 1 to 3 months; however, an untreated infection can lead to development of painful inguinal lymphadenopathy. The lymph nodes will ulcerate and form *buboes* (pus-filled abscesses) in about 25% of cases. Once a patient has been identified, treatment should be offered.

Pathogenesis

Chancroid is caused by the gram-negative bacterium *H. ducreyi. H. ducreyi* enters the skin through a break in the epithelium. Minor trauma such as that experienced during sexual intercourse can lead to transmission. Once the bacteria have entered the body, they recruit a host of inflammatory cells to the infected area.[46] The bacteria also set up a response that causes the secretion of interleukin-6 (IL-6) and interleukin-8 (IL-8) from cells of both the epidermis and dermis. IL-8, in turn, induces polymorphonuclear leukocytes (PMNs) and macrophages to form abscesses, giving rise to the intradermal pustules. IL-6 stimulates CD4 cell activity in the area through the upregulation of T-cell interleukin-2 (IL-2) receptor expression. The formation of the characteristic ulcers seen in chancroid is caused by the cytolethal distending toxin (HdCDT) in *H. ducreyi* leading to apoptosis and necrosis of human cells.[47]

Screening

There is no recommended regular screening for chancroid. Patients are screened based on the appearance of the ulcer as well as the presence of other symptoms. For any patient presenting with a genital ulcer, chancroid should be a part of the differential diagnosis. If the patient has traveled to areas where the disease is more prevalent, screening for the presence of an ulcer should be considered.

Focused History and Physical Examination

The patient may report painful papules, pustules, or ulcers. If ulcers are present, the patient usually experiences dyspareunia. The patient may complain of flulike symptoms such as fever or weakness. Question the patient regarding travel to areas where disease prevalence is high and contact with someone in the sex industry.[48]

Generally small, painful papules appear within 3 to 7 days of exposure. These rapidly break down into shallow, soft, painful ulcers with ragged, undermined edges and a red border (Fig. 15.13). Ulcers may vary in size. Deep erosion can lead to marked tissue destruction. The inguinal lymph nodes become tender, enlarged, and form a bubo. The skin over the abscess is erythematous and can break down to form a sinus. As the lymph nodes drain, the infection can spread to other areas of skin, resulting in new lesions.[48]

Diagnosis

The definitive diagnosis of chancroid is made with culture. *H. ducreyi* requires a special culture medium and is not always available in clinics. If possible, a sample of

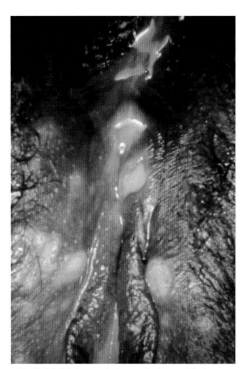

Figure 15.13 Multiple, nonindurated chancroid ulcers must be differentiated from ulcers caused by herpes simplex and syphilis. Chancroid ulcers cause discomfort and may be associated with inguinal lymphadenopathy. The diagnosis is made by culturing *Haemophilus ducreyi* from the ulcer. (From Baggish MS, Karram MM. *Atlas of Pelvic Anatomy and Gynecologic Surgery.* Elsevier; 2021.)

pus from a bubo or exudate from the edge of an ulcer yields the best results. Serological testing for syphilis and HIV and cultures for HSV should be performed as a part of the differential diagnosis to exclude these causes of genital ulcers.[48] If testing is not available, a probable diagnosis can be made. The presence of painful genital ulcers and suppurative inguinal adenopathy strongly support the diagnosis. If the following criteria are met, the patient should be treated for chancroid[6]:

- Presence of one or more painful genital ulcers
- Clinical appearance of the ulcer
- Regional lymphadenopathy with or without suppuration
- Absence of evidence confirming syphilis performed at least 7 days after the onset of symptoms
- Negative culture or HSV PCS test from the exudate

NOT TO BE MISSED

Chancroid is an uncommon infection in the United States. The true incidence of chancroid is unclear because of the difficulty identifying and/or the lack of access to testing for *H. ducreyi*.

Management

PATIENT-CENTERED CARE: HIV patients are more likely to experience treatment failure and may need to be treated for a longer period.

Pharmacological

Once the diagnosis is made, the patient should be treated with antibiotics. Successful treatment cures the disease and resolves the clinical symptoms. Partner treatment prevents reinfection and further spread of the disease. All sexual contacts within 10 days of the beginning of symptoms should be treated. Box 15.6 outlines the treatment for chancroid. Even with adequate treatment, scarring caused by draining lymph nodes can occur. If large fluctuant nodes are present, consider incision and drainage. There is no effective nonpharmacological alternative for treatment.

Patients should be examined 3 to 7 days post-treatment. The lesions should be showing clinical improvement. If there is no improvement, consider the following:[6]

- Incorrect diagnosis
- Co-infection with another STI

BOX 15.6   Recommended Treatment for Chancroid

- Azithromycin 1 g orally in a single dose
  OR
- Ceftriaxone 250 mg IM is single dose
  OR
- Ciprofloxacin 500 mg orally twice a day for 3 days*
  OR
- Erythromycin base 500 mg orally twice a day for 7 days*

* Some resistance has been seen worldwide.
From U.S. Centers for Disease Control and Prevention. Sexually transmitted infections treatment guidelines, 2021. *MMWR Morbid Mortal Wkly Rep.* 2021;70(4):1–187.

- HIV status
- Incorrect use of medication
- Resistance to the antibiotic provided

❗ SAFETY ALERT

Ciprofloxacin is low risk to the fetus but can be toxic if breastfeeding; alternative therapy should be prescribed.

Education and Counseling

Education should be aimed at prevention. To date, there is no effective vaccine for the prevention of chancroid. Emphasize avoidance of high-risk sexual activities, including unprotected sexual intercourse or sexual intercourse with high-risk individuals. As with all STIs, condom use and limiting the number of sexual partners are important prevention strategies. Patients who are traveling to a high-risk area should be informed and counseled of the signs and symptoms of the disease. Patients should abstain from intercourse until 7 days after completion of therapy and only if the partner has been treated. Treatment of partners regardless of symptoms is recommended. All partners within 10 days of the onset of symptoms should be treated.[6]

Herpes Simplex Virus

Epidemiology

HSV is among the most prevalent of the STIs.[49,50] HSV-1 is usually acquired in childhood. It is contracted by exposure to oral secretions that contain the virus and can lead to oral herpes, usually referred to as *fever blisters*. HSV-2 is commonly seen in the urogenital tract, and the most common transmission is by sexual contact. HSV is not a reportable STI and can be subclinical, so the real prevalence is not known.[27]

HSV-1 and HSV-2 can both cause genital herpes. Most cases of recurrent genital herpes are caused by HSV-2. From 2015 to 2016, the seroprevalence of HSV-2 in the United States was approximately 12% among patients 14 to 49 years of age.[51] Seroprevalence appears to increase with age, and it is greater among females compared with males (21% vs 12%). Prior HSV-1 infection does not appear to affect the rate of HSV-2 acquisition.[6] Most patients with genital herpes are undiagnosed. This is either caused by the mild or unrecognized infection; because of this, prevention is more difficult as a patient can spread the disease without awareness of it.[6]

Pathogenesis

HSV belongs to the alpha herpesvirus group. The virus is approximately 160 nm in diameter and has a linear, double-stranded DNA genome. HSV-1 prefers the oral epithelium, while HSV-2 prefers the genital epithelium, but there is a crossover with the virus. The majority of genital herpes cases are associated with HSV-2, but an increasing number are associated with HSV-1. HSV infection is mediated by attachment via ubiquitous receptors to cells, including sensory neurons. This can lead to the establishment of latency period and the reactivation of the virus.[52]

HSV-1 and HSV-2 have the following unique biological properties:[52]

- *Neurovirulence:* Capacity to invade and replicate in the nervous system
- *Latency:* Establishment and maintenance of latent infection in nerve cell ganglia proximal to the site of infection
- *Reactivation:* Reactivation and replication of latent HSV, always in the area supplied by the ganglia in which latency was established

These properties are responsible for the fact that HSV can become a chronic recurring problem and help establish the need for suppression therapy in some female patients. Cellular immunity is an important defense against HSV, therefore people with impaired T-cell immunity are more at risk for transmission and recurrence.[53] HSV is a human disease with humans as the only natural reservoirs. There are no vectors involved in transmission.[54] HSV is transmitted by close personal contact. Infection occurs when there is inoculation of the virus into susceptible mucosal surfaces or through small cracks in the skin. Because the virus is readily inactivated at room temperature and by drying, personal contact with the active virus is necessary for transmission.[6] There is no routine screening recommended for HSV.

Focused History and Physical Examination

There are three types of genital HSV infections:

- *Primary:* No preexisting antibodies to either HSV-1 or HSV-2
- *Non-primary:* Presence of antibodies for either HSV-1 or HSV-2 and develops an infection with the other strain
- *Recurrent:* Reactivation of the strain from a previous infection

Signs and symptoms may vary according to the type of infection involved. Most symptoms are seen with a primary infection; however, the symptoms can range from mild to severe to almost no symptoms at all. It is important to remember that many patients with HSV are asymptomatic. The symptoms seen in a primary infection are usually more severe than repeat infections and are as follows:

- Systemic symptoms (67%)
  - Fever
  - Headache
  - Malaise
  - Myalgia
- Local pain and itching (98%)
- Dysuria (63%)
- Tender lymphadenopathy (80%) [54]

More than 87% of seropositive patients have no previous diagnosis of genital herpes.[55] Symptomatic patients can have one or more lesions that are not the typical painful presentation, so the lesion is either missed or misdiagnosed. Before the lesions appear, many patients experience prodromal symptoms. These include flulike symptoms.[55,56] The patient may also experience mild tingling at the site of the lesion up to 48 hours before lesion appearance or a shooting pain in the buttocks, legs, or hips up to 5 days beforehand. The average incubation period after exposure is 4 days (range, 2 to 12 days).[55] Up to 60% of infected individuals will asymptomatically shed the virus.[56]

Nonprimary first-episode infection is usually associated with fewer lesions. There are also fewer systemic symptoms than with a primary infection. Because there are antibodies against one HSV type, there may be some protection against the development of symptoms as well as the severity of the symptoms. Although not well studied, a 1999 study showed that with a prior HSV-1 infection, there was a threefold increased likelihood of asymptomatic infection.[57] Recurrences of genital HSV are common. These infections seem to be less severe than both primary and nonprimary infections. The average duration of lesions in a recurrent infection is generally shorter. With a primary infection, the average length of the lesion is around 19 days as opposed to 10 days for a recurrent infection. The duration of viral shedding is usually 2 to 5 days.[54]

Physical examination may reveal the appearance of multiple vesicular lesions with some that may have ruptured to form shallow ulcers (Fig. 15.14). They are usually painful to touch. The lesions appear to progress from vesicles to pustules to ulcers. Once the ulcer has formed, the lesion will crust over and heal. The average time it takes an ulcer to crust and heal is within 7 days of ulcer formation. Lesions appear in multiple stages at the same time.[56]

> **PATIENT-CENTERED CARE:** To prevent transmission to the neonate, all pregnant patients should be asked about a history of genital herpes at the first prenatal visit and should be questioned about symptoms and examined for lesions at the beginning of labor. If present, a cesarean delivery may be considered.

Diagnosis

The CDC recommends that a clinical diagnosis be confirmed with type-specific laboratory testing. If a patient is positive for HSV, then testing for HIV should be performed. The preferred method of testing is with cell culture and PCR. This is a part of the testing for all patients presenting with genital ulcer disease. Because the viral culture sensitivity can be low, especially with recurrent infection, and it declines rapidly as the lesions heal, PCR is the test of choice to diagnose genital herpes. See Table 15.12 for a comparison of available tests.[6] Although serological testing provides information on previous infections, is not recommended in the general population. Patients at high risk may choose to be tested. It should be considered in the following situations:[6]

- Recurrent infection with negative HSV PCR or culture
- Atypical presentation with negative HSV PCR or culture
- Previous clinical diagnosis without laboratory confirmation
- A patient with a partner with a positive diagnosis of herpes

> **PATIENT-CENTERED CARE:** Asymptomatic patients who test positive for HSV-2 infection on type-specific serology testing should be counseled in the same way as those with symptoms.

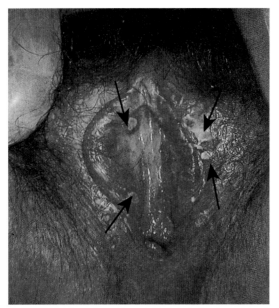

Figure 15.14 Herpes simplex ulcers seen on the vulva *(arrows)*. (From Habif TP. *Clinical Dermatology: A Color Guide to Diagnosis and Therapy.* Mosby; 2004.)

Management

Pharmacological

Although there is no cure for genital herpes, antiviral therapy can offer some benefits to symptomatic patients. The drugs choices are acyclovir, valacyclovir, and famciclovir.

Although these drugs suppress the virus and help control symptoms, they do not eradicate the virus or affect the risk, frequency, or severity of recurrence. Topical antivirals are not very effective against genital herpes

TABLE 15.12 Diagnostic Test for Herpes Simplex Virus

	Tzanck Smear	Virus Culture	Immunofluorescence Assay	Polymerase Chain Reaction
Sensitivity	Low	Low	Low	Highest available
Specificity	Low	High	High	High
Viral typing	No	Yes	No	Yes
Comments	Lacks sensitivity and specificity, so not recommended	Sensitivity declines as lesions heal. Better test at beginning of outbreak with high viral shedding	Lacks sensitivity, so not recommended	Recommended, especially for central nervous system infections

Modified from U.S. Centers for Disease Control and Prevention. Sexually transmitted infections treatment guidelines, 2021. *MMWR Morbid Mortal Wkly Rep.* 2021;70(4):1–187.

and are not recommended. The dose needed is dependent on the type of infection presenting. See Table 15.13 for recommended treatment for primary and recurrent infections. Treatment is recommended for the first case as symptoms can become severe and prolonged.[6]

NOT TO BE MISSED

The medications available to treat genital herpes help speed healing of ulcers in patients who have just been infected or those who are having repeat outbreaks, but they do not cure the disease.

! SAFETY ALERT

The CDC recommends that patients with an allergic or adverse reaction to the three approved antivirals be desensitized to the drugs as there are no other effective treatments available.

Although recurrence can occur with both HSV-1 and HSV-2, it is more likely to occur with HSV-2. If the patient is experiencing recurrence, suppression therapy can be offered.[6] Suppression therapy has the added benefit of decreasing the risk of HSV-2 transmission to partners.[58] Because the incidence of recurrence decreases over time, it is recommended that the patient should be counseled on discontinuation. If the patient has a recurrence while off, then suppression therapy can be restarted. There is no laboratory monitoring needed for patients on suppression therapy. Box 15.7 identifies the recommended suppression therapies.[6] There are no effective nonpharmacological treatments for genital herpes.

TABLE 15.13 Treatment for Genital Herpes

First Clinical Episode*	Episodic Therapy for Recurrent
• Acyclovir 400 mg orally 3 times a day for 7–10 days OR • Valacyclovir 1 g orally twice a day for 7–10 days OR • Famciclovir 250 mg orally 3 times a day for 7–10 days	• Acyclovir 800 mg orally twice a day for 5 days OR • Acyclovir 800 mg orally 3 times a day for 2 days OR • Valacyclovir 500 mg orally twice a day for 3 days OR • Valacyclovir 1 g orally once a day for 5 days OR • Famciclovir 125 mg orally twice a day for 5 days OR • Famciclovir 1 g orally twice a day for 1 day OR • Famciclovir 500 mg orally once, followed by 250 mg orally twice daily for 2 days

*Can extend treatment longer than 10 days if healing is incomplete.
Modified from U.S. Centers for Disease Control and Prevention. Sexually transmitted infections treatment guidelines, 2021. *MMWR Morbid Mortal Wkly Rep.* 2021;70(4):1–187.

Education and Counseling

Both the patient and partner should be counseled to help the patient cope with the diagnosis, prevent transmission, identify any concerns, and identify any misconceptions.

BOX 15.7 Recommended Suppression Therapy for Genital Herpes

- Acyclovir 400 mg orally twice a day
  OR
- Valacyclovir 500 mg orally once a day*
  OR
- Valacyclovir 1 g orally once a day
  OR
- Famciclovir 250 mg orally twice a day

* may be less effective than other regimens in those experiencing 10 or greater episodes/year.

NOT TO BE MISSED

It is possible to spread HSV even if there are no visible ulcers. It is not possible to contract HSV by touching doorknobs, toilet seats, or other objects. It is sexually transmitted.

Patient education addresses the natural history of their infection with emphasis on viral shedding, the potential for clinical recurrence, and sexual transmission even in the absence of symptomatic infection. Suppression therapy should be discussed as an option to prevent recurrence. Because it is possible to transmit the virus during asymptomatic periods, all present and future partners must be aware of the HSV status before continuing or initiating a sexual relationship. The possibility for asymptomatic viral shedding that can lead to transmission of the disease is much more common in patients with HSV-2. Condoms may help reduce the risk of transmission and should be used with all sexual encounters whether or not lesions are present.[59] Once prodromal symptoms or lesions have appeared, patients should avoid sexual intercourse until the lesions are gone. This is critical to reducing transmission as the condom is not 100% effective in preventing herpes transmission, even if used correctly.[6]

PATIENT-CENTERED CARE: Immunocompromised patients, such as those with HIV infection, may have prolonged and severe episodes. Suppressive therapy is recommended.

Syphilis

Epidemiology

Syphilis is a systemic infection caused by the bacterium *Treponema pallidum*. Most new cases of syphilis are sexually acquired; however, it can also be passed from the mother to the fetus during pregnancy. The disease is divided into stages based on the clinical manifestations. If not adequately treated, syphilis can cause serious health problems. The rates of all types of syphilis are increasing. The rates of both primary and secondary (P&S) syphilis have increased by 11.2%.[27] During 2019, there were 129,813 reported new diagnoses of syphilis (all stages). Syphilis is more prevalent in males and especially MSM. Although this group accounts for the largest group, the rate in females has also risen. Rates in females have increased by 178.6% since 2015.[27] The incidence of congenital syphilis has increased to 44.5 cases per 100,000 live births in 2019; the number of reported cases in the United States increased to 1870.[27]

Pathogenesis

Syphilis is usually classified in four stages: *primary, secondary, latent,* and *tertiary. T. pallidum* is the causative organism of syphilis. Identified in 1905, it is a bacterium from the order Spirochaetales. *T. pallidum* is approximately 10 to 13 microns long but only 0.15 microns in width, making it too small to be visualized by direct microscopy.[60] The organism, however, can be seen with darkfield microscopy, which shows *T. pallidum* as a delicate, corkscrew-shaped organism with tightly wound spirals (Fig. 15.15). Its characteristic rotary motion with flexing and back-and-forth movements is sufficient to make a diagnosis.

Because the organism cannot be cultured, there is some limitation on the information that is available on

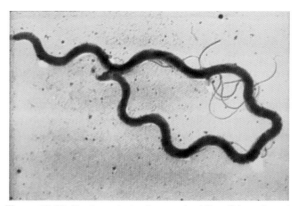

Figure 15.15 Electron photomicrograph of *T. pallidum,* the spirochete that causes syphilis, (From U.S. Centers for Disease Control and Prevention. *STD Clinical Slides;* 2020. https://www.cdc.gov/std/training/clinicalslides/default.htm.)

the pathogenesis of *T. pallidum*. The infection initiates when the organism gains access to subcutaneous tissue. This is usually by a microscopic abrasion in the skin or mucosal tissue. The spirochete evades host immune responses and establishes the initial ulcerative lesion at the site of entrance to the body. It also infects the regional draining lymph nodes. Incubation time from exposure to development of primary lesions averages 3 weeks but can range from 10 to 90 days.[61] The characteristic lesion of primary syphilis develops after an incubation period of 3 to 6 weeks. Histologically, it is characterized by mononuclear leukocytes infiltration, macrophages, and lymphocytes. During this stage, the spirochete can be isolated from the surface of the ulceration or the overlying exudate of the chancre.

Whether or not it is treated, healing of the chancre occurs within 3 to 12 weeks with considerable residual fibrosis. Secondary syphilis develops about 4 to 10 weeks after the appearance of the primary lesion. During this stage, the spirochetes multiply and spread throughout the body. The manifestations, both skin and systemic, are varied and help make the diagnosis. Latent syphilis is a stage at which the features of secondary syphilis have resolved but the patient remains seropositive. The disease is still present, and some patients will experience recurrence of the infectious skin lesions of secondary syphilis. Two-thirds of patients with latent syphilis will remain asymptomatic, and one-third go on to develop tertiary syphilis. Tertiary syphilis mainly affects the cardiovascular system (80% to 85%) and the CNS (5% to 10%) and develops over months to years involving slow tissue damage related to chronic inflammation. Syphilis should be treated at any stage to prevent the damage associated with disease progression.[61]

Screening
Screening for syphilis is based on risk factors. The USPSTF strongly recommends that clinicians screen individuals at increased risk and all pregnant patients for syphilis infection.[62,63]

Focused History and Physical Examination
Sometimes called the *great pretender,* the manifestations of syphilis (particularly advanced syphilis) are nonspecific and may mimic other diseases. Development of a timeline for the course of symptoms is needed to provide a diagnosis that leads to a diagnosis of the current stage of the disease. The following are typically included in the history:[61]

- History of syphilis
- Known contact
- Typical signs and symptoms over the past 12 months
- Most recent serological test

Obtain a thorough sexual and social history for the patient and partners, including exposure to blood products or intravenous (IV) drug use. Diagnosis of the stage of syphilis is based on the signs and symptoms (Table 15.14).[6,61,64]

Primary syphilis presents mainly with a chancre at the site of inoculation. The chancre usually begins as a single, painless papule that rapidly becomes eroded and indurated, with a surrounding red areola (Fig. 15.16). The chancre can appear in a number of places, so a complete examination of all possible areas of inoculation is needed. The primary lesion is usually associated with regional lymphadenopathy. The nodes are usually discrete, firm, mobile, and painless. There is no change in the overlying skin. The lesion is highly infectious, and if a dark-field examination is to be performed for diagnostic purposes, the specimen is obtained from this site.

Secondary syphilis may present in many different ways but usually includes a localized or diffuse mucocutaneous rash (Fig. 15.17). The rash maybe macular, papular, pustular, or a combination of all seen at one time. Generalized nontender lymphadenopathy may be noted.[61]

Latent syphilis can be early (<1 year after infection) or late (>1 year after infection). Latent syphilis is not contagious. The disease is asymptomatic during this stage. Diagnosis is made by detection on serological tests. The patient may have missed the symptoms during the P&S stage or have been a treatment failure. Syphilis may remain latent permanently if not diagnosed and treated. If latent syphilis is diagnosed, it should be treated with antibiotics as relapses with contagious skin or mucosal lesions can occur.[61,64]

Tertiary syphilis is a slowly progressive disease that causes end-stage organ damage. It may affect any organ. The disease is generally not contagious at this stage. Examples of organ manifestations include the following:[61,64]

- CNS
  - Impaired balance
  - Paresthesia
  - Incontinence
  - Impotence

TABLE 15.14	**Syphilis by Stages**[6,61,64]			
Stage	**Incubation**	**Common Manifestations**	**Other Manifestations**	**Diagnostic Test**
Primary	10–90 days	Contagious Chancre (small painless skin ulcer)	Regional lymphadenopathy	Darkfield of lesion (80%) Nontreponemal test (78%–86%) Treponemal-specific test (76%–84%)

Secondary	1–3 months	Contagious
		Diffuse rash
		Condyloma lata
		Lymphadenopathy
		Arthralgia
		Fatigue
		Fever
		Weight loss
		Renal system
		   Glomerulonephritis
		   Nephrotic syndrome
		CNS symptoms
		   Headache
		   Cranial neuropathy
			CNS symptoms
			Iritiis
			Uveitis
			Annular syphilis
			Pustular lesions
			Alopecia
			Ulceronodular syphilis
				Darkfield of lesion (80%)
				Nontreponemal test (100%)
				Treponemal-specific test (100%)

Latent Early Late	<1 year >1 year	Not contagious No symptoms No symptoms	None None	Nontreponemal test (95%–100%) Treponemal-specific test (97%–100%)
Tertiary	Months to years	Not contagious Late neurosyphilis*	Cardiovascular Gummatous lesions	Nontreponemal test (71%–73%) Treponemal-specific test (94%–96%)
Neurosyphilis		Contagious depending on stage Hyperreflexia Seizures Personality changes Cognitive changes Neuropathy	Visual changes Hearing changes Aphasia Paresis Loss of bladder or bowel function	Cerebrospinal fluid examination

*Can develop at any stage.

- Focal neurological findings, including
  - Sensorineural hearing
  - Vision loss
- Cognitive changes
- Cardiovascular
  - Chest pain
  - Back pain
  - Symptoms related to aortic aneurysms

Neurosyphilis can occur at any stage and can be asymptomatic or symptomatic. If asymptomatic, there are no signs or symptoms, but cerebrospinal fluid (CSF) abnormalities are demonstrable. These include the following:

- Possible pleocytosis
- Elevated protein
- Decreased glucose
- Reactive CSF Venereal Disease Research Laboratory (VDRL) test

Symptomatic neurosyphilis can present as meningitis. This usually develops between 6 months to several

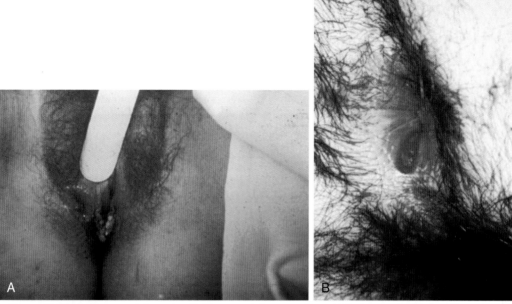

Figure 15.16 A, Chancre of the vulva. **B,** Chancre of the anus. (From U.S. Centers for Disease Control and Prevention. *STD Clinical Slides;* 2020. https://www.cdc.gov/std/training/clinicalslides/default.htm.)

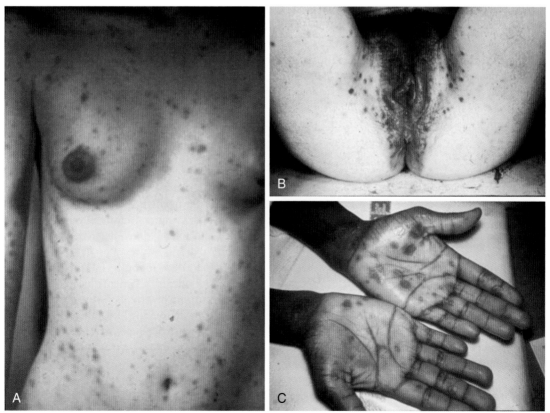

Figure 15.17 A–B, Secondary syphilis: papulo-pustular rash. **C,** Rash on hands. (From U.S. Centers for Disease Control and Prevention. *STD Clinical Slides;* 2020. https://www.cdc.gov/std/training/clinicalslides/default.htm.)

years of initial infection. Patients present with the following typical symptoms of meningitis:

- Headache
- Nausea and vomiting
- Photophobia
- Cranial nerve abnormalities

Although there may be other presentations of neurosyphilis, this is the most common.[61,64] The physical findings also vary by stage (see Table 15.14). The physical examination should include a complete inspection and palpation of the following:

- Oral cavity
- Lymph nodes
- Skin of torso
- Palms of hands and soles of feet
- Genitalia and perianal areas
- Neurological examination
- Abdomen

If tertiary syphilis is expected, the examination should include the aforementioned assessments as well as a complete examination of the system that is thought to be affected.[64]

Diagnosis

Three diagnostic tests are used for syphilis. The dark-field microscopic test uses the exudate or tissue from the lesion to detect the organism. Molecular tests detect *T. pallidum* in tissue or lesion exudate. Serological tests provide a presumptive diagnosis. There are two types of serological tests:[6]

- Nontreponemal test (NT)
  - VDRL
  - Rapid plasma reagin (RPR)
- Treponemal test (TT)
  - Fluorescent treponemal antibody absorbed (FTA-ABS) test
  - Immunoassay (EIA)
  - Chemiluminescence immunoassay
  - Immunoblot
    - Rapid treponemal assay
  - *T. pallium* passive particle agglutination (TP-PA)

One type of serological test alone is not sufficient for a diagnosis. It is a two-step process that requires one test from each type to be performed. The NT is completed first and, if positive, is followed by a TT. The NT for antibodies correlates well with the activity of the disease. A quantitative test should be performed. The NT is used to follow treatment response. A fourfold change in titer is needed to show clinical improvement.

The diagnosis of neurosyphilis is dependent on the use of several tests as one test alone is insufficient to make the diagnosis. Patients with the following test results are considered to have neurosyphilis:[6]

- Reactive serological test
- Abnormal cell count and protein in CSF
- Reactive CSF VDRL with or without clinical manifestations

Management

Pharmacological. Penicillin G is the treatment of choice for all stages of syphilis. The goals of treatment for early syphilis (primary, secondary, and early latent) are to prevent long-term problems associated with infection. Early treatment is necessary to reduce

---

NOT TO BE MISSED

A CSF examination should be performed in patients with syphilis and neurological symptoms.

---

transmission. Treatment and follow-up are based on the stage. See Table 15.15 for recommended treatment and follow-up for uncomplicated syphilis. Treatment for more complicated patients can be accessed from the CDC. Treatment of sexual partners is important. Transmission occurs during primary, secondary, and early latent phases. All partners within 90 days of diagnosis should be treated presumptively for primary syphilis, even if their serological test is negative. If the contact was greater than 90 days ago, treat as if the serological test is positive.[6]

Single-dose treatment for early syphilis has been reviewed and found to be effective in a large randomized clinical trial.[65] Cure rates of clinical disease are high at 90% to 100% for both HIV-uninfected and HIV-infected individuals.[66] Patients should be monitored clinically and with laboratory testing to help ensure adequate response to therapy (see Table 15.15). There is no effective nonpharmacological treatment for syphilis.

CLINICAL SURVIVAL TIP Patients with latent syphilis should undergo follow-up serological testing at 6, 12, and 24 months to assess an adequate response to treatment.

TABLE 15.15 Treatment and Follow-up for Syphilis[6]

Stage	Treatment	Follow-up
Primary and Secondary	Recommended regimen for adults* 　Benzathine penicillin G 2.4 million units IM in a single dose	Clinical and serological evaluation at 6 and 12 months More frequent if needed
Latent	Early latent syphilis 　Benzathine penicillin G 2.4 million units IM in a single dose Late latent syphilis or latent syphilis of unknown duration 　Benzathine penicillin G 7.2 million units total, administered as 3 doses of 2.4 million units at 1-week intervals	Quantitative nontreponemal serological tests at 6, 12, and 24 months CSF examination if: • A sustained (>2-week) fourfold increase • Initially high titer (>1:32) fails to decline • Signs or symptoms develop
Tertiary	Tertiary syphilis with normal CSF examination 　Benzathine penicillin G 7.2 million units total, administered as 3 doses of 2.4 million units IM each at 1-week intervals	Rule out neurosyphilis with a CSF examination before therapy Cardiovascular syphilis: managed in consultation with an infectious disease specialist. Limited information is available concerning clinical response and follow-up of patients who have tertiary syphilis.
Neurosyphilis	Recommended regimen 　Aqueous crystalline penicillin G 18–24 million units per day, administered as 3–4 million units IV every 4 hours or continuous infusion, for 10–14 days Alternative regimen* 　Procaine penicillin G 2.4 million units IM once daily PLUS 　Probenecid 500 mg orally four times a day, both for 10–14 days	CSF examination every 6 months until the cell count is normal Consider retreatment if cell count has not decreased after 6 months or the CSF cell count or protein is not normal after 2 years
Pregnancy	Recommended regimen 　Pregnant women should be treated with the penicillin regimen appropriate for their stage of infection	Coordinated prenatal care and treatment are vital Serological titers repeated at 28–32 weeks and at delivery Serological titers can be checked monthly in female patients at high risk for reinfection

*Ensures compliance with therapy.
Modified from U.S. Centers for Disease Control and Prevention. Sexually transmitted infections treatment guidelines, 2021. *MMWR Morbid Mortal Wkly Rep.* 2021;70(4):1–187.

> **PATIENT-CENTERED CARE:** Penicillin is the drug of choice to treat syphilis. Patients with an allergic or adverse reaction to penicillin should be desensitized to the drugs and treated, especially pregnant patients.

Education and Counseling

The primary goals of education and counseling are prevention. Patient counseling with syphilis should include the following:

• Nature of the disease
• Transmission
• Treatment and follow-up
• Risk reduction

When discussing the nature of the disease, it is important to inform the patient that symptoms will disappear even without treatment, but the disease is still present and can cause long-term problems if untreated. Syphilis should be treated whether or not it is symptomatic to prevent transmission and limit morbidity. Correct and consistent use of latex condoms can reduce the risk of syphilis. However, condoms are not 100% effective, as a syphilis lesion outside of the area covered by a latex condom can still allow transmission. Education should include partner-based interventions including partner notification and treatment.

When treating syphilis, the possibility of a Jarisch-Herxheimer reaction should be discussed. This is a self-limiting reaction to antitreponemal therapy and is not an allergic reaction to the penicillin. The patient might experience the following:

- Fever
- Malaise
- Nausea and vomiting
- Chills
- Exacerbation of secondary rash

Jarisch-Herxheimer symptoms usually appear within 24 hours of treatment, and symptom management is suggested. Rest, fluids, and antipyretics are useful. Although self-limiting, the reaction can pose a problem for pregnant patients as it can precipitate labor. Pregnant patients should be instructed to see their obstetrical care provider and to be aware of the signs and symptoms of labor.[6]

Human Papillomavirus

Epidemiology

Because HPV is a nonreportable disease and most infections are brief, asymptomatic, or subclinical, the incidence and prevalence estimates on genital HPV infection are limited. The estimated annual incidence of sexually transmitted HPV infections is 3 million cases, with an estimated $775 million spent annually in direct medical costs to treat conditions associated with genital HPV infection.[27] There are about 150 HPV types, over 40 of which can infect the genital area.[6] HPV types are classified by their association with cancer. Nononcogenic or low-risk HPV types (HPV 6 or 11) are associated with benign or low-grade abnormalities of cervical cells, anogenital warts, and recurrent respiratory papillomatosis.[67]

Oncogenic, or high-risk, HPV types (16 and 18) can cause intraepithelial neoplasia of the anogenital region. Affected areas in females include the cervix, vulva, vagina, and anus.[68]

NOT TO BE MISSED

HPV-6 and HPV-11 are responsible for most cases of anogenital warts.

HPV is associated with some oropharyngeal cancers. Most HPV infections are self-limiting and are asymptomatic or unrecognized. Most sexually active individuals become infected with HPV at least once in their lifetime. The body's immune system will clear most HPV infections within 2 years of infection. This occurs in about 90% of infections, but some infections can persist and lead to long-term problems. Because of the nature of the complications and the fact that the disease is so prevalent, the CDC recommends vaccination against HPV.[6] The clinical presentation of condylomata acuminata is apparent in 1% of the sexually active population. Molecular studies indicate that 10% to 20% of females 15 to 49 years of age have been exposed to HPV.[69]

Pathogenesis

HPV is a group of non-enveloped, double-stranded DNA viruses belonging to the family Papovaviridae. Over 200 types of HPV have been identified, with more than 40 that can be transmitted through sexual contact and cause anogenital warts. With HPV, gene intensification and viral assembly occurs as epithelium in the basal layer of the skin matures.[70] Koilocytosis, a characteristic viral change associated with HPV, can be detected both cytologically and histologically. This is why the Pap smear works so well to identify the presence of HPV. Abnormal pap smears in females 30 years of age or older, if not accompanied by HPV cotesting, can be followed with an HPV DNA test to determine further diagnostics and treatment. Although persistent HPV infection is important to the development of cervical cancer, 5.5% to 11% of cervical cancers are not associated with HPV.[71] Host issues that are not completely understood are also important in the development of cervical cancer. Table 15.16 provides a list of the known HPV viruses and their risk of the development of cancers.[70]

Screening

Because much of HPV is self-limiting and does not cause major problems, routine screening for HPV is not recommended in the 21- to 29-year age group. Female patients should be followed with a routine Pap smear, a Pap smear with HPV cotesting, or HPV testing alone (see Chapter 24) and managed according to the results.[6]

> **PATIENT-CENTERED CARE:** Latent HPV may become active, particularly with pregnancy and immunosuppression.

TABLE 15.16	Human Papillomavirus Type as Related to Cancer Risk	
Risk	**Type**	**Comments**
Low oncogenic risk	6, 11, 40, 42, 43, 44, 54, 55, 61, 70, 72, 81	Associated with genital condyloma and low-grade squamous intraepithelial lesion
High oncogenic risk	16, 18, 31, 33, 35, 39, 45, 51, 52, 56, 58, 59, 66, 68	Associated with high-grade squamous intraepithelial lesion and invasive carcinoma
Unclear oncogenic risk	26, 53, 73, 82	

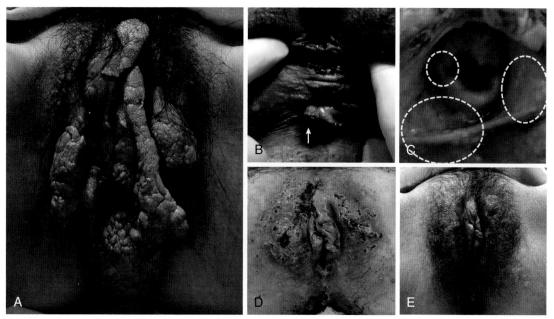

Figure 15.18 Anogenital warts. (From Lee SR, Jeon JH, Jeong K, Chung HW. Giant vulvar verruciform xanthoma can mimic a common vulvar mass, genital warts. Arrow and encircled areas denote warts in difficult to see background. *Am J Obstet Gynecol.* 2017;216[4]:422.e1–422.e2.)

Focused History and Physical Examination

The clinical history and presentation of HPV infection vary according to the anatomic area involved. Anogenital warts are usually asymptomatic, or the patient may have noticed a growth. The growths are most often described as painless bumps, but there may be some pruritus and discharge. Lesions usually involve multiple lesions instead of a single lesion and involve more than one area of the genitalia. Although anogenital warts have a long incubation period, two-thirds of individuals who have sexual contact with a partner who has genital warts develop lesions within 3 months. Oral, vaginal, cervical, and anal lesions are possible. To guide the physical examination, a history of oral, vaginal, and anal intercourse should be obtained. Anogenital warts (condylomata acuminata) appear as exophytic cauliflower-like (Fig. 15.18) lesions that are usually found near moist surfaces. Usual areas of appearance are the perianal area, vaginal introitus, vagina, labia, and vulva.[69]

Findings that suggest anogenital warts are single or multiple soft, smooth or papillated papules or plaques limited to the anogenital area. Color may vary from that of the skin. Because the infection may occur simultaneously in more than one site, a complete examination of the genital area and perianal skin is needed. A careful inspection and palpation of the vulva, perineum, perianal skin, mons pubis, and crural folds should be performed. If the patient engages in oral-genital sex, an examination of the mouth and throat should be performed. All lesions should be described as to appearance, size, and location. It is important to rule out the presence of other STIs by looking for evidence of ulcerations, adenopathy, vesicles, and discharge. An inspection for irregularities in shape, form, or color that may suggest melanoma or malignancy should be performed. Warts may appear in the urethra, vagina, and cervix, so inspection of these areas is needed.[69]

Diagnosis

Diagnosis is usually made by visual inspection. If the lesions are atypical, the diagnosis can be confirmed with a biopsy. Consider biopsy if the patient is immunocompromised and has an uncertain diagnosis, is unresponsive to standard therapy, or experiences worsening of the disease during therapy.[6]

> **CLINICAL SURVIVAL TIP** If there is uncertainty about the diagnosis of a lesion, a biopsy should be performed.

Although it has been suggested that the application of 3% to 5% acetic acid to the affected area may cause the area to turn white, diagnosis using this method is not recommended by the CDC. A mucosal change alone without a discrete lesion would not be treated with the current available therapy, so the results of the test would not influence clinical management. HPV testing is not recommended for anogenital warts as the test results do not confirm the diagnosis and do not guide treatment.[6]

Management

The goal of treatment is to remove the warts and reduce symptoms. Although the warts will resolve spontaneously in most patients, they can cause distress to the patient, so removal is indicated. The available therapies for treatment reduce but probably do not eliminate the infection. It is unknown if treatment that reduces the viral DNA of the HPV reduces its transmission.[6] Once the patient has cleared the lesions, follow-up should be performed in 3 months to assess recurrence. If lesions have returned or did not completely resolve, consider the use of another recommended therapy.

> **NOT TO BE MISSED**
>
> Primary indications for treatment of anogenital warts are bothersome symptoms *and/or* psychological distress.

Pharmacological

There are several effective treatments for anogenital warts, with no evidence to suggest that one of the recommended treatments is superior to the other. The decision of treatment modality is based on the following:

- Wart size
- Number of warts
- Location of warts
- Patient preference
- Cost of treatment
- Provider experience with treatment
- Convenience to patient
- Adverse effects

The CDC recommends treatments that are either patient or provider applied. See Box 15.8 for CDC recommendations for external anogenital warts. There is no clear advantage of one treatment. Table 15.17 provides a comparison of the recommended treatments.

Nonpharmacological Treatment

The nonpharmacological treatments for HPV are cryotherapy and surgical removal. Both require specialized

> **BOX 15.8   U.S. Centers for Disease Control and Prevention Recommended Treatment for External Anogenital Warts**
>
> **Patient-Applied**
> - Imiquimod 3.75% or 5% cream* †
> - *OR*
> - Podofilox 0.5% solution or gel
> - *OR*
> - Sinecatechins 15% ointment†
>
> **Provider-Administered**
> - Cryotherapy with liquid nitrogen or cryoprobe
> - *OR*
> - Surgical removal either by tangential scissor excision, tangential shave excision, curettage, laser, or electrosurgery
> - *OR*
> - Trichloroacetic acid (TCA) or bichloroacetic acid (BCA) 80%–90% solution
>
> * Imiquimod is a patient-applied, topically active immune enhancer that stimulates production of interferon and other cytokines.
> † Might weaken condoms and vaginal diaphragms.
> From U.S. Centers for Disease Control and Prevention. Sexually transmitted infections treatment guidelines, 2021. *MMWR Morbid Mortal Wkly Rep.* 2021;70(4):1–187.

TABLE 15.17	Comparison of Treatments for External Genital Warts			
Treatment	**Dosage**	**Side Effect**	**Comments**
Podofilox 0.5% Solution Gel	Twice daily for 3 days, then no treatment for 4 days. Repeat up to 4 times. Apply with a cotton swab. Apply with a finger.	Treatment	Total area treated should not exceed 10 cm Total amount limited to 0.5 mL per day Contraindicated in pregnancy because of toxicity Patient applied
Imiquimod 5% **Imiquimod 3.75% Both**	Apply 3 times a week for up to 16 weeks. Apply nightly for up to 8 weeks. Apply at bedtime, wash with soap and water 6–10 hours after treatment.	Mild to moderate redness of skin, irritation	Topical immune enhancer Human data in pregnancy limited, but animal data suggest it is safe Patient applied
Sinecatechins (green tea extract)	Apply 3 times a day using a finger to ensure coverage with a thin layer. Do not wash off, and use no longer than 16 weeks.	Erythema (15%) Pruritis/burning, pain ulceration edema induration and vesicular rash	Avoid sexual contact while ointment is on skin Not recommended for HIV-infected patients Safety in pregnancy is not known Patient applied
Trichloracetic acid (TCA) **Bichloracetic acid (BCA)**	Apply small amount to the wart, and allow to dry. Will develop a white frost to tissue. Can be repeated weekly.	Skin irritation, burns, swelling and pain	Caustic agent that chemically coagulates the wart If burning is excessive, wash off, or apply sodium bicarbonate to neutralize Data are limited on these preparations
Cryotherapy	Liquid nitrogen	Pain Necrosis Blistering	Destroys by thermally induced cytolysis Requires proper training Might want to use local anesthesia to reduce pain with treatment
Surgical removal	Either by tangential scissor excision, tangential shave excision, curettage, or electrosurgery	Pain, bleeding, and infection	Can eliminate in a single visit Requires clinical training Anesthesia required

Modified from U.S. Centers for Disease Control and Prevention. Sexually transmitted infections treatment guidelines, 2021. *MMWR Morbid Mortal Wkly Rep.* 2021;70(4):1–187.

equipment and education. Both are effective and a part of the CDC recommendations for treatment. Treatment for non-external warts recommended by the CDC are cryotherapy, surgical removal, and either trichloroacetic or bichloroacetic acid 80% to 90% solution.[6]

Education and Counseling

Counseling and education are viewed from three perspectives. First, HPV is vaccine preventable. Vaccines are safe and effective against some of the viral strains that cause both anogenital warts and cancer. When used consistently and correctly, condoms can lower the transmission of HPV and HPV-related disease. Although they lower transmission, not all areas that are infected may be covered. Because skin-to-skin

transmission is possible, condoms might not provide complete prevention. Transmission can also be affected by sexual behavior, so limiting sexual partners is recommended. As with all STIs, abstaining from sexual activity is the most effective method for preventing the acquisition of HPV.

The second area of education and counseling includes general knowledge related to HPV. It is important to inform patients how common this infection is and that most sexually active individuals will get HPV during their lifetime.[6] Because most individuals do not develop active lesions or the lesions go undiagnosed, it is not possible to determine which partner was the one to transmit the infection in any given relationship. Although some HPV viruses are carcinogenic, the majority of infections are self-limiting and clear spontaneously. The types that cause anogenital warts are not the same as those that cause cancer. There are no tests to determine if the virus will clear or progress, so awareness of possible long-term problems and testing for cervical cancer should be a part of the routine care of female patients. Although there is no treatment to eradicate the virus from the body, there are effective treatments for the precancerous lesions. HPV in pregnancy does not affect the ability to maintain the pregnancy, but not all treatment options are available to the pregnant patient. Rarely, transmission to the infant during vaginal delivery can occur.

Patients with anogenital warts may be counseled that untreated lesions may resolve on their own, usually within 1 year. The types of HPV that cause anogenital warts are not the same as those that cause cervical cancer, therefore anogenital warts alone do not require more frequent Pap smears.[6] Even though the warts are self-limiting, many females find them to be psychologically distressing and should be counseled accordingly. Sexual partners should be informed and counseled on HPV. If indicated, they should be examined and treated as appropriate. The CDC makes no recommendation regarding whether all future sexual partners should be informed of a prior infection because duration of persistent virus after the warts have disappeared is unknown.[6]

Human Immunodeficiency Virus

According to the CDC, approximately 1.2 million individuals in the United States are living with HIV, including about 161,800 who are unaware of their status. Almost 40% of new HIV infections are transmitted by individuals who are living with undiagnosed HIV. For those who are living with undiagnosed HIV, testing is the first step in maintaining a healthy life and reducing the spread of HIV (www.cdc.gov/hiv/testing/index.html).

The CDC recommends HIV testing/screening for adolescents and adults between 13 and 64 years of age at least once during their lifetime. HIV screening is recommended for all pregnant patients using an opt-out approach. Patients whose initial screening test is negative should have repeat testing in the third trimester. Screening for patients 65 years of age and older is indicated if there is an increased risk of infection (e.g., new sexual partner). HIV screening should be performed yearly; however, patients who engage in high-risk behaviors should be tested more frequently.

Focused History and Physical Examination

Obtaining an inclusive sexual history is a substantial or essential part of a health care assessment that can have a dual effect. The history provides detailed background information that is used to establish a behavior risk profile that will be used to guide the health care provider. In addition, this profile may also help the patient understand behavior that may not have otherwise been viewed as risky.

Human Immunodeficiency Virus Screening

There are three types of HIV tests: antibody tests, combination tests (antibody/antigen tests), and NAATs. What makes these tests different is their ability to detect a different serological window of detection. It can take 3 to 12 weeks before a person has enough antibodies to detect HIV.

The enzyme-linked immunosorbent assay (ELISA) is the most commonly used antibody test. The Rapid HIV test is another antibody test that is becoming more commonly used because results are available in as little as 15 minutes.

The combination test, also known as the fourth-generation test, is not only able to detect and confirm the presence of HIV-1 infection; it is also able to detect the p24 antigen, HIV antibodies, and qualitative HIV-1 RNA.

NAATs are able to detect HIV in the blood 7 to 28 days after a patient has been infected. However, this test is not commonly used when screening for HIV screening because of cost.

A positive HIV screening assay requires confirmation. The HIV Western blot and the indirect immunofluorescence assay are no longer a recommended confirmatory test. The HIV treatment guidelines recommend additional testing with an immunoassay that can differentiate HIV-1 from HIV-2 antibodies on all specimens with an initial reactive assay (Fig. 15.19).

NOT TO BE MISSED

Specimens that are reactive on the initial immunoassay and nonreactive or indeterminate on the antibody differentiation assay should proceed to HIV-1 NAAT for confirmation.

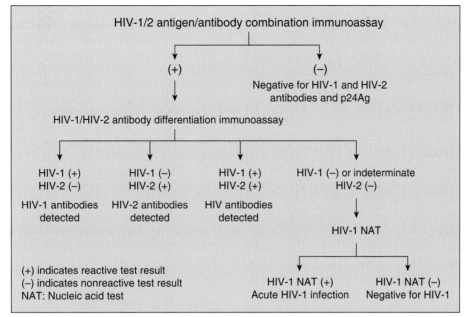

Figure 15.19 Immunoassay that differentiates HIV-1 from HIV-2 antibodies. (From Deresinski S. *New Recommendations for HIV Testing.* Relias Media–Continuing Medical Education Publishing; 2014. https://www.reliasmedia.com/articles/17142-new-recommendations-for-hiv-testing.)

Diagnosis

Acute HIV-1 infection occurs immediately after infection and is characterized by an initial surge of viremia. Although anti–HIV-1 antibodies are undetectable, HIV-1 RNA or p24 antigen is present. Recent infection is generally considered the phase up to 6 months after infection during which detectable anti–HIV-1 antibodies develop. Signs and symptoms a patient may experience during this phase are fever, lymphadenopathy, skin rash, myalgia, arthralgia, headache, diarrhea, oral ulcers, leucopenia, thrombocytopenia, and transaminase elevation.

Management

There is currently no cure for HIV infection. However, the advancements in highly active antiretroviral therapy (HAART) have decreased morbidity, and the virus can be managed as a chronic disease. Once-a-day regimens of combination medications are common and highly effective. Long-acting injectable therapies are currently being studied in clinical trials.

> ### NOT TO BE MISSED
>
> In general, ART regimens for treatment-naïve patients should consist of two NRTIs combined with a third active antiretroviral from one of three classes including integrase strand transfer inhibitors (INSTIs), nonnucleoside reverse transcriptase inhibitors (NNRTI), or protease inhibitors (PIs) with a booster, which can be cobicistat or ritonavir.

Preexposure Prophylaxis

Preexposure prophylaxis (PrEP) is a combination of two HIV medications (tenofovir and emtricitabine), known as Truvada and Descovy, that are taken as a daily regimen. PrEP is for people who are at a very high risk for HIV. Truvada is approved for daily use to help lower the risk of getting HIV from sex by more than 90% and from intravenous drug use by more than 70%. The federal guidelines also recommend PrEP for couples who are in a serodiscordant relationship.

KEY POINTS

- Vaginitis and STIs are two of the most common problems treated in the primary care of female patients, especially reproductive-age females. It is important that all clinicians be familiar with the diagnosis and treatment of these conditions.
- Vaginitis should be treated, and the risk factors for the conditions should be addressed so they can be prevented if possible.
- BV is the most common of the vaginal infections and can be difficult to prevent as it is related to the vaginal environment.
- Trichomoniasis is an STI, and the patient and partner should be treated.
- VVC can cause severe itching and can be an early warning sign of diabetes in females with persistent and repeated infections.
- The rate of STIs is still increasing in the United States, and one of the major goals of care is prevention.
- Prevention is based mainly on behavioral changes that reduce the risk of transmission.
- Some STIs are vaccine preventable, and the clinician should encourage all patients to follow the CDC guidelines for prevention.
- Control of STIs is dependent on the proper diagnosis and adequate treatment. Treatment recommendations of CDC should be used.

REFERENCES

1. Vaginitis, Gor HB. (2021). Medscape; 2021. https://emedicine.medscape.com/article/257141-overview#a5.
2. Clinic, Cleveland (2021). Consult QD. *The Art and Science of Diagnosing Vaginitis.* https://consultqd.clevelandclinic.org/the-art-and-science-of-diagnosing-vaginitis/.
3. Sobel, J. D. (2022). *Vaginal Discharge (Vaginitis): Initial Evaluation. UpToDate.* https://www.uptodate.com/contents/approach-to-women-with-symptoms-of-vaginitis/.
4. Carr, P. L., Felsenstein, D., & Friedman, R. H. (1998). Evaluation and management of vaginitis. *J Gen Intern Med*, 13(5), 335–346.
5. U.S. Centers for Disease Control and Prevention. (2000). *Tracking the Hidden Epidemics; Trends in STIs in the United States.* https://stacks.cdc.gov/view/cdc/6468.
6. U.S. Centers for Disease Control and Prevention. (2021). Sexually transmitted infections treatment guidelines, 2021. *MMWR Morbid Mortal Wkly Rep*, 70(4), 1–187.
7. Goje, O. (2021). *Overview of Vaginitis.* Merck Manual. http://www.merckmanuals.com/professional/gynecology-and-obstetrics/vaginitis,-cervicitis,-and-pelvic-inflammatory-disease-pid/overview-of-vaginitis.
8. Frobenius, W., & Bogdan, C. (2015). Diagnostic value of vaginal discharge, wet mount and vaginal pH: An update on the basics of gynecologic infectiology. *Geburshilfe und Freuenheilkunde*, 75(4), 355–366.
9. Paladine, H. L., & Desai, U. A. (2018). Vaginitis: diagnosis and treatment. *Am Fam Physician*, 97(5), 321–329.
10. Kinney, R. G., & Spach, D. H. (Self-Study STI Modules for Clinicians—Vaginitis. https://www.std.uw.edu/go/comprehensive-study/vaginitis/core-concept/all.
11. Koumans, E. H., Sternberg, M., Bruce, C., et al. (2007). The prevalence of bacterial vaginosis in the United States, 2001–2004: Association with symptoms, sexual behaviors and reproductive health. *Sex Transm Dis, 34*, 864–869.
12. McCance, K. L., & Huether, S. E. (2006). *Pathophysiology: The Biologic Basics for Disease in Adults and Children* (5th ed.). St. Louis: Elsevier Mosby.
13. Amsel, R., Totten, P. A., Spiegel, C. A., Chen, K. C., Eschenbach, D., & Holmes, K. K. (1983). Nonspecific vaginitis: Diagnostic criteria and microbial and epidemiologic associations. *Am J Med*, 74(1), 14–22.
14. Webb, L. (2021). Probiotics for preventing recurrent bacterial vaginosis. *JAAPA*, 34(2), 19–22.
15. U.S. (2021). Centers for Disease Control and Prevention. *Trichomoniasis Statistics.* https://www.cdc.gov/std/trichomonas/stats.htm.
16. Sobel, J. D. (2021). *Trichomonas: Clinical Manifestations and Diagnosis.* UpToDate. https://www.uptodate.com/contents/trichomoniasis.
17. Carcio, H. A., & Secor, R. M. (2015). *Advanced Health Assessment of Women* (3rd ed.). New York: Springer Publishing Company.
18. Morris, S. R. (2020). Trichomoniasis. Merck Manual. https://www.merckmanuals.com/professional/infectious-diseases/sexually-transmitted-infections-stis/trichomoniasis.
19. U.S. Centers for Disease Control and Prevention. *Expedited Partner Therapy in the Management of Sexually Transmitted Diseases.* https://stacks.cdc.gov/view/cdc/6804#:~:text=Expedited%20partner%20therapy%20%28EPT%29%20is%20the%20practice%20of,therapy%20%28PDPT%29%2C%20although%20other%20methods%20may%20be%20employed.
20. Berg, A. O., Heidrich, F. E., Fihn, S. D., et al. (1984). Establishing the cause of genitourinary symptoms in women in a family practice: comparison of clinical examination and comprehensive microbiology. *JAMA, 251*, 620–625.

21. Sobel, J. D., & Mitchell, C. (2021a). *Candida Vulvovaginitis: Clinical Manifestations and Diagnosis*. UpToDate. https://www.uptodate.com/contents/candida-vulvovaginitis-clinical-manifestations-and-diagnosis.

26. Sobel, J. D., Chaim, W., Nagappan, V., & Leaman, D. (2003). Treatment of vaginitis caused by Candida glabrata: Use of topical boric acid and flucytosine. *Am J Obstet Gynecol*, *189*, 1297–1300.

22. Sobel, J. D. (2021b). Candida Vulvovaginitis: Treatment. *UpToDate*. https://www.uptodate.com/contents/candida-vulvovaginitis-treatment#!.

23. Krapf, J. M. (2021). Vulvovaginitis. *Medscape*. http://emedicine.medscape.com/article/2188931-overview.

24. Hardy, J. (Candida glabrata. http://www.hardydiagnostics.com/wp-content/uploads/2016/05/Candida-glabrata.pdf.

25. Rietmeijer, K. (2021). *Prevention of Sexually Transmitted Infections*. UpToDate. https://www.uptodate.com/contents/prevention-of-sexually-transmitted-infections.

26. Adimora, A. A., & Schoenbach, V. J. (2005). Social context, sexual networks, and racial disparities in rates of sexually transmitted infections. *J Infect Dis*, *191*(suppl 1), S115–S122.

27. U.S. Centers for Disease Control and Prevention. (2021). *Sexually Transmitted Disease Surveillance 2019*. https://www.cdc.gov/std/statistics/2019/std-surveillance-2019.pdf.

28. Underwood, J. M., et al. (2020). Youth risk behavior surveillance—United States, 2019. *MMWR Morbid Mortal Wkly Rep*, *69*(1), 1–88.

29. Crepaz, N., Marks, G., Liau, A., et al. (2009). Prevalence of unprotected anal intercourse among HIV-diagnosed MSM in the United States: a meta-analysis. *AIDS*, *23*(13), 1617–1629.

30. Johnson, W. D., Diaz, R. M., Flanders, W. D., et al. (2008). Behavioral interventions to reduce risk for sexual transmission of HIV among men who have sex with men. *Cochrane Database Syst Rev* 16(3), CD001230.

31. Meyers, D., Wolff, T., Gregory, K., Marion, L., et al. (2008). USPSTF recommendation for STI screening. *Am Fam Phys.*, *15*(77), 819–824.

32. Weller, S., & Davis, K. (2002). Condom effectiveness in reducing heterosexual HIV transmission. *Cochrane Database Syst Rev* (1): CD003255.

33. Warner, L., Stone, K. M., Macaluso, M., et al. (2006). Condom use and risk of gonorrhea and Chlamydia: a systematic review of design and measurement factors assessed in epidemiologic studies. *Sex Transm Dis*, *33*(1), 36–51.

34. Holmes, K. K., Levine, R., & Weaver, M. (2004). Effectiveness of condoms in preventing sexually Transmitted infections. *Bull World Health Organ*, *82*(6), 454–461.

35. Hernandez-Romieu, A. C., Siegler, A. J., Sullivan, P. S., et al. (2014). How often do condoms fail? A cross-sectional study exploring incomplete use of condoms, condom failures and other condom problems among black and white MSM in southern USA. *Sex Transm Infect*, *90*(8), 602–607.

36. Steiner, M. J., Cates, W., Jr., & Warner, L. (1999). The real problem with male condoms is nonuse. *Sex Transm Dis*, *26*(8), 459–462.

37. U.S. Centers for Disease Control and Prevention. (*Condom Effectiveness: External (Sometimes Called Male) Condom Use*. https://www.cdc.gov/condomeffectiveness/external-condom-use.html?CDC_AA_refVal=https%3A%2F%2Fwww.cdc.gov%2Fcondomeffectiveness%2Fmale-condom-use.html.

38. Wiyeh, A. B., Mome, R. K. B., Mahasha, P. W., Kongnyuy, E. J., & Wiysonge, C. S. (2020). Effectiveness of the female condom in preventing HIV and sexually transmitted infections: a systematic review and meta-analysis. *BMC Public Health*, *20*(1), 319.

39. Mayo Clinic. *Female Condom*. https://www.mayoclinic.org/female-condom/img-20006654.

40. U.S. Centers for Disease Control and Prevention. (Condom Effectiveness: Internal (Sometimes Called Female) Condom Use. https://www.cdc.gov/condomeffectiveness/internal-condom-use.html.

41. Mantell, J. E., Kelvin, E. A., Exner, T. M., et al. (2009). Anal use of the female condom: does uncertainty justify provider inaction? *AIDS Care*, *21*(9), 1185–1194.

42. U.S. Centers for Disease Control and Prevention. (2021). *National Overview—Sexually Transmitted Disease Surveillance, 2019*. https://www.cdc.gov/STI/statistics/2019/overview.htm#:~:text=In%202019%2C%20129%2C813%20cases%20of,11.2%25%20during%202018%E2%80%932019.

43. U.S. Centers for Disease Control and Prevention. (2017). *Antibiotic Resistant Gonorrhea Basic Information*. https://www.cdc.gov/std/gonorrhea/arg/basic.htm.

44. U.S. Preventive Services Task Force. (2021). *Chlamydia and Gonorrhea: Screening*. https://www.uspreventiveservicestaskforce.org/uspstf/recommendation/chlamydia-and-gonorrhea-screening.

45. U.S. Centers for Disease Control and Prevention. Expedited Partner Therapy in the Management of Sexually Transmitted Diseases. https://stacks.cdc.gov/view/cdc/6804#:~:text=Expedited%20partner%20therapy%20%28EPT%29%20is%20the%20practice%20of,therapy%20%28PDPT%29%2C%20although%20other%20methods%20may%20be%20employed.

46. Li, W., Katz, B. P., Bauer, M. E., & Spinola, S. M. (2013). Haemophilus ducreyi infection induces activation of

the NLRP3 inflammasome in nonpolarized but not in polarized human macrophages. *Infect Immun*, 81(8), 2997–3008.

47. Wising, C., Azem, J., Zetterberg, M., Svensson, L. A., et al. (2005). Induction of apoptosis/necrosis in various human cell lineages by Haemophilus ducreyi cytolethal distending toxin. *Toxicon*, 45(6), 767–776.

48. Morris, S. R. (2020). Chancroid. *Merck Manual*. https://www.merckmanuals.com/en-pr/professional/infectious-diseases/sexually-transmitted-infections-stis/chancroid.

49. Satterwhite, C. L., Torrone, E., Meites, E., et al. (2013). Sexually transmitted infections among US women and men: Prevalence and incidence estimates, 2008. *Sex Transm Dis*, 40(3), 187–193.

50. Smith, J. S., & Robinson, N. J. (2002). Age-specific prevalence of infection with herpes simplex virus types 2 and 1: A global review. *J Infect Dis*, 186(Suppl 1), S3–S28.

51. McQuillan, G., Kruszon-Moran, D., Flagg, E. W., & Paulose-Ram, R. (2018). Prevalence of Herpes Simplex Virus Type 1 and Type 2 in Persons Aged 14–49: United States 2015–2016. U.S. Centers for Disease Control and Prevention. *NCHS Data Brief* (304), 1–8.

52. Schiffer, J., & Corey, L. (2015). Herpes simplex virus. In J. E. Bennett, R. Dolin, & M. J. Blaser (Eds.), *Principles and Practice of Infectious Diseases* (8th ed) *Vol 2*. (pp. 1713–1730). Philadelphia: Elsevier.

53. Mark, K. E., Wald, A., Margaret, A. S., et al. (2008). Rapidly cleared episodes of herpes simplex virus reactivation in immunocompetent adults. *J Infect Dis*, 198(8), 1141–1149.

54. Albrecht, M. A. (2021). Epidemiology, Clinical Manifestation, and Diagnosis of Genital Herpes Simplex Virus Infections. *UpToDate*.

55. U.S. Centers for Disease Control and Prevention. *Genital Herpes – CDC Detailed Fact Sheet*. https://www.cdc.gov/std/herpes/stdfact-herpes-detailed.htm.

56. Roett, M. A., Mayor, M. T., & Uduhiri, K. A. (2012). Diagnosis and management of genital ulcers. *Am Fam Phys.*, 85(3), 254–262.

57. Langenberg, A. G., Corey, L., Ashley, R. L., et al. (1999). A prospective study of new infections with herpes simplex virus type 1 and type 2. Chiron HSV Vaccine Study Group. *N Engl J Med*, 341(19), 1432–1438.

58. Corey, L., Wald, A., Patel, R., et al. (2004). Once-daily valacyclovir to reduce the risk of transmission of genital herpes. *N Engl J Med*, 350(1), 11–20.

59. Wald, A., Langenberg, A. G. M., Krantz, E., et al. (2005). The relationship between condom use and herpes simplex virus acquisition. *Ann Intern Med*, 143(10), 707–713.

60. Musher, D. M. (1990). Biology of treponema pallidum. In K. K. Holmes, P. D. Mardh, P. F. Sparling, et al. (Eds.), *Sexually Transmitted Diseases* (p. 205). New York: McGraw-Hill.

61. Chandrasekar, H. C. (2017). Syphilis. *Medscape*. https://emedicine.medscape.com/article/229461-overview#a5.

62. U.S. Preventive Services Task Force. (2022). *Screening for Syphilis Infection in Nonpregnant Adolescents and Adults US Preventive Services Task Force Reaffirmation Recommendation Statement*. https://jamanetwork.com/journals/jama/fullarticle/2796685#:~:text=Screening%20for%20syphilis%20infection%20in%20nonpregnant%20adults%20and,Services%20Task%20Force%20Procedure%20Manual.%20Updated%20May%202021.

63. U.S. Preventive Services Task Force. (2018). *Syphilis Infection in Pregnant Women: Screening*. https://www.uspreventiveservicestaskforce.org/uspstf/recommendation/syphilis-infection-in-pregnancy-screening.

64. Mattei, P. L., Beachkofsky, T. M., Gilson, R. T., & Wisco, O. J. (2012). Syphilis: a reemerging infection. *Am Fam Phys.*, 86(5), 433–440.

65. Clement, M. E., Okeke, N. L., & Hicks, C. B. (2014). Treatment of syphilis: a systematic review. *JAMA*, 312(18), 1905–1917.

66. Rolfs, R. T., Joesoef, M. R., Hendershot, E. F., et al. (1997). A randomized trial of enhanced therapy for early syphilis in patients with and without human immunodeficiency virus infection. The Syphilis and HIV Study Group. *N Engl J Med*, 337(5), 307–314.

67. Lacey, C. J., Lowndes, C. M., & Shah, K. V. (2006). Chapter 4: Burden and management of non-cancerous HPV-related conditions: HPV-6/11 disease. *Vaccine*, 24, S35–S41.

68. Parkin DM. Bray F. Chapter 2: The burden of HPV-related cancers. Vaccine. 2006;24 Suppl 3:S3/11–25.

69. Gearhart, P. A. (2017). Human Papillomavirus (HPV). *Medscape*. https://emedicine.medscape.com/article/219110-overview.

70. PathologyOutlines.com. HPV. http://www.pathologyoutlines.com/topic/cervixHPV.html.

71. Xing, B., Guo, J., Sheng, Y., Wu, G., & Zhao, Y. (2021). Human papillomavirus-negative cervical cancer: A comprehensive review. *Front Oncol*, 17(10), 606335.

16

Menstrual Disorders

Sarah B. Freeman

OBJECTIVES

- Describe the physiological components of a normal menstrual cycle and how a malfunction of one component may lead to a menstrual disorder.
- Use the PALM-COEIN acronym (*p*olyp, *a*denomyosis, *l*eiomyoma, *m*alignancy, *c*oagulopathy, *o*vulatory, *e*ndometrial, *i*atrogenic, and *n*ot otherwise classified) to organize an approach to diagnosing abnormal uterine bleeding (AUB) in the primary care setting.

- Classify bleeding patterns associated with AUB, and demonstrate an understanding of different evaluation techniques.
- Based on the patient's type and severity of bleeding, construct an appropriate management protocol for the most common menstrual disorders including first-line treatments and any emergent findings.
- Evaluate when a patient with AUB needs more specialized care, and make the appropriate referral.

INTRODUCTION

Menstrual disorders are problems that affect a female's menstrual cycle. They may include one or more of the following:

- Cycle-related symptoms
  - Premenstrual syndrome (PMS)
  - Premenstrual dysphoric disorder (PMDD)
  - Dysmenorrhea
- Amenorrhea
- Heavy periods

The normal menstrual cycle is a coordinated cycle of stimulatory and inhibitory effects that result in the release of a mature oocyte. A variety of factors contribute to the regulation of the cycle. A complete discussion of the physiology of the menstrual cycle is found in Chapter 2. In order to discuss abnormality in the menstrual cycle it is important to define the normal menstrual cycle. Menarche generally takes place between 12 and 15 years of age, and menopause generally begins between 45 and 55 years of age. The normal cycle is 21 to 35 days with the luteal phase having less variation in length (12 to 14 days). The average menstrual flow lasts between 4 and 6 days, however, between 2 and 8 days are considered normal. Average blood loss is about 50 mL per cycle, though 20 to 80 mL is within normal limits[1-3] (Table 16.1).

Not all bleeding is related to menstruation, and the clinician must be able to define bleeding that is a part of menstruation as well as bleeding that occurs outside of menstruation. The most common types of this bleeding are as follows:

- Intermenstrual-irregular bleeding (usually light) occurring between normal menstrual periods
- Postcoital bleeding

TABLE 16.1	**Characteristics of the Normal Menstrual Cycle**	
Characteristics	**Normal**	**Variations**
Regularity	+/− 2 to 20 days	Irregular: Varying lengths of bleeding-free intervals exceeding 20 days within a 90-day period Amenorrhea: No bleeding in a 90-day period
Frequency	24 to 38 days	Infrequent: One to two episodes of >38 days in a 90-day period Frequent: More than four episodes of <24 days in a 90-day period
Duration	Up to 8 days	Shortened: No clinical entity associated with shortened menses other than amenorrhea Prolonged: >8 days
Volume	Up to 80 mL (used in research)	Clinical definition is subjective; defined as a volume that does not interfere with a female's quality of life

Modified from Singh S, Best C, Dunn S, et al. Abnormal uterine bleeding in premenopausal women. *J Obstet Gynaecol Can.* 2015;35(5):S5–S6.

- Premenstrual/postmenstrual spotting-bleeding that occurs (usually regularly) for one or more days before or after the recognized cycle[4]

> **PATIENT-CENTERED CARE:** When approaching patients complaining of a menstrual disorder, patients must understand that some degree of irregularity can be part of a normal physiological process.

Age is important when assessing bleeding. Bleeding can also occur outside of the reproductive age of females, and this may also need to be evaluated. Bleeding outside of normal reproductive life is defined as follows:[4]
- Precocious: Menstruation; bleeding occurring before 9 years of age
- Postmenopausal: Bleeding occurring more than 1 year after cessation of menses

There are times in which irregular cycles can be expected. A female may experience irregular menstrual cycles at both ends of reproductive life. During adolescence, the interval from the first cycle to the second cycle may be outside the normal parameters. Immaturity of the hypothalamic-pituitary-ovarian axis during the early years after menarche often results in anovulation, and cycles may be somewhat long.

By year 3 after menarche, 60% to 80% of menstrual cycles are within the normal range.[5] Irregular bleeding is a hallmark of perimenopause. The progression through menopause normally leads to lengthening of the frequency and shortening of the duration of the cycles.

A complete discussion of menopause can be found in Chapter 13. Though there are parameters and guidelines available to help classify and diagnose menstrual disorders, the patient is the expert in her own cycle and is the best source for what constitutes abnormal.

ABNORMAL UTERINE BLEEDING

AUB is a term that encompasses most menstrual disorders. It describes any diagnosis referring to irregularity in the timing, frequency, amount, or duration of uterine bleeding. AUB is one of the most common gynecological complaints of reproductive-age females seen in the primary care setting. It affects 11% to 13% of reproductive-age females at any given time, and the prevalence increases with age. By 36 to 40 years of age, 24% of females may present with AUB. AUB affects one-third of females in their lifetime, and one-half of these individuals do not seek treatment, even with health care access.[6] The economic impact and the effect on a patient's quality of life are two of the parameters for determining treatment.

AUB can be caused by a wide variety of local and systemic diseases or related to medications. Common causes are as follows:
- Genital tract disorders
  - Uterus
  - Cervix
  - Vulva
  - Vagina
- Pregnancy related
- Trauma including sexual abuse
- Drugs
- Systemic disease

The history and physical examination are dependent on the suspected cause. Most common causes may vary by age (Table 16.2). When discussing AUB, there has been much confusion related to the varied use of terminology to describe AUB symptoms. This has led to difficulties in many areas, including documenting symptoms. The International Federation of Gynecology and Obstetrics Menstrual Disorders Committee (FIGO MDC) used an evidence-based approach to develop parameters of normal menstrual bleeding.[2-3] The current terminology is as follows:

- *Abnormal uterine bleeding:* An overarching term used to describe any symptomatic variation. This term covers the full range of symptoms of abnormal bleeding.

TABLE 16.2 Causes of Abnormal Uterine Bleeding by Age

Age	Cause
Prepubescence	Foreign body Trauma—consider sexual abuse Tumor—ovarian Precocious puberty
Menarche (within the first few years)	Hypothalamic immaturity Coagulation disorders Stress
Reproductive age (may also occur in the prepubescent female)	Ovulatory dysfunction Pregnancy Cancer Structural problems Endocrine dysfunction Infection Coagulation disorders Medications (e.g., antipsychotics, selective serotonin reuptake inhibitors)
Perimenopause	Anovulation Structural problems Cancer
Menopause	Cancer Structural problems Hormone therapy

- *Bleeding:* Bloody discharge from the vagina that requires the use of protection
- *Spotting:* Bloody discharge from the vagina that does not require protection
- *Bleeding/spotting episode:* Number of consecutive days of bleeding or spotting
- *Bleeding/spotting-free intervals:* Number of days between bleeding and spotting episodes
- *Bleeding spotting segments:* One bleeding and spotting episode and the immediate spotting-free interval that follows it
- *Reference:* Number of consecutive days used in that analysis (usually 90)
- *Acute AUB:* An episode of uterine bleeding in a nonpregnant female of reproductive age that requires intervention to prevent further blood loss
- *Chronic abnormal uterine bleeding:* Bleeding from the uterus that is abnormal in frequency, regularity, duration, and/or volume and has been present for at least the majority of the past 6 months[7-8]

CLINICAL SURVIVAL TIP Understanding the physiology of menstruation is critical to diagnosing and managing AUB.

When examining normal menstrual physiology, there are several points at which the system can be altered leading to abnormal bleeding. Given the number of possible causes, it is important to have an organized approach to the diagnosis of abnormal uterine bleeding. In 2010, FIGO formally accepted and disseminated their system for classifying abnormal uterine bleeding, which uses the PALM-COEIN acronym. The American College of Obstetricians and Gynecologists adopted this structure in 2011, and it has replaced the older terms (e.g., *menorrhagia, metrorrhagia*) for a more formulaic and less subjective diagnostic vocabulary.

The classification system is divided into nine basic categories that are arranged according to the PALM-COEIN acronym. The components of the PALM group (*p*olyp, *a*denomyosis, *l*eiomyoma, *m*alignancy) are structural entities that are visually measurable using imaging techniques and/or histopathology. The components of the COEIN group (*c*oagulopathy, *o*vulatory, *e*ndometrial, *i*atrogenic, and *n*ot otherwise classified) are nonstructural entities that cannot be defined by imaging or histopathology (Fig. 16.1). This classification

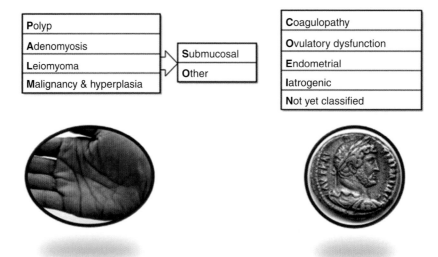

Polyp
Adenomyosis
Leiomyoma
Malignancy & hyperplasia

Submucosal
Other

Coagulopathy
Ovulatory dysfunction
Endometrial
Iatrogenic
Not yet classified

Figure 16.1 PALM-COEIN classification system for abnormal uterine bleeding. The basic system comprises four categories that are defined by visually objective structural criteria (PALM: *p*olyp, *a*denomyosis, *l*eio-myoma, *m*alignancy and hyperplasia), four that are unrelated to structural anomalies (COEI: *c*oagulopathy, *o*vulatory, *e*ndometrial, *i*atrogenic), and one reserved for entities that are *n*ot otherwise classified (N). The leiomyoma category (L) is subdivided into patients with at least one submucosal myoma (LSM) and those with myomas that do not affect the endometrial cavity (LO). (From Munro MG, Critchley HO, Broder MS, et al. FIGO classification system (PALM-COEIN) for causes of abnormal uterine bleeding in nongravid women of reproductive age. *Int J Gynaecol Obstet.* 2011;113[1]:3–13.)

system should be kept in mind while doing the history and physical examination as it can provide a guide for the assessment.[8]

The history and physical examination will help determine the cause and guide the management of the patient presenting with AUB. Several initial questions must be answered to further guide the evaluation (Fig. 16.2). A complete menstrual history provides a starting point for gathering information about the bleeding. All female patients must be accessed for the following:

- Age of menarche
  - Prior history of menstrual problems and irregularity
  - Heavy bleeding
  - Spotting
  - Intermenstrual bleeding
- Dysmenorrhea
- Other symptoms associated with the menstrual cycle

As causes are age-related, the reproductive age should be used to guide the history. In reproductive-age female patients, it is important to assess for the following:
- Date of last menstrual period (LMP)
- Date of previous menstrual period (PMP)

- Current cycle length and any variation from the patient's normal cycle
  - Interval between periods
  - Regularity over at least the past year
  - Number of days both on average and for the past two cycles
- Any heavy or intermenstrual bleeding
- Current other symptoms related to the cycle
  - Dysmenorrhea
  - PMS/PMDD symptoms

For postmenopausal patients, it is important to collect information on age of LMP, previous and current use of hormone therapy, and history of postmenopausal bleeding.

> **CLINICAL SURVIVAL TIP** It is important to rule out un-suspected pregnancies and endometrial cancer in the evaluation of AUB.

Evaluation of the amount of bleeding is subjective and difficult to assess. The following questions can help quantify blood loss:
1. How often to you change your pad or tampon during peak flow?

2. How many pads to you use during a typical cycle, and how has this changed?
3. Do you have to change pads at night?
4. Do you pass clots; if so, how large are they?

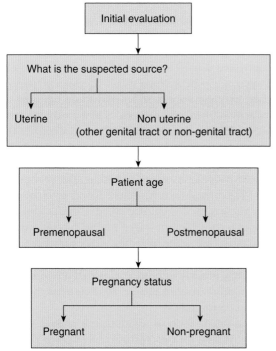

Figure 16.2 Things to consider during the initial evaluation of possible uterine bleeding.

For the typical female, pads/tampons are changed every 2 hours, and the average female uses fewer than 21 pads/tampons per cycle. The patient very rarely needs to get up during the night to change a pad, and clots are usually less than 1 inch in diameter.[9] Variation from this pattern is considered to be abnormal. Estimating blood loss is difficult because patients change pads with different amounts of blood on them. Figure 16.3 may be useful in estimating the amount of blood loss.[10]

The general history should be guided by the menstrual cycle history. A gynecological history should include the following:

- Sexual history: To help determine the patient's risk for pregnancy or sexually transmitted infections.
- History of obstetrical or gynecological surgery
  - Prior cesarean delivery increases the likelihood of a cesarean scar defect.[11]
  - Prior myomectomy increases possibility that uterine fibroids are responsible.
- Contraceptive history
  - Combined hormonal contraception (CHC) can lead to unscheduled bleeding
  - Progestin-only pills (POPs) can cause irregular uterine bleeding or amenorrhea.
  - Progestin implants may cause either irregular bleeding or less frequently, amenorrhea
  - Intrauterine device (IUD) changes menstrual flow.

Feminine Pad	Type	Score	Tampon	Type	Score	Extraneous	Type	Score
	Day	1 mL		Light	0.25 mL		Light	1 mL
				Medium	0.5 mL			
	Night	1 mL		Heavy	1.0 mL			
				Super	1.0 mL			
	Day	2 mL		Light	0.5 mL		Moderate	3 mL
				Medium	1.0 mL			
	Night	3 mL		Heavy	1.5 mL			
				Super	2.0 mL			
	Day	3 mL		Light	1.0 mL			
				Medium	1.5 mL			
	Night	6 mL		Heavy	3.0 mL			
				Super	4.0 mL			
	Day	4 mL		Light	3.0 mL		Heavy	5 mL
				Medium	4.0 mL			
	Night	10 mL		Heavy	8.0 mL			
				Super	12.0 mL			

Figure 16.3 Estimated blood loss during menstruation. (From Dasharathy SS, Mumford AZ, Pollack NJ, et al. Menstrual bleeding patterns among regularly menstruating women. *Am J Epidemiol*. 2012;175[6]:536–545.)

- Levonorgestrel IUDs typically cause an initial period of irregular spotting or bleeding followed by a gradual decrease in menstrual flow.
  - Copper IUDs can increase both the amount and duration of menstrual flow.

There are areas outside of the reproductive system that should also be explored, depending on age and other symptoms. Thyroid disorders can be associated with abnormal bleeding. Ask about both the symptoms of thyroid disease as well as a family history. Bleeding disorders can also cause abnormal bleeding. Heavy menstrual flow is common in females with bleeding disorders; up to 15% to 20% of female patients presenting with heavy bleeding may have some type of bleeding disorder, most commonly von Willebrand disease or a possible platelet function defect.[12]

Medications can cause AUB in several different ways. Anticoagulants may result in heavy or prolonged uterine bleeding, and a variety of other medications can cause amenorrhea. General history areas that might help suggest a possible cause are discussed in the following sections.

PHYSICAL EXAMINATION

A focused physical examination should be performed that is geared to rule out all suspected causes of AUB. Vital signs should be assessed, and a complete pelvic examination should be performed on all patients presenting with AUB. Other assessments should be based on the information discovered in the history. Before performing a pelvic examination, the clinician should conduct a general inspection that includes the following:

- Signs of severe volume depletion: Helps confirm the patient's history of very heavy bleeding and/or the need for prompt immediate inpatient care.
- Obesity: Often a risk factor for both polycystic ovarian syndrome (PCOS) and endometrial cancer.
- Signs of androgen excess: Signs of PCOS (hirsutism, acne, clitoromegaly, male pattern balding, or Acanthosis nigricans)
- Ecchymosis: Sign of trauma or bleeding disorder
- Purpura: Sign of trauma or bleeding disorder

As with the history, considering the PALM-COIEN system can help guide the pelvic examination. All potential sites of genital bleeding should be considered. Assessment of the vulva, vagina, cervix, urethra, anus, and perineum should be considered. Any abnormal findings along the genital tract such as mass, laceration, ulceration, friable area, vaginal or cervical discharge, or foreign body should be noted.

Assess for the size and contour of the uterus. Limited uterine mobility should be noted. If present, this finding suggests that pelvic adhesions or a pelvic mass is present. An enlarged uterus may be caused by pregnancy, uterine leiomyomas, adenomyosis, or uterine malignancy. A boggy, globular, tender uterus is typical of adenomyosis. Leiomyomas usually cause the uterus to be firm and the enlargement to be asymmetrical. Uterine enlargement caused by pregnancy is softer and more uniform. An enlarged uniformly shaped uterus in a postmenopausal patient with bleeding suggests endometrial cancer. Tenderness may present in females with pelvic inflammatory disease (PID) and endometriosis.

If the patient is currently bleeding, the volume and site of bleeding should be noted. Blood or blood clots in the vaginal vault should be noted. Patients who present with a complaint of heavy vaginal bleeding should be assessed for acute bleeding. The presence of an adnexal mass or tenderness should be noted. Ovarian cancer may present with intermenstrual bleeding as the only symptom. Any suspicious adnexal mass should be worked up promptly.[13]

If indicated, a breast examination should be performed to assess for galactorrhea as it suggests the presence of hyperprolactinemia. A patient complaining of a milky discharge from either breast (while not pregnant, postpartum, or breastfeeding) may need a prolactin (PRL) level to rule out a pituitary tumor.

> **CLINICAL SURVIVAL TIP** Patients who are hemodynamically unstable or who have copious, ongoing blood flow from the uterus or other genital tract site should be evaluated and possibly referred for management to an emergency department.

Diagnostic Workup

NOT TO BE MISSED

Most reproductive-age females with AUB should be evaluated initially with the following tests: human chorionic gonadotropin (hCG), complete blood count (CBC), hemoglobin, and/or hematocrit. Additional tests may be performed to assess for particular etiologies.

Initially AUB should be evaluated with the following tests:

- hCG
- CBC including a hemoglobin and/or hematocrit
- Ferritin level (dependent on the patient's history and assessment)

Sexually active patients who present with uterine bleeding should have a pregnancy test. If positive, the patient should be referred for further evaluation and care. Postmenopausal patients and those at increased risk who present with bleeding must be evaluated for endometrial or other gynecological malignancy.[14] Patients with heavy or prolonged bleeding should be evaluated for anemia with a hemoglobin and/or hematocrit. You may also consider a ferritin level as it can help identify female patients who, although not currently anemic, are at risk because of depleted iron stores.[15] A CBC can also be useful if you suspect the following:

- Bleeding disorder: platelet count
- Infection: white blood cell count with differential

Additional testing depends on information obtained on the history and physical examination. It is performed to rule out specific problems.

Endocrine tests should be performed if indicated by the history or physical examination. Reasons to perform endocrine testing are as follows:

- Thyroid function tests to assess for thyroid disease
  - Most often associated with amenorrhea
  - Ovulatory dysfunction: thyroid-stimulating hormone (TSH)
  - Heavy menstrual bleeding (HMB) is associated with hypothyroidism
- PRL level should be measured in patients who report the following:
  - Anovulatory bleeding
  - Amenorrhea
  - Galactorrhea
  - Medications that can cause hyperprolactinemia
  - Antipsychotics
  - Selective serotonin reuptake inhibitors (SSRIs)
- Testosterone levels
  - To assess for signs of androgen excess

- Follicle-stimulating hormone (FSH) or luteinizing hormone (LH)
  - Suspected anovulatory bleeding and amenorrhea
  - Menopause
- Estrogen levels
  - Primary ovarian insufficiency (POI; also known as *premature ovarian failure*)
  - Estrogen-secreting ovarian tumor
  - Rare etiology of AUB, but should be considered if an adnexal mass is present.

Coagulation tests should be ordered if bleeding disorders are suspected. These disorders are most common in young reproductive-age females. Up to 15% to 24% of female patients presenting with HMB may have some type of bleeding diathesis.[16-17] A bleeding disorder should be suspected if heavy or prolonged menses began at menarche. Other signs are a family history of coagulopathy, easy bruising, and prolonged bleeding from mucosal surfaces or taking medications associated with an increased bleeding tendency.[18] Tests to consider to rule out bleeding disorders are as follows:

- Partial thromboplastin time
- Prothrombin time
- Activated partial thromboplastin time
- Fibrinogen

EMB is needed in a subset of females to rule out endometrial neoplasia. Indications for EMB vary by age group (Table 16.3).[19-20] In general, all females older than 45 years of age who present with both intermenstrual and/or heavy bleeding should have an EMB to rule out endometrial cancer. Nineteen percent of cases of endometrial cancer occur in females 45 to 54 years of age compared with 6% in those 35 to 44 years of age.[20-23]

The decision to refer for pelvic imaging should be based on suspected diagnosis as well as patient age, history, and symptoms. Several factors will help guide the decision to refer. If the abdominal and/or bimanual pelvic examination findings include an enlarged or globular uterus or adnexal mass, imaging may be appropriate.

TABLE 16.3   Risk for Endometrial Cancer[19-20]

Risk Factors	Relative Risk (RR)	
Increased age	1.4% in females 50 to 70 years of age	
Early menarche	2%	
Unopposed estrogen therapy	2%–10% (dependent on years of therapy)	
Late menopause (after 55 years of age)	2%	
Nulliparity	2%	
Polycystic ovarian syndrome	3%	
Obesity	Type 1	Type 2
BMI 25–29.9 kg/m2	1.5%	1.2%
BMI 30.0–34.9 kg/m2	2.5%	1.7%
BMI 30.0–34.9 kg/m2	4.5%	2.2%
BMI >40 kg/m2	7.1%	3.1%
Lynch syndrome (hereditary nonpolyposis colorectal cancer)	13% to 71% lifetime risk	

BMI, Body mass index; *Type 1 and Type 2*, classification of endometrial cancer.

Pelvic ultrasonography is the first-line imaging study in female patients with AUB. A transvaginal examination should be performed unless there is a reason to not perform the vaginal study. Transvaginal ultrasonography (TVUS) can be used to detect structural abnormalities, including most polyps. It can also be used to detect areas of focal thickening in the endometrium. This focal thickening may indicate a small intrauterine mass such as an endometrial polyp or submucous leiomyomas. Saline infusion sonography is a technique in which sterile saline is instilled into the endometrial cavity and TVUS is performed.[24] This procedure allows for an architectural evaluation of the uterine cavity to detect lesions that may be missed or poorly defined by TVUS. If direct visualization of the endometrial cavity is needed, a hysteroscopy is performed. Referral for these procedures should be performed based on your clinical judgement.

ABNORMAL UTERINE BLEEDING/HEAVY MENSTRUAL BLEEDING

To avoid missing any problem, the PALM-COIEN system provides a framework for the assessment and diagnosis. Primary care management of the most common presentation will be discussed.

NOT TO BE MISSED

Uterine structural abnormalities that cause AUB (e.g., polyps, fibroids, adenomyosis) may require referral for surgical management.

POLYPS

The first diagnosis to consider is polyps. Endometrial polyps are one of the most common causes of abnormal genital bleeding. They are referred to as *AUB-P* in the nomenclature recommended by FIGO.[8]

They occur in both premenopausal and postmenopausal females and are hyperplastic overgrowths of endometrial glands and stroma. Most endometrial polyps are benign, but malignancy can occur in some females.[25] The common presenting symptom is AUB that is reported by the patient as either intermenstrual bleeding or spotting. Patients with a suspected endometrial polyp should be referred for evaluation with pelvic imaging or hysteroscopy. Treatment is usually surgical removal.[26-27]

NOT TO BE MISSED

Endometrial polyps are more likely to be malignant in postmenopausal females with bleeding.

ADENOMYOSIS

Adenomyosis (AUB-A) refers to the presence of endometrial glands and stroma within the uterine muscle. The endometrial tissue causes both hypertrophy and hyperplasia of the surrounding myometrium. This can cause diffuse globular enlargement of the uterus that must be differentiated from pregnancy. The incidence of AUB-A is unknown because a positive diagnosis is determined by microscopic examination of the uterus after removal.[28] The diagnosis of adenomyosis is suggested by the following characteristic clinical manifestations:[28]

- HMB
- Dysmenorrhea
- Uniformly enlarged uterus
- Absence of endometriosis or leiomyomas.

Suspected AUB-A should be referred for diagnosis and treatment. The definitive treatment for adenomyosis is hysterectomy.

LEIOMYOMAS

Uterine leiomyomas (AUB-L) are the most common pelvic tumor in females. Incidence by 50 years of age is >80% for Black females and almost 70% for White females.[29] Leiomyomas may also be referred to as *fibroids* or *myomas*. Leiomyomas are benign tumors arising from the smooth muscle cells of the myometrium. They are seen mostly in reproductive-age females and typically present with the following:[30]

- Heavy or prolonged menstrual bleeding
- Pelvic pressure and pain
- Reproductive dysfunction
  - Infertility
  - Obstetrical complications

The FIGO classification of leiomyoma is AUB-L, and this is further divided into two subcategories that are based on the location of the tumor:[8]

- Submucosal (AUB-LSM)
- Other (AUB-LO)
  - Intramural
  - Subserosal
  - Other

Heavy and/or prolonged menses is the typical bleeding pattern with leiomyomas and the most common fibroid symptom.[31] Heavy uterine bleeding may be responsible for associated problems, such as iron deficiency. The presence and degree of uterine bleeding are determined, in large part, by the location of the fibroid; size is of secondary importance. Submucosal myomas (AUB-S) protrude into the uterine cavity and frequently cause HMB.[32]

With AUB-LO, the bleeding pattern can vary. If the tumors are intramural, they are commonly associated with heavy and prolonged bleeding, while subserosal tumors do not usually cause heavy bleeding. The subserosal tumors are more frequently associated with increased pain.

Uterine leiomyomas are a clinical diagnosis based on pelvic examination and imaging. The indication for pelvic imaging typically includes symptoms of AUB, pelvic pain or pressure, or infertility and an enlarged, firm, irregular uterus on pelvic examination. TVUS is the most widely used imaging modality for evaluating leiomyomas because of its availability and cost-effectiveness. The diagnosis is typically made based on a pelvic ultrasound findings that confirm the presence of a uterine tumor.[33] Treatment can be instituted if the ultrasound examination is positive for the tumors.

There are several treatment options used for the management of leiomyomas (Fig. 16.4). The major goal of treatment is the relief of symptoms.[34] The type and timing of any intervention should be individualized, based on factors such as the following:[35]

- Type and severity of symptoms
- Size of the myoma(s)
- Location of the myoma(s)
- Reproductive plans and obstetrical history

Any complication such as anemia should also be managed. Expectant therapy is used when bleeding is not severe and anemia is not present. TVUS should be performed as a baseline, and the patient should be seen yearly to evaluate any progression of the tumor. If HMB begins or anemia develops, then other treatment options should be considered. Progression of the size of the tumor on pelvic examination requires further imaging and, again, other treatment options must be considered.[36]

For the primary care office, medical management can be instituted. Table 16.4 lists the current medical options for management of leiomyomas. If the disease continues to progress, the patient should be referred for evaluation for surgical management.[34-37]

MALIGNANCY AND HYPERPLASIA (AUB-M)

Malignancy of the reproductive tract may present with HMB. A discussion of these disorders is found in Chapter 20.

HMB-COEIN

HMB usually refers to heavy bleeding related to ovulatory cycles. HMB must be treated when quality of life is affected, or it causes anemia. The impact on quality of life can be related to the following:

- Need to change pads or tampons frequently
- Bleeding that stains clothing or bedding
- Avoidance of activities because of bleeding

When addressing nonstructural causes of bleeding, the COEIN acronym is used. These letters stand for *coagulopathy*, *ovulatory* dysfunction, *endometrial*, *iatrogenic*, and *not* otherwise classified:

- Coagulopathy (AUB-C): The term *coagulopathy* is used to encompass systemic disorders that result in

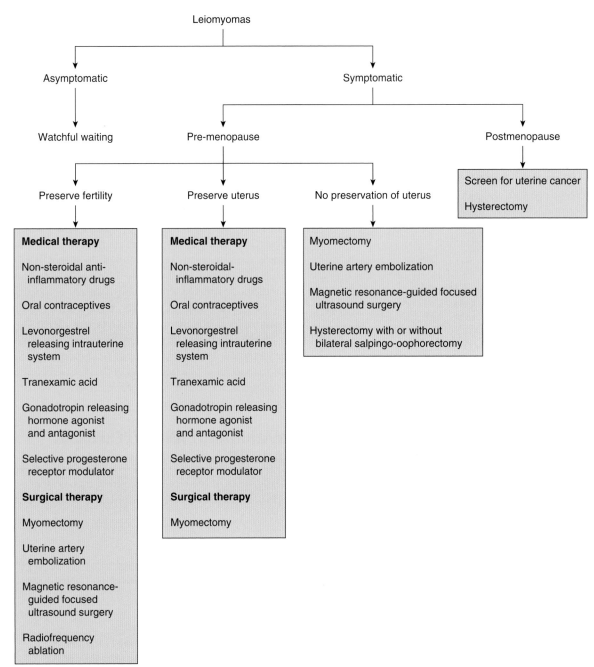

Figure 16.4 Treatment option for leiomyomas (Modified from De La Cruz MS, Buchanana EM. Uterine fibroids: diagnosis and treatment. *Am Fam Physician.* 2017;95[2]:100–107; American College of Obstetricians and Gynecologists' Committee on Practice Bulletins—Gynecology. Management of Symptomatic Uterine Leiomyomas: ACOG Practice Bulletin, Number 228. *Obstet Gynecol.* 2021;137[6]:e100–e115; Stewart EA. Uterine fibroids. *Lancet.* 2001;357[9252]:293–298; Mas A, Tarazona M, Carrasco JD, Estaca G, Cristobal I, Monleon J. Updated approaches for the management of uterine fibroids. *Int J Womens Health.* 2017;9:607–617.)

TABLE 16.4 Medical Management of Leiomyomas

Drugs	Mechanism of Action	Advantages	Disadvantages	Fertility Preserved
Gonadotropin-releasing hormone antagonists with add-back therapy Elagolix: 300 mg BID with 1 mg estradiol and 0.5 mg norethindrone acetate daily Relugolix (under FDA review) Gonadotropin- releasing hormone agonist Leuprolide acetate depot: 3.75 mg/month intramuscularly 11.25 mg/3 months Goserelin acetate: 3.6 mg/month subcutaneously 10.8 mg subcutaneous implant every 3 months Histrelin: 50 mcg implant every 12 months Triptorelin: 3.75 mg/month; 11.25 mg/3 months; 22.5 mg/6 months Nafarelin acetate: twice-daily intranasal spray	Suppress gonadotropins and ovarian sex hormones Cause amenorrhea	Decrease blood loss Improve pain and bulk symptoms Decrease blood loss and improve anemia Reduce uterine size	Hot flushes Headaches Expense Menopausal symptoms Bone loss	Yes
Oral contraceptives: multiple brands Take daily for 21 day and 7 days off	Work to stabilize the endometrium	Reduce blood loss	Do not decrease uterine size	Yes
Levonorgestrel-releasing intrauterine device: Kyleena, Liletta, Mirena. Change every 3 to 5 years depending on device chosen	Likely stabilizes the endometrium	Reduce blood loss and decrease volume of leiomyomas	Irregular bleeding pattern	Yes
Selective progesterone receptor modulators Ulipristal acetate: oral, 5 mg or 10 mg once daily for 13 weeks Mifepristone: 5–50 mg/day for 3–6 months	Decrease size of tumors	Decrease blood loss Not associated with hypoestrogen state	Headaches Breast tenderness Not FDA approved for treatment of leiomyomas Not used long term Abortive agent in larger doses	Yes
Tranexamic acid Lysteda: 1300 mg 3 times daily (3900 mg/day) Cyklokapron: 1000 mg to 1500 mg three to four times daily	Antifibrinolytic agent	Reduces blood loss Can be used while trying to become pregnant	Does not decrease size of tumor Contraindicated with history of venous thromboembolism or elevated risk of thrombosis	Yes
Nonsteriodal antiinflammatory drugs Multiple drugs in this class can be used	Antiinflammatory and prostaglandin inhibitor	Not well studied but reduces blood loss Relieve pain	Does not reduce size of tumor	Yes

Continued

Drugs	Mechanism of Action	Advantages	Disadvantages	Fertility Preserved
Progestin implants, injections, and pills	Endometrial atrophy	Improve bleeding and can lead to amenorrhea	Irregular bleeding and spotting	Yes
Implants		May decrease uterine size	DMPA (prolonged use) bone loss	
Nexplonon: change every 3 years				
DMPA 150 mg IM every 3 months				
Progestin-only pills: take daily				

TABLE 16.4 Medical Management of Leiomyomas—cont'd

FDA, U.S. Food and Drug Administration.
Developed from De La Cruz MS, Buchanana EM. Uterine fibroids: diagnosis and treatment. *Am Fam Physician*. 2017;95(2):100–107. American College of Obstetricians and Gynecologists' Committee on Practice Bulletins—Gynecology. Management of Symptomatic Uterine Leiomyomas: ACOG Practice Bulletin, Number 228. *Obstet Gynecol*. 2021;137[6]:e100–e115. Stewart EA. Uterine fibroids. *Lancet*. 2001;357[9252]:293–298; Mas A, Tarazona M, Carrasco JD, Estaca G, Cristobal I, Monleon J. Updated approaches for the management of uterine fibroids. *Int J Womens Health*. 2017;9:607–617; Moroni R, Vieira C, Ferriani R, Candido-Dos-Reis F, Brito L. Pharmacological treatment of uterine fibroids. Ann Med Health Sci Res. 2014;4(Suppl 3):S185–S192.

abnormal bleeding. If this is suspected, patients must be referred for diagnosis and treatment.

- Ovulatory dysfunction (AUB-O): Ovulatory dysfunction occurs when a patient is either anovulatory or has infrequent ovulation. AUB-O is irregular, nonovulatory (noncyclic) bleeding. Although bleeding may be infrequent in some patients with AUB-O, it can be prolonged and heavy in others. Hemorrhage may occur. The etiology of AUB-O should be identified. Once identified, treatment should target the underlying cause. Both thyroid disease and hyperprolactinemia are common causes of AUB-O, and treatment of these conditions may restore normal cyclic menses. One of the most common etiologies of AUB-O is PCOS.[38] Treatment goals for AUB-O are as follows:
  - Establish a regular bleeding pattern
  - Establish amenorrhea
  - Prevent heavy bleeding
  - Prevent endometrial hyperplasia/cancer.[38]

Females with ovulatory dysfunction may attempt ovulation induction if pregnancy is desired.[14] Medical management is discussed later in this chapter.

- Endometrial causes (AUB-E): Endometrial causes of AUB are seen in females with predictable menses and suggests normal ovulation. It can present as both HMB and intermenstrual bleeding. The diagnosis should be considered in the absence of other definable causes. Most often, the cause of such bleeding is a primary disorder of the endometrium. Patients with AUB-E should be referred for definitive diagnosis and management.

- Iatrogenic bleeding (AUB-I): This category includes AUB caused by medical devices as well as medications. Management is the recognition and removal of the cause.

- Not otherwise classified (AUB-N): This category may encompasses several entities that contribute to or cause uterine bleeding. These have either been poorly defined, inadequately examined, and/or are extremely rare. If unable to classify the bleeding in one of the aforementioned categories, the patient is labeled AUB-N and referred for further workup.[8]

Because the treatment of HMB and AUB-O may differ depending on cause, you may need to differentiate between ovulatory and anovulatory bleeding. Anovulatory bleeding is most likely to have the following characteristics:

- Irregular, often infrequent menses with bleeding ranging from excessive to minimal
- Estrogen-dominant/progesterone-deficient status

Fourteen percent of females with recurrent anovulatory cycles develop endometrial hyperplasia or cancer. Management is aimed at not only relieving symptoms but at preventing the development of long-term problems.[39]

Ovulatory bleeding occurs at regular intervals, and flow and/or duration are excessive. Duration is usually greater than 7 days.

TREATMENT OPTION: HMB/AUB-O

Management of abnormal bleeding can be either medical or surgical. Consideration for treatment of reproductive-age females with abnormal bleeding with a benign etiology should be based on the following factors:

- Etiology
- Severity of bleeding
  - Anemia
  - Interference with daily activities
- Associated symptoms and issues
  - Pelvic pain
  - Infertility
- Contraceptive needs and plans for future pregnancy
- Medical comorbidities
- Underlying risk for venous thromboembolic disease and/or arterial thrombotic events
- Patient preferences and access to the following:
  - Medical versus surgical
  - Short-term therapy versus long-term therapy[22]

> **! SAFETY ALERT**
>
> If malignancy is suspected, then immediate referral is needed.

There are a number of both medical and surgical treatment options available. This chapter will cover both hormone and non-hormone medical treatment. Hormone options include the following:

- Combined hormonal contraception (CHC)
- Levonorgestrel intrauterine system (LNG-IUS)
- Cyclic oral progestin

The comparative efficacies of different therapies for HMB/AUB have been evaluated. The most effective medical approach when compared in efficacy of endometrial ablation is the LNG-IUS. The use of the LNG-IUS reduces blood loss by 71% to 95%. Cyclical oral progestin treatment reduces bleeding by 87%, while estrogen-progestin contraceptive use results in a 20% to 69% reduction. Non-hormone options include the following:

- Nonsteroidal antiinflammatory drugs (NSAIDS)
- Antifibrinolytics (tranexamic acid)

In systematic reviews that included observational studies and randomized trials of females with HMB, use of tranexamic acid and NSAIDs reduced menstrual blood loss by 26% to 54% and 10% to 52%, respectively.[22,40-43] Table 16.5 provides a summary of the medical treatment for AUB. If the patient needs surgical intervention, she should be referred to a gynecologist.

POLYCYSTIC OVARIAN SYNDROME

PCOS is an important cause of menstrual irregularity and is the leading cause of AUB-O. It is the most common endocrinopathy among reproductive-age females in the United States. The prevalence of PCOS is between 6.5% and 8% of reproductive-age females. It should always be ruled out if the abnormal bleeding presents as missed or infrequent menses.[44,45] It is important to remember that PCOS is a syndrome that reflects multiple etiologies and has a variety of clinical presentations. Its key features are AUB caused by ovulatory dysfunction and hyperandrogenism. PCOS affects multiple systems and requires a comprehensive approach to both diagnosis and treatment. There are many complications associated with PCOS including diabetes, cardiovascular disease, and endometrial cancer.

The pathogenesis of PCOS is multifactorial and involves a complex alteration of the hormone balance in affected females (Fig. 16.5). PCOS is thought to be a complex genetic trait, similar to those that are associated with cardiovascular disease, type 2 diabetes mellitus, and metabolic syndrome. There are interactions between multiple genetic variants and environmental factors that foster its development. The inherited basis of PCOS was established by both studies performed with twins and reports showing an increased prevalence of PCOS in females with a first-degree relative affected by the disorder.[46-48]

PCOS is characterized clinically by AUB in the form of oligomenorrhea/amenorrhea and hyperandrogenism. Other risk factors associated with cardiovascular disease may also be present, such as obesity, glucose intolerance, dyslipidemia, fatty liver, and obstructive sleep apnea. Clinical features and complications include the following:

- Menstrual dysfunction
  - Delayed menarche
  - Oligomenorrhea (fewer than nine menstrual periods in 1 year)
  - Amenorrhea (no menstrual periods for 3 or more consecutive months)

TABLE 16.5 **Medical Management of Heavy Menstrual Bleeding/Abnormal Uterine Bleeding**

Treatment	Mechanism	Advantages	Disadvantages	Contraceptive Effect
Combined hormonal contraception (CHC; oral, transdermal, vaginal) Cyclic dosing Non-cyclic dosing	Suppresses the hypothalamic-pituitary-ovarian axis Endometrial atrophy	Reduces dysmenorrhea and premenstrual syndrome (PMS)	Breast tenderness, mood changes, breakthrough bleeding Rarely VTE, stroke, or myocardial infarction	Yes
Levonorgestrel intrauterine system (LNG-IUS) Can use up to 5 years with one device	Local suppression of proliferation of the endometrium and vascularity	Reduces dysmenorrhea 80% with amenorrhea after first year Does not require the patient to do anything daily	Irregular bleeding the first year, breast tenderness, acne	Yes
Cyclic progesterone Medroxyprogesterone acetate (MPA): 5–10 mg for 10–14 days Norethindrone (NET): 5 mg daily for 5–19 days	Suppresses endometrial proliferation	Effective as short-term therapy to reduce heavy bleeding	Not tolerated long term as well as LNG-IUS Caution in patients with hepatic dysfunction Weight gain, headaches	No
Antifibrinolytics Tranexamic acid: 3 tablets three times a day; begin the first day of menses, and continue for 5 days	Reversible blockage of plasminogen and inhibition of fibrinolysis	Reduce menstrual blood loss	Indigestion, diarrhea, headaches, leg cramps Use with caution in patients at risk for VTE and renal disease More expensive than other oral therapies	No
NSAIDS Naproxen 500 mg twice a day for 4–5 days Ibuprofen 600–1200 mg daily for 4–5 days Mefenamic acid 500 mg twice a day for 4–5 days	Reduce prostaglandin levels by inhibiting cyclooxygenase and decreasing the ratio of prostacyclin to thromboxane	Reduce overall pain	Indigestion, exacerbation of asthma, gastritis, increase risk of gastrointestinal bleeding	No

VTE, Venous thromboembolism.
Modified from Matthews ML, Abnormal uterine bleeding in reproductive-aged women. *Obstet Gynecol Clin North Am.* 2018;45(1):103–115; Committee on Practice Bulletins—Gynecology. Practice Bulletin No. 136: Management of abnormal uterine bleeding associated with ovulatory dysfunction. Obstet Gynecol. 2013;122:176. Reaffirmed 2018.; Association of Professors of Gynecology and Obstetrics [APGO] Educational Series on Women's Health Issues. *Clinical Management of Abnormal Uterine Bleeding.* Association of Professors of Gynecology and Obstetrics; 2006; Sweet MG, Schmidt TA, Weiss PM, Madsen KP. Evaluation and management of abnormal uterine bleeding in premenopausal women. *Am Fam Physician.* 2012;85(1):35–43; Matteson KA, Rahn DD, Wheeler TL 2nd, et al. Nonsurgical management of heavy menstrual bleeding: a systematic review. Obstet Gynecol. 2013;121:632–643; Kaunitz AM, Meredith S, Inki P, et al. Levonorgestrel-releasing intrauterine system and endometrial ablation in heavy menstrual bleeding: a systematic review and meta-analysis. Obstet Gynecol. 2009;113:1104–1116; Abu Hashim H, Alsherbini W, Bazeed M. Contraceptive vaginal ring treatment of heavy menstrual bleeding: a randomized controlled trial with norethisterone. Contraception. 2012;85:246–252; Singh S, Best C, Dunn S, Leyland N, Wolfman WL; Clinical Practice – Gynaecology Committee. Abnormal uterine bleeding in pre-menopausal women. *J Obstet Gynaecol Can.* 2013;35(5):473–475.

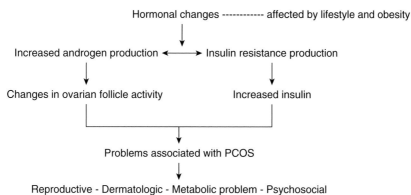

Figure 16.5 Pathology of polycystic ovarian syndrome *(PCOS).*

- Infertility
- Endometrial hyperplasia
- Endometrial cancer
- Hyperandrogenism
  - Acne
  - Hirsutism, thick, pigmented body hair in a male distribution
  - Male-pattern hair loss
  - Elevated serum androgen concentrations
- Polycystic ovaries seen on TVUS
- Metabolic issues/cardiovascular risks
  - 40% to 85% of females overweight or obese compared with age-matched controls
  - Insulin resistance
  - 30% of females with lean body type
  - 70% of females with overweight/obese body type
- Increased risk for type 2 diabetes
- Other
  - Nonalcoholic steatohepatitis
  - Sleep apnea
- Mood disorders
  - Depression
  - Anxiety
  - Impaired quality of life
  - Eating disorders/binge eating[44,49-53]

The diagnostic workup should begin with a thorough history and physical examination. The clinical presentation of PCOS is variable. Patients may be asymptomatic, or they may have multiple gynecologic, dermatologic, or metabolic manifestations. Clinicians should focus on the following:[44,53,54]

- Patient's menstrual history
- Fluctuations in the patient's weight and menses

- Cutaneous findings
  - Hair growth and distribution
  - Acne
  - Alopecia
  - Acanthosis nigricans: velvety, hyperpigmented plaques on the skin, usually occurring in the folds of the neck or axillae
  - Skin tags

A complete physical examination should be performed because of the metabolic effects of PCOS. Attention should be given to the inspection for signs of excessive androgens such as skin and hair abnormalities.

NOT TO BE MISSED

Once the diagnosis of PCOS is made, cardiometabolic risk assessment should include measurement of blood pressure and body mass index (BMI), fasting lipid profile, and glucose testing.

Patients suspected of having PCOS should be questioned regarding the presence of associated metabolic problems.[44] Many female patients with irregular menses and symptoms of androgen excess can be diagnosed based on the history and physical examination alone. Diagnostic workup usually includes an assessment of androgen levels as well as TVUS of the ovaries to assess for the typical cyst seen in most patients with PCOS. Total serum testosterone is a measure of androgen level that is usually used. Levels may vary by laboratory, so normal values may be different depending on the method used to evaluate.[55] PCOS is confirmed when other conditions that mimic PCOS are excluded. Other laboratory assessment may be needed to rule out other causes of the symptoms. Some tests to consider are as follows:[44]

- FSH/LH
- Thyroid testing
- Adrenal function studies

Although several groups have developed criteria for the diagnosis of PCOS, most expert groups use the Rotterdam criteria in the diagnosis of PCOS. The criteria are as follows:

- Oligo-ovulation and/or anovulation
- Clinical and/or biochemical signs of hyperandrogenism
- Polycystic ovaries (by ultrasound examination)

Two of the three criteria are required to make the diagnosis.[56-58] Table 16.6 provides a comparison of all current diagnosis methods used.[58-61]

Treatment goals for the management of PCOS relate to not only symptom relief but also prevention of long-term problems associated with the syndrome. Goals include the following:[56,57,62]

- Reduction of androgen levels and management of androgen excess symptoms
- Protection of the endometrium to prevent endometrial hyperplasia and cancer
- Management of underlying metabolic abnormalities and reduction of risk factors for type 2 diabetes and cardiovascular disease
- Contraception if the patient does not want to become pregnant. Females with oligomenorrhea ovulate intermittently, and unwanted pregnancy may occur.
- Ovulation induction for those pursuing pregnancy

As with all chronic diseases, treatment begins with lifestyle changes. Normalization of weight in the overweight patient can help reduce the insulin resistance. A low-glycemic/low-fat diet can help lower insulin resistance as well as lower blood pressure, triglycerides, and C-reactive protein.[63] Weight loss can result in a decrease in the androgen level as well as an increase in ovulatory function. As little as 5% to 10% reduced body mass has been shown to increase ovulation in females with PCOS.[64-66] Exercise not only increases weight loss but also improves insulin resistance, so it is an important part of any lifestyle recommendation.

NOT TO BE MISSED

Combined oral contraceptive pills remain the first-line treatment of hyperandrogenism in females who do not desire pregnancy.

There are several classes of drugs used to treat PCOS. The aim of drug therapy is to reduce both the symptoms and long-term problems by affecting the underlying pathophysiology. Table 16.7 provides a summary of the current recommended treatment for PCOS.[45,54,57,58,63,68] Patients who desire pregnancy should be referred to a reproductive endocrinologist for treatment.

AMENORRHEA

Amenorrhea (absence of menses) can be a transient, intermittent, or permanent condition resulting from dysfunction in the hypothalamus, pituitary, ovaries,

TABLE 16.6 **Criteria for Diagnosing Polycystic Ovarian Syndrome**		
NIH Consensus Criteria (1990)[60]	**Rotterdam Criteria (2003)[58,59]**	**AES Definition (2008)[61]**

Menstrual irregularity
  Oligomenorrhea
  Anovulation
Clinical and/or biochemical signs of hyperandrogenism
Exclusion of NCCAH and androgen-secreting tumors
All are required
	Oligomenorrhea and/or anovulation
	Clinical and/or biochemical signs of hyperandrogenism
	Polycystic ovaries seen on ultrasound examination (not a reliable discriminator in adolescents or patients within 8 years of menarche)
	Exclusion of other conditions that mimic PCOS
	Two out of three are required
		Clinical and/or biochemical signs of hyperandrogenism
		  Ovarian dysfunction
		  Oligomenorrhea
		  Anovulation
		  Polycystic ovaries seen on ultrasound examination
		Exclusion of other androgen excess or ovulatory disorders
		All are required

AES, Androgen Excess Society; *NCCAH,* non-classic congenital adrenal hyperplasia; *NIH,* National Institutes of Health; *PCOS,* polycystic ovarian syndrome.

TABLE 16.7 Pharmacological Management of Polycystic Ovarian Syndrome

Drug	Purpose	Mechanism of Action	Dosage	Common Side Effects
Combined hormonal contraception	Regulate menses Decrease androgens Protect the endometrium from unopposed estrogen stimulation	Suppress both luteinizing hormone and ovarian androgens Increase sex-hormone–binding globulin, which decreases free testosterone	One daily for 21/24 days, then 4–7 days hormone free	Breast tenderness Breakthrough bleeding Mood swings
Progestins (medroxy-progesterone)	Increase regularity Protect the endometrium from unopposed estrogen stimulation	Transform proliferative endometrium to secretory endometrium and cause withdrawal bleeding	5–10 mg orally for 10–14 days every 1–3 months	Breakthrough bleeding Mood swings
Biguanide (metformin)	Increases regularity Decreases androgens Lowers insulin levels	Decreases hepatic glucose levels, secondarily reducing insulin levels May have a direct effect on steroidogenesis	500 mg three times daily (1500 mg daily) and 850 mg twice daily (1700 mg daily)	Gastrointestinal problems Diarrhea Abdominal pain
Anti-androgen (spironolactone)	Decreases androgens	Inhibits androgen from binding to androgen receptor cells	25–200 mg a day	Hyperkalemia Headache Fatigue

uterus, or vagina. Amenorrhea can be classified in several ways. Physiological amenorrhea is considered normal, and although it is not considered a disease, it may require some health care intervention. Physiological amenorrhea is present three times in a females life: during pre-puberty, pregnancy, and menopause.

NOT TO BE MISSED

Pregnancy is the most common cause of secondary amenorrhea in reproductive-age females and should be excluded based on a sensitive pregnancy test.

Amenorrhea can also be considered pathological. Pathological amenorrhea can be either primary (absence of menarche by 15 years of age or thereafter) or secondary (absence of menses for more than 3 months in females with previous regular menstrual cycles or 6 months in females with irregular menses).[67,68] Secondary amenorrhea is present in 3% to 4% of reproductive-age females.[69] Approximately 0.3% of females experience primary amenorrhea[69] and should be referred to a gynecologist for a complete workup and management. This chapter will discuss the evaluation and management of secondary amenorrhea.

It is important to remember that a single missed menstrual period may not need to be worked up, but amenorrhea lasting 3 months or longer and oligomenorrhea (fewer than nine menstrual cycles per year or cycle length greater than 35 days) require investigation. The etiological and diagnostic considerations for oligomenorrhea are the same as for secondary amenorrhea.

The single leading cause of amenorrhea in reproductive-age females is pregnancy, and all sexually active females should have pregnancy ruled out as the initial part of any workup. Because no method of contraception is 100% effective, even current contraceptive users should have a pregnancy test performed. If pregnant, the management is discussion of options (see Chapter 10) and referral as desired by the patient.

When assessing for the etiology of secondary amenorrhea, it is important to look at the hypothalamic-pituitary-ovarian axis and rule out causes within each of these areas. Common causes are as follows:[68,70-75]

- Hypothalamic amenorrhea (associated with low estrogen and low FSH/LH)

- Hypothalamic hypogonadism
- Stress
- Eating disorder (anorexia nervosa)
- Athlete's amenorrhea
- Exercise
- Stress
- Diet
- Pituitary amenorrhea
  - Pituitary tumor (associated with low estrogen and FSH/LH)
  - Hyperprolactinemia (associated with high PRL and low estrogen FSH/LH)
  - Prolactinoma
  - Drugs (especially antipsychotics)
  - Primary hypothyroidism (also high TSH)
  - Sheehan syndrome (pituitary atrophy after postpartum hemorrhage)
- Ovarian amenorrhea (associated with low estrogen and high FSH/LH)
  - Gonadal dysgenesis
  - POI (premature ovarian failure)
  - PCOS (normal FSH, high LH, and possible high androgen levels; estrogen levels can be normal to high)
- Outflow tract (hormone levels are normal; may occur post–endometrial surgery)
  - Cervical stenosis
  - Asherman syndrome

Estimated frequencies of the different causes of secondary amenorrhea include the following:[68,76,77]

- Hypothalamic: 35% (almost all functional hypothalamic amenorrhea)
- Pituitary: 17% (13% hyperprolactinemia, 1.5% "empty sella," 1.5% Sheehan syndrome, 1% Cushing syndrome)
- Ovary: 40% (30% PCOS, 10% POI)
- Uterus: 7% (Asherman syndrome or intrauterine adhesions)
- Other: 1%
  - Cervical stenosis
  - Ovarian or adrenal tumors
  - Endocrine disorders such as thyroid problems

A pregnancy test is recommended as a first step in evaluating any patient with secondary amenorrhea. This can be performed before seeing the patient, and the results will guide the rest of the evaluation. If the patient is not pregnant, a complete history with a review of selected systems to assess risk factors and symptoms

that might suggest any of the major causes of secondary amenorrhea should be performed. The history should include the following questions:

- Has there been stress, change in weight, diet, or exercise habits, or is there an eating disorder or illness (suggests functional hypothalamic amenorrhea)?
- Is the patient taking any drugs that might cause or be associated with amenorrhea?
- Are there any signs of hyperandrogenism such as hirsutism, acne, or a history of irregular menses (suggests PCOS)?
- Are there symptoms of hypothalamic-pituitary disease, including headaches, visual field defects, fatigue, or polyuria and polydipsia (suggests a pituitary tumor)?
- Are there any symptoms of estrogen deficiency, including hot flashes, vaginal dryness, poor sleep, or decreased libido (suggests premature ovarian failure)?
- Has the patient had galactorrhea (suggests hyperprolactinemia)?
- Is there a history of obstetrical catastrophe, severe bleeding, dilatation and curettage, or endometritis or other infection that might have caused scarring of the endometrial lining (suggests Asherman syndrome)?

> **CLINICAL SURVIVAL TIP** A complete understanding of the menstrual cycle is necessary for the clinician to diagnose and manage secondary amenorrhea.

A complete menstrual history that includes the onset of breast development (thelarche), the appearance of pubic hair (pubarche), and the first menses (menarche) should be performed. Bleeding patterns now and in the past should be recorded, along with the number of periods in the past 12 months. In older patients, any signs or symptoms of menopause should be noted. Are there other symptoms associated with the menses that might suggest ovulatory cycles?

Once the history is complete, a physical examination should be performed. The physical examination is guided by the history and should include the following[56,68,70-73]:

- Height and weight
  - A BMI greater than 30 kg/m^2 is observed in 50% or more females with PCOS.
  - BMI less than 18.5 kg/m^2 may indicate functional hypothalamic amenorrhea caused by an eating

disorder, strenuous exercise, or a systemic illness associated with weight loss.

- Skin and hair inspection
  - Hirsutism, acne, striae, and acanthosis nigricans are signs of androgen excess and PCOS
  - Dry skin and hair can be a sign of thyroid disease
- Breasts
  - Evidence of galactorrhea can be a sign of pituitary problems
- Vulvovaginal examination
  - Signs of estrogen deficiency can be related to premature ovarian failure or physiological amenorrhea caused by natural menopause
- Head and neck
  - Parotid gland swelling and/or erosion of dental enamel would suggest an eating disorder
  - An enlarged thyroid gland suggests thyroid disease
- Other as indicated in history

After ruling out pregnancy, the initial laboratory evaluation for females with secondary amenorrhea should include the following:[77]

- FSH
  - POI
- Serum PRL
  - Hyperprolactinemia
- TSH
  - Thyroid disease
- Estradiol (E2)
  - Need to take into account that levels change across the menstrual cycle, so values vary.

Testing can be performed on any day of the cycle in the presence of prolonged amenorrhea, but if there has been a recent cycle, a test on days 2 to 4 would provide the best information. Follow-up testing should be based on initial results as well as the results of the history and physical examination.

Clinical evidence of hyperandrogenism (hirsutism, acne, alopecia) requires additional testing. Total testosterone should be measured as a part of the initial laboratory tests. Many clinicians also measure serum dehydroepiandrosterone sulfate (DHEAS) concentration as well as free testosterone. With hyperandrogenism, the likely cause of the secondary amenorrhea is PCOS.[61,62]

Further assessment of estrogen status may need to be performed to help with interpreting the FSH and E2 values. Estrogen status over time can be assessed with a progestin challenge test (PCT). This test involves giving medroxyprogesterone 10 mg for 10 days. Withdrawal bleeding confirms that there has been endogenous estrogen exposure without ovulation.[71]

Absence of bleeding can be caused by either hypoestrogenism or an outflow tract disorder. If there is an absence of bleeding, an estrogen/progestin withdrawal test can be performed. This test is performed by administering oral conjugated estrogens 0.625 mg/day or their equivalent (oral estradiol 1 mg/day, transdermal estradiol 0.05 mg) for 35 days and then adding a progestin (typically medroxyprogesterone 10 mg/day) from days 26 to 35. If no bleeding occurs in response to this test, the patient may have an outflow tract problem and must be referred for further diagnosis and treatment.

A measure of endometrial thickness on pelvic ultrasound examination (<4 mm is consistent with hypoestrogenism) can be performed, but it is not routinely performed as the PCT can provide the same information and is more cost-effective.[79,80] Figure 16.6 provides a stepwise method for the evaluation of secondary amenorrhea.

Management of secondary amenorrhea depends on the desires of the patient. Some general goals of treatment include the following:

- Correct the underlying pathology, if possible
- Help the patient achieve fertility, if desired
- Prevent complications of the disease process such as
  - Osteoporosis
  - Endometrial cancer
  - Androgen level problems

Hypothalamic amenorrhea can be caused by multiple factors. Treatment is dependent on cause. Lifestyle changes that emphasize adequate calorie intake and a balance of calories with exercise are important. Athlete's amenorrhea can cause problems for the female patient, therefore lifestyle modification is the first line of treatment. It is important to remember that many athletic females are reluctant to modify their behavior for fear of it affecting their athletic ability. These patients may need to be referred for more in-depth therapy. Cognitive behavioral therapy has been shown to be effective in restoring ovulation cycles in some females.[72]

Nonathletic females who are underweight or who appear to have nutritional deficiencies should have nutritional counseling. These patients are likely to have an eating disorder such as anorexia nervosa or bulimia and require a multidisciplinary team specializing in the

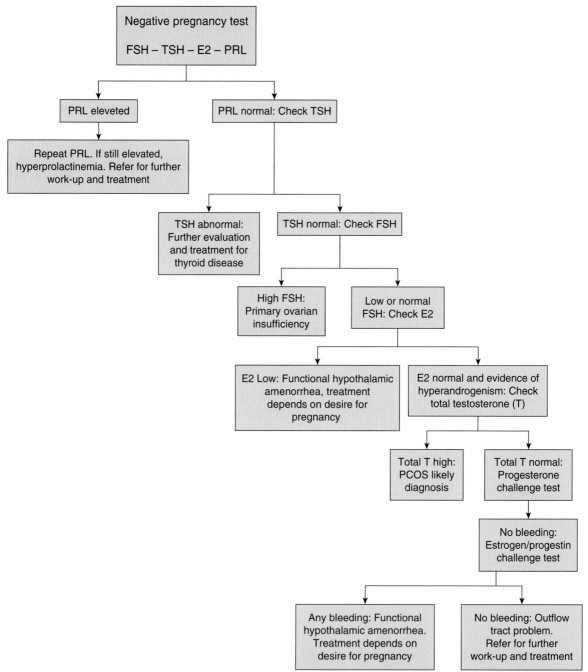

Figure 16.6 Interpretation of workup for amenorrhea for the non-pregnant female patient (Modified from McIver B, Romanski SA, Nippoldt TB. Evaluation and management of amenorrhea. *Mayo Clin Proc.* 1997;72[12]:1161–1169.)

assessment and treatment of eating disorders. Referral is needed for these patients. Stress can be a large factor in hypothalamic amenorrhea, therefore stress-reduction technique counseling is a critical part of treatment.[70]

If the amenorrhea is caused by hyperprolactinemia or thyroid disease, these causes should be managed appropriately. The patient should be referred for management if necessary. If amenorrhea is a result of drug use, the need for the drug should be evaluated in relationship to the problem of the amenorrhea. If the drug is necessary and the patient must be left on it, management should be related to the patient's desire for regular menses or pregnancy.

NOT TO BE MISSED

Females with secondary amenorrhea may ovulate sporadically and may still be at risk for pregnancy.

Patients with functional hypothalamic amenorrhea who are having intermittent ovulation should be managed according to their desire for pregnancy. If pregnancy is desired, the patient should be referred for treatment. Another key factor is whether the patient desires to have regular withdrawal bleeding. If regular bleeding is desired, there are three options available:
- CHC
- Hormone replacement therapy given cyclically
- Monthly progestin withdrawal

As the reproductive needs change, treatment may need to be changed to meet the patient's current desires.[72,77] Female patients with POI should receive estrogen therapy for prevention of bone loss. If the patient is having intermittent ovarian function and does not wish to become pregnant, combined oral contraceptives should be used. If no ovarian function is present, hormone replacement doses of estrogen and progestin are appropriate.[73]

PATIENT-CENTERED CARE: As age and reproductive desires change, management must be adjusted to meet these needs.

PCOS management is discussed earlier in the chapter. Patients desiring pregnancy should be referred for evaluation and management.

▐ KEY POINTS

- Understanding of the menstrual cycle is necessary to the diagnosis and management of female patients with menstrual disorders.
- The normal cycle is 21 to 35 days, with the luteal phase having less variation in length (12 to 14 days). The average menstrual flow lasts between 4 and 6 days.
- Treatment of AUB depends on the desire of the patient for future pregnancy. Medical options that treat the symptoms and preserve reproductive ability are needed.
- AUB is a common gynecological complaint. AUB can be caused by a wide variety of local and systemic diseases. The most common etiologies are conditions associated with pregnancy, structural uterine pathology (e.g., fibroids, endometrial polyps, adenomyosis), ovulatory dysfunction, bleeding disorders, or neoplasia.
- Age is a criterial factor when determining the management of female patients with AUB.
- Endometrial sampling should be performed in nonpregnant female patients with AUB and an increased risk of endometrial hyperplasia or cancer.
- Treatment should not be initiated until the etiology of AUB has been evaluated and premalignant or malignant disease excluded. Empiric treatment without evaluation may miss a primary etiology that must be corrected or mask symptoms of neoplastic disease.
- The goal of initial therapy is to control the bleeding, treat anemia (if present), and restore quality of life. Initial therapy is typically pharmacological.
- The initial treatment for female patients with AUB is CHC.
- Pregnancy is a common cause of secondary amenorrhea and should be excluded based on a sensitive pregnancy test (hCG).
- Initial laboratory testing for female patients with amenorrhea without hyperandrogenism should include serum PRL, FSH, and TSH to test for hyperprolactinemia, ovarian failure, and thyroid disease, respectively. If hyperandrogenism is present, then total testosterone should be performed to help confirm the diagnosis of PCOS.
- Combined estrogen-progestin oral contraceptives are the first-line pharmacological therapy for female patients with PCOS for the management of both hyperandrogenism and menstrual dysfunction and for providing contraception.

REFERENCES

1. Faucher M, Schuiling K. Normal and abnormal uterine bleeding. In: Schuiling KD, Likis FE, eds. *Women's Gynecologic Health.* Boston: Jones and Bartlett Publishers; 2013.
2. Fraser IS, Critchley HO, Munro MG, Broder M. Can we achieve international agreement on terminologies and definitions used to describe abnormalities of menstrual bleeding? *Hum Reprod.* 2007;22:635.
3. Fraser IS, Critchley HO, Munro MG, et al. A process designed to lead to international agreement on terminologies and definitions used to describe abnormalities of menstrual bleeding. *Fertil Steril.* 2007;87:466.
4. Singh S, Best C, Dunn S, et al. Abnormal uterine bleeding in premenopausal women. *J Obstet Gynaecol Can.* 2015;35(5):S5–S6.
5. American Academy of Pediatrics Committee on Adolescence; American College of Obstetricians and Gynecologists Committee on Adolescent Health Care, Diaz A, Laufer MR, Breech LL. Menstruation in girls and adolescents: using the menstrual cycle as a vital sign. *Pediatrics.* 2006;118(5):2245–2250.
6. Agency for Healthcare Research and Quality. *Primary Care Management of Abnormal Uterine Bleeding—Comparative Effectiveness Review Number 96.* AHRQ Publication No.13-EHC025-EF; 2013.
7. Fraser IS, Critchley HO, Broder M, Munro MG. The FIGO recommendations on terminologies and definitions for normal and abnormal uterine bleeding. *Semin Reprod Med.* 2011;29:383.
8. Munro MG, Critchley HO, Broder MS, et al. FIGO classification system (PALM-COEIN) for causes of abnormal uterine bleeding in nongravid women of reproductive age. *Int J Gynaecol Obstet.* 2011;113(1):3–13.
9. Warner PE, Critchley HD, Lunsden MA, et al. Menorrhagia I: measured blood loss, clinical features, and outcome in women with heavy periods: a survey with follow-up data. *Am J Obststet Gynecol.* 2004;190:1216.
10. Dasharathy SS, Mumford AZ, Pollack NJ, et al. Menstrual bleeding patterns among regularly menstruating women. *Am J Epidemiol.* 2012;175(6):536–545.
11. Tower AM, Frishman GN. Cesarean scar defects: an under-recognized cause of abnormal uterine bleeding and other gynecologic complications. *J Minim Invasive Gynecol.* 2013;20:562.
12. Kouides PA, Byams VR, Philipp CS, et al. Multisite management study of menorrhagia with abnormal laboratory haemostasis: a prospective crossover study of intranasal desmopressin and oral tranexamic acid. *Br J Haematol.* 2009;145:212.

13. Shaw JA. *Menorrhagia Clinical Presentation.* Updated December 20, 2018. https://emedicine.medscape.com/article/255540-clinical#b4.
14. Pinkerton JV. *Abnormal Uterine Bleeding due to Ovulatory Dysfunction (AUB-O).* Merck Manual; 2017. https://www.merckmanuals.com/professional/gynecology-and-obstetrics/menstrual-abnormalities/abnormal-uterine-bleeding-due-to-ovulatory-dysfunction-aub-o.
15. Matthews ML. Abnormal uterine bleeding in reproductive-aged women. *Obstet Gynecol Clin North Am.* 2018;45(1):103–115.
16. Kouides PA, Byams VR, Philipp CS, et al. Multisite management study of menorrhagia with abnormal laboratory haemostasis: a prospective crossover study of intranasal desmopressin and oral tranexamic acid. *Br J Haematol.* 2009;145:212.
17. Committee on Adolescent Health Care, Committee on Gynecologic Practice. Committee Opinion No. 580: von Willebrand disease in women. *Obstet Gynecol.* 2013;122:1368. Reaffirmed 2018.
18. Philipp CS, Faiz A, Dowling N, et al. Age and the prevalence of bleeding disorders in women with menorrhagia. *Obstet Gynecol.* 2005;105:61.
19. Risk factors for endometrial cancer. UpToDate; 2021. https://www.uptodate.com/contents/image/print?imageKey=OBGYN%2F62089.
20. Setiawan VW, Yang HP, Pike MC, et al. Type I and II endometrial cancers: have they different risk factors? *J Clin Oncol.* 2013;31:2607.
21. Committee on Practice Bulletins—Gynecology. Practice Bulletin No. 128: diagnosis of abnormal uterine bleeding in reproductive-aged women. *Obstet Gynecol.* 2012;120:197. Reaffirmed 2016.
22. Committee on Practice Bulletins—Gynecology. Practice Bulletin No. 136: management of abnormal uterine bleeding associated with ovulatory dysfunction. *Obstet Gynecol.* 2013;122:176. Reaffirmed 2018.
23. Reed SD, Newton KM, Clinton WL, et al. Incidence of endometrial hyperplasia. *Am J Obstet Gynecol.* 2009;200:678.e1.
24. Khan F, Jamaat S, Al-Jaroudi D. Saline infusion sonohysterography versus hysteroscopy for uterine cavity evaluation. *Ann Saudi Med.* 2011;31:387.
25. Lee SC, Kaunitz AM, Sanchez-Ramos L, Rhatigan RM. The oncogenic potential of endometrial polyps: a systematic review and meta-analysis. *Obstet Gynecol.* 2010;116:1197.
26. Preutthipan S, Herabutya Y. Hysteroscopic polypectomy in 240 premenopausal and postmenopausal women. *Fertil Steril.* 2005;83:705.
27. Nathani F, Clark TJ. Uterine polypectomy in the management of abnormal uterine bleeding: a systematic review. *J Minim Invasive Gynecol.* 2006;13:260.

28. Taran FA, Stewart EA, Brucker S. Adenomyosis: epidemiology, risk factors, clinical phenotype and surgical and interventional alternatives to hysterectomy. *Geburtshilfe Frauenheilkd*. 2013;73(9):924.

29. Baird DD, Dunson DB, Hill MC, et al. High cumulative incidence of uterine leiomyoma in black and white women: ultrasound evidence. *Am J Obstet Gynecol*. 2003;188:100.

30. Stewart EA. Clinical practice. Uterine fibroids. *N Engl J Med*. 2015;372:1646.

31. Committee on Practice Bulletins—Gynecology. Practice Bulletin No. 128. Diagnosis of abnormal uterine bleeding in reproductive-aged women. *Obstet Gynecol*. 2012;120:197. Reaffirmed 2016.

32. Wegienka G, Baird DD, Hertz-Picciotto I, et al. Self-reported heavy bleeding associated with uterine leiomyomata. *Obstet Gynecol*. 2003;101:431.

33. Dueholm M, Lundorf E, Hansen ES, et al. Accuracy of magnetic resonance imaging and transvaginal ultrasonography in the diagnosis, mapping, and measurement of uterine myomas. *Am J Obstet Gynecol*. 2002;186:409.

34. De La Cruz MS, Buchanana EM. Uterine fibroids: diagnosis and treatment. *Am Fam Physician*. 2017;95(2):100–107.

35. American College of Obstetricians and Gynecologists' Committee on Practice Bulletins—Gynecology. Management of Symptomatic Uterine Leiomyomas: ACOG Practice Bulletin, Number 228. *Obstet Gynecol*. 2021;137(6):e100–e115.

36. Stewart EA. Uterine fibroids. *Lancet*. 2001;357(9252):293–298.

37. Mas A, Tarazona M, Carrasco JD, Estaca G, Cristobal I, Monleon J. Updated approaches for the management of uterine fibroids. *Int J Womens Health*. 2017;9:607–617.

38. Association of Professors of Gynecology and Obstetrics [APGO]. Educational Series on Women's Health Issues. *Clinical Management of Abnormal Uterine Bleeding*. Association of Professors of Gynecology and Obstetrics; 2006.

39. Sweet MG, Schmidt TA, Weiss PM, Madsen KP. Evaluation and management of abnormal uterine bleeding in premenopausal women. *Am Fam Physician*. 2012;85(1):35–43.

40. Matteson KA, Rahn DD, Wheeler 2nd TL, et al. Non-surgical management of heavy menstrual bleeding: a systematic review. *Obstet Gynecol*. 2013;121:632–643.

41. Kaunitz AM, Meredith S, Inki P, et al. Levonorgestrel-releasing intrauterine system and endometrial ablation in heavy menstrual bleeding: a systematic review and meta-analysis. *Obstet Gynecol*. 2009;113:1104–1116.

42. Abu Hashim H, Alsherbini W, Bazeed M. Contraceptive vaginal ring treatment of heavy menstrual bleeding: a randomized controlled trial with norethisterone. *Contraception*. 2012;85:246–252.

43. Singh S, Best C, Dunn S, Leyland N, Wolfman WL, Clinical Practice – Gynaecology Committee. Abnormal uterine bleeding in pre-menopausal women. *J Obstet Gynaecol Can*. 2013;35(5):473–475.

44. Williams T, Mortada R, Porter S. Diagnosis and treatment of polycystic ovary syndrome. *Am Fam Physician*. 2016;94(2):106–113.

45. Azziz R, Woods KS, Reyna R, et al. The prevalence and features of the polycystic ovary syndrome in an unselected population. *J Clin Endocrinol Metab*. 2004;89:2745–2759.

46. Vink JM, Sadrzadeh S, Lambalk CB, Boomsma DI. Heritability of polycystic ovary syndrome in a Dutch twin-family study. *J Clin Endocrinol Metab*. 2006;91:2100–2004.

47. Legro RS, Driscoll D, Strauss 3rd JF, et al. Evidence for a genetic basis for hyperandrogenemia in polycystic ovary syndrome. *Proc Natl Acad Sci U S A*. 1998;95:14956–14960.

48. Kahsar-Miller MD, Nixon C, Boots LR, et al. Prevalence of polycystic ovary syndrome (PCOS) in first-degree relatives of patients with PCOS. *Fertil Steril*. 2001;75:53–58.

49. Randeva HS, Tan BK, Weickert MO, et al. Cardiometabolic aspects of the polycystic ovary syndrome. *Endocr Rev*. 2012;33:812–814.

50. Ecklund LC. Endocrine and Reproductive effects of polycycstic ovarian syndrome. *Obstet Gynecol Clin North Am*. 2014;42(1):55–65.

51. Setji TL, Holland ND, Sanders LL, et al. Nonalcoholic steatohepatitis and nonalcoholic fatty liver disease in young women with polycystic ovary syndrome. *J Clin Endocrinol Metab*. 2006;91(5):1741–1747.

52. Vgontzas AN, Legro RS, Bixler EO, et al. Polycystic ovary syndrome is associated with obstructive sleep apnea and daytime sleepiness: role of insulin resistance. *J Clin Endocrinol Metab*. 2001;86(2):517–520.

53. Kavitha A, Veena KS, Sirisha K, et al. A short review on polycycstic ovary syndrome. *Innovare J Med Sci*. 2016;4(2):6–10.

54. Mani H, Davies MJ, Bodicoat DH, et al. Clinical characteristics of polycystic ovary syndrome: investigating differences in white and South Asian women. *Clin Endocrinol (Oxf)*. 2015;83(4):542–549.

55. Pinola P, Piltonen TT, Puurunen J, et al. Androgen profile through life in women with polycystic ovary syndrome: a Nordic Multicenter Collaboration Study. *J Clin Endocrinol Metab*. 2015;100:3400–3407.

56. Legro RS, Arslanian SA, Ehrmann DA, et al. Diagnosis and treatment of polycystic ovary syndrome: an Endocrine Society clinical practice guideline. *J Clin Endocrinol Metab*. 2013;98:4565–4592.

57. Teede HJ, Misso ML, Costello MF, et al. Recommendations from the international evidence-based guideline for the assessment and management of polycystic ovary syndrome. *Fertil Steril*. 2018;110:364–379.

58. Rotterdam ESHRE/ASRM-Sponsored PCOS consensus workshop group. Revised 2003 consensus on diagnostic criteria and long-term health risks related to polycystic ovary syndrome (PCOS). *Hum Reprod.* 2004;19:41–47.

59. Neven ACH, Laven J, Teede HJ, Boyle JA. A summary on polycystic ovary syndrome: diagnostic criteria, prevalence, clinical manifestations, and management according to the latest international guidelines. *Seminars Reprod Med.* 2018;36(1):5–12.

60. Zawadski JK, Dunaif A. Diagnostic criteria for polycystic ovary syndrome: Towards a rational approach. In: Givens JR, Haseltine FP, Merriam GE, Dunaif A, eds. *Polycystic Ovary Syndrome (Current Issues in Endocrinology and Metabolism).* Boston: Blackwell Scientific Inc; 1992:377.

61. Azziz R, Carmina E, Dewailly D, et al. The Androgen Excess and PCOS Society criteria for the polycystic ovary syndrome: the complete task force report. *Fertil Steril.* 2009;91:456.

62. American College of Obstetricians and Gynecologists' Committee on Practice Bulletins—Gynecology. ACOG Practice Bulletin No. 194: Polycystic Ovary Syndrome. *Obstet Gynecol.* 2018;131(6):e157–e171.

63. Pereira MA, Swaidslun J, Goldfine AB, Rifai N, Ludwig DS. Effects of a low-glycemic load diet on resting energy expenditure and heart disease risk factors during weight loss. *JAMA.* 2004;292(20):2482–2490.

64. Pasquali R, Antenucci D, Casimirri F, et al. Clinical and hormonal characteristics of obese amenorrheic hyperandrogenic women before and after weight loss. *J Clin Endocrinol Metab.* 1989;68:173–179.

65. Kiddy DS, Hamilton-Fairley D, Bush A, et al. Improvement in endocrine and ovarian function during dietary treatment of obese women with polycystic ovary syndrome. *Clin Endocrinol (Oxf).* 1992;36:105–107.

66. Huber-Buchholz MM, Carey DG, Norman RJ. Restoration of reproductive potential by lifestyle modification in obese polycystic ovary syndrome: role of insulin sensitivity and luteinizing hormone. *J Clin Endocrinol Metab.* 1999;84:1470–1474.

67. Deligeoroglou E, Athanasopoulos N, Tsimaris P, et al. Evaluation and management of adolescent amenorrhea. *Ann N Y Acad Sci.* 2010;1205:23–32.

68. Practice Committee of the American Society of Reproductive Medicine. Current evaluation of amenorrhea. *Fertil Steril.* 2006;86:S148–S155.

69. Vickers H, Gray T, Jha S. Amenorrhoea. *InnovAiT.* 2018;11(2):80–88.

70. Gordon CM, Ackerman KE, Berga SL, et al. Functional hypothalamic amenorrhea: an Endocrine Society Clinical Practice Guideline. *J Clin Endocrinol Metab.* 2017;102(5):1413–1439.

71. Klein DA, Poth MA. Amenorrhea: an approach to diagnosis and management. *Am Fam Physician.* 2013;87(11):781–788.

72. Committee on Adolescent Health Care. Committee Opinion No. 702: Female Athlete Triad. *Obstet Gynecol.* 2017;129(6):e160–e167.

73. Welt CK. Primary ovarian insufficiency: a more accurate term for premature ovarian failure. *Clin Endocrinol (Oxf).* 2008;68(4):499–509.

74. Frellick M. Endocrine Society Issues Hypothalamic Amenorrhea Guideline. *Medscape Medical News.* 2017;30. http://www.medscape.com/viewarticle/877950.

75. Shrivastava Priyanka S, Anubha V, Kumar SR. Secondary Amenorrhea: Causes, Management and Outcome Using Algorithmic Approach. *IOSR-JDMS.* 2017;16(5):87–91.

76. Reindollar RH, Novak M, Tho SP, McDonough PG. Adult-onset amenorrhea: a study of 262 patients. *Am J Obstet Gynecol.* 1986;155:531–543.

77. Laufer MR, Floor AE, Parsons KE, et al. Hormone testing in women with adult-onset amenorrhea. *Gynecol Obstet Invest.* 1995;40:200–203.

78. Nakamura S, Douchi T, Oki T, et al. Relationship between sonographic endometrial thickness and progestin-induced withdrawal bleeding. *Obstet Gynecol.* 1996;87:722–725.

79. Rebar RW, Connolly HV. Clinical features of young women with hypergonadotropic amenorrhea. *Fertil Steril.* 1990;53:804–810.

17

Vulvar Dermatology and Conditions of the Vulva

Susan E. Hoffstetter

OBJECTIVES:

Vulvar dermatoses:
- Obtain a vulvar history, and perform a vulvar examination.
- Develop a plan to diagnose common vulvar disorders: lichen simplex chronicus (LSC), lichen sclerosus (LS), and lichen planus (LP).
- Explain the role of vulvar biopsy in diagnosis.
- Formulate a plan for the initial treatment strategies for vulvar dermatoses, including when to refer.

- Integrate diagnosis, management, therapies, treatments, and evaluation of vulvar dermatoses into practice.

Vulvodynia:
- Differentiate generalized and localized vulvodynia.
- Describe risk factors and comorbidities of vulvodynia.
- Formulate a multiple level of treatment for vulvodynia, including self-management, pharmacological therapies, and nonpharmacological options, and integrate it into practice as necessary.

INTRODUCTION

The vulva, inclusive of the labia majora, minora, clitoris with hood, perineal body, and vestibule, is often overlooked by clinicians during routine pelvic examinations. Inspection and assessment of normal structures, skin pigmentation, and normal variants of the vulvar structures and pigmentation are critical to enhance the clinician's skill in the identification of abnormalities. Patient-reported symptoms should be validated and given consideration in a comprehensive differential diagnosis list.

This chapter is divided into two sections. The first section includes the fundamentals of obtaining a complete vulvar history, information on how to perform a comprehensive examination, and a review of three common vulvar dermatoses: LSC, LS, and LP.

Later in the chapter, the difficult clinical problem of vulvodynia will be discussed. Vulvodynia has been described since the 1880s as an "excessive sensibility of the nerves supplying the mucous membranes of the vulva"[1] or "super-sensitivities" of the vulva.[2] It was described as

burning vulvar syndrome by the International Society for the Study of Vulvovaginal Disease (ISSVD) in 1975. A variety of terms have been used to label vulvar pain, including *essential vulvodynia, dysesthetic vulvodynia, vulvar vestibulitis syndrome, vulvar dysesthesia, provoked vulvar dysesthesia,* or *spontaneous vulvar dysesthesia.* The ISSVD established the classification of *generalized vulvodynia* or *localized vulvodynia* and then subdivided each type into *provoked, unprovoked,* or *mixed.*[3] The term *vestibulitis* has been discarded.[4]

FOCUSED HISTORY

In obtaining a vulvar history, the patient's health literacy level must be taken into consideration. It would be helpful to simplify medical terminology and use language that the patient can understand. Misinformation and self-diagnosis are a source of concern and fear for many female patients and their partners. During history taking, it is critical to listen to patients closely and address their concerns directly. Take care not to formulate a diagnosis or plan of care prematurely.

For the clinician, a vulvar history may be challenging to obtain. Female patients are often unfamiliar with names of body parts, have not visualized the vulvar tissues, or have limitations in visualization as a result of body habitus. It may be helpful to use a vulvar image to educate and identify location of symptom(s), lesions, or area/s of concern (Fig. 17.1). Female patients often present with photos on their digital devices, which is helpful when symptoms, lesions, or areas of concern are intermittent or resolution has occurred before the office visit.

A comprehensive history of patients with any type of vulvar concern should include sexual function, physical or sexual violence/abuse or a previous history of violence/abuse, and psychiatric diagnosis such as anxiety, depression, and obsessive compulsive disorder. Life changes, stressors, hormonal changes (childbirth, lactation, and menopause), and caregiver status are noteworthy. Comorbid conditions that may increase the risk for some types of vulvar diseases include fibromyalgia, irritable bowel syndrome, interstitial cystitis, and Hashimoto thyroiditis. It is important to assess for correlation of onset of symptomatology with new or changing medical or psychological issues.

> **NOT TO BE MISSED**
>
> A comprehensive history of patients with any type of vulvar concern should include sexual function, physical or sexual violence/abuse or a previous history of violence/abuse, and psychiatric diagnosis such as anxiety, depression, and obsessive-compulsive disorder.

> **CLINICAL SURVIVAL TIP:** Comorbid conditions that can increase the risk for some types of vulvar diseases include fibromyalgia, irritable bowel syndrome, interstitial cystitis, and Hashimoto's thyroiditis.

Symptoms

Common vulvar symptoms include itching, burning, pain, lesions, bumps, or ulcerations. Listen for the words used to describe symptoms, such as *tingling, itchy, burning, pins-and-needles sensation, on fire, cut glass,* or *razorblade sensation.* To the trained clinician, the patient will inform you of the diagnosis by a description of symptoms. It is critical to assess if the presenting symptom(s) is new, intermittent, cyclic, or long-standing and if the areas involved are focused in one area or generalized.

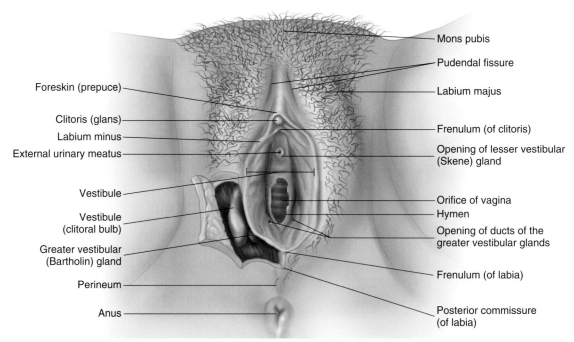

Figure 17.1 External female genitalia (vulva). (From Patton KT, Thibodeau GA. *The Human Body in Health and Disease.* 6th ed. St. Louis, Mosby; 2014.)

Using a Likert 10-point rating scale (0 = absence of symptom to 10 = highest level of symptom), have the patient rate the level of symptom or discomfort. It is helpful to establish a baseline number score to evaluate improvement over time.

> **CLINICAL SURVIVAL TIP:** Many of the symptoms of vulvar disease are similar, so be sure to listen to how the patient describes the symptoms.

It is worthwhile to attempt to identify the patient's aggravating and alleviating factors for the symptom(s). Common aggravating factors can include scented detergents, soaps, over-the-counter feminine hygiene products, clothing, exercise, sitting, and sexual activity. Sometimes cyclic triggers occur with menses or aggravating factors from previous therapies or medications. Stress can be an aggravating factor for some female patients related to employment, family trauma, and monetary distress. Ask if the patient awakens from sleep with symptoms. If the patient has an intimate or sexual partner, ask if the partner has symptoms or contributes to the onset of symptoms. The identification of aggravating factors is critical to optimize the condition of the vulvar tissues. Alleviating factors can include bathing, medications, and use of over-the-counter products.

PHYSICAL EXAMINATION

Evaluate the vulva in a systematic manner. Look for differences in pigmentation. Note skin texture and changes to the normal vulvar structures. Be cautious not to misinterpret the pigmentation changes of vitiligo with other white/leukoplakia dystrophies. There are usually no symptoms with vitiligo, and there is no change in skin texture or loss of structures.

Next, consider infection or inflammatory conditions. If lesions are present, classify them as an *ulcer, blister, or papule.* Note if the surface or contour of the lesion is flat or raised or if there are changes to the normal architecture of the vulva. Note if there is any type of exudate or crusting from the lesion or in the affected area. Attempt to establish the length of time the lesion has been present and if the area is changing or increasing in the area. Consider the pigmentation of the lesion: skin-colored, erythematous, leukoplakia, or dark to black. If you are

suspicious that the lesion is a melanoma, referral to dermatology is advised. Determine if other symptom(s) such as itching, pain, and burning are present. Evaluate the quality and texture of the skin: smooth, rough, thinning, parchment like, or presence of fissures, cuts, or skin tears. Be careful not to misinterpret normal physiological changes or normal variants with abnormal changes. In postmenopausal patients, be sure to recognize the physiological changes of menopause including dry and thinning tissues, loss of adipose tissues in the mons and labia, and pale pigmentation of the vestibular tissues. Figure 17.2 demonstrates typical atrophic changes to the vulva caused by menopause. It is helpful for the clinician to instruct the patient on performing a vulvar self-examination while performing a careful inspection and assessment. The use of a handheld mirror is essential to patient instruction.

> **CLINICAL SURVIVAL TIP:** Be careful not to misinterpret normal physiological changes or normal variants with abnormal changes. In postmenopausal patients, be sure to recognize the physiological changes of menopause including dry and thinning tissues, loss of adipose tissues in the mons and labia, and pale pigmentation of the vestibular tissues.

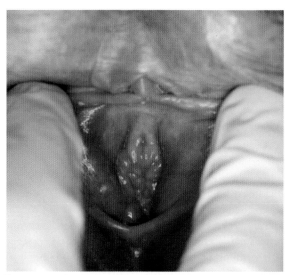

Figure 17.2 Severe atrophy of the vulvar vestibule with subsequent prominent urethral meatus. (From Goldstein AT, King MA. Ospemifene may not treat vulvar atrophy: a report of two cases. *Sex Med.* 2016;4[3]:e217–e220.)

The vulva should be inspected for any lesions or abnormalities suggestive of a premalignant or malignant condition. If any abnormal or suspicious areas are identified, a biopsy (see Clinical Survival Tip) is indicated. A vulvar colposcopy has limited value and risks symptom flare as a result of the caustic effect of acetic acid.[5] A referral to a vulvar specialist or gynecological oncologist should be considered if biopsy results warrant or the expected response to prescribed therapies does not occur.

CLINICAL SURVIVAL TIP
- Informed consent is required.
- A punch biopsy is a clean procedure, not a sterile procedure.
- A punch biopsy will leave a scar.
- Look for the greatest area of change; obtain the whole lesion if possible.
- Samples obtained from the edge, the thickest portion, or the area with the most irregular color change will yield the best pathology results.
- Stabilize the skin with the thumb and forefinger; stretch slightly perpendicular to the skin tension lines.
- Hold the punch perpendicular to the skin, and rotate it into the skin with firm, constant pressure.
- Avoid a back-and-forth twisting motion.
- Do not remove the punch to check your progress as this would result in a ragged wound and a shredded biopsy sample.
- When the punch reaches the subcutaneous fat, there is a less resistance.
- Remove the punch, and apply downward finger pressure at the sides of the wound to pop up the core.
- Grasp the specimen with forceps, and cut it off at the base.

A vaginal examination including a wet prep and yeast culture should be performed. If microscopy is not an option, the clinician can use the Affirm probe (Becton Dickinson Microbiology Systems, Sparks, MD), a rapid test for detection of the nucleic acid (RNA) of *Candida albicans*, *Trichomonas vaginalis*, and *Gardnerella vaginalis* (as a marker for bacterial vaginosis).

It is important to rule out infectious or inflammatory diseases such as candidiasis, recurrent vaginitis, herpes simplex virus, or a desquamative inflammatory vaginitis. Normal findings such as atrophy should be considered in lactating and postmenopausal populations.

A speculum examination is not always required, as a Q-tip inserted vaginally is adequate to collect a specimen for wet-mount analysis. A yeast culture is the gold standard for identification of yeast and offers species identification with drug sensitivities to guide treatment for persistent infections.[6] The yeast culture can be obtained from areas on the labia, on the vestibule, and from the vaginal canal. Any abnormal conditions identified should be treated.

CLINICAL SURVIVAL TIP: Be sure and rule out infections and inflammation of the vagina when patients present with vulvar symptoms.

VULVAR DERMATOSES

Lichen Simplex Chronicus

LSC is a common vulvar disease. It accounts for approximately 35% of female patients in vulvar specialty clinics.[12] It is characterized by epithelial thickening and hyperkeratosis created by a persistent rubbing and scratching (the *chronic itch-scratch cycle*). Patients will scratch because scratching feels good! Over time, the skin becomes thickened with accentuations of normal skin markings (lichenification). These skin changes are seen mainly on the labia majora but can be found on the hood of the clitoris, interlabial sulci, outer aspect of the labia minora, and perianal tissues.[7]

The gross appearance of the involved tissues are elevated and ill-defined. Accentuations of normal skin markings (lichenification) occur. Hypopigmentation or hyperpigmentation will occur, and the skin can appear dusky red with slight hyperkeratosis to grayish white. The skin is thickened with increased hyperkeratosis, fissures and excoriations, and hair loss caused by scratching (Fig. 17.3).[7]

Symptoms, which can last for years, include itching and scratching. Heat, sweat, rubbing from tight clothes, persistent pad use, and contact irritants including fragrant soaps, laundry products, and topical products play a role in the persistence of symptoms. LSC can also develop secondary to other conditions such as candidiasis, psoriasis, LS, lichen planus, or neoplasia. Patients with a history of allergies, eczema, hay fever or asthma can be more susceptible to LSC.[7]

Diagnosis can be made by clinical assessment and vulvar biopsy. Treatment of LSC includes the use of

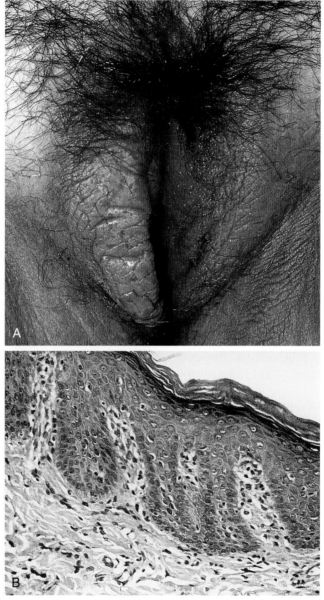

Figure 17.3 A. Lichen simplex chronicus manifesting in the right labium majus. There is thickening and accentuation of skin markings, with surface excoriation caused by recent scratching. B. Histopathology: pronounced acanthosis, orthokeratosis, hypergranulosis, papillary dermal fibrosis and perivascular chronic inflammation (From Stevens A, Dalziel KL. Vulvar dermatoses. In: Robboy SJ, Anderson MC, Russell P, eds. *Pathology of the Female Reproductive Tract*. Edinburgh: Churchill Livingstone; 2002.)

medium- to low-level corticosteroid ointment. The goal of the topical corticosteroid is to stop the itching and scratching to allow the skin to heal. Topical steroid use twice daily until the itching stops followed with a slow taper normally leads to resolution of LSC. Gentle care of the vulvar skin using baking soda soaks, a skin protectant, and a skin emollient are helpful for symptom relief. For some patients, hydroxyzine at bedtime can be beneficial to alleviate the itching, which can disrupt sleep. Treatment of contributing factors, such as infections (e.g., candidiasis) and the elimination of contact irritants, are critical to successful treatment outcomes.[7]

Lichen Sclerosus

LS is a chronic lymphocytic-mediated inflammatory mucocutaneous disease. The etiology of LS is unknown but is considered multifactorial. There is a genetic link for LS with a familial occurrence in 22% of cases.[8] Auto-antibodies in the basement membrane occur in 44% to 74% of females, which is supportive of an autoimmune etiology.[9] The prevalence of LS is 1:70 to 1:1000.[10] Approximately 15% of LS cases occur in prepubescent females. In postmenopausal females, the incidence of LS is 1:30.[11] Twenty percent of female patients with LS will have another auto-immune disease such as thyroid (most common) vitiligo, systemic lupus erythematosus, alopecia, or rheumatoid arthritis.[12]

LS can occur on any part of the body; 80% of females with LS of the skin will have genital involvement. With LS, there is a 4% risk of developing vulvar squamous cell carcinoma.[13] LS can be patchy or generalized on the vulva, clitoris/periclitoral area, perineal body, or gluteal cleft, but it does *not* involve the vagina. The most common symptom of vulvar LS is pruritus, which can be severe for 30% to 50% of patients.[14] Other symptoms include burning pain/soreness, dyspareunia, and external dysuria. Interestingly, some patients are asymptomatic.

Gross appearance of the involved vulvar tissues includes a markedly thin epidermis with a layer of hyperkeratosis. Classic lesions have ivory white skin and "cigarette paper," parchment-or cellophane-like tissues that extend around the vulvar to anal region in a figure-of-eight or keyhole configuration. The skin can have excoriations, erosions, thickening, or scarring (Fig. 17.4). Pigmentation changes range from a white/leukoplakia, silvery hue to erythematous. Phimosis or burying of the clitoris can occur. The obliteration of labia minora and periclitoral structures will occur over time; it is possible to lose all normal vulvar structures if treatment is inadequate or nonexistent. Introital stenosis may occur, preventing coital activity.

A diagnosis by punch biopsy is advised to obtain histological confirmation (Fig. 17.5). Punch biopsies should be taken in areas that are thickened, ulcerated, indurated, or fissured with the greatest change in color or texture. Biopsies can differentiate benign versus neoplastic lesions to diagnose or confirm an abnormality and to help focus treatment.

Treatment of vulvar LS is twofold and consists of symptomatic relief and slowing of disease progression

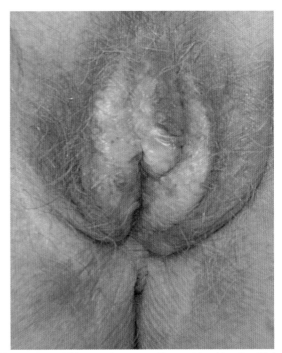

Figure 17.4 Lichen sclerosus. (From *Hutchison's Clinical Methods: An Integrated Approach to Clinical Practice.* 25th ed. Elsevier; 2023.)

with prevention of scarring, prevention of loss of structure, and early recognition of squamous cell carcinoma. Topical corticosteroids are the mainstay of treatment and are effective in reducing symptoms and improving histopathological findings. Testosterone in petrolatum is no longer used, as it is ineffective and has many side effects. Topical estrogen is not a treatment for LS.[14] Most published data on treatment consist of the use of ultra-high-potency corticosteroids such as clobetasol propionate 0.05%. For initial treatment of LS, the ultra-high-potency corticosteroids reduce patient symptoms quickly and effectively, and they stop disease progression. However, long-term management of LS can be maintained with lower-potency topical corticosteroids. Medium-potency triamcinolone 0.1% ointment for long-term management was shown to be effective with satisfactory patient symptom control/relief, no increase in vulvar cancer occurrence, and no increase in disease progression.[15] Vulvar skin care guidelines are an essential component of a successful treatment plan. These include removing all contact irritants and using baking soda soaks, emollients (e.g., natural vegetable-based oils), olive oil, and

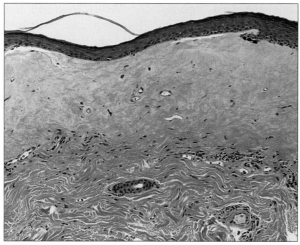

Figure 17.5 Histology of lichen sclerosus. Homogenized papillary dermis with lymphocytic infiltrate beneath the zone is a classic finding. A flattened dermal-epidermal junction is also seen. (From Bolognia JL, Jorizzo JL, Rapini RP, Schaffer JV. *Dermatology*. Mosby Elsevier; 2008.)

skin protectants (e.g., A&D ointment or petroleum jelly). Caution reproductive-age patients regarding the potential degradation of latex condoms from petroleum jelly.

SAFETY ALERT

Caution reproductive-age patients regarding the potential degradation of latex condoms from petroleum jelly.

SAFETY ALERT

- Use warm water to wash the vulva. Dry thoroughly with a clean towel. (If the vulva is very irritated, you can try drying it with a blow dryer set on cool.)
- The vagina cleanses itself naturally in the form of normal, vaginal discharge. Avoid using douches unless prescribed by your provider. These products can upset the natural balance of organisms.
- Wear cotton underwear, especially if prone to vulvar irritation.
- Use a mild soap for cleansing.
- Avoid the use of tampons for prolonged periods because of the risk for toxic shock syndrome.
- Avoid feminine hygiene products, which can irritate the vulva; these include sanitary pads, feminine sprays and deodorants, scented oils, bubble baths, bath oils, talc, and powder.

Lichen Planus

LP is a papulo-squamous disease of the skin and mucous membranes. It is an erosive or desquamative disease that is a chronic, destructive, and debilitating condition.[16] LP can occur on the vulva or in the vagina, mouth, or esophagus. Prevalence rates of vulvovaginal LP are unknown, but it is estimated to affect 0.5% to 2% of the population. The prevalence of oral LP in females is 1%, and 60% to 70% of these females will develop vulvar LP. Approximately 70% of females with vulvar LP have vaginal involvement. The highest incidence of occurrence is between 50 and 60 years of age. A 3% to 5% risk of vulvar squamous cell carcinoma exists for females with LP.[17]

The etiology of LP is considered to be a T-cell–mediated cutaneous hypersensitivity reaction in the skin and mucous membranes. It is an auto-immune disorder with antibodies found in the basement membrane in 61% of affected females and circulating antibodies found in 41% of affected females. There is a genetic *HLA DQB1 0201* allele found with LP. Other considerations in the development of LP are from environmental chemicals, drugs, and a history of hepatitis C virus.[17]

Symptoms of LP include soreness, pruritus, "raw" sensations, burning pain that can be severe, dyspareunia, and vaginal bleeding. Patients can experience external dysuria as the urine burns the raw tissues. Some patients will have a malodorous, mucopurulent vaginal discharge that is composed of a large component of white blood cells in an alkaline vaginal pH. Theories directly link this discharge to LP or to an inflammatory vaginitis with an autoimmune component.[17]

The diagnosis of LP can be made if the classic finding of Wickham striae is present. Wickham striae appear as a fine, subtle white interlacing papule made of gray-white, lacy strands of hyperkeratosis. In cases of severe disease, there is erosion in the vestibule surrounded by white epithelium (Fig. 17.6). A biopsy with immunofluorescence can be helpful, but results can be nonspecific, therefore clinical correlation is critical.

Vaginal involvement is associated with denuding of vaginal epithelium. The vaginal mucosa is sharply demarcated with erythematous patches and associated exudates. Distinct erythematous patches from the introitus to the apex of the vaginal fornices can occur, and some patients will have involvement of the portico of the cervix. Stenosis and synechiae can cause obliteration of the vaginal canal precluding sexual function.

Vulvar treatment includes a combination of vulvar skin care guidelines and topical corticosteroids. Medium-potency topical corticosteroid ointments can be applied to vulvar and vestibular areas. Depending on the level of disease and symptomatology, a burst of oral prednisone 20 up to 60 mg/day for 2 to 6 weeks can be given. In more advanced or symptomatic patients, tacrolimus 0.1% ointment (a macrolide immune system modulator) can be considered.[17]

Vaginal treatment includes the use of 25-mg hydrocortisone suppositories. The use of vaginal dilators should be considered to help restore and/or maintain vaginal patency and allow for continued sexual function. The level of disease within the vagina, patient choice, and motivation are important factors to consider in managing vaginal LP. If the oral mucosa is involved, referral to a dental/oral surgeon is suggested. Triamcinolone acetonide paste can be prescribed.[17]

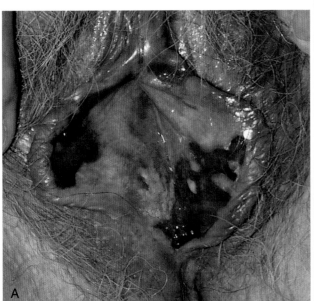 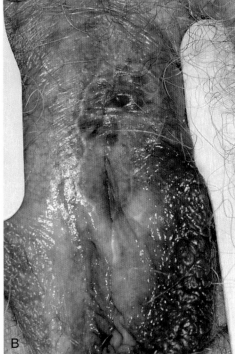

Figure 17.6 Lichen planus. **A,** Eroded ulcers in the vulva. **B,** Lacy reticulated pattern of lichen planus with periclitoral scarring in a 71-year-old female patient who has had oral lichen planus for 10 to 15 years, cutaneous lichen planus of the arms and legs for 18 months, and bouts of erosive vaginal lichen planus with scarring and partial vaginal stenosis. (From Fisher BK, Margesson LJ. *Genital Skin Disorders: Diagnosis and Treatment.* St. Louis: Mosby; 1998.)

> **CLINICAL SURVIVAL TIP:** If the oral mucosa exhibits the presence of LP, referral to a dental/oral surgeon is suggested.

Vulvar Cancer

In the United States, vulvar cancer accounts for about 4% of cancers of the female reproductive organs and 0.6% of all cancers in females. Less than 20% of vulvar cancers occur in females younger than 50 years of age, and greater than 50% occur in females older than 70 years of age.[13] The majority of females with vulvar cancer have a keratinizing squamous cell carcinoma that is not related to human papillomavirus (HPV) and normally found in older females. Paget disease is a rare adenocarcinoma found mainly in females 70 years of age and older. There is an increased risk of vulvar cancer with conditions such as LS, LP, chronic inflammatory skin conditions, and high-risk HPV infection.

Symptoms of vulvar cancer include a visible lesion, mass, or ulceration. Tenderness, itching, burning, or pigmentation changes can occur. Some patients will be asymptomatic in the early stages of vulvar cancer. A physical examination is imperative to visualize any abnormal lesion, mass, or areas of pigmentation change. Diagnosis is made by vulvar biopsy; 90% of vulvar cancers are squamous cell carcinoma[72] (Fig. 17.7). Treatment is managed by oncologists who specialize in gynecological cancers. If a melanoma is suspected, then referral to dermatology is advised.

VULVODYNIA

Vulvodynia is chronic vulvar discomfort or pain lasting 3 months or longer. It causes significant physical and psychological distress affecting quality of life for patients and their partners. Vulvodynia is characterized by burning, stinging, irritation, or rawness of the female genitalia in which there is no infection, skin disease, or neoplasia of the vulva or vagina and no specific clinically identifiable neurological disorder as the etiology of these symptoms.[4] A diagnosis of vulvodynia is made by exclusion. A study by Sadownik[18] found that presenting symptoms included dyspareunia (71%), history of recurrent yeast infection (64%), vulvar burning (57%), vulvar itching (46%), and problems with sexual response (33%).[19]

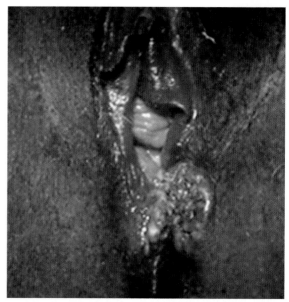

Figure 17.7 Vulvar cancer. (From Cecil RL, Goldman L, Schafer AI. *Goldman's Cecil Medicine*. Elsevier Saunders; 2012.)

NOT TO BE MISSED

Vulvodynia is a chronic pain condition that affect the patient's quality of life.

The classification of vulvodynia is based on the site of the pain, whether it is localized or generalized, and whether the pain is provoked, unprovoked, or mixed.[20] *Provoked* refers to any touch or stimulation that elicits pain (sexual or nonsexual). *Unprovoked* refers to pain that occurs in the absence of touch or stimulation, and *mixed* refers to pain that varies with or without touch or stimulation. Localized and generalized vulvodynia can be provoked, unprovoked, or mixed.

Localized vulvodynia or vestibulodynia is pain that is caused by touching a localized area of the vulva, commonly occurring in the region of the vestibular glands. It can also occur at the clitoris, clitorodynia, or on one side of the vulva (hemi-vulvodynia). The pain has been described as *burning, stinging, tearing, throbbing, razor blades* or *cut glass*. Patients with localized vulvodynia have dyspareunia or avoid sex because of the pain at the introitus. The pain can last for hours to days after sexual touch, intercourse, or attempts at intercourse. Inserting or wearing tampons can be painful. Patients may not be able to engage in routine exercise or activities such as riding a bicycle or wearing tight clothing or jeans because of pain. Patients can be relatively pain free if the painful areas are not touched. Localized vulvodynia is further subdivided into *primary vestibular* pain during the first attempt at vaginal penetration versus *secondary vestibular* pain after a period of normal function. A recent study showed that primary and secondary vulvodynia had different histological features, indicating that they may be different entities.[21]

> **PATIENT-CENTERED CARE:** There is no way to describe the pain caused by vulvodynia. The pain has been described as *burning, stinging, tearing, throbbing, razor blades,* or *cut glass.*

Generalized vulvodynia is pain and burning on or around the vulva including the mons pubis, labia majora, labia minora, vestibule, and perineum. Patients with generalized vulvodynia describe burning, stinging, rawness, or aching in the vulva. The pain may be constant or intermittent. It may range from mild discomfort to severe pain that can prevent daily activities. Symptoms may be diffuse or in different areas at different times. Patients may have good days and bad days. The area hurts most of the time, even when nothing is touching it. Sitting may be uncomfortable. Some patients report increased vaginal discharge with the pain. Urination may contribute to the pain and burning. Sexual touch or intercourse is possible at times for some patients.

Prevalence and Risk Factors

Vulvodynia affects females of all age groups from adolescence through menopause.[22] The prevalence of vulvodynia is about 8.3% to 16% of females in the United States.[19,23] A National Institutes of Health study estimates that 13 million females may suffer from symptoms at some point in their lifetime[19] and that 6% have symptoms before 25 years of age.[22] These prevalence rates are believed to be greatly underreported because of the absence of visible abnormalities of the vulva. Forty percent of symptomatic females remain undiagnosed.[20]

Risk factors for the development of vulvodynia include repeated urogenital infections (i.e., bacterial vaginosis, candidiasis, condyloma, trichomoniasis, and urinary tract infections). Multiple infections compound the risk of vulvodynia, with an odds ratio (OR) >8 with three or more infections reported in the 12 months before the onset of vulvodynia.[24] A review by Goldstein found that females who take oral contraceptive pills (OCPs) have an increased risk of developing vestibulodynia; furthermore, those taking OCPs containing 20 mcg of ethinyl estradiol were more likely to develop vestibulodynia than those taking OCPs containing higher doses of ethinyl estradiol.[25]

Etiology

The etiology of vulvodynia is unknown. Theories suggest a multifactorial etiology including embryonic derivation,[26,27] chronic inflammation,[28] genetic immune factors,[29,30] nerve pathways,[31-34] abnormal response to environmental factors (e.g., infection, irritants, or trauma), hormonal changes,[35] HPV, or oxalates.[36,37] The pathophysiology suggests that vulvodynia is a chronic disorder of the nerves that supply the vulva. The painful tissue has been shown to have nerve fiber proliferation or neural hyperplasia.[31,32,33] Chronic inflammation, such as contact irritants, recurrent vulvovaginal infections, hormonal changes, and chronic skin conditions, acts as a trigger. Normal sensations are perceived as abnormal, which results in heightened sensitivity.

Comorbidities With Psychological Diagnosis and Chronic Pain Conditions

A relationship has been shown between comorbid pain conditions. In a study by Reed et al., approximately 1940 females were screened for interstitial cystitis, irritable bowel syndrome, fibromyalgia, and vulvodynia.[38] Prevalence ranged from 7.5% to 11.8%. However, 27% screened positive for multiple conditions. The presence of vulvodynia was significantly associated with other pain syndromes (p-value <.001; OR 2.3 to 3.3). Other associated conditions include recurrent yeast infections and chronic fatigue syndrome.[39,40]

The chronic nature of vulvodynia can negatively affect the patient's self-image and lead to psychological disorders such as depression and anxiety. Vulvodynia is not considered a psychopathological condition.[22,41] However, in a study by Tribo et al.,[42] more than 50% of females report depression and/or anxiety as a presenting symptom. Further studies have shown that the odds of having vulvodynia are four times more likely in females with an antecedent mood or anxiety disorder. Vulvodynia has also been associated with new or recurrent mood and anxiety disorders, with an OR of 1.7.[43]

Females with vulvodynia may also experience significant sexual, psychological, and relationship problems. Many may benefit from psychological support, sex therapy, and/or counseling. The cycle of pain caused by vulvodynia may ultimately lead to avoidance of all sexual activities: fear of pain and anticipation of pain during sexual intercourse, partial avoidance of sexual intimacy and activity, sexual arousal disorder, loss of libido, problems with orgasm/anorgasmic disorders, phobic avoidance of sexual activities, and subsequent relationship difficulties.

Evaluation and Physical Examination

The evaluation of the patient with vulvodynia should include a comprehensive medical history noting any association of life changes, stressors, new medical conditions, childbirth and lactation, menopausal status, surgeries, and previous failed therapies with the onset of symptoms or the association of symptom flares. Identification of possible contact irritants by patient recall includes all products that come in contact with the vulvar skin. The identification is critical to optimize the condition of the vulvar tissues. Common irritants include scented detergents, soaps, and over-the-counter feminine hygiene products.

Q-tip testing should be used to identify areas on the vulva or areas in which the patient is symptomatic (Fig. 17.8). The Q-tip should touch lightly and in a consistent pattern starting with the outer thighs, mons, labia majora, inner labial folds, labia minora, posterior fourchette, vestibule, and in the region of the peri-urethral and Bartholin glands. For the vestibule, the left and right sides should be examined separately rather than trying to spread the labia and examine both sides at once. Instruct the patient to classify areas as painless or as mild, moderate, or severe pain, or have the patient apply a number value based on a Likert 10-point pain scale (0 = no pain to 10 = most severe level of pain). A diagnosis of localized vulvodynia can be made if the patient experiences discrete areas of pain, and a diagnosis of generalized vulvodynia can be made if the patient experiences pain in a broad area. If no pain, tenderness, or burning is elicited with Q-tip testing, vulvodynia would not be considered in a differential diagnosis for patient symptoms.[20]

NOT TO BE MISSED

To identify specific symptomatic areas on the vulva, perform the Q-tip test. The Q-tip should touch lightly and in a consistent pattern starting with the outer thighs, mons, labia majora, inner labial folds, labia minora, posterior fourchette, vestibule, and in the region of the peri-urethral and Bartholin glands. There is no way to describe the pain caused by vulvodynia. The pain has been described as *burning, stinging, tearing, throbbing, razor blades* or *cut glass.*

Treatment
Management Goals

Vulvodynia is a chronic pain condition that presents management challenges for both the clinician and patient. Symptom resolution is not often a realistic outcome. The primary goals of treatment are symptom reduction, improvement in quality of life, some level of sexual function, and return to activities of daily living. Patient understanding and acceptance of treatment goals is critical. Treatments can be a slow and frustrating. Just as there is no single identified etiology for vulvodynia, there is no single treatment that is effective for symptom relief for all patients.

In 2016, the American College of Obstetrician and Gynecologists published Committee Opinion Number 673 on persistent vulvar pain, which stated a few important points to remember when treating patients with vulvodynia.[45]

- Persistent vulvar pain is a complex disorder that frequently is frustrating to the patient and clinician.

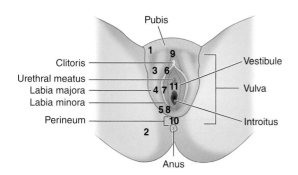

Figure 17.8 Q-tip test for vulvodynia. Perform a check clockwise: 1 to 2 inner thigh, 3 to 5 labia majora, 6 to 8 interlabial sulcus, 9 clitoris and hood, 10 perineum, and 11 vestibule. (Redrawn from Shah M, Hoffstetter S. Vulvodynia. *Obstet Gynecol Clin North Am.* 2014;41[3]:453–464.)

It can be difficult to treat, and rapid resolution is unusual.

- Vulvar pain can be caused by a specific disorder, or it can be idiopathic. Idiopathic vulvar pain is called *vulvodynia*.
- Optimal treatment remains unclear. An individualized multidisciplinary approach to address all physical and emotional aspects should be considered. It is important to begin any treatment approach with a detailed discussion, including an explanation of the diagnosis and determination of realistic treatment goals.

Initial treatment steps must include self-management strategies to maximize tissue quality and eliminate possible contributing factors for vulvar pain. The addition of pharmacological agents, as tolerated in increasing dosages and combinations, are needed to maximize the response. Nonpharmacological approaches are equally important to offer holistic care to these patients.

Self-Management Strategies

Education regarding the implementation of strict vulvar care/hygiene is essential to eliminate the possibility of contact irritants as an etiology or a trigger for vulvar symptoms. Adherence to vulvar hygiene has been shown to be an effective initial strategy to reduce vulvar complaints of burning, itching, pain, and dyspareunia. Dyes, perfumes, or enzymes in any product that comes in contact with the vulvar tissues should be considered a source of irritation. This includes laundry detergents, fabric softeners, body soaps, feminine hygiene products, non-cotton underwear, and over-the-counter vaginal products.[46]

To reduce symptoms, bathing the vulva in a mild baking soda solution can be soothing. This is a simple treatment that patients can use to attenuate their symptoms that does not require the use of medications. Lukewarm water is recommended, as hot water can exacerbate vulvar symptoms. Caution should be exercised if using the bathtub for the sitz bath, as residue from cleaning products can serve as a contact irritant. Ice packs applied for 2 to 3 minutes at a time can offer relief and can be applied to the vulva for short periods without harm.[20] To improve the quality of the vulvar skin, vegetable oil or olive oil may be used to serve as an emollient. These oils may be used liberally and may be effective in providing comfort and reduce symptoms. A&D ointment or Vaseline can serve as a barrier to

protect the skin and can be applied one to two times daily as desired.

Pharmacological Strategies

In selecting a vehicle for delivery of topical medications, ointments provide a better mode of delivery than creams. Ointments have a lower risk of causing a symptom flare compared with creams. Creams contain more preservatives and stabilizers, which can act as a contact irritant and cause burning on application.[20]

> **CLINICAL SURVIVAL TIP:** Ointments are preferred over creams as a vehicle for delivery of topical medications because creams contain more preservatives and stabilizers, which can act as a contact irritant and cause burning on application.

Topical Medications

Local anesthetics such as lidocaine ointment can provide temporary relief from the pain to enable intercourse if applied topically to painful areas of contact, normally at the introitus, a few minutes before coitus. In 2003, Zolnoun advised overnight use of topical lidocaine to allow for healing, and a significant decrease in pain with sexual activity was found.[47] Benzocaine is not advised as it can produce contact irritation and risk a flareup of symptoms.[20] The use of topical antidepressants such as doxepin 5% cream, gabapentin 2% to 6%, or amitriptyline 2% mixed with baclofen 2% in a water-washable base can be applied by fingertip to the affected areas.[71]

Pain Medications

Narcotic pain medications should be used with caution in patients with vulvodynia, as they do not effectively treat the pain of vulvodynia and have a high risk of addiction. Tramadol and hydrocodone/acetaminophen combinations have been used as a short-term therapy for vulvodynia flares.

Pain Modulators

The use of neuropathic pain modulators including tricyclic antidepressants (e.g., amitriptyline or desipramine) can help decrease neuropathic chronic pain by a central action that alters the transmission of pain impulses to the brain through the dorsal horn.[50] In a small study funded by the National Institute of Child Health and Human Development (NICHD), amitriptyline with or without topical triamcinolone was no more effective than self-management approaches in managing vulvar pain.[51] A randomized, controlled trial of oral desipramine and topical lidocaine alone or in combination was not superior to placebo.[52] Other antidepressants, such as duloxetine and venlafaxine, have also been used, but there are little data to support their use. Research is evaluating the use of gabapentin, a drug that helps control epileptic seizures, for patients with provoked vestibulodynia in a randomized, controlled trial.[53]

The newest anticonvulsant utilized for chronic pain is pregabalin. A small retrospective chart review showed improvement in symptoms.[54] There is a small open-label trial with lamotrigine that has shown a decrease in pain at 8 weeks.[55] Topiramate has also been used, but little supportive data are available. Hydroxyzine and cetirizine have been used to reduce pruritus. For some patients, combinations of the neuropathic pain medications (i.e., amitriptyline, gabapentin, and pregabalin) can also be used, as they have different mechanisms of action. Neuropathic pain medications should not be discontinued suddenly; dosages should be weaned before discontinuation (Table 17.1).

TABLE 17.1   Pharmacological Strategies

TOPICAL PREPARATIONS			
Drug Name	**Directions for Use/Dosing**	**Side Effects**	**Purpose or Data to Support Use**
Lidocaine 5% ointment	Apply as needed in a small amount. Systemic absorption is possible with frequent or excessive use.	Erythema	Temporary relief before coitus (short-term use only).[70]
Doxepin	In a water-soluble base		Data supporting treatment are limited.[71]
Gabapentin	In a water- soluble base		Data supporting treatment are limited.[71]
Amitriptyline 2% with baclofen 2%	In a water-soluble base. Apply 1–3 times a day.	Irritation, erythema, rash	Topical has fewer side effects than systemic.[70]
ORAL NEUROPATHIC PAIN MODULATORS			
Antidepressants Amitriptyline	10 mg at bedtime; increase by 10 mg every 3–4 weeks. Maximum dose 150 mg a day.	Drowsiness, dizziness, dry mouth, constipation, weight gain, urinary retention, tachycardia, blurred vision, confusion	Not widely used because of side effects.[70]
Desipramine	Same dosing as amitriptyline	Drowsiness, dizziness, blurred vision, dry mouth, constipation, tachycardia, urinary retention, diaphoresis, weakness, nervousness, rash, seizures, tinnitus, anxiety, confusion	No difference between desipramine and placebo in a large National Institutes of Health trial.[70]

Continued

TABLE 17.1	**Pharmacological Strategies—cont'd**			
ORAL NEUROPATHIC PAIN MODULATORS				
	Duloxetine	Start with 20 mg a day and increase to 60 mg daily for symptom control		Off-label use to treat chronic pain. Effectiveness not tested in studies.[70]
	Venlafaxine	Start with a 37.5-mg dose. Maximum dose 150 mg a day.	Headache, nausea, somnolence, weight loss, anorexia, constipation, anxiety, vision changes, diarrhea, dizziness, dry mouth, insomnia, weakness, sweating, hypertension	Off-label use to treat chronic pain. Effectiveness not tested in studies.[70]
Anticonvulsants	Gabapentin	Start with 100–300 mg at bedtime, and advance as tolerated in divided doses twice a day to three times a day. Common doses range from 300–1800 mg. Maximum dose 3600 mg.	Dizziness, somnolence, ataxia, fatigue, nystagmus, tremor, diplopia, rhinitis, blurred vision, nausea, vomiting, nervousness, dysarthria, weight gain	No more effective than placebo in one controlled study.[70]
	Pregabalin	Start with 50–75 mg a day. Common dose range is 75–150 mg (in one or two 75-mg doses). Maximum dose 600 mg a day.		Used in neuropathic pain.[71]
Other Agents				
	Topamax	Use only if above therapies are not successful. Start at 25 mg once a day to twice a day. Maximum dose is 200 mg twice a day.	Dose related. Fatigue, paresthesia, tremor, asthenia, confusion, dizziness, diplopia, difficult concentration, memory problems, nervousness	Little data to support use.
	Lamictal			One clinical trial to support its use after above therapies unsuccessful.
	Hydroxyzine	25 mg at bedtime as needed to reduce pruritus		For pruritus only.
	Zyrtec	10 mg once a day to reduce pruritus		For pruritus only.

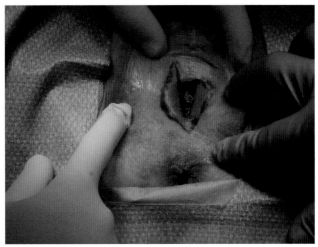

Figure 17.9 Outline of surgical excision area to treat vulvodynia. (From Shah M, Hoffstetter S. Vulvodynia. *Obstet Gynecol Clin North Am.* 2014;41[3]:453–464.)

Nonpharmacological Strategies

Nonpharmacological strategies can be used as an adjunct to any of the above therapies. Psychological treatment can provide techniques for relaxation or coping with pain or an opportunity to explore other conditions that may relate to the pain.[20] Couples therapy and sexual therapy are additional options that may benefit both the patient and partner. A randomized, controlled trial found that females who had cognitive behavioral therapy reported a 30% decrease in vulvar pain that occurs with intercourse.[56]

There has been limited research on hypnotherapy for vulvodynia.[57] A case report showed resolution of localized vulvodynia after 12 psychotherapy sessions, 8 of which included hypnosis. Some small pilot studies have shown that acupuncture treatment for localized vulvodynia was well tolerated, and quality-of-life measurements were higher after completing treatment and at 3-month follow-up.[58-60] Association of oxalates and vulvar pain has been theorized. High levels of oxalate in the urine can be reduced with diet and calcium citrate. It is a treatment recommended with little evidence to support its use or effectiveness.[61]

Surgery

Vestibulectomy, surgical excision of the vulvar vestibule, is an option taken cautiously for patients with localized vulvodynia after failure of other attempted therapies. Success rates vary from 60% to 85% at short-term follow-up.[62-64] The area of excision is outlined in Figure 17.9.

VAGINISMUS

Vaginismus, involuntary spasm of the pelvic floor muscles, is a common secondary finding with vulvodynia. Evaluation and management is necessary to improve patient outcomes.[66] To assess for vaginismus, using one digit, palpate the muscular attachments along the pubic arch and the insertion of the levator ani and coccygeus muscles. Palpate the levator muscles at the 4 o'clock and 8 o'clock positions to determine if it reproduces any discomfort or tenderness. If pressure elicits tenderness or pain and/or muscles are in a state of contracture, a diagnosis of vaginismus is made. Referral to a pelvic floor physical therapist is beneficial once the vestibular pain scores are improved.

Nonpharmacological Strategies

Nonpharmacological treatment for vaginismus includes physical therapy with pelvic floor exercises and biofeedback. The patient's control of specific body responses enables relaxation of pelvic muscles, which may result in subsequent pain reduction. Clinical experience has found increased success with physical therapy when Q-tip pain scores are decreased at initiation of therapy.

Physical therapists must be specifically trained in pelvic floor and biofeedback for optimum results. Use of transcutaneous electrical nerve stimulation is an emerging treatment.[45] Success rates of 60% to 80 % have been reported with pelvic floor–trained physical therapists.[67]

Vaginal dilators can be helpful to overcome the tension in the pelvic floor muscles and are available in varying sizes. Patients can use the dilator before attempts with intercourse to accommodate penetration when symptoms allow a return to sexual activity. Hypnosis has been tried with some limited success.[57]

Pharmacological Strategies

Pharmacological treatments include vaginal valium inserted at bedtime and topical baclofen. Research studies are ongoing with Botox injections.[68,69]

█ SUMMARY

Vulvar symptoms are similar in vulvar conditions. The use of vulvar biopsy is an important tool for an accurate diagnosis. If possible, biopsy should be sent to a gynecological pathologist. If there is a poor response to therapy, a repeat biopsy is advised.

The standard treatment for vulvar dystrophies includes vulvar skin care guidelines with the removal of all contact irritants in conjunction with topical corticosteroids. Consider medium-potency corticosteroid ointments to achieve treatment goals and symptom control, and use ultra-high-potency corticosteroids if necessary. Ointments are more easily tolerated compared with creams on sensitive vulvar skin.

Vulvodynia causes significant physical and psychological distress and affects quality of life in female patients and their families. Patients with vulvodynia often seek care from several providers in an attempt to find resolution of their symptoms; 60% of patients consulted three or more physicians in seeking a diagnosis, and 40% remain undiagnosed.[18] Spontaneous remission has occurred in some patients, but the majority of patients have had multiple attempts with medical management without 100% resolution of symptoms. Referral to clinics specializing in vaginal and vulvar disease should be encouraged to optimize management strategies and maximize the quality of life for these patients and their partners. Concurrent emotional and psychological support may be invaluable.

█ KEY POINTS

- Patients can have more than one type of vulvar skin condition: LS, LSC, and/or LP.
- Refer the patient if there is no improvement in the disease or symptoms.
- Consider vulvar psoriasis as a diagnosis with erythematous tissue.
- Vitiligo does not cause anatomical change, therefore it should not be confused with LS.
- Paget disease is a rare adenocarcinoma that is found mainly in females >70 years of age.

- Older female patients should have a vulvar examination as the risk for abnormal findings increases with age.
- It is important to focus on successful management of symptoms rather than a cure.
- Patient education is essential in facilitating shared decision making between the patient and health care provider.

REFERENCES

1. Thomas TG. *Practical Treatise on the Diseases of Women.* Philadelphia: Henry C. Leason; 1880:145.
2. Skene AJC. Diseases of the external organs of generation. In: *Treatise on the Diseases of Women.* New York: D. Appleton & Co.; 1888:77–99.
3. Moyal-Barracco M, Lynch PJ. 2003 ISSVD terminology and classification of vulvodynia: a historical perspective. *J Reprod Med.* 2004;49(10):772–777.
4. Haefner HK. Report of the international society for the study of vulvovaginal disease terminology and classification of vulvodynia. *J Low Genit Tract Dis.* 2007;11(1): 48–49.

5. Balgia BS, ed. *Principles & Practice of Colposcopy*. New Dehli: JP Medical Publishers; 2011:195–206.
6. Geiger AM, Foxman B, Sobel J. Chronic vulvovaginal candidiasis: characteristics of women with candida albicans, candida glabrata and no candida. *Genitourinary Med*. 1995;71(5):304–307.
7. Margesson L, Haefner H. *Vulvovaginal Disorders: Lichen Simplex Chronicus*. International Society for the Study of Vulvovaginal Disease Publication; 2015.
8. Higgins CA, Cruickshank ME. A population-based case-control study of aetiological factors associated with vulval lichen sclerosus. *J Obstet Gynaecol*. 2012;32(3):271–275.
9. Chi CC, Kirtschig G, Baldo M, Lewis F, Wang SH, Wojnarowska F. Systematic review and meta-analysis of randomized controlled trials on topical interventions for genital lichen sclerosus. *J Am Acad Dermatol*. 2012;67(2):305–312.
10. Eva LJ. Screening and follow up of vulval skin disorders. *Best Pract Res Clin Obstet Gynaecol*. 2012;26(2):175–188.
11. Jones RW, Scurry J, Neill S, MacLean. Guidelines for the follow-up of women with vulvar lichen sclerosus in specialist clinics. *Am J Obstet Gynecol*. 2008;198(5):496.
12. Thorstensen KA, Birenbaum DL. Recognition and management of vulvar dermatologic conditions: lichen sclerosus, lichen planus, and lichen simplex chronicus. *J Midwifery Wom Health*. 2012;57(3):260–275.
13. American Cancer Society. Key Statistics for Vulvar Cancer. https://www.cancer.org/cancer/vulvar-cancer/about/key-statistics.html#:~:text=Key%20Statistics%20for%20Vulvar%20Cancer%20In%20the%20United,vulvar%20cancer%20at%20some%20point%20during%20their%20life.
14. Margesson L. *Vulvovaginal Disorders: Lichen Sclerosus*. International Society for the Study of Vulvovaginal Disease Publication; 2015.
15. Lefevre C, Hoffstetter S, Meyer S, Gavard J. Management of lichen sclerosus with triamcinolone ointment: effectiveness in reduction of patient symptom scores. *J Low Genit Tract Dis*. 2011;15(3):205–209.
16. McPherson T, Cooper S. Vulval lichen sclerosus and lichen planus. *Dermatol Ther*. 2010;23(5):523–532.
17. Margesson L. *Vulvovaginal Disorders: Lichen Planus*. International Society for the Study of Vulvovaginal Disease Publication; 2015.
18. Sadownik LA. Clinical profile of vulvodynia patients. A prospective study of 300 patients. *J Reprod Med*. 2000;45:679–684.
19. Harlow BL, Stewart EG. A population-based assessment of chronic unexplained vulvar pain: have we underestimated the prevalence of vulvodynia? *J Am Med Women's Assoc*. 2003;58:82–88.
20. Haefner HK, Collins ME, Davis GD, et al. The vulvodynia guideline. *J Low Genit Tract Dis*. 2005;9:40–51.
21. LeClair C, Goetsch M, Korcheva V, et al. Differences in primary compared with secondary vestibulodynia by immunohistochemistry. *Obstet Gynecol*. 2011;117(6):1307–1313.
22. Metts JF. Vulvodynia and vulvar vestibulitis: challenges in diagnosis and management. *Am Fam Physician*. 1999;59(6):1547–1562.
23. Reed BD, Harlow SD, Sen A, et al. Prevalence and demographic characteristics of vulvodynia in a population-based sample. *Am J Obstet Gynecol*. 2012;206(2):170. e1–170.e1709.
24. Nguyen RH, Swanson D, Harlow BL. Urogenital infections in relation to the occurrence of vulvodynia. *J Reprod Med*. 2009;54(6):385–392.
25. Goldstein A, Krapf J, Belkin Z. *Do Oral Contraceptives Pills Cause Vulvodynia? Time to Finally End the Controversy*. International Pelvic Pain Society; 2014.
26. McCormack WM. Two urogenital sinus syndromes. Interstitial cystitis and focal vulvitis. *J Reprod Med*. 1990;35(9):873–876.
27. Fitzpatrick CC, DeLancey JO, Elkins TE, McGuire EJ. Vulvar vestibulitis and interstitial cystitis; a disorder of urogenital sinus-derived epithelium. *Obset Gynecol*. 1993;81(5 Pt 2):860–862.
28. Sloan S, Reynold L, Gall S, et al. Chronic inflammation in vestibular tissue is normal. *Int J Gynecol Pathol*. 1999;18:360–366.
29. Goetsch MF. Vulvar vestibulitis: prevalence and historic features in a general gynecologic practice population. *Am J Obstet Gynecol*. 1991;164(6 Pt 1):1609–1614. discussion 1614–1616.
30. Foster DC, Piekarz KH, Murant TI, et al. Enhanced synthesis of pro inflammatory cytokines by vulvar vestibular fibroblasts: implications for vulvar vestibulitis. *Am J Obstet Gynecol*. 2007;196(4):346e1–346e8.
31. Bohm-Starke N, Hilliges M, Falconer C, Rylander E. Increased intraepithelial innervation in women with vulvar vestibulitis syndrome. *Gynecol Obstet Invest*. 1998;46(4):256–260.
32. Tympanidis P, Terenghi G, Dowd P. Increased innervation of the vulvar vestibule in patients with vulvodynia. *Br J Dermatol*. 2003;148(5):1021–1027.
33. Weström LV, Willén R. Vestibular nerve fiber proliferation in vulvar vestibulitis syndrome. *Obstet Gynecol*. 1998;91(4):572–576.
34. Krantz KE. Innervation of the human vulva and vagina. *Obstet Gynecol*. 1959;12:382–396.
35. Eva LJ, MacLean AB, Reid WM, et al. Estrogen receptor expression. *Am J Obstet Gynecol*. 2003;189:458–461.

36. Greenstein A, Militscher I, Chen J, et al. Hyperoxaluria in women with vulvar vestibulitis syndrome. *J Reprod Med.* 2006;51(6):500–502.

37. Harlow BL, Abenhaim HA, Vitonis AF, Harnack L. Influence of dietary oxalates on the risk of adult onset vulvodynia. *J Reprod Med.* 2008;53(3):171–178.

38. Reed BD, Harlow SD, Sen A, et al. Relationship between vulvodynia and chronic comorbid pain conditions. *Obstet Gynecol.* 2012;120(1):145–151.

39. Gardella B, Parru D, Nappi R, et al. Interstitial cystitis is associated with vulvodynia and sexual dysfunction a case control study. *J Sex Med.* 2011;8(6):1726–1734.

40. Carric D, Shere K, Peters K. The relationship of interstitial cystitis/painful bladder syndrome to vulvodynia. *Urol Nurs.* 2009;29(4):233–238.

41. Bornstein J, Zarfati D, Abramovici H. Vulvar vestibulitis: physical or psychosexual problem? *Obstet Gynecol.* 1999;93:876–880.

42. Tribo MJ, Andio O, Ros S, et al. Clinical characteristics and psychopathological profile of patients with vulvodynia: an observational and descriptive study. *Dermatology.* 2008;216(1):24–30.

43. Khandker M, Brady SS, Vitonis AF, et al. The influence of depression and anxiety on risk of adult onset vulvodynia. *J Women's Health.* 2011;20(10):1445–1451.

44. Deleted in proofs.

45. American College of Obstetricians and Gynecologists. *Persistent Vulvar Pain. Committee Opinion Number 673. September 2016.* Washington, DC: American College of Obstetricians and Gynecologists; 2016.

46. Lifits-Podorozhansky YM, Podorozhansky Y, Hoffstetter S, Gavard JA. Role of vulvar care guidelines in the initial management of vulvar complaints. *J Low Genit Tract Dis.* 2012;16(2):88–91.

47. Zolnoun DA, Hartmann KE, Steege JF. Overnight lidocaine ointment for treatment of vulvar vestibulitis. *Obstet Gynecol.* 2003;102:84–87.

48. Deleted in proofs.

49. Deleted in proofs.

50. Reed BD, Caron AM, Gorenflo DW, Haefner HK. Treatment of vulvodynia with tricyclic antidepressants: efficacy and associated factors. *J Low Genit Tract Dis.* 2006;10(4):245–251.

51. Brown CS, Wan J, Bachmann G, Rosen R. Self-management, amitriptyline, and amitriptyline plus triamcinolone in the management of vulvodynia. *J Women's Health.* 2009;18:163–169.

52. Foster DC, Kotok MB, Huang LS, et al. Oral desipramine and topical lidocaine for vulvodynia: a randomized controlled trial. *Obstet Gynecol.* 2010;116:583–593.

53. Brown C. A Controlled Trial of Gabapentin in Vulvodynia: Biological Correlates of Response. NIH Project 1R01HD065740-01A1. National Institutes of Health.

54. Aranda J, Edwards L. Lyrica for the Treatment of Vulvodynia: A Retrospective Chart Review. Presented at the 2007 International Society for the Study of Vulvovaginal Disease World Congress, (Vancouver, BC. Unpublished manuscript).

55. Meltzer-Brody SE, Zolnoun D, Steege JF, et al. Open label trial of lamotrigine focusing on efficacy in vulvodynia. *J Reprod Med.* 2009;54:171–178.

56. Bergeron S, Binik YM, Khalifé S, et al. A randomized comparison of group cognitive-behavioral therapy, surface electromyographic biofeedback, and vestibulectomy in the treatment of dyspareunia resulting from vulvar vestibulitis. *Pain.* 2001;91:297–306.

57. Kandyba K, Binik YM. Hypnotherapy as a treatment for vulvar vestibulitis syndrome: a case report. *J Sex Marital Ther.* 2003;29:237–242.

58. Danielsson I, Sjorg I, Ostman C. Acupuncture for the treatment of vulvar vestibulitis: a pilot study. *Acta Obstet Gynecol Scan.* 2001;80:437–441.

59. Aung SKH. Sexual dysfunction: a modern medical acupuncture approach. *Med Acupuncture.* 2002;13(2):7–9.

60. Powell J, Wojinarowska F. Acupuncture for vulvodynia. *J R Soc Med.* 1999;92:579–581.

61. Harlow BL, Abenhaim HA, Vitonis AF, Harnack L. Influence of dietary oxalates on the risk of adult onset vulvodynia. *J Reprod Med.* 2008;53(3):171–178.

62. McCormack WM, Spence M. Evaluation of the surgical treatment for vulvar vestibulitis. *Eur J Obstet Gynecol Reprod Biol.* 1999;86:135–138.

63. Haefner HK. Critique of new gynecologic surgical procedures: surgery for vulvar vestibulitis. *Clin Obstet Gynecol.* 2000;43:689–700.

64. Goldstein A, Klingman D, Christopher K, et al. Surgical treatment of vulvar vestibulitis syndrome: outcome assessment derived from a postoperative questionnaire. *J Sex Med.* 2006;3:923–931.

65. Deleted in proofs.

66. Abramov L, Wolman I, David MP, et al. Vaginismus: an important factor in the evaluation and management of vulvar vestibulitis syndrome. *Gynecol Obstet Invest.* 1994;38(3):194–197.

67. Haefner HK. *Vulvodynia. Vulvovaginal Disease Update 2013.* Durham, NC: International Society for the Study of Vulvovaginal Disease; 2013:157.

68. Pelletier F, Parratte B, Penz S, et al. Efficacy of high doses of botulinum toxin A for treating of provoked vestibulodynia. *Br J Dermatol.* 2011;164:617–622.

69. Petersen CD, Giraldi A, Lundvall L, et al. Botulinum toxin type A—a novel treatment for provoked vestibulodynia? Results from a randomized placebo controlled double blinded study. *J Sex Med*. 2009;9:2523–2537.

70. National Vulvodynia Association. Vulvodynia Treatments. https://www.nva.org/learnpatient/medical-management/.

71. Spadt SK, Kingsberg S. *Vulvar pain of unknown cause (vulvodynia): Treatment*. 2022. UpToDate.

72. Eifel PJ, Berek JS, Markman MA. Cancer of the cervix, vagina, and vulva. In: DeVita Jr VT, Lawrence TS, Rosenberg SA, eds. *Cancer: Principles and Practice of Oncology*. 9th ed. Philadelphia: Lippincott Williams & Wilkins; 2011:1311–1344.

Pelvic Pain

Natasha Seth-McCoy

OBJECTIVES

- Compare and contrast key characteristics of acute and chronic pelvic pain.
- Describe the differential diagnosis for acute and chronic pelvic pain.
- Identify the appropriate diagnostic workup for pelvic pain.
- Describe the appropriate treatment for pelvic pain.
- Identify when to consult, collaborate, or refer patients with pelvic pain.

INTRODUCTION

Pelvic pain is a common reason female patients seek medical advice. The diagnosis of pelvic pain in female patients can be challenging because many symptoms and signs are insensitive and nonspecific.[1] It is important to obtain a thorough history and physical examination to promptly diagnose the patient and to properly manage the pain in the event that it could be life-threatening. Pelvic pain can be acute or chronic. This chapter discusses each type of pelvic pain in detail.

ACUTE PELVIC PAIN

Definition

Acute pelvic pain is defined as lower abdominal pain or pelvic pain lasting for less than 3 months.[2] The duration of pain can vary. It can last for a few hours or for days, and it often has a sudden onset. Over one-third of reproductive-age females will experience nonmenstrual pelvic pain.[3]

Pathophysiology

Acute pelvic pain can arise from somatic pain, visceral pain, a combination of somatic and visceral pain, and neurogenic pain. Somatic pain is localized pain that results from the activation of peripheral nociceptors without injury to the peripheral nerve or central nervous system. The origin of this pain can be subcutaneous tissue, abdominal or pelvic muscles, peritoneal, or skeletal (Box 18.1). Visceral pain occurs from activation of nociceptors in the pelvis, chest, abdomen, or intestines (Box 18.2). Pain occurs when the internal organs or tissues are injured. Visceral pain is diffuse, not localized, pain, and it is not clearly defined. The pain is often described as feeling *deep, achy, dull,* or *squeezing*. Neurogenic pain arises from the nervous system. Neurogenic pain in the pelvis is caused by injury to the sensory nerves (e.g., herpes, syphilis, tumors, diabetes, multiple sclerosis).

Differential Diagnosis for Acute Pelvic Pain

Females of reproductive age may experience acute pelvic pain as a result of gastrointestinal, urinary, gynecological, and other disorders (Table 18.1).

Pregnant females may also experience pelvic pain. The pregnant patient may have the same differential diagnoses as a patient of reproductive age, but there are additional diagnoses specific to pregnancy. Pregnancy-specific diagnoses include corpus luteum cyst, ectopic pregnancy, miscarriage, labor, uterine rupture (previous cesarean scar), placental abruption, endometritis (postpartum), ovarian vein thrombosis (postpartum), and diastasis of the pubic symphysis.

BOX 18.2 Visceral Pain

- Menstrual pain
- Endometriosis
- Ovulation
- Injury to the gallbladder, bladder, kidney, or intestines
- Constipation
- Indigestion
- Ischemic uterine fibroids
- Appendicitis

The differential diagnosis for adolescent patients would also include an imperforated hymen and transverse vaginal septum. The differential diagnosis for postmenopausal patients would be the same as for reproductive-age patients with the exclusion of pregnancy or menstrual-related disorders.

NOT TO BE MISSED

Females of reproductive age may experience acute pelvic pain due to gastrointestinal, urinary, gynecological, and other disorders.

History

The history and physical examination narrow the differential diagnosis and allow the provider to choose the proper test, as many of the diagnoses considered in acute pelvic pain require confirmatory testing.[1] A history of present illness including a pain history (past and present), location, onset and duration, and characterization of the pain (sharp, deep, intermittent) should be obtained as well as a thorough review of systems to narrow the gap for the differential diagnosis.[2]

The age of the patient is pertinent because it can be indicative of certain conditions. In younger female patients, some of the common conditions include sexually transmitted infections (STIs), pelvic inflammatory disease (PID), and ectopic pregnancy. In adolescent female patients, the pain could be related to congenital uterine or vaginal anomalies that hinder menstrual flow. Appendicitis is seen more in adolescents and adults younger than 30 years of age. Diverticulitis is seen more in adults older than 40 years of age.

It is important to obtain a descriptive pain assessment including prior history of pain. Determine where the pain is located and whether it radiates. Ascertain the event in which the pain originated and whether it was sudden or gradual in nature. Ask about the duration and onset of the pain. If the pain had a sudden onset, consider a diagnosis of appendicitis or an ectopic pregnancy. It is important to obtain a description of the pain (dull, sharp, colicky, cyclic). The pain could be cyclic in nature, which typically presents as ovulation pain (mittelschmerz). Identify the severity of the pain. You can also use a pain scale to assess the intensity of pain. If the patient has had this pain in the past, ask about the prior evaluation and treatment plan.[2]

Inquire about any associating factors such as nausea, vomiting, fever, or chills. If a fever is present, then an infectious etiology is suggested, such as PID, tuboovarian abscess, pyelonephritis, or appendicitis. Identify if the patient is experiencing dysuria, frequency, or hematuria, which is indicative of a urinary tract infection. Ask about purulent vaginal discharge, odor, or bleeding that is commonly seen with an STI. Dizziness, syncopal episodes, cramping, and heavy vaginal bleeding are associated with ectopic pregnancy and threatened abortion. Endometriosis can cause dyspareunia or dysmenorrhea.[2]

Obtain a thorough obstetrical/gynecological history. The history should include the last menstrual cycle, duration and frequency of the menstrual cycle, and amount of menstrual flow (heavy, light). Ask about the current method of contraception. Inquire about sexual history including new partners and mode of intercourse (oral, vaginal, and anal). Discuss any history of sexually transmitted infections and treatment received. Inquire about the patient's last pap smear and the results. Review all prior pregnancies and complications if noted.

Discuss past medical and surgical history. There is an increased risk for bowel obstruction with abdominal surgery. Previous pelvic surgery (tubal ligation) or

TABLE 18.1	**Differential Diagnoses of Acute Pelvic Pain**		
Gastrointestinal	**Urinary**	**Gynecological**	**Other**
Irritable bowel syndrome	Pyelonephritis	Pelvic inflammatory disease	Dissecting aortic aneurysm
Bowel obstruction	Cystitis	Tubo-ovarian abscess	Sickle cell crisis
Gastritis	Ureterolithiasis	Ovarian torsion	Opioid-seeking behavior
Hernia		Ruptured hemorrhagic ovarian	
Appendicitis		cyst	
Diverticulitis		Ectopic pregnancy	
		Endometriosis	
		Endometritis	
		Ovulation	

history of a prior ectopic pregnancy is a predisposing factor for an ectopic pregnancy.

Obtain a social history. Ask about alcohol, drug, and tobacco use. Discuss if there is a history of domestic abuse (trauma to the abdomen).

NOT TO BE MISSED

It is important to obtain a thorough history and physical examination to promptly diagnose the patient and to properly manage the pain in the event that it could be life-threatening.

PHYSICAL EXAMINATION

The physical examination should be initiated with a general assessment of how the patient appears. Vital signs should be obtained to assess for fever, tachycardia, or hypotension. These findings could be suggestive of an infectious process or shock related to blood loss.

An abdominal examination should start with an inspection. Observe for visible signs of distension, trauma, scars, ecchymosis, hernia, or erythema. Auscultate the abdomen for bowel sounds because the absence of bowel sounds can signify peritonitis. Ask the patient to point where the pain is located. Palpate the abdomen for signs of tenderness or masses. Observe for rebound tenderness or involuntary guarding.

Pelvic Examination

A pelvic examination is a very important aspect of the evaluation process for the female patients with pelvic pain. Inspect the external genitalia for lesions, rashes, or swollen areas. Examine the Bartholin and Skene glands for tenderness or swelling. Perform a speculum examination. Evaluate the vagina and the cervix for abnormal discharge, lesions, polyps, ulcerations, masses, or blood. If the cervix is friable and discharge is noted, then this could be indicative of STI or PID. Cervical cultures for chlamydia and gonorrhea and a wet mount from the posterior vaginal fornix should be obtained.

A bimanual examination should be performed after the speculum has been removed. The cervix should be assessed for cervical motion tenderness. The uterus and adnexa should be palpated for size and symmetry. An enlarged uterus can signify pregnancy or fibroids. Enlarged palpable adnexa could be suggestive of an ectopic pregnancy, ovarian neoplasm, or cyst. If indicated, a rectovaginal examination should be performed.[2]

CLINICAL SURVIVAL TIP Palpate beginning in areas where there is no pain and progressing toward areas the patient has identified as painful will allow for patient cooperation in obtaining a complete abdominal and pelvic examination.

Laboratory Testing

Laboratory values are useful in giving direction to a potential diagnosis. All female patients should have a pregnancy test performed. If the urine pregnancy test is positive, then a blood quantitative beta human chorionic gonadotropin (hCG) test should be ordered. A positive pregnancy test could indicate a normal pregnancy or an abnormal pregnancy (ectopic pregnancy, molar pregnancy, threatened abortion). A complete blood count with differential can be useful, especially if the cause of the acute pelvic pain is unclear. An elevated white blood cell count can signify an infectious process. A urinalysis and urine culture can be performed to look for a possible bladder infection. Blood cultures can be obtained if there is a suspicion for sepsis. Finally, evaluation of the cervix and vagina for chlamydia, gonorrhea, trichomoniasis, and bacterial vaginosis can be helpful in patients with risk factors for and/or symptoms of infection.[2]

NOT TO BE MISSED

In the evaluation of pelvic pain, all female patients should have a pregnancy test performed.

⚠ SAFETY ALERT

Pelvic pain in a patient with a positive pregnancy test can indicate an ectopic pregnancy, which constitutes a gynecological emergency.[4]

Imaging

The goal of imaging is to make the most accurate diagnosis using the least amount of radiation; therefore transvaginal ultrasonography is the imaging modality of choice in the initial evaluation of pelvic pain.[1] Ultrasonography can also be used to assess nongynecological diagnoses such as appendicitis and urinary obstruction.

Magnetic resonance (MRI) and computed tomography (CT) of the abdomen/pelvis can be useful if the etiology of the pelvic pain is still unclear. Ultrasonography and MRI are safe during pregnancy.

An abdominal x-ray can be used for evaluation of a possible bowel obstruction or perforation. An abdominal x-ray is not a diagnostic test used for gynecological evaluation.

Laparoscopy

Laparoscopic evaluation of the pelvis may be necessary to make the correct diagnosis if other, less invasive testing has been inconclusive or if there is a life-threatening medical emergency. It is also used as a treatment option when imaging determines its use or if significant symptoms persist without responding to initial treatments.[2]

NOT TO BE MISSED

Laparoscopic evaluation of the pelvis may be necessary to make the correct diagnosis if other, less invasive testing has been inconclusive or if there is a life-threatening medical emergency.

CHRONIC PELVIC PAIN

Definition

Chronic pelvic pain is defined as pain that occurs in the pelvis that last for 6 months or longer. The pain can be constant or intermittent. Chronic pelvic pain can be functionally debilitating.

Pathophysiology

Chronic pelvic pain generally arises from either a visceral source such as the reproductive, genitourinary, and gastrointestinal tracts or from a somatic source such as the pelvic bones, ligaments, muscles, and fascia.[5] Somatic pain may be superficial or deep pain that is described as localized, sharp, or dull. Visceral pain arises from the internal organs and is transmitted through the sympathetic tracts of the autonomic nervous system, and it is usually described as dull or poorly localized.[5]

Differential Diagnosis

It is best to categorize chronic pelvic pain differential diagnoses in either gynecological or nongynecological classifications. The gynecological classifications are as follows:
- Endometriosis
- Adenomyosis
- PID
- Pelvic adhesions
- Ovarian tumor (malignant or benign)
- Leiomyoma (fibroids)
- Dysmenorrhea
- Uterovaginal prolapse
- Dyspareunia, vulvar pain, mittelschmerz
  The nongynecological classifications are as follows:
- Urinary (interstitial cystitis, calculi)
- Gastrointestinal (irritable bowel syndrome, diverticulitis, chronic constipation, celiac disease, colon cancer)
- Musculoskeletal (fibromyalgia, abdominal muscle strain, diastasis of the pubic symphysis)
- Neurologic (nerve injury associated with pelvic surgery)

- Psychosocial (opiate dependency, physical/sexual abuse, depression)

History

Obtaining a thorough history is advantageous in evaluating a patient who presents with chronic pelvic pain. The history should focus on the characteristics of pain, including quality, duration, and modifying factors as well as its association with menses, sexual activity, urination, defecation, and radiation treatment.[6] The COLDERR acronym (character, onset, location, duration, exacerbation, relief, radiation) can be used to obtain a general understanding of the patient's history of present illness.[7]

Character: What does the pain feel like? (sharp, dull, crampy)

Onset: Was the pain onset sudden or gradual? Is it cyclic or constant?

Location: Is the pain localized or diffuse?

Duration: How long has the pain been present, and has it changed over time?

Exacerbation: Which activities and movements make the pain worse?

Relief: Which medications, activities, and positions make the pain better?

Radiation: Does the pain radiate anywhere (back, groin, flank)?

Domestic violence, physical abuse, and sexual abuse should be addressed because they are associated with chronic pelvic pain. Inquire about unintentional weight loss, postmenopausal vaginal bleeding, irregular vaginal bleeding, or postcoital bleeding because this can be a sign of malignancy.

A thorough review of systems should be obtained to exclude other nongynecological diagnosis. Ask questions about bowel habits in regard to frequency, consistency, associated pain, or blood in stool. Inquire about urological habits such as frequency, dysuria, hematuria, or nocturia. Review the patient's past surgical history to establish if the pain is related to previous surgeries.

Physical Examination

The physical examination can identify areas of tenderness and the presence of masses or other anatomical findings that aid in the diagnosis.[6] The physical examination should be initiated with vital signs that includes temperature, blood pressure, pulse, and respiratory rate to assess for instability. The clinician should inspect the abdomen for visible signs of distension, trauma, scars, ecchymosis, hernia, or erythema. The clinician should also auscultate the abdomen for bowel sounds and palpate the abdomen for tenderness, masses, or peritoneal signs. Percussion and palpation should also be performed for organomegaly. Palpation can help with pain mapping by identifying the location of the pain, especially when the pain is described as being felt "all over."

A pelvic examination consists of inspection of the external genitalia, a speculum examination, a bimanual examination, and a rectal examination if needed. The external genitalia should be inspected for lesions or masses. The clinician should palpate the external genitalia and note if there is tenderness or swelling. A speculum examination should also be performed to visualize the vaginal wall, inspect the cervix for discharge or lesions, and inspect the vaginal cuff if a hysterectomy has been performed. A bimanual examination should be performed after the speculum examination. The bimanual examination allows the clinician to assess for cervical motion tenderness, mobility of the uterus, and the size and position of the uterus. The clinician should palpate the ovaries for masses or tenderness. A rectal examination can be performed to assess the tightness of the anal sphincter, tenderness, masses, or presence of stool.

Screening and Diagnostic Tests

The selected screening and tests should be based on the patient's history and physical assessment. It may be appropriate to obtain a serum beta hCG level to rule out pregnancy; a complete blood count; urinalysis and urine culture; erythrocyte sedimentation rate; and vaginal swabs to test for gonorrhea and chlamydia.[6]

Imaging

Transvaginal ultrasonography is useful during the initial evaluation to investigate any pelvic masses or nodules found during the physical examination and to reassure the patient if no significant abnormalities are discovered. MRI and CT can be used to evaluate findings that were noted on the ultrasound examination.

Treatment

Treatment of pelvic pain should be based on the underlying cause of the pain.[8] Treatment can be medical or surgical management. Medical management may include antiinflammatory drugs, narcotics, antidepressants, ion channel blockers, hormone medications, and antibiotics.

Nonsteroidal antiinflammatory drugs (NSAIDs) usually are a safe category to start with; however, there are contraindications to these drugs, especially in patients with gastrointestinal disorders.[9] Acetaminophen can be used in patients who have gastrointestinal disorders because it does not cause harm to the gastric mucosa. NSAIDS include ibuprofen, naproxen sodium, ketorolac, mefenamic acid, and celecoxib.

Narcotic pain medications should be used only for acute pelvic pain; however, patients with chronic pain may be candidates for narcotic therapy in some instances under careful supervision.[9] When using narcotics, it is imperative to obtain a narcotic contract. Any patient with a history of drug use or current drug use is not a candidate for narcotic therapy.

Antidepressants such as tricyclic antidepressants, selective serotonin reuptake inhibitors (SSRIs), serotonin-norepinephrine reuptake inhibitors (SNRIs), and ion channel blockers can be used for neuropathic pain as well as depression. Tricyclic antidepressants include amitriptyline, imipramine, and desipramine. SSRIs include paroxetine, fluoxetine, and citalopram. SNRIs include venlafaxine and duloxetine.

Ion channel blockers including gabapentin, pregabalin, lamotrigine, phenytoin, mexiletine, and carbamazepine can be used.

Hormone medications can be used when the pain is associated with the menstrual cycle. Continuous or cyclic low-dose oral contraceptive pills or gonadotropin-releasing hormone agonists should be considered, even if the cause is thought to be irritable bowel syndrome,

interstitial cystitis, or pelvic congestion syndrome because these conditions also respond to hormone treatment.[6]

Antibiotics are used if an infectious process is the source of pelvic pain.

Surgical management may be necessary and has been shown to be helpful in reducing chronic pelvic pain that is unrelieved by any other measure.[5] Some of the common surgeries are lysis of adhesions, presacral neurectomy, total abdominal hysterectomy, and ablative therapy for endometriosis.[8]

Other therapies include neurostimulation, physical therapy, and psychotherapy.

NOT TO BE MISSED

Treatment of pelvic pain should be based on the underlying cause of the pain.

Referral

A referral should be made for the patient with pelvic pain if the patient requires diagnostic procedures, surgical management, or medical management that is out of the clinician's scope of practice or if the diagnosis or management is unclear. Because a multidisciplinary treatment approach will benefit most patients with pelvic pain, the referring provider should stay engaged in the care of the patient and coordinate the plan of care with any subspecialists involved.[6]

KEY POINTS

- Pelvic pain is a common complaint for female patients.
- A thorough history and physical examination is key to the diagnosis and prevention of a life-threatening condition.
- Patients may experience acute pelvic pain as a result of gastrointestinal, urinary, gynecological, or other disorders.
- All patients with pelvic pain require pregnancy testing in the initial workup.
- Chronic pelvic pain is either cyclic or noncyclic.
- Treatment for pelvic pain depends on the underlying cause.

REFERENCES

1. Kruszka PS. Evaluation of acute pelvic pain in women. *Am Fam Physician.* 2010;82(2):141.
2. Stratton P. *Evaluation of Acute Pelvic Pain in Nonpregnant Adult Women.* UpToDate; 2021.
3. Bhavsar AK, Gelner EJ, Shorma T. Common questions about the evaluation of acute pelvic pain. *Am Fam Physician.* 2016;93(1):41.
4. Walker JJ. Ectopic pregnancy. *Clin Obstetrics Gynecol.* 2007;50(1):89–99.
5. Schuiling KD, Likis FE. *Women's Gynecologic Health.* Sudbury, MA: Jones and Bartlett; 2006.
6. Ortiz DD. Chronic pelvic pain in women. *Am Fam Physician.* 2008;77(11):1535–1542.
7. Gibbs RS, Karlan BY, Haney AF, Nygaard I. *Danforth's Obstetrics and Gynecology.* 10th ed. Philadelphia: Lippincott; 2008.
8. Tu FF, As-Sanie S. *Chronic Pelvic Pain in Adult Females: Treatment.* UpToDate; 2022.
9. Steege J, Siedhoff M. Chronic pelvic pain. *Obstet Gynecol.* 2014;124(3):616–629.

19

Managing Musculoskeletal Problems

Sarah B. Freeman and Kimberly Gray

OBJECTIVES

- Discuss the epidemiology and pathogenesis of the two most common musculoskeletal problems (osteoporosis and pelvic organ relaxation/prolapse) seen in a women's health practice.
- Understand the risk factors leading to osteoporosis and pelvic organ relaxation/prolapse.

- Develop a plan of care for the screening, prevention, and treatment of osteoporosis.
- Identify and develop a plan of care for pelvic relaxation/pelvic prolapse syndromes that includes referral for surgery as indicated.

INTRODUCTION

Although females and males experience the same musculoskeletal problems, there are two conditions that are commonly seen in the typical women's health care practice. Pelvic relaxation and pelvic prolapse are unique to females. These conditions are related to childbearing as well as the hormone changes that accompany aging. Early identification of loss of muscle tone (pelvic relaxation) and early treatment can help prevent the progression that leads to pelvic organ prolapse (POP).

Osteoporosis is also a disease that affects females at a much greater rate than males and is associated with a decrease in hormone production that is normally seen as a part of menopausal changes. Postmenopausal osteoporosis is one of the leading skeletal diseases in females, and it can lead to a decrease in quality of life. It is also a leading cause of loss of independence in females as a result of changes in mobility related to both vertebral and hip fractures. Taking measures to decrease the amount of bone loss as well as preventing falls that lead to fracture are an important part of providing good care to females. Both of these conditions will be discussed in this chapter.

OSTEOPOROSIS

Osteoporosis is often a silent disease. It is the most common bone disease in females and many times is not recognized until after a fracture has occurred. Osteoporosis is characterized by low bone mass, deterioration of bone tissue, and disruption of bone architecture. This causes a compromise of bone strength and an increase in the risk of fracture. It is an important issue in the health of female patients because bone loss occurs as hormone levels decline, therefore all females experience a degree of bone loss. Promotion of good bone health and preventive strategies to help maximize bone health and minimize bone loss are an important part of the provision of health care to female patients.

Epidemiology

Osteoporosis is a major health concern affecting both males and females. More than 10 million individuals have osteoporosis, and 80% of these individuals are females. Another 43.3 million have low bone density (osteopenia) and are at increased risk for development of the disease. Each year, more than 1.5 million fractures of the back, wrists, and hips are attributed to this disease. Osteoporosis is more common in females and is the main cause of bone fractures in postmenopausal females and older adults. Because females lose up to 20% of their bone mass in the 5 to 7 years following menopause, about 1 in 6 postmenopausal females have osteoporosis.[1,2]

Ethnicity as well as some lifestyle issues affect the development of this disease. Table 19.1 shows the effect of ethnicity on bone loss and osteoporosis. This table is for females at 50 years of age, and it is important to note that prevalence of the disease increases with age.

More significant than the number of females with disease is the number of females with fractures caused by the disease. Osteoporosis is the leading cause of vertebral, hip, and wrist fractures in females older than 50 years of age. According to the National Osteoporosis Foundation, osteoporosis is responsible for more than 2 million fractures yearly:

- 297,000 hip fractures
- 547,000 vertebral fractures
- 397,000 wrist fractures
- 135,000 pelvic fractures
- 675,000 fractures at other sites

Fracture can be a major cause of loss of mobility and chronic pain, and this has a great impact on quality of life. During their lifetime, about one-half of White, Asian, and Hispanic females and one-third of African American females older than 50 years of age will experience an osteoporosis-related fracture. Further examination reveals the following:

- 1 in 4 will develop a vertebral deformity.[3]
- 1 in 7 will experience a hip fracture.[4]
- Risk increases steadily as bone density declines.[2]
- Risk of hip fracture is equal to a female's combined risk of breast, uterine, and ovarian cancer.[2]

Table 19.2 lists the long-term effects associated with fracture, including the many economic problems associated with these fractures. Treatment of osteoporosis-related fractures has resulted in over $17 billion in annual direct costs. Other annual economic costs are as follows:

- Hospital admissions (over 430,000 yearly)
- Medical visits (about 2.5 million yearly)
- Nursing home admissions (180,000 yearly)
- Loss of income resulting from morbidity and mortality[5]

NOT TO BE MISSED

Osteoporosis is a major health problem for females and a leading cause of pain and disability for postmenopausal females.

TABLE 19.1 Females and Osteoporosis[5]

Ethnicity	% With Osteoporosis	% With Osteopenia	Total %
White (non-Hispanic) and Asian	20	50–65	70–85
Hispanic	10–20	49–56	59–71
Native American	12	45	57
African American	5–10	35–38	40–48

TABLE 19.2 Impact of Fractures[5]

Both Hip and Vertebral	Impact of Hip Fracture	Vertebral Fracture
• Acute and chronic pain • Depression • Decrease in social interaction • Limits on mobility • Anxiety caused by fear of another fracture	• Increased mortality (10% to 20% die within 1 year of fracture) • Increased risk of other fractures (10% have a second fracture in 1 year) • Loss of function (60% do not regain full function) • Loss of independence (25% require long-term nursing home care)	• Height loss • Kyphosis • Respiratory or gastrointestinal problems caused by skeletal changes • Limited ability to reach objects as a result of a change in ability to stretch

Pathophysiology

Bone remodeling (removing old bone and replacing it with new bone) is a normal process that helps maintain a healthy skeleton capable of supporting the body. Osteoporosis is a disease of the bone that is caused by an imbalance in this process. When the normal processes of bone turnover are out of balance, the body is unable to produce bone at the rate that it is lost. As females age and their hormone levels decline, osteoclast activity (cells that break down old bone tissue) exceeds osteoblast activity (cells that build new bone tissue). This leads to a loss of bone tissue and a change in architecture of the bone (Fig. 19.1), which increases bone fragility and, when coupled with other changes associated with age, leads to an increase in risk of fractures (Fig. 19.2). These fractures occur when there is too much stress placed on the weakened bone.[6] As bone density decreases, fracture rates increase (Fig. 19.3).

Risk Factors for Osteoporosis and Fracture

An important part of providing care is the identification and management of risk factors. When discussing osteoporosis, it is important to remember that there are two types of risk factors: those that are modifiable and those that are not. Table 19.3 examines these risk factors. If modifiable risk factors are present, the patient must be counseled on how to positively affect these factors. Risk factor modification must occur early to prevent excessive bone loss.

Although it is never too late to try and modify these factors, early intervention is critical to preventive therapy. Chronic health conditions as well as medications can affect the development of osteoporosis. If possible, switching to a medication that does not affect bone should be accomplished; if not, early detection and treatment are indicated. Control of long-term diseases may also have a positive impact on the development of osteoporosis, and patients should be assisted in developing strategies to maximize control of these disorders.

To determine the risk of fracture, the World Health Organization (WHO) developed a risk factor tool that can be used to help determine the need for intervention or further testing and to educate the patient regarding specific risk factors. The Fracture Risk Assessment Tool (FRAX) is an online tool that provides clinicians a way

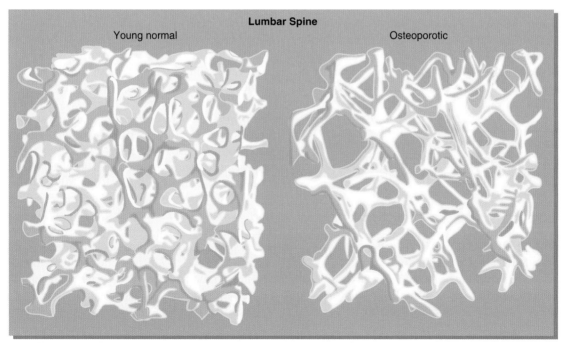

Figure 19.1 Healthy bone versus osteoporotic bone. (Reprinted from Ralph Müller, Peter Rüegsegger, Micro-Tomographic Imaging for the Nondestructive evaluation of Trabecular Bone Architecture, 61–79, Copyright (2021), with permission from IOS Press. The publication is available at IOS Press through http://dx.doi.org/10.3233/978-1-60750-884-7-61)

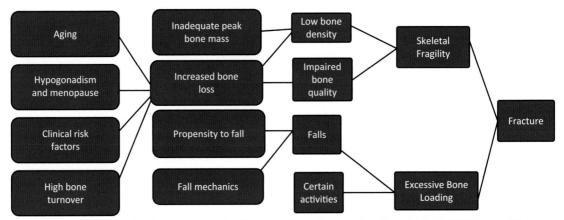

Figure 19.2 Factors that increase the risk of fracture. (From Cosman F, deBeur SJ, LeBoff MS, et al. Clinician's guide to prevention and treatment of osteoporosis. *Osteoporos Int.* 2014;25[10]:2359–2381.)

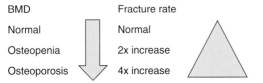

Figure 19.3 Rate of increase of fracture related to bone mineral density *(BMD).*

to quantify the risk of developing a hip or other osteoporotic fracture over the next 10 years. It is most effective in patients in the 50–70-year-old age range and is accurate in the quantification of risk in both White and non-White females.[7,8] Table 19.4 illustrates one of the FRAX tools that can be used to assess fracture risk.

> **PATIENT-CENTERED CARE:** Control of long-term diseases may also have a positive impact on the development of osteoporosis, and patients should be assisted in developing strategies to help them maximize control of these disorders.

Screening and Diagnosis
History and Physical Examination
Diagnosis and screening begin with a history and physical examination. Evaluation includes the following:[6,7]
- Rule out diseases that mimic osteoporosis.
- Determine the cause(s) of osteoporosis.
- Identify factors that contribute to the development and progression of osteoporosis.
- Determine the severity of the disease.

- Determine the risk of fracture, and develop a plan to prevent it.
- Provide appropriate prevention and/or treatment.

The assessment of risk factors (see Table 19.3) is an important place to begin. Risk assessment is not something that should wait until menopause but should be done on adult female patients as part of their routine physical examination so preventive measures can be taken before the significant bone loss seen at menopause. Menstrual history is important when assessing the likelihood of development of postmenopausal osteoporosis. The date of the last menses can provide the information needed to begin screening because bone loss accelerates in the first few years following menopause.

Another important part of the history is looking for secondary causes of osteoporosis. The most common form of osteoporosis in females is postmenopausal osteoporosis; there are other causes (Table 19.5), and it is important to identify these causes and treat them. It is important to remember that osteoporosis may be present without any symptoms. Symptoms usually occur only after a fracture has occurred. Early factures, especially those that occur in the spine, may go unnoticed as the pain is either minimal or attributed to a muscle injury to the back. Clinicians must be aware of the presenting signs and symptoms of vertebral fracture:[9]
- Acute pain following a fall or minor trauma
- Localized pain typically identifiable at the vertebral level
  - Mid or lower thorax
  - Upper lumbar spine
- Description of pain is

TABLE 19.3	**Risk Factors for Osteoporosis and Osteoporotic Fractures**[6]	
Nonmodifiable	**Modifiable**	**Possible to Affect**
Age	Lifestyle	Chronic diseases*
Race: White/Asian	• Smoking	• Endocrine disorders
Gender: Female	• Excessive vitamin A intake	• Diabetes
Family history of fracture: First-degree	• Low calcium intake	• Thyroid disease
relative	• High alcohol intake: >3 drinks per day	• Adrenal disorders
Family history of osteoporosis	• Vitamin D deficiency	• Gastrointestinal disorders
Genetic disorders	• Decreased physical activity, especially	• Malabsorption
• Cystic fibrosis	weight-bearing exercise	• Inflammatory bowel disease
• Homocystinuria	Weight <127 lb	• Celiac disease
• Marfan syndrome	Low hormone levels	• Chronic liver disease
• Hemochromatosis	• Menopause	• Renal disease
Inability to bear weight such as para-	• Amenorrhea	• Medical condition that predisposes
plegia	• Eating disorders	to fall: poor vision
	• Fall risk	Use of some medications

*Control of disease may affect the development of osteoporosis.
BMI, Body mass index.

- Sharp
- Nagging
- Dull
- Movement exacerbates pain and causes it to radiate to the abdomen.
- Pain may be accompanied by paravertebral muscle spasms that worsen with activity.
- Pain may be chronic with multiple fractures and severe kyphosis.

On physical examination, a patient who has experienced compression fracture of the vertebra may present with the following:[10]

- Point tenderness over the involved vertebra
- Dowager hump (thoracic kyphosis with exaggerated cervical lordosis)
- Lumbar lordosis
- Decreased height
  - 2 to 3 cm per fracture
  - Progressive kyphosis

Pain is the most common presenting symptom of all other fractures. Once a patient has had a hip fracture, there may be some difficulty with weight bearing on the affected side as well as limited range of motion. It is important during assessment to determine if the fracture was caused by a low-impact injury. Fractures that are worse than the injury that causes them may result from poor bone mass, and these patients should be worked up for osteoporosis. Screening includes the following:[11]

- Quantify bone mass using imaging to help determine action.
- Identify previous fractures and risk for future fractures using history, physical examination, and imaging.
- Identify the risk of fracture unrelated to bone mass per the history.

Once the screening history and physical examination has been performed, laboratory testing and imaging should be considered. This will provide the clinician with information that will inform the plan of care.

First, if appropriate, it is helpful to rule out secondary causes. Table 19.6 describes tests that should be considered when the clinician suspects a secondary cause of osteoporosis. Further testing may be needed based on the results of the initial test. If a secondary cause or contributing condition is identified, proper management of both the condition and the osteoporosis is required.

> **CLINICAL SURVIVAL TIP** Screen all female patients older than 65 years of age and younger females if the estimated 10-year fracture risk equals or exceeds that of a White female with no risk factors.

When deciding who should be screened using imaging, several organizations have published recommendations. Table 19.7 lists these organizations and their recommendations. All of the organizations recognize the importance of screening in postmenopausal female

TABLE 19.4 Fracture Index Assessment Tool for Postmenopausal Females[37]

Question/Answer	Index Value
What is your current age in years?	0
1. <65	1
2. 65–69	2
3. 70–74	3
4. 75–79	4
5. 80–84	5
6. >85	
Have you broken any bones after 50 years of age?	1
	0
1. Yes	
2. No/don't know	
Has your mother had a hip fracture after 50 years of age?	1
	0
1. Yes	
2. No/don't know	
Do you weight 125 pounds or less?	1
1. Yes	0
2. No	
Do you need to use your arms to assist yourself in standing up from a chair?	2
	0
1. Yes	
2. No	
If you have a current bone mineral density (BMD) assessment, what was your total hip T-score?	0
	2
	3
1. >–1	4
2. –1 to –2	
3. –2 to –2.5	
4. <–2.5	

If there is no BMD assessment and a total FRACTURE Index score of ≥4, evaluate further, including a BMD. If there is a current BMD assessment and a total FRACTURE Index score of ≥6, consider intervention. (From An Assessment Tool for Predicting Fracture Risk in postmenopausal women D. M. Black, M. Steinbuch, L. Palermo, P. Dargent-Molina, R. Lindsay, M. S. Hoseyni & O. Johnell in *Osteoporosis International* (2001).12, 519–528)

patients after 65 years of age and all female patients who have had a fragility fracture. Bone mineral density (BMD) is recommended as the first-line test for the diagnosis and screening of osteoporosis. Bone density is the amount of mineral content that is present at the measured site. There are several potential uses for BMD testing, and it should be considered a necessary screening for female patients older than 65 years of age. BMD testing includes the following:[12]

- Diagnose both osteoporosis and osteopenia.
- Establish the severity of bone loss.
- Determine fracture risk.
- Identify patients who need pharmacological intervention, and monitor the effectiveness of therapy.

BMD correlates well with bone strength and quality and has been shown to be an excellent predictor of fracture risk. The risk of fracture increases exponentially with a decrease in BMD. The lower the bone mass, the higher the risk of fracture. The definition of *osteoporosis* as established by the WHO is based on the comparison of bone density to that of a young person when measured at the spine, hip, or forearm and is reported as a T-score (Table 19.8).[6]

The most common method used for measurement of bone density is dual-energy x-ray absorptiometry (DEXA). Although other measures are used, DEXA is considered the gold standard for diagnosing osteoporosis. Although it is presently the best test, it has some limitations. One of the biggest problems in interpretation for the postmenopausal female is the presence of osteoarthritis. Osteoarthritis at both the hip and spine can lead to an increase in bone density without an increase in bone strength. This causes the DEXA measurement to be inaccurate as a predictor of fracture risk for these patients. Additionally, the presence of osteomalacia, a disease that affects bone mineralization, can lead to a false low score as it underestimates bone mass.[7]

There is an increased fracture risk with the diagnosis of both osteopenia and osteoporosis (see Fig. 19.3), and intervention necessitates consideration. There is a twofold increase in fracture rate with osteopenia and a fourfold increase with osteoporosis.[6] BMD testing is covered by Medicare for a wide range of reasons. Testing can be done every 2 years in the following circumstances:[13]

- Radiographic evidence of osteoporosis, osteopenia, vertebral fracture
- Estrogen deficiency with proven risk of osteoporosis
- Long term glucocorticoid therapy using doses of or greater than 5mg of prednisone for 3 months or longer
- Primary hyperparathyroidism
- To monitor response to therapy

> **! SAFETY ALERT**
>
> There is an increased risk of fracture with the diagnosis of both osteopenia and osteoporosis.

TABLE 19.5   Causes of Secondary Osteoporosis* [6,29]

Endocrine	Nutrition	Chronic Diseases	Drugs	Others
Thyroid disorders	Alcoholism	Chronic renal failure	Antiepileptic drugs	Spinal cord injury
Adrenal disorders	Anorexia nervosa	Rheumatoid arthritis[†]	Aromatase inhibitors	Seizure disorders[†]
Diabetes (types 1 and 2)	Malabsorption syndrome	Systemic lupus erythematosus	Immunosuppressants	Some malignancies
Hypogonadism	Calcium deficiency	Chronic liver disease	Glucocorticoids	
Porphyria	Vitamin D deficiency	Chronic obstructive lung disease[†]	Gonadotropin-releasing hormones	
Growth hormone deficiency	Total parenteral nutrition	Human immunodeficiency virus/acquired immunodeficiency syndrome	Heparin	
	Gastric bypass surgery	Organ transplant[†]	Lithium	
			Selective serotonin reuptake inhibitors	
			Thiazolidinedione	
			Depo-Provera	
			Loop diuretics	
			Proton pump inhibitors	

*Partial list.
[†]May be caused by medication used.

TABLE 19.6   Laboratory Tests to Exclude Secondary Causes of Osteoporosis* [6,12,30]

Test	Excludes
Complete blood count Serum protein electrophoresis	Malignancies
Complete blood chemistry	Calcium problems, renal function, diabetes, liver disease, nutritional problems
Vitamin D levels	Vitamin D deficiency
Thyroid-stimulating hormone	Thyroid disease
Serum tryptase	Mast cell disease
Serum parathyroid hormone	Hyperparathyroidism (primary or secondary)
Estradiol: Consider in premenopausal or perimenopausal patients; not necessary in postmenopausal patients	Hypogonadism
24-hour urinary cortisol	Adrenal disease

*Other diseases may need to be considered based on the results of the test performed.

Treatment

Once testing has been completed, a plan of care can be developed for the patient. Care is based on the history and physical examination as well as the BMD. There are several goals for the treatment of bone mass. First and foremost is the protection of bone density and the deceleration of bone loss. Additionally, a goal of any therapy is the maintenance of maximum mobility. If mobility impairment has already occurred, the plan should include ways to preserve mobility as well as restore what has been lost, if possible. Treatment is aimed at prevention of morbidity and maintenance of function.

Recall that osteoporosis is one of the leading causes of loss of independence, and the aim of management is to preserve quality of life. Treatment of low BMD includes both nonpharmacological and pharmacological therapy. There are also universal recommendations for all patients to help to prevent or delay bone loss.

Nonpharmacological/Universal

The National Osteoporosis Foundation and the American Association of Clinical Endocrinologists (AACE) have universal recommendations for all females for the prevention and management of osteoporosis (Fig. 19.4). These

TABLE 19.7   Recommendation for Osteoporosis Screening for Females in the United States[15,31,32]

Organization	Recommendation

American Association of Clinical Endocrinologists	Females 65 years of age and older
	All postmenopausal females:
	  With a history of fracture without major trauma
	  With osteopenia identified radiographically
	  Starting or taking long-term systemic glucocorticoid therapy
	Other perimenopausal or postmenopausal females with risk factors for osteoporosis if willing to consider pharmacological interventions:
	  Low body weight (<127 lb)
	  Long-term systemic glucocorticoid therapy (≥3 months)
	  Family history of osteoporotic fracture
	  Early menopause
	  Current smoking
	  Excessive consumption of alcohol
	  Secondary osteoporosis

American College of Obstetricians and Gynecologists	Postmenopausal females 65 years of age and older Postmenopausal females younger than 65 years of age who are at increased risk of osteoporosis as determined by a formal clinical risk assessment tool Screen every 2 years unless development of additional risk factors
National Osteoporosis Foundation	Females 65 years of age and older regardless of risk factors Younger menopausal females and females in the menopausal transition with clinical risk for fractures Females who had a fracture at 50 years of age or older Females with conditions or taking medication associated with low bone mass or bone loss
U.S. Preventive Services Task Force	Females 65 years of age or older Females younger than 65 years of age whose fracture risk is ≥ that of a 65-year-old White female with no additional risk factors.

TABLE 19.8   World Health Organization Definition of Osteoporosis Using Bone Mineral Density[6,11]

Interpretation	T-Score	Meaning of Score
Normal	−1.0	BMD is within 1 SD of normal (that of a young adult).
Osteopenia	−1.0 to −2.5	BMD is 1 to 2.5 SD of normal (also known as *low bone mass*).
Osteoporosis	−2.5 or greater	BMD is 2.5 SD or more below the normal. If the patient has already sustained a fracture, the diagnosis is severe osteoporosis.

BMD, Bone mineral density; *SD*, standard deviation.

nonpharmacological interventions should be encouraged throughout the lifespan and should be considered a part of all routine care. Lifestyle is important in the prevention of osteoporosis, and the promotion of a bone-healthy lifestyle is especially important in the care of female patients. The universal recommendations are as follows:[2,6,12]

- Counsel on the risk of osteoporosis.
- Discuss the impact of osteoporotic fractures.
- Provide dietary counseling including the following:
  - Adequate total calcium intake (1200 mg/day for females 51 years of age and older)
  - Supplement if diet inadequate

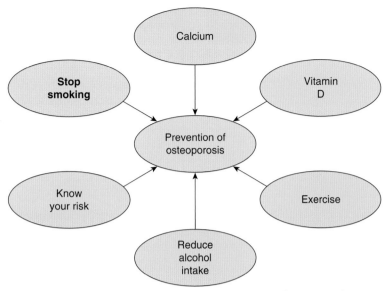

Figure 19.4 Universal measures for the prevention of osteoporosis.

- Adequate vitamin D intake (800–1000 IU/day)
- Supplement if necessary for patients who are 50 years of age and older
- Weight-bearing and muscle-strengthening exercises
  - Improve agility, strength, posture, and balance
  - Maintain or improve bone strength
  - Reduce the risk of fractures
- Fall prevention measures
  - Home safety assessment
  - Balance training exercises
  - Correct vitamin D insufficiency
  - Avoid central nervous system depressant medications
  - Monitor antihypertensive medication
  - Correct vision
- Avoidance of tobacco
- Avoidance of excessive alcohol intake (no more than one drink per day for females)
- Adequate protein intake (0.8 g/kg)

NOT TO BE MISSED

Fall risk assessments should be performed and an exercise program that includes weight bearing and muscle strengthening is recommended for all females older than 65 years of age.

Another nonpharmacological measure is the prevention of falls. Fall prevention is critical to the prevention of fracture. Falls are the precipitating cause of most fractures, thus assessing the patient's risk of falls and examining measures to prevent falls are important in the management of osteoporosis. Although all patients must be counseled on fall risk and prevention, it is especially important for patients who are predisposed to falls. Female patients who are older and frail are at high risk for falls. Box 19.1 contains a list of conditions that increase the likelihood of a fall. Data show that some fall prevention measures reduce the risk of falls.

Females at risk for falls might want to consider the use of a hip protector. Although they do not affect the risk of falling, they reduce the risk of fracture from a fall. Hip protectors are tights with padded shields covering both hips that patients wear under their clothing. Patient acceptability has been a barrier to the widespread use of hip protectors in part because of the bulk of the pads, which creates a bulging appearance at both hips.[12]

Physical therapy may also be beneficial to patients, especially those with kyphosis and back pain. It is also useful for patients with an unstable gait and can aid in preventing falls. The therapy should focus on weight-bearing exercise as well as back strengthening and balance training. Referral is needed for most

BOX 19.1 Factors That Increase Risk for Falls[35]

Intrinsic Factors
- Advanced age
- Previous falls
- Muscle weakness
- Gait and balance problems
- Poor vision
- Postural hypotension
- Chronic conditions including arthritis, stroke, incontinence, diabetes, Parkinson's, dementia

Extrinsic Factors
- Lack of stair handrails
- Poor stair design
- Lack of bathroom grab bars
- Dim lighting or glare
- Obstacles and tripping hazards
- Slippery or uneven surfaces
- Psychoactive medications
- Improper use of assistive device

BOX 19.2 Fall Prevention Measures[36]

- Do balance and strength training exercises
- Talk with your health care provider about medication side effects
- Make your home safer by using night lights, installing grab bars in the bathroom, and securing carpet to the floors
- Get your vision and hearing checked regularly
- Stand up slowly to avoid dizziness
- Use a cane or walker for extra stability

physical therapy and should be offered to the appropriate patients.[12] Fall prevention measures are shown in Box 19.2.

Pharmacological Management

Postmenopausal female patients who meet the following parameters should be considered for pharmacological intervention:
- A clinical or morphometric fracture of either the vertebrae or hip
- T-score of <2.5 at the femoral neck or spine once secondary causes have been eliminated
- BMD between −1.0 and −2.5 at the femoral neck or spine and a 10-year probability of hip fracture of >3%
- BMD between −1.0 and −2.5 at the femoral neck or spine and a 10-year probability of any major osteoporotic fracture of >20% based on the U.S. adapted WHO FRAX algorithm.[12]

The purpose of treatment is to prevent further bone loss and to have a positive impact on bone density. This is accomplished to decrease the occurrence of fracture and help preserve function. There are a number of classes of drugs used in the treatment of osteoporosis (Table 19.9). These FDA-approved options affect the rate of bone turnover by inhibiting bone resorption and can be used for prevention and/or treatment.
- Bisphosphonates
- Selective estrogen receptor modulator/estrogen agonist/antagonist
- RANK ligand inhibitors
- Calcitonin
- Parathyroid hormone (PTH)
- Estrogen
- Romosozumab

Over time, these drugs may cause an increase in bone mass of between 5% and 10% at the lumbar spine, thus stabilizing bone mass. Although not enough of an increase to restore normal bone density is achieved, it does improve bone mass and has a protective effect against fracture.[6,11,12] The decision on which drug to utilize is based on clinical information obtained from the patient and the patient's ability to tolerate the drug. Figure 19.5 provides a suggested treatment plan based on the recommendations of AACE and the American College of Endocrinology (ACE).[12]

> **CLINICAL SURVIVAL TIP** All drug therapy must be accompanied with lifestyle change in order to maximize therapeutic effect.

Bisphosphonates. There are several different drugs within this class. These drugs are considered the first-line treatment for both prevention and treatment of bone density problems because they have a relatively low risk profile and are very cost-effective.[6] Bisphosphonates can be given either orally or intravenously

TABLE 19.9 Medications for the Treatment of Osteoporosis[6,12,33,34]

Medication	Indication and Dosage	Fracture Reduction	Contraindications	Adverse Events
Bisphosphonates				
Alendronate Fosamax Binosto	Prevention: 5 mg/day 35 mg/week Treatment: 10 mg/day 70 mg/week	Vertebral[‡] Nonvertebral[†] Hip[‡]	Abnormalities of the esophagus Inability to sit up for 30 minutes Hypersensitivity Uncorrected hypocalcemia Not recommended if CrCl <35 mL/min	Esophagitis Abdominal pain Diarrhea Musculoskeletal pain Dyspepsia Dysphagia Flulike symptoms (rare) Atypical femoral fracture Jaw osteonecrosis (rare)
Risedronate Actonel Atelvia	Prevention and Treatment: 5 mg/day 35 mg/week 75 mg/two consecutive days each month 150 mg/month	Vertebral[‡] Nonvertebral[†] Hip[‡]	Inability to sit up for 30 minutes Hypersensitivity Uncorrected hypocalcemia Not recommended if CrCl <35 mL/min	Esophagitis Abdominal pain Diarrhea Musculoskeletal pain Dyspepsia, dysphagia Flulike symptoms (rare) Atypical femoral fracture Jaw osteonecrosis (rare)
Ibandronate Boniva	Prevention and Treatment: 150 mg/month Treatment: 3 mg every 3 months IV	Vertebral[‡] Nonvertebral[*] Hip[§]	Hypersensitivity Uncorrected hypocalcemia Not recommended if CrCl <35 mL/min	Esophagitis Abdominal pain Diarrhea Musculoskeletal pain Dyspepsia, dysphagia Flulike symptoms (rare) Atypical femoral fracture Jaw osteonecrosis (rare)
Zoledronic acid Reclast	Prevention and Treatment: 5 mg every 2 years IV Treatment: 5 mg/year IV	Vertebral[‡] Nonvertebral[†] Hip[†]	Hypersensitivity Hypocalcemia Not recommended if CrCl <35 mL/min	Acute phase: fever, flulike symptoms, headache, arthralgia/myalgia Jaw osteonecrosis Transient increase in creatinine Atrial fibrillation Hypocalcemia Atypical femoral fracture
Selective Estrogen Receptor Modulators				
Raloxifene Evista	Prevention and Treatment: 60 mg/day	Vertebral without previous fracture[‡] Vertebral with previous fracture[†] Nonvertebral[§] Hip[§]	Pregnancy Breastfeeding History of deep venous thrombosis Hypersensitivity	
Calcitonin				
Calcitonin-salmon Miacalcin Fortical	Treatment: 200 IU/day nasal spray 100 IU or IM every day SQ	Vertebral[*] Nonvertebral[§] Hip[§]	Hypersensitivity	Nausea Flushing With nasal spray: rhinitis

Continued

TABLE 19.9 Medications for the Treatment of Osteoporosis[6,12,33,34]—cont'd

Medication	Indication and Dosage	Fracture Reduction	Contraindications	Adverse Events
Parathyroid Hormones				
Teriparatide Forteo	Treatment: 20 mcg/day SQ	Vertebral[‡] Nonvertebral[‡] Hip[¶]	Paget disease Prior therapeutic radiation to the skeleton Skeletal malignancies (primary or metastases) Hypercalcemia if pregnant or breast-feeding Unexplained elevated alkaline phosphatase Hypersensitivity	Orthostatic hypotension Increased serum calcium Increased urinary calcium Increased serum uric acid BLACK BOX WARNING *Shown to increase the incidence of osteosarcoma in male and female rats, dependent on dose and duration*
Abaloparatide Tymlos	Treatment: 80 mcg/day SQ	Vertebral[‡] Nonvertebral[‡] Hip[¶]	Paget disease Prior therapeutic radiation to the skeleton Skeletal malignancies (primary or metastases) Hypercalcemia if pregnant or breast-feeding Unexplained elevated alkaline phosphatase Hypersensitivity	Orthostatic hypotension Increased serum calcium Increased urinary calcium Increased serum uric acid BLACK BOX WARNING *Shown to increase the incidence of osteosarcoma in male and female rats, dependent on dose and duration*
RANK Ligand Inhibitors				
Denosumab Prolia Xgeva	Treatment: 60 mg/6 months SQ	Vertebral[‡] Nonvertebral[†] Hip[†]	Hypocalcemia	Pain in back, extremity, and musculoskeletal Hypertriglyceridemia Cystitis Infectious disease Rash Hypocalcemia Aseptic necrosis of jaw (rare) Atypical femoral fracture

Continued

TABLE 19.9 Medications for the Treatment of Osteoporosis[6,12,33,34]—cont'd

Medication	Indication and Dosage	Fracture Reduction	Contraindications	Adverse Events
Estrogens				
Estrogen Over 30 brand names	Multiple doses either PO or transdermally	Vertebral[‡] Nonvertebral[†] Hip[‡]	Known or suspected pregnancy History of thromboembolic disorder Estrogen-dependent neoplasia Breast cancer in most patients Liver dysfunction or disease (either active or in the past year) Stroke or MI	Bloating Breast tenderness Uterine bleeding Breast cancer Increased rate of MI, stroke, venous thromboembolism, and pulmonary embolism Possible problems: dementia, gallbladder disease, hypercalcemia, visual abnormities
Miscellaneous Bone Resorption Inhibitors				
Romo- sozumab Evenity	Prevention: 210 mg SQ monthly	Vertebral[‡] Nonvertebral[†] Hip[*]	Stroke or MI in the past year Hypocalcemia Kidney disease	Osteonecrosis Headache Joint pain

[*]<40%
[†]40 to 50%
[‡]<50%
[§]No impact
[¶]No data
All doses are PO unless stated otherwise.
IV, Intravenously; *MI*, myocardial infarction; *PO*, orally; *SQ*, subcutaneously;
Modified from National Center for Health Statistics. NCHS Data Brief. No. 405. March 2021. *Osteoporosis or Low Bone Mass in Older Adults: United States, 2017–2018.* https://www.cdc.gov/nchs/data/databriefs/db405-H.pdf; Burge R, Dawson-Hughes B, Solomon DH, Wong JB, King A, Tosteson A. Incidence and economic burden of osteoporosis-related fractures in the United States, 2005–2025. *J Bone Mineral Res.* 2007;22:465–475; Camacho PM, Petak SM, Brinkley N, et al. American Association of Clinical Endocrinologists and American College of Endocrinology clinical guidelines for the diagnosis and treatment of postmenopausal osteoporosis—2016. *Endrocrine Practice.* 2016; 22(Suppl 4):1–42; Lewiecki, EM, Dinavahi, RV, Lazaretti-Castro, M, et al. One year of romosozumab followed by two years of denosumab maintains fracture risk reductions: Results of the FRAME extension study. *J Bone Mineral Res.* 2019;34(3):419–428; Allen, S, Forney-Gorman, A, Homan, M, Kearns, A, Kramlinger, A, Sauer, M. Institute for Clinical Systems Improvement. *Diagnosis and Treatment of Osteoporosis.* (2017). //www.icsi.org/wp-content/uploads/2019/01/Osteo.pdf.

(IV). The most likely adverse reaction is related to gastrointestinal problems. For maximum absorption and to minimize difficulties, the pills must be taken first thing in the morning, on an empty stomach (defined as an overnight fast) and with a full glass of water. Patients must remain upright after administration for at least 30 minutes to reduce the risk of gastrointestinal complaints. If unable to take in the oral form, some of the medications are available for IV administration. One advantage to the non-oral route is the frequency of administration. Ibandronate is given every 3 months, and zoledronic acid is given every 1 to 2 years depending on the patient's reaction to the drug. The most common adverse event reported with IV administration is flulike symptoms. It is recommended that the patient be pretreated with acetaminophen to reduce the occurrence of this side effect.[6,12,13]

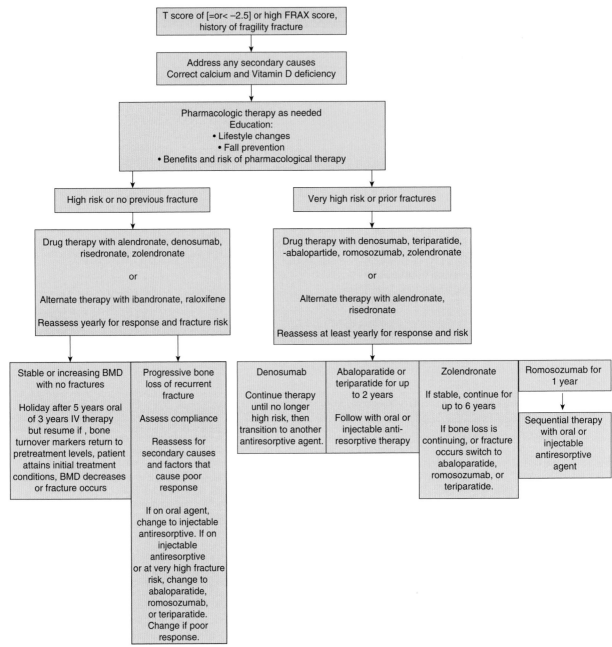

Figure 19.5 American Association of Clinical Endocrinologists/American College of Endocrinology clinical practice guidelines for the diagnoand treatment of postmenopausal osteoporosis–2020 update. (Modified from Camacho PM, Petak SM, Binkley N, et al. American Association of Clinical Endocrinologists and American College of Endocrinology Clinical Practice Guidelines for the Diagnosis and Treatment of Postmenopausal Osteoporosis—2016. Executive Summary. *Endocr Pract.* 2016;22[9]:1111–1118.)

> **CLINICAL SURVIVAL TIP** Bisphosphonates are the first-line pharmacological therapy for the treatment of osteoporosis.

Selective Estrogen Receptor Modulators. Selective estrogen receptor modulators (SERMs) are not widely tolerated by females because of the increase in vasomotor symptoms that are associated with menopause. A 6% increase in the development of hot flashes in females taking this class of drugs has been demonstrated.[1] There is, however, an advantage to using SERMs in a subset of females at risk for breast cancer. Raloxifene, the only drug in this class approved by the U.S. Food and Drug Administration (FDA), is also approved for the prevention of breast cancer; it can provide an added benefit for these patients. Raloxifene has no data to support a positive effect on hip and nonvertebral fractures, making it a better choice for prevention as opposed to treatment. There is also a quick loss of benefits when the drug is discontinued, and most of the gains in BMD are lost within 2 years of discontinuation.[6,12,13]

> **PATIENT-CENTERED CARE:** Raloxifene offers the advantage of contributing to breast cancer prevention in females at high risk for breast cancer; it may be the drug of choice for these patients for the prevention of osteoporosis.

RANK Ligand Inhibitors. This monoclonal antibody is used to reduce the development of mature osteoclasts as well as decrease the function of mature osteoclasts, thereby affecting the rate of bone turnover. It is usually used for patients who have already developed osteoporosis, and has a low side-effect/high safety profile. Because BMD returns rapidly to pretreatment levels once the medication is discontinued, it is recommended that the drug not be discontinued without providing another treatment method.[12]

Calcitonin. Calcitonin is approved for use in females who are at least 5 years postmenopausal. It has a good safety profile and can be given using multiple routes of administration; this offers additional choices for patients. Although it has a good safety profile, the efficacy profile is lower than most other treatment options.

As it has only been shown to affect vertebral fracture, it may have limited use in patients who are at increased risk for fractures. Because of hypersensitivity, it is recommended that the patient be skin tested if there is a suspicion of sensitivity to the drug.[12]

> **CLINICAL SURVIVAL TIP** If patients cannot tolerate or their symptoms do not improve with bisphosphonate therapy, a RANK ligand inhibitor or PTH can be used to prevent osteoporotic fracture.

Parathyroid Hormone. PTHs are approved for the treatment of osteoporosis. Although well tolerated, they are very expensive. PTH provides good protection against both vertebral and nonvertebral fractures; however, there is no data on protection against hip fracture. PTH increases BMD dramatically but is only approved for use for 2 years. Once 2 years has been reached and the drug is discontinued, there is a rapid decrease in BMD; it is recommended that another form of therapy be started. Most commonly, a bisphosphonate is started.[3,6,12]

> **! SAFETY ALERT**
>
> Prescribing estrogen for the prevention of osteoporosis should only be considered when other medications cannot be used and there is significant risk for development of osteoporosis.[12]

Estrogen. Estrogen is approved for the prevention of osteoporosis only and not for treatment. Data on fracture prevention and estrogen have been shown to be effective in preventing all types of fractures associated with osteoporosis. It is important to remember that a patient with an intact uterus will also need to be prescribed progestin to protect against endometrial cancer and prolonged unopposed estrogen stimulation of the endometrium. Estrogen prescribed for the management of vasomotor symptoms in early menopause has the added effect of protecting against bone loss. There is controversy regarding the use of estrogen because of possible cardiovascular and breast effects. These factors must be considered when prescribing the drug, and, as with all drugs, the risk-to-benefit ratio should be considered. When estrogen is appropriate for long-term therapy, it can be used alone or in combination with other classes of drugs used to treat osteoporosis.[6,12]

> **! SAFETY ALERT**
>
> It is important to remember that a patient with an intact uterus will also need to be prescribed progestin to protect against endometrial cancer and prolonged unopposed estrogen stimulation of the endometrium.

> **CLINICAL SURVIVAL TIP** The current recommendation is to prescribe estrogen at the lowest possible dose for the shortest period necessary.

Romosozumab. This osteoanabolic drug stimulates bone formation and inhibits bone resorption. It is given subcutaneously and can provide mild injection site reactions and hypersensitivity reactions. Romosozumab is not recommended for females who are at high risk for cardiovascular disease, especially those with a recent heart attack or stroke.[14]

> **! SAFETY ALERT**
>
> Romosozumab is not recommended for females who are at high risk for cardiovascular disease, especially those with a recent heart attack or stroke.

Combined Use of Therapies. There are little to no data on the use of more than one drug for the prevention and management of osteoporosis. Although studies have shown an additive effect on bone density, there are no studies that show an improved reduction of fractures. Because combined therapy increases the cost as well as the side-effect profile, it is not currently recommended that combined therapy be used. The exception to this is the use of combined therapy in a patient who has a suboptimal response to single-drug therapy or one who is on therapy for other reasons, such as on raloxifene for the prevention of breast cancer. In these cases, adding another agent that treats osteoporosis should be considered.[12]

Sequential Use of Therapeutic Agents. Treatment using an antiresorptive agent (denosumab, bisphosphonates, or raloxifene) is recommended after discontinuation of anabolic agents (abaloparatide, romosozumab, teriparatide) to prevent fracture efficacy and BMD loss. Additionally, it is possible to switch from a bisphosphonate to an anabolic agent; however, following denosumab with an anabolic agent is not recommended because of hip BMD loss.[15]

Long-Term Treatment. The concern with long-term treatment involves the development of osteonecrosis of the jaw and atypical femoral fracture. Osteonecrosis of the jaw is a rare condition that is associated with high-dose bisphosphonate therapy. The majority of data are from patients undergoing cancer therapy. The medication dosage for this therapy is 10 times higher than for osteoporosis therapy. Considered a rare occurrence, atypical femoral fracture is associated with a greater than 5-year treatment with bisphosphonate therapy. Both must be evaluated in relationship to the benefit of preventing the common fractures associated with osteoporosis, and the benefits outweigh the risk of the rare fractures for most patients. Other areas of concern are patients with preexisting cardiovascular disease caused by the increased risk of new-onset atrial fibrillation. Careful consideration of the drug choice can help to minimize health risk.

Bisphosphonate drugs have a cumulative effect on the bone and can provide protection after they have been discontinued. Because of this, bisphosphonate holidays can be given after 5 years of therapy. In the patient at lower risk for fracture, no other drugs are needed during the holiday, and the drug can be restarted if bone loss begins again. For patients at a high risk for fracture, it is recommended that the patient remain on therapy with these drugs for 10 years. There are no risk-to-benefit data on using these drugs beyond 10 years, but one may consider use of another drug after this time.[12] PTHs can be used for a maximum of 2 years. When discontinued, another treatment should be administered as bone loss begins within 1 year of discontinuation.[12]

Summary

Osteoporosis is a major health concern for the postmenopausal patient. For these patients, prevention begins early with the promotion of diet and exercise to maximize bone density and continues with screening. Screening for risk factors and potential occult fracture symptoms should be part of the routine care provided for female patients. When appropriate, imaging in the form of DEXA is performed and pharmacological agents are added to the universal lifestyle recommendations.

PELVIC RELAXATION SYNDROMES/PELVIC ORGAN PROLAPSE

Pelvic relaxation is a general term used to refer to problems related to a loss of muscle tone in the lower pelvic region and vagina. The term comprises a number of differing syndromes (Table 19.10).[16] Defined as a condition affecting females both during and after the reproductive years, POP causes bladder and bowel problems as well as chronic pelvic pain and has a negative impact on quality of life. Pelvic relaxation is characterized by a prolapse of the pelvic organs into the vaginal area and beyond. Most involved are the bladder (cystocele), rectum (rectocele), and uterus (uterine prolapse). Cystocele is discussed in Chapter 22 along with urinary tract problems, their most common manifestation. This chapter will provide a general overview and conservative management approaches for rectocele and uterine prolapse.

The general symptoms of POP are as follows:[17]

- Aching type of pain
  - Vagina
  - Lower back
  - Lower abdomen
  - Groin
- Pressure or heaviness in the vagina
- Feeling of "something falling out"
- Bladder control problems worsened by
  - Heavy lifting
  - Coughing
  - Sneezing
- Frequent urinary tract infections
- Difficulty with bowel movements

The symptoms presented by the patient are related to the area of prolapse as well as the severity. Table 19.11 lists the general and syndrome-specific causes of pelvic relaxation.[17,18]

> ### NOT TO BE MISSED
> Relaxation of the supportive structures of the pelvic floor leads to several syndromes known together as *POP.*

Epidemiology

More than one-third to one-half of females in the United States have a form of POP, and of these, about one-fourth have more than one.[19] By 50 years of age, one-half of all females are affected. The number of females reporting symptoms seems to be an underestimation of the females experiencing the problem. Many females are embarrassed to bring up the symptoms, so it is important to ask routine questions concerning the presence or absence of these disorders. An estimated 200,000 females undergo surgery annually to correct POP.[20] There is an 11% to 19% lifetime risk of the need for a surgical intervention for POP.[20] Because POP is more like to occur as females age, the rate of occurrence and surgery is expected to increase as the population ages.

> ### NOT TO BE MISSED
> Childbirth, aging, and lack of estrogen are major factors that affect the pathophysiology of POP.

Pathophysiology

The pathophysiology of POP is related to a weakening of both the muscles and ligaments that support the pelvic floor. The muscular support of the pelvis is the pelvic diaphragm, and the major muscles are the levator ani and the coccygeus muscle. Any weakness in these muscles can lead to prolapse of the interior structures into

TABLE 19.10	Definition of Pelvic Organ Prolapse[16]
Cystocele	Herniation of the bladder against the anterior vaginal wall with possible protrusion into the vaginal canal. The bladder may be visible in the vaginal opening.
Cysto-urethrocele	Herniation of the bladder neck as well as the bladder into the anterior vaginal wall.
Rectocele	Herniation of the lower segment of the large intestine against the posterior vaginal wall with possible protrusion into the vaginal canal. If it includes the small intestine, it is called an *enterocele.*
Uterine prolapse	Descent of the uterus into the vaginal canal. May descend to outside of the vagina.
Vaginal prolapse	Bulging of the top portion of the vagina into the lower vagina.

TABLE 19.11 Causes of Pelvic Relaxation[17,18]		
General	**Rectocele**	**Uterine Prolapse**
Childbirth	Chronic constipation	Pelvic tumors
Vaginal delivery	Increased intraabdominal pressure	Fibroids
Obesity		
Aging/menopause		
Injury caused by pelvic surgery		
Chronic straining		
Chronic obstructive pulmonary disease		
Asthma		
Reactive airway disease		
Congenital weakness of the pelvic support system		
Spinal cord injury		
Muscular atrophy conditions		
Race (higher in White individuals)		

the vagina and beyond. Further support is provided to the female pelvic organs by a group of ligaments. The broad ligament is a flat sheet of peritoneum that supports the uterus, fallopian tubes, and ovaries. It extends from the lateral pelvic walls on both sides and encloses the internal female organs completely. The broad ligament is divided into the following three sections:

- The *mesometrium* surrounds the uterus and is the largest subsection of the broad ligament.
- The *mesovarium* is associated with the ovaries.
- The *mesosalpinx* is associated with the fallopian tubes.

The round ligament originates at the uterine horns and attaches to the labia majora, passing through the inguinal canal. Because of its location, pelvic pain may develop as the uterus descends and causes increased pressure on the ligament. The cardinal ligaments originate from the side of the cervix and the lateral vaginal fornix. They attach on the lateral pelvic wall at the level of the ischial spines, providing uterine support laterally. The uterosacral ligaments are bilateral fibrous tissue bands that attach the cervix to the sacrum, thus providing support to help hold the uterus in place. The pubocervical ligaments are also bilateral and attach the cervix to the posterior surface of the pubic symphysis. This further supports the uterus within the pelvic cavity.[21] These supporting structures have the following functions:[20]

- Support pelvic organs
- Prevent urinary and fecal leakage
- Prevent POP
- Help regulate abdominal pressure
- Enhance sexual function and pleasure

In the normal individual, the pelvic floor supports much of the weight of the pelvic organs, and the pelvic ligaments stabilize these structures. When the levator ani is damaged and unable to adequately support the weight of the pelvic organs, an increased amount of pressure is placed on the ligaments. The ligaments are not designed to carry this increased load, and they weaken over time, allowing the bladder, rectum, small bowel, or uterus to descend into the vagina. This resulting prolapse of pelvic structures leads to the syndromes associated with pelvic relaxation.[22] Fig. 19.6 demonstrates various POPs.

Diagnosis and Screening for Pelvic Organ Prolapse

One of the most important diagnostic tools is a thorough history. When evaluating for POP, it is important to take a history that includes the signs and symptoms of all syndromes associated with pelvic relaxation. Table 19.12 lists the symptoms that are common to all presentations of POP and those that are specific to either uterine prolapse or rectocele.

Physical examination is the same for all POP syndromes. The examination should include an abdominal examination to exclude an abdominal or pelvic tumor responsible for the prolapse. The pelvic examination is used not only to determine the presence of POP but also to access the severity of the problem. The external genitalia is examined, and it should be noted if any of the internal structures are visible. If not visible on the first inspection, the labia should be separated and reassessed for internal structures. Again, if no internal structures

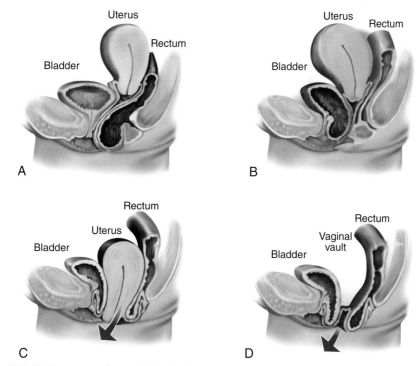

Figure 19.6 Pelvic organ prolapse. A. Rectocele (rectal prolapse). B. Cystocele (bladder prolapse). C. Uterine prolapse. D. Vaginal vault prolapse. (From Badylak S. *Host Response to Biomaterials: The Impact of Host Response on Biomaterial Selection.* Waltham, MA: Academic Press; 2015: XX.)

TABLE 19.12 Signs and Symptoms of Pelvic Organ Prolapse[18,23]

General	Uterine Prolapse	Rectocele
Pelvic pressure and fullness	Mass of budging in the vagina	Difficulty with defecation
Perception of something falling out	Feel as if sitting on a small ball	Constipation
Bearing down sensation	Low back pain	Fecal incontinence
Symptoms worsen when standing or	Tissue protrusion from the vagina	Incomplete empting of the rectum
lifting and improve when lying down	Recurrent urinary tract infections	Straining to defecate
Pain with intercourse	Unusual vaginal discharge	Manual assistance with defecation
	Urinary retention	

are seen with this assessment, have the patient bear down, and observe if any of the tissues become visible. It is also important to note the presence or absence of urine or fecal leakage.

Once the external examination is complete, a vaginal examination is performed. Visualization of the vagina for the presence or absence of prolapse is best accomplished with a single-blade (Sims) speculum. This allows for a clear view of the vaginal wall and complete visualization of any abnormalities. To retract

the anterior wall and better visualize the posterior wall, the clinician places the blade against the anterior vaginal wall and then presses upward with gentle traction. The presence of a rectocele is noted by bulging of the posterior vaginal wall. Once the wall is inspected with the patient relaxed and the presence or absence of a bulge is noted, have the patient bear down, and note any changes that occur.[23]

To evaluate for a cystocele, the clinician repeats the procedure on the posterior wall of the vagina. The cervix should be clearly visualized to assess for uterine prolapse. If this cannot be done with the single-blade speculum, use a double-blade speculum, and again note the cervical position with the patient both relaxed and while bearing down.[24] The degree of prolapse is then determined and recorded (Table 19.13).[25,26]

A bimanual examination is performed to help determine both vaginal tone and degree of prolapse. To begin the examination, the patient is instructed to squeeze the clinician's fingers once they are inserted in the vagina. The clinician should note the firmness of the muscle grip on the fingers. The clinician then palpates the vaginal walls for the presence or absence of a bulge and determines its location. Then the location of the cervix is determined in relationship to the hymeneal ring. The findings should be described, and the assessment should include not only the presence or absence of POP, but the severity of the disorder. There are no routine laboratory or imaging studies required. Further workup is based on presenting symptoms and the necessity to rule out other problems.

> **CLINICAL SURVIVAL TIP** The use of a single-blade speculum provides the most accurate information for diagnosing cystoceles and rectoceles.

Treatment

Treatment of POP is based on the severity of symptoms. Conservative treatment consists of lifestyle changes, pelvic floor muscle training, and mechanical support. If the condition worsens or conservative treatment does not improve symptoms and patient quality of life, the patient should be referred for surgical repair. Referral is indicated for stage 4 prolapse or if symptoms of the disorder are contributing to poor quality of life. Referral should be made any time the patient requests an evaluation for surgical repair or the POP has led to complications.

> **CLINICAL SURVIVAL TIP** Treatment is based on symptoms and the degree of impact on quality of life.

> **PATIENT-CENTERED CARE:** Conservative management is recommended in patients who do not fit the criteria for surgery or are poor surgical risks.

Lifestyle Changes. The major lifestyle change that can affect the symptoms of POP is weight loss. Obesity, especially abdominal obesity, leads to increased intraabdominal pressure, which can lead to worsening of the POP. The loss of any amount of weight can improve symptoms as well as slow the progression of the prolapse. Return to normal BMI is ideal, but any amount of weight loss can benefit the patient. Symptoms can also be improved by avoiding or controlling anything that increases the symptoms. The patient should avoid straining and heavy lifting as well as treat any chronic coughing. Of course, if the coughing is caused by smoking, education and assistance in smoking cessation are warranted. Lifestyle change alone may be enough for the management of mild POP.

Pelvic Floor Muscle Training. Along with other lifestyle changes, exercise is also important. Pelvic floor exercises help strengthen the muscle and control the symptoms. Kegel exercises are used to strengthen the pelvic floor muscles and should be taught to the patient. There are many ways to teach Kegel exercises, and patients should begin early as they may also help to prevent POP. To perform Kegel exercises, instruct the patient to first tense the muscles in the pelvic floor for

TABLE 19.13 **Staging for Pelvic Organ Prolapse**[25,26]	
Baden Walker System	**POP-Quantification System**
Grade Description	*Grade Description*
0: Normal position at the site	0: No prolapse
1: Descent halfway to the hymen	1: >1 cm above the hymen
2: Descent to the hymen	2: <1 cm proximal or distal to the hymen
3: Descent halfway past the hymen	3: >1 cm below the plane of the hymen, but no further than 2 cm less than the length of the vagina
4: Maximal descent for the site	4: Complete vaginal eversion

a count of 3, and then relax them for a count of 3. Ten repetitions are considered a set.

The goal is to increase the amount of time the muscles can be held tense. As muscle strength improves, the count is held longer for a count of 10. The goal should be to complete three sets of ten repetitions every day. Biofeedback, electrical stimulation, and vaginal weights can be used along with Kegel exercises to enhance muscle strength.

Biofeedback for pelvic floor muscle retraining helps patients improve the strength of pelvic floor muscles and has been shown to improve bowel or bladder function related to POP. To provide electrical stimulation, electrodes are placed close against a muscle, and a current is passed to stimulate contraction of the muscles. The electrical stimulation can artificially activate muscle fibers to contract. This assists the weak pelvic floor muscles to tighten. Biofeedback is used when a patient has trouble voluntarily contracting the muscle. It can also assist with the ability to hold the contraction longer, thus helping increase muscle strength.

Vaginal weights are also used to aid in the development and effectiveness of pelvic floor strengthening. Weights are placed in the vagina. Then the patient is instructed to perform Kegel exercises and to try to lift the weight toward the top of the vagina. Once this is accomplished in the recumbent position, the patient can try standing and perform the lift against gravity.

> **CLINICAL SURVIVAL TIP** Patients can be referred to a physical therapist for help with pelvic floor conditioning.

Mechanical Support. Mechanical support is provided with the use of a pessary. The purpose of the pessary is to restore the prolapsed organ to its normal anatomical position. Several different types of pessaries are available. Information on the different types of pessaries can be found in Chapter 22.

The patient must be fitted for a pessary. The size and type of pessary required is determined during the vaginal examination. Pessaries with a supportive function, such as ring pessaries, are used for stages I and II POP, while space-filling pessaries, such as cube pessaries, are used for stages III and IV POP.[27] Figure 19.7 describes the considerations based on clinical experience that may be used to help determine the appropriate pessary to prescribe.[25] Many times it is a matter of trial and error; if the patient has trouble with one type of pessary, another can be tried.

When fitting a pessary, the clinician must follow the following steps:
- Ensure that the bladder is empty.
- Ensure that a finger can be swept between the pessary and the wall of the vagina.
- Fit the patient with the largest pessary that does not cause discomfort.
- Have the patient walk around and void to ensure that the pessary is a proper fit and does not fall out or cause urinary retention.[26]

Patients who are able to remove and reinsert the pessary on their own will have the choice to remove it weekly for cleaning. It can be cleaned with soap and water and replaced in the vagina. Although not mandatory with all pessaries, sexually active patients may prefer to remove the pessary before intercourse. There is no consensus on the follow-up regimen, and it may vary depending on the following:[26]
- Patient's ability to remove and insert the pessary
- Extent of prolapse
- Health of the vaginal epithelium

> **CLINICAL SURVIVAL TIP** There are many shapes and sizes of pessaries available to help the clinician provide individual care.

There is no consensus on how often the patient should be seen, but a follow-up examination should be performed in 2 to 3 weeks to assess how the pessary is performing. The clinician should always ask about vaginal discharge, pain, bleeding, or any discomfort as well as difficulty removing and replacing the pessary. The clinician should remove the pessary and assess the vaginal wall for lesions. If present, the pessary must be discontinued until the vaginal lesion heals. If the patient is doing well, a checkup every 6 to 12 months is warranted.

When the pessary cannot be removed regularly by the patient, follow-up examinations are usually performed at 2- to 3-month intervals. At these visits, the pessary is removed. Along with a vaginal examination to check for lesions and bruising, the pessary is examined for discoloration, cracking, and deformation. It is cleaned and replaced in the vagina.[26-28] Although they are rare, side effects and complications can be seen with a pessary. The most common side effects include vaginal discharge and odor. These should be managed, and if recurrent, the pessary should be taken out and cleaned

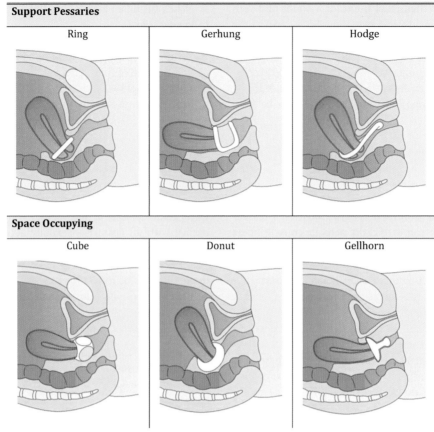

Figure 19.7 Different types of support and space-occupying pessaries. (From Oliver R, Thakar R, Sultan AH. The history and usage of the vaginal pessary: a review. *Eur J Obstet Gynecol Reprod Biol.* 2011;156[2]:125–130.)

more frequently to determine if this decreases the symptoms. Serious complications from pessaries are rare and include the following:[28]

- Vesicovaginal fistula
- Rectovaginal fistula
- Erosion
- Impaction
- Vaginal strictures

Serious complications should be referred for treatment.

Summary

With the aging population, both osteoporosis and POP are conditions that are frequently seen by the clinician in a primary care office. Knowing how to assess and provide first-line treatment is essential to the provision of the female patient's health. As important as treatment, providing referrals to patients is an integral part of primary care management. There are several points to remember when assess and treating these disorders.

KEY POINTS

- Osteoporosis
  - Osteoporosis is a silent disease that affects 1 in 6 females.
  - All females should be assessed for risk factors, and bone health lifestyle changes should be encouraged.

- The goal of treatment is bone preservation and fall prevention.
- Screening with DEXA should begin at 65 years of age in low-risk females and earlier if risk factors are present.

- Adequate calcium and vitamin D intake and weight-bearing exercise should be discussed with all female patients as preventive measures against bone loss.
- All drug therapy must be accompanied with lifestyle changes to maximize therapeutic effect.
- Bisphosphonates are the first-line pharmacological therapy for the treatment of osteoporosis.
- POP
  - POP is cause by a weakening in the support structures of the pelvis.
  - POP is prolapse of the bladder, rectum, uterus, and or vagina.
  - These may occur together or alone.
  - By 50 years of age, 50% of females have some degree of POP, which can affect quality of life.
  - Ask about signs and symptoms of POP at routine visits as many patients feel uncomfortable bringing up the subject.
  - There are multiple approaches to the nonsurgical treatment of POP, and these should be offered to patients.
  - If the treatment cannot be successfully done in the primary care setting, the clinician should refer the patient for specialized care.
  - Musculoskeletal problems for females provide a challenge for primary care clinicians, and assessment for treatment or referral is a part of routine care.

REFERENCES

1. National Center for Health Statistics. NCHS Data Brief. No. 405. March 2021. *Osteoporosis or Low Bone Mass in Older Adults: United States, 2017–2018.* https://www.cdc.gov/nchs/data/databriefs/db405-H.pdf.
2. Bone Health and Osteoporosis Foundation. What Women Need to Know. https://www.nof.org/preventing-fractures/general-facts/what-women-need-to-know/.
3. Chesnut 3rd CH, Silverman S, Andriano K, et al. A randomized trial of nasal spray salmon calcitonin in postmenopausal women with established osteoporosis: the prevent recurrence of osteoporotic fractures study. PROOF Study Group. *Am J Med.* 2000;109:267–276.
4. Ettinger B, Black DM, Mitlak BH, et al. Reduction of vertebral fracture risk in postmenopausal women with osteoporosis treated with raloxifene: results from a 3-year randomized clinical trial. Multiple Outcomes of Raloxifene Evaluation (MORE) Investigators. *J Am Med Assoc.* 1999;282:637–645.
5. Burge R, Dawson-Hughes B, Solomon DH, Wong JB, King A, Tosteson A. Incidence and economic burden of osteoporosis-related fractures in the United States, 2005–2025. *J Bone Mineral Res.* 2007;22:465–475.
6. Cosman F, deBeur SJ, LeBoff MS, et al. Clinician's guide to prevention and treatment of osteoporosis. *Osteoporosis Int.* 2014;25(10):2359–2381.
7. Kanis JA, Hans D, Cooper C, et al. Interpretation and use of FRAX in clinical practice. *Osteoporosis Int.* 2011;22:2395–2411.
8. Watts NB, Lewiecki EM, Miller PD, Baim S. National osteoporosis Foundation 2008 clinicians' guide to prevention and treatment of osteoporosis and the World health organization fracture risk assessment tool (FRAX): what they mean to the bone densitometrist and bone technologist. *J Clin Densitom.* 2008;11(4):473–477.
9. Sweet MG, Sweet JM, Jeremiah MP, Galazka SS. Diagnosis and treatment of osteoporosis. *Am Family Physician.* 2009;79(3):93–200.
10. Bethel M. *Osteoporosis. Practice Essentials.* Medscape; 2017. Updated January 20, 2021 http://emedicine.medscape.com/article/330598-overview.
11. Kanis JA, Delmas P, Burckhardt C, et al. Guidelines for diagnosis and management of osteoporosis. *Osteoporosis Int.* 1997;7:390–406.
12. Camacho PM, Petak SM, Brinkley N, et al. American Association of Clinical Endocrinologists and American College of Endocrinology clinical guidelines for the diagnosis and treatment of postmenopausal osteoporosis—2020 update. *Endocrine Practice.* 2020;26(5):564–570.
13. Medstar Health. *Osteoporosis: Screening and Managment. Clinical Practice Guidelines.* 2021. www.medstarfamilychoicedc.com/-/media/project/mho/mfcdc/pdf/clinical-practice-guidelines/osteoporosis-screening-and-management-final-october-2021.pdf.
14. Management of Osteoporosis in Postmenopausal Women: The 2021 Position Statement of The North American Menopause Society Editorial Panel. Management of osteoporosis in postmenopausal women: the 2021 position statement of the North American Menopause Society. *Menopause.* 2021;28(9):973–997.
15. Camacho PM, Petak SM, Binkley N, et al. American association of clinical Endocrinologists/American College of Endocrinology clinical practice guidelines for the diagnosis and treatment of postmenopausal osteoporosis—2020 update. *Endocr Pract.* 2020;26(5):564–570.
16. Gale Encyclopedia of Medicine. *Pelvic Relaxation.* The Gale Group; 2008.
17. McNeely SG. *Overview of Pelvic Organ Prolapse.* Merck Manuals; 2022. https://www.merckmanuals.com/professional/gynecology-and-obstetrics/pelvic-organ-prolapse-pop/?autoredirectid=1135.

18. Barsoom RS, Sinert RH. *Uterine Prolapse in Emergency Medicine Treatment & Management.* Medscape; 2018. https://emedicine.medscape.com/article/797295-treatment.

19. Lawrence JM, Lukacz ES, Nager CW, Hsu JW, Luber KM. Prevalence and co-occurrence of pelvic floor disorders in community-dwelling women. *Obstet Gynecol.* 2008;111(3):678–685.

20. Rogers RG, Fashokun TB. *Pelvic Organ Prolapse in Females: Epidemiology, Risk Factors, Clinical Manifestations, and Management.* UpToDate; 2022. https://www.uptodate.com/contents/pelvic-organ-prolapse-in-females-epidemiology-risk-factors-clinical-manifestations-and-management.

21. Whitehead C. *Ligaments of the Female Reproductive Tract.* Teach Me Anatomy; 2016. http://teachmeanatomy.info/pelvis/female-reproductive-tract/ligaments/.

22. Cespedes RD, Cross CA, McGuire EJ. Pelvic prolapse: diagnosing and treating cystoceles, rectoceles, and enteroceles. *Medsc Wom Health.* 1998;3(4):3.

23. Shaw HA. *Rectocele.* Medscape; 2017. Updated July 15, 2022 http://emedicine.medscape.com/article/268546-overview.

24. Fashokun, TB, Rogers, RG. (2023). Pelvic organ prolapse in women: Diagnostic evaluation. https://www.uptodate.com/contents/pelvic-organ-prolapse-in-women-diagnostic-evaluation.

25. Kuncharapu I, Majeroni BA, Johnson DW. Pelvic organ prolapse. *Am Family Physician.* 2010;81(9):1111–1117.

26. Doshani A, Teo RE, Mayne CJ, Tincello DG. Uterine prolapse. *Br Med J.* 2007;335(7624):819–823.

27. Choi KW, Hong JY. Management of pelvic organ prolapse. *Korean J Urol.* 2014;55(11):693–702.

28. Jones KA, Harmanli O. Pessary use in pelvic organ prolapse and urinary incontinence. *Rev Obstet Gynecol.* 2010;3(1):3–9.

29. Gronholz MJP. Diagnosis and management of osteoporosis-related fracture: a multifactorial osteopathic approach. *J Am Osteopathic Assoc.* 2008;108:575–585.

30. Elam, EW. (2022). *Osteoporosis workup.* https://emedicine.medscape.com/article/330598-worku.

31. American College of Obstetricians and Gynecologists' Committee on Clinical Practice Guidelines–Gynecology. Osteoporosis prevention, screening, and diagnosis: ACOG clinical practice guideline No. 1. *Obstetrics Gynecol.* 2021;138(3):494–506.

32. National Osteoporosis Foundation. *Health Care Professionals Toolkit*; 2019. https://static1.squarespace.com/static/5d7aabc5368b54332c55df72/t/5dd2e2a92e1e1821e328308e/1574101724294/HCP+Toolkit-with+graphics.pdf.

33. Prescribing Information for Abaloparatide. *Radius Health Inc*; 2017. https://www.accessdata.fda.gov/drugsatfda_docs/label/2017/208743lbl.pdf.

34. Lewiecki EM, Dinavahi RV, Lazaretti-Castro M, et al. One year of romosozumab followed by two years of denosumab maintains fracture risk reductions: results of the FRAME extension study. *J Bone Mineral Res.* 2019;34(3):419–428.

35. Centers for Disease Control and Prevention. (2017). *Risk factors for falls (Fact sheet).* https://www.cdc.gov/steadi/pdf/steadi-factsheet-riskfactors-508.pdf.

36. National Institutes of Health, National Institute on Aging. (n.d.). *Six Tips To Help Prevent Falls.* https://www.nia.nih.gov/health/infographics/six-tips-help-prevent-falls.

37. An Assessment Tool for Predicting Fracture Risk in postmenopausal women D. M. Black, M. Steinbuch, L. Palermo, P. Dargent-Molina, R. Lindsay, M. S. Hoseyni &O. Johnell in *Osteoporosis International.* (2001).12, 519–528.

20

Reproductive Cancers

Aimee Chism Holland

OBJECTIVES

- Identify gynecological cancer types diagnosed in females across the lifespan.
- Develop a plan for screening for gynecological cancers based on current guidelines.

- Translate risk factors, signs, and symptoms associated with common gynecological cancers into a plan of care.
- Examine current treatment options for gynecological cancers.

INTRODUCTION

Cancer occurs when abnormal cells grow and divide in the body. *Metastasis* is the term used to describe the process of abnormal cells spreading to different parts of the body. The location where cancer cells originate is used to differentiate the name given for a specific cancer diagnosis. For example, if a cancer cell originated in the ovary but spread to the surrounding organs and tissues, then it is called *ovarian cancer*. Although the exact cause of gynecological cancers is not always known, factors associated with genetics, behavior, and the environment can influence a patient's risk of developing these cancers. The prognosis is optimal, and treatment is most effective when the cancer is diagnosed in an early stage. Prevention is key; therefore the goal of the clinician should be preventive care.

NOT TO BE MISSED

Prognosis is optimal, and treatment is most effective when cancer is diagnosed in an early stage.

The three most common cancers in females in the United States include breast cancer, lung cancer, and colorectal cancer.[1] More females are diagnosed with breast cancer than any other cancer, followed by lung

cancer and then colorectal cancer.[1] More females die from lung cancer, followed by breast cancer and then colorectal cancer.[1]

Gynecological cancer is the term used to describe a cancer that develops in a female's reproductive organ. There are five types of gynecological cancers, which we will describe in this chapter. These include cervical, endometrial, ovarian, vulvar, and vaginal cancers. Breast cancer is not considered a gynecological cancer because it does not originate in a female reproductive organ.

CLINICAL SURVIVAL TIP
Breast cancer is not considered a gynecological cancer because it does not originate in a female reproductive organ.

The American College of Obstetricians and Gynecologists (ACOG) recommends performing a hereditary cancer risk assessment to identify individuals at increased risk of developing certain types of gynecological cancers.[2] The Society of Gynecologic Oncology (SGO) recommends offering genetic counseling to individuals with a known risk for inherited predisposition to cancer. The purpose of genetic counseling and genetic testing is to help improve cancer prevention and early detection. The SGO published the Genetics Toolkit in 2016 for health care providers to determine who should be referred for genetic counseling.[3]

Once a patient is diagnosed with a gynecological cancer, a referral to a gynecology oncologist or general oncologist is necessary to determine if it has spread. This process is referred to as *staging*. Staging helps determine the best treatment for optimal prognosis based on current research. Staging is determined based on two different systems. The FIGO system is based on the International Federation of Gynecology and Obstetrics guidelines,[4] and the tumor, nodes, and metastasis (TNM) system is based on the American Joint Committee on Cancer guidelines.[5]

> **CLINICAL SURVIVAL TIP** The FIGO system is based on the International Federation of Gynecology and Obstetrics guidelines, and the TNM system is based on the American Joint Committee on Cancer guidelines.

CERVICAL CANCER

Cervical cancer is defined as cancer cells that originate in the cervix. There are three main types of cervical cancer. These include squamous cell carcinoma, adenocarcinoma, and mixed adenosquamous carcinoma. Squamous cell carcinoma is the most common type of cervical cancer, accounting for 80% to 90% of cervical cancer cases diagnosed. Adenocarcinoma is diagnosed in 10% to 12% of cases.[6] Mixed adenosquamous carcinoma is rarely diagnosed.

No female in the United States should die from cervical cancer because it is a preventable cancer.[6] Cervical cancer is considered a cancer that can be successfully treated when it is diagnosed early.[6] The primary cause of cervical cancer is human papillomavirus (HPV). Persistent HPV infections lead to cervical intraepithelial neoplasia (CIN) that can develop into cervical cancer. The most common high-risk HPV types associated with the majority of cervical cancer cases include strands 16 and 18.[6] HPV 16 and HPV 18 account for 70% of cervical cancer and CIN cases.[6] HPV can be prevented with vaccination. More than 90% of cervical neoplasia cases arise in the squamous cells of the transformation zone (SCJ),[14] the area of the cervix where squamous cells and columnar cells meet.

> **NOT TO BE MISSED**
>
> Cervical cancer is preventable and can be successfully treated when diagnosed early. The primary cause of cervical cancer is HPV.

Cervical cancer is most commonly diagnosed in females with a median age of 50 years.[23] The highest incidence of cervical cancer in the United States is found in Caucasian females followed by Hispanic females (Fig. 20.1).[8]

> **CLINICAL SURVIVAL TIP** Risks factors for HPV, CIN, and cervical cancer include the following:[6]
> - Early age of sexual debut
> - Early age with first full-term pregnancy (<17 years of age)
> - Cigarette smoking
> - Immunosuppression
> - In utero diethylstilbestrol (DES) exposure
> - Prior abnormal cervical cytology
> - Multiple sex partners or sex partner with multiple partners
> - No condom use with coitus
> - Overweight or obesity
> - Diet low in fruits and vegetables
> - Long-term oral contraceptive pill use
> - Intrauterine device use
> - Low socioeconomic status
> - Family history of cervical cancer
> - Not following cervical cancer screening guidelines

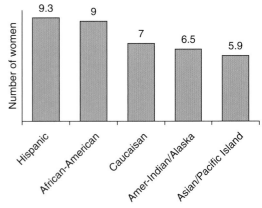

Figure 20.1 Cervical cancer statistics (race per 100,000 women). (Data from U.S. Cancer Statistics Working Group. *U.S. Cancer Statistics Data Visualizations Tool*, based on 2020 submission data (1999–2018): U.S. Department of Health and Human Services, Centers for Disease Control and Prevention and National Cancer Institute; June 2021. www.cdc.gov/cancer/dataviz.)

Signs and symptoms of cervical cancer vary with each stage of the diagnosis. During the early stage of cervical cancer, patients are usually asymptomatic. During the middle stages, patients may observe abnormal vaginal bleeding and malodorous discharge. Signs and symptoms are most observable during the later stages and include pelvic pain, back pain, bladder pain, fatigue, anemia secondary to heavy bleeding, weight loss, anorexia, constipation, malodorous discharge, and lower extremity edema. The cervix changes in appearance with the progression of cervical cancer. A healthy, nonpregnant cervix will appear firm and does not bleed when touched. However, with cervical cancer the appearance and firmness changes to one that easily bleeds and is spongy or soft to the touch.

The American Society for Colposcopy and Cervical Pathology (ASCCP), ACOG, the American Cancer Society (ACS), and the American Society for Clinical Pathology published the most current cervical cancer screening recommendations in 2012. Table 20.1 includes the screening guidelines for females across the lifespan.[9]

If the Pap test is abnormal, appropriate follow-up and possibly further evaluation is needed based on the patient's age, Pap test results, and if cotesting with HPV was performed. The ASCCP algorithms for management of abnormal cervical cancer screening tests are recommended for managing abnormal Pap test results.[10] Colposcopy may be indicated for the following abnormal Pap smear findings:[11]

- Unsatisfactory results with HPV identified
- Negative results with HPV identified in females 30 years of age and older
- Atypical squamous cells of undetermined significance (ASC-US) results with HPV identified
- Atypical squamous cells, cannot rule out high-grade squamous intraepithelial lesion (ASC-H) results
- Low-grade squamous intraepithelial lesion (LSIL) results
- High-grade squamous intraepithelial lesion (HSIL) results
- Atypical glandular cells (AGC) results

Colposcopy is the standard of care for screening the cervix when a Pap test identifies abnormal cells. A colposcopy is a procedure that may include one or more cervical biopsies along with an endocervical curettage. A colposcope magnifies abnormal cells so a biopsy site can be identified. The primary purpose of colposcopy is to detect and treat abnormal cervical cells before they progress to cervical cancer.[12] A colposcopy is recommended with abnormal cytology screening and the presence of high-risk HPV types. This procedure is performed based on abnormal cervical cytology management guidelines published by the ASCCP. Clinicians often use the smart phone application version of the ASCCP algorithms to manage abnormal Pap test and colposcopy findings.

> **CLINICAL SURVIVAL TIP** A colposcopy is recommended with abnormal cytology screening and the presence of high-risk HPV types.

TABLE 20.1   Cervical Cancer Screening Guidelines[9,22]

Age Range	Screening Recommendation
Younger than 21 years of age	Do not screen for cervical cancer.
21–29 years of age or ≥25 years of age	Perform a Pap test (cytology) every 3 years. Perform high-risk HPV testing every 3 years.
30–64 years of age	Perform cotesting with Pap test and HPV screen every 5 years (preferred) or cytology alone every 3 years (acceptable)
≥65 years of age	Stop screening if there are adequate prior negative cytology reports.

HPV, Human papillomavirus

Cervical tissue biopsies are referred to as *histology pathology.* Histology pathology findings are considered the gold standard of care for diagnosing cervical cancer. Cervical cancer is clinically staged based on clinical examination instead of surgical findings.

Clinicians can attend a comprehensive colposcopy course to learn the basic steps for performing colposcopy-guided procedures. After attending an initial workshop, preceptor guidance should be utilized until demonstrating competency. Advanced practice nurses should consult with each State Board of Nursing to confirm approved procedures and requirements for performing them.

The oncologist determines which treatment the patient requires. Future fertility desires are considered when the treatment is planned.

ENDOMETRIAL CANCER

Endometrial cancer is defined as a malignancy that originates in the endometrium of the uterus. It is most commonly diagnosed in postmenopausal females in their early 60s. However, the diagnosis has been made in females across the lifespan following the initiation of menstruation with ongoing unopposed estrogen exposure. Incidence rates for endometrial cancer are highest in White females followed by African-American females.[13] However, mortality rates are highest in African-American females followed by White females.[13]

Educating patients about risk factors and preventive measures is an important role of the clinician.

Lynch syndrome is a rare autosomal genetic disorder associated with an increased risk for endometrial, colorectal, and ovarian cancers.[8] Between 5% and 9% of females younger than 50 years of age who are diagnosed with endometrial cancer also have a diagnosis of Lynch syndrome.[8] The ACOG recommends collecting an endometrial biopsy every 1 to 2 years starting between 30 and 35 years of age for females diagnosed with Lynch

syndrome.[2] An endometrial biopsy should also be collected when changes in routine menstrual cycle patterns are observed.[8] In addition, the ACOG recommends that females with Lynch syndrome undergo prophylactic hysterectomy and bilateral salpingo-oophorectomy once childbearing is completed and a colonoscopy every 1 to 2 years starting at 20 years of age.[8]

Cowden syndrome is another autosomal dominant condition associated with an increased lifetime risk for endometrial cancer.[2] Cowden syndrome is also a risk factor for developing breast and thyroid cancers.[2] Peutz-Jeghers syndrome is another rare condition associated with an increased risk of endometrial cancer. It is also associated with an increased risk of cervical, breast, and colon cancers.[2]

Preventive measures of endometrial cancer include using contraceptive measures, maintaining a healthy body weight, and prescribing progesterone with estrogen in menopausal females taking hormone therapy. In young females with a diagnosis of polycystic ovarian syndrome (PCOS), ensure that routine menses take place. In menopausal females taking hormone therapy, ensure that they receive combined estrogen and progesterone treatment. Educate all patients to return for evaluation with irregular spotting or bleeding, especially postmenopausal patients.

Signs and symptoms of endometrial cancer include postmenopausal bleeding, abnormal uterine bleeding (AUB) in reproductive-age females, intermittent vaginal spotting, unusual vaginal discharge, pelvic pain, or an enlarged uterus.

Currently, there are no routine screening guidelines or tests specifically for endometrial cancer evaluation as there are for breast and cervical cancers. The definitive screening tests used to diagnose endometrial cancer include endometrial biopsy and/or hysteroscopy with dilation and curettage (D&C).

The endometrial biopsy is a very successful office procedure for detecting endometrial cancer if an adequate amount of tissue is collected (Fig. 20.2). Additional testing is recommended if an inadequate tissue sample is collected, if there are inconsistencies observed between the biopsy and imaging, or if symptoms persist despite a negative biopsy result.[15]

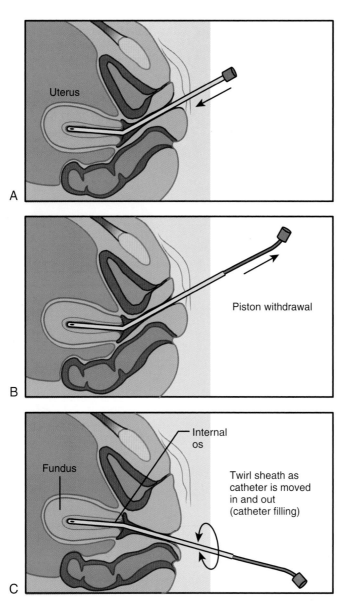

Figure 20.2 Endometrial biopsy. **A,** Pipelle is inserted into the uterus through the cervical os (curve in pipelle as drawn is exaggerated in this flexible instrument). **B,** Withdraw piston to create a vacuum for suctioning tissue. **C,** Twirling and moving catheter 2-3cm within uterine cavity (without withdrawing from uterus) allows tissue to be dislodged and vacuum draws tissue into pipelle for collection. (Redrawn with permission from Renee L. Cannon.)

A hysteroscopy with D&C is considered the gold standard for assessing AUB and diagnosing endometrial cancer because it provides a more comprehensive sample of the uterine lining compared with endometrial biopsy. A D&C procedure should be considered in patients whose office endometrial biopsy is negative or inadequate, endometrial thickness is 5 mm or greater in postmenopausal females, or when there is a high suspicion of malignancy.[15]

A pelvic ultrasound examination and a Pap test can be helpful for identifying risk factors associated with endometrial cancer but are not considered screening tests for it. An endometrial stripe thickness greater than 5 mm observed on ultrasonography in a menopausal patient is considered indicative for further evaluation.[15] Endometrial cells in postmenopausal patients and AGCs present on a Pap test are other reasons for further evaluation of endometrial cancer. Neither of these tests should be ordered to make the diagnosis of endometrial cancer.

Surgery remains the primary treatment option for endometrial cancer. For patients with an invasive tumor, an aggressive histological subtype, and/or advanced stage, adjuvant treatment in the form of either chemotherapy or radiation therapy may be necessary. Future fertility desires are considered when the treatment is planned.

NOT TO BE MISSED

Treatment for endometrial cancer may consist of the following options:
- Progesterone hormone therapy
- Surgery: total abdominal hysterectomy with bilateral salpingo-oophorectomy (TAH-BSO)
- Radiation therapy
- Chemotherapy

PATIENT-CENTERED CARE: When considering treatment options for endometrial cancer, the patients' fertility desires must be considered.

OVARIAN CANCER

Ovarian cancer is a malignancy that originates in the ovaries. It is the most lethal type of the reproductive cancers with the highest mortality rate. Postmenopausal White females are predominantly diagnosed with ovarian cancer. Epithelial-type ovarian cancer accounts for the majority of diagnosed cases.[16] Other types of ovarian cancer types include germ cell, stromal cell, and nonspecific mesenchymal type.

NOT TO BE MISSED

Ovarian cancer is the most lethal type of the reproductive cancers with the highest mortality rate.

Ovarian cancer is difficult to diagnose in an early stage because there are subtle signs and symptoms experienced (Fig. 20.3). For this reason, educating patients about protective measures, risk factors, and signs and symptoms of ovarian cancer is imperative.

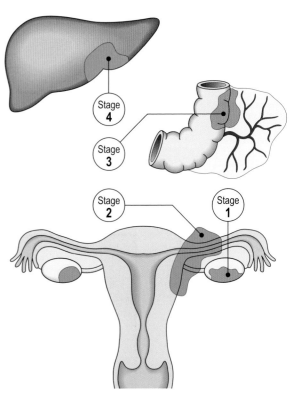

Figure 20.3 Ovarian cancer staging. Stage 1: The tumor is limited to the ovary. Stage 2: There is involvement of other pelvic structures. Stage 3: Intraabdominal spread beyond the pelvis occurs. Stage 4: Distant metastases occurs. (From Cross SS. *Underwood's Pathology: A Clinical Approach.* Elsevier/Churchill Livingstone; 2019.)

NOT TO BE MISSED

Protective measures against ovarian cancer include the following:

- Breastfeeding history
- Multiparity
- Hysterectomy
- Bilateral tubal ligation (BTL)
  Risk factors for ovarian cancer include the following:
- Family history of ovarian cancer
- Family history of *BRCA1* or *BRCA2* gene mutations
- Nulligravid
- Early menarche
- Late menopause
- Endometriosis

Early signs and symptoms of ovarian cancer are subtle and include mild abdominal discomfort, mild

NOT TO BE MISSED

Late-stage signs and symptoms of ovarian cancer include the following:

- Increased abdominal girth
- Abdominal bloating and discomfort
- Unexplained vaginal bleeding
- Gastrointestinal symptoms
- Urinary frequency
- Fatigue
- Weight loss
- Liver ascites
- Pleural effusion

bladder or rectum pressure, and vague digestive symptoms. Later signs and symptoms are often obvious.

Hereditary breast and ovarian syndrome (HBOS) is caused by *BRCA1* and *BRCA2* mutations.[2] HBOS carries an increased risk for developing ovarian cancer along with other cancers including breast cancer, pancreatic cancer, uterine cancer, and melanoma. In addition to increasing the risk for endometrial cancer, Lynch syndrome is also responsible for a proportion of hereditary ovarian cancers.[8] Another risk factor for ovarian cancer is Peutz-Jeghers syndrome. Peutz-Jeghers syndrome is a rare condition associated with an increased risk for other cancers, including cervical, endometrial, breast, and colon cancers[2] (Table 20.2).

Females with a *BRCA1* mutation have a 39% to 46% lifetime risk of developing ovarian cancer, while females with a *BRCA2* mutation have a lifetime risk of 12% to 27%.[2] Females with a *BRCA2* mutation also have an increased risk of developing breast cancer. The prevalence of *BRCA* mutations is 1 in 40 in females of Ashkenazi Jewish descent and approximately 1 in 500 in the general non-Jewish U.S. population.[2]

There are no recommended guidelines for routine ovarian cancer screening in low-risk females as there are for cervical and breast cancers. No proven screening method has been identified for early ovarian cancer detection. Females who carry the *BRCA1* mutation should be screened annually with a transvaginal ultrasound examination and a serum cancer antigen 125 (CA-125) test. Patients who experience ovarian cancer

TABLE 20.2   Summary of Syndromes With Malignant Manifestations Associated With Breast and Ovarian Cancer[2]

Syndrome	Breast Cancer	Ovarian Cancer	Endometrial Cancer	Colon Cancer	Other Types of Cancer
Hereditary breast and ovarian cancer	X	X			Pancreatic, proatate, and melanoma
Lynch		X	X	X	Gastric, ureteral, biliary, pancreatic, glioblastoma, renal pelvis
Li-Fraumeni	X			X	Sarcomas, brain, adrenocortical
Cowden	X		X	X	Benign mucocutaneous lesions, thyroid, gastrointestinal hamartomas
Peutz-Jeghers	X	X		X	Cervical adenoma malignum, gastrointestinal hamartomas, pancreatic, gastric, small bowel
Hereditary diffuse gastric cancer	X				Gastric, colorectal

Reprinted with permission from Hereditary cancer syndromes and risk assessment. ACOG Committee Opinion No. 793. American College of Obstetricians and Gynecologists. *Obstet Gynecol* 2019;134:e143–9.

signs and symptoms should receive diagnostic screening with pelvic ultrasonography, computed tomography (CT), or magnetic resonance imaging (MRI) along with a serum CA-125 test. Serum CA-125 is not a reliable test for detecting ovarian cancer. The choice of treatment depends primarily on the surgical staging of the disease. The oncologist determines which treatment the patient requires.

NOT TO BE MISSED

Treatment for ovarian cancer may consist of the following options:
- Surgery (TAH-BSO)
- Chemotherapy
- Possible radiation therapy

CLINICAL SURVIVAL TIP There are no recommended guidelines for routine ovarian cancer screening in low-risk females as there are for cervical and breast cancers. No proven screening method has been identified for early ovarian cancer detection.

VULVAR CANCER

Vulvar cancer is a malignancy that originates in the vulva. The primary type of vulvar cancer is squamous cell carcinoma. Vulvar cancer is not very common and is diagnosed most commonly in postmenopausal females.

Preventive measures include completing the HPV vaccine series and smoking cessation. Risk factors for vulvar cancer include HPV infection, vulvar intraepithelial neoplasia (VIN), cigarette smoking, lichen sclerosis, early sexual debut, and immunodeficiency.

Common signs and symptoms of vulvar cancer include changes in skin color pigmentation and texture, itching, bleeding, discharge, pain, and burning.[17] Visual inspection of the vulva is an important part of the gynecology annual examination. A vulvar biopsy is recommended to screen pigmented lesions in postmenopausal females and in reproductive-age females with failed medical management of topical treatments.[18] The vulvar biopsy is the definitive diagnostic test used to make the diagnosis of vulvar cancer. CT, MRI, or chest radiography may also be ordered to screen for metastasis.

Treatment is recommended with the presence of VIN. Wide local excision is often performed if the area is suspicious for malignancy. If the area is not suspicious for malignancy, then surgical therapy, laser ablation, or medical therapy is performed.

Because there is a lifetime risk of recurrent VIN and vulva cancer after resolution in previously diagnosed individuals, routine monitoring should take place. If normal findings are present at 6 and 12 months following treatment, then monitoring should continue to take place annually. See Figure 17.7 in for an image of vulvar cancer.

VAGINAL CANCER

Vaginal cancer is defined as a malignancy that originates in the vagina. The main types of vaginal cancer include squamous cell cancer, adenocarcinoma, melanoma, and sarcoma. The most common type of vaginal cancer is invasive squamous cell cancer, accounting for approximately 70 in 100 cases of vaginal cancer.[19] Adenocarcinoma is most common in females younger than 30 years of age who were exposed to DES in utero.[19]

The primary causes of vaginal cancer include HPV infection, DES exposure in utero, and cigarette smoking. Vaginal cancer is very rare in the United States and is most commonly diagnosed in postmenopausal females.[19] Preventive measures include completing the HPV vaccination series, limiting the number of lifetime sexual partners, and smoking cessation. Risk factors for vaginal cancer include DES exposure in utero, squamous cell cancer of the cervix or vulva, and cervical cancer risk factors.[19]

There are no signs or symptoms routinely experienced during the early stages of vaginal cancer.

Diagnostic testing is routinely performed to diagnose vaginal cancer. Key elements utilized to diagnose vaginal cancer include pelvic inspection at the annual examination. Vaginal cytology, vaginal colposcopy, and vaginal biopsy are performed when indicated.

Vaginal cancer is clinically staged and based on the physical examination, cystoscopy, proctoscopy, radiography, biopsy, and fine-needle aspiration. Potential treatment options for vaginal cancer include laser surgery, excisional surgery, radiation therapy, neoadjuvant chemotherapy, or a combination of these options.

TABLE 20.3   Common Signs and Symptoms of Gynecological Cancers[6,15-17,19]

Symptoms	Cervical Cancer	Ovarian Cancer	Endometrial Cancer	Vulvar Cancer	Vaginal Cancer
Bleeding or discharge	X	X	X	X	X
Pain or pressure sensation		X	X	X	
Abdominal or back pain		X			
Bloating or flatulence		X			
Changes in bowel habits		X			X
Vulvar itching or burning				X	
Changes in vulvar skin				X	

NOT TO BE MISSED

Late-stage signs and symptoms of vaginal cancer include the following:

- Vaginal bleeding
- Vaginal discharge
- Presence of a mass or lesion
- Blood in urine or stool
- Constipation
- Pelvic pain
- Abdominal pain
- Weight loss
- Fatigue

CONCLUSION

The five types of cancer that make up the gynecological cancers include cervical, endometrial, ovarian, vulvar, and vaginal cancers. Primary care clinicians should be very familiar with the common signs and symptoms reviewed in this chapter for each gynecological cancer as reviewed in Table 20.3. Education is an important component to prevention and early detection of cancer. Therefore clinicians are encouraged to educate patients about genetic screening, prevention, risk factors, common signs and symptoms, and treatment options for each cancer type when appropriate.

KEY POINTS

- Prevention of cancer should be the main goal of the clinician when caring for patients.
- Cancers found in the early stages have a more favorable prognosis, and treatments work optimally.
- Cervical cancer is preventable when the patient is protected by the HPV vaccine and receives screening per recommendations.
- Any abnormal vaginal bleeding in females 45 years of age and older should be considered cancer until proven otherwise.
- Because ovarian cancer is difficult to diagnose in an early stage, it is imperative to teach the patient both prevention and signs and symptoms.
- Vulvar and vaginal cancers are rare in the United States.

REFERENCES

1. U.S. Department of Health and Human Services. (n.d.). *Cancer stat facts: Common cancer sites*. NIH, National Cancer Institute Surveillance, Epidemiology, and End Results Program. https://seer.cancer.gov/statfacts/html/common.html.
2. American College of Obstetricians and Gynecologists. Hereditary cancer syndromes and risk assessment. *Obstet Gynecol*. 2015;125(6):1538–1543.
3. Society of Gynecologic Oncology. *Genetics Toolkit*; 2020. https://www.sgo.org/genetics/genetics-toolkit/.
4. International Federation of Gynecology and Obstetrics. *FIGO Cancer Report*; 2015:13(S2). http://obgyn.onlinelibrary.wiley.com/hub/issue/10.1002/ijgo.2015.131.issue-S2/.
5. American Joint Committee on Cancer. *Eighth Edition Staging Rules*; 2018. https://www.facs.org/quality-programs/cancer-programs/american-joint-committee-on-cancer/staging-education/rules/.

6. American Society for Clinical Oncology. 2020. *HPV and cancer.* Cancer.Net. https://www.cancer.net/navigating-cancer-care/prevention-and-healthy-living/hpv-and-cancer#:~:text=HPV%20causes%20nearly%20all%20cervical,%2D16%20or%20HPV%2D18.

7. U.S. Centers for Disease Control and Prevention. (n.d.). Cancer Statistics at a Glance. United States Cancer Statistics: Data Visualizations. https://gis.cdc.gov/Cancer/USCS/#/AtAGlance/.

8. U.S. Centers for Disease Control and Prevention. *HPV-Associated Cervical Cancer Rates by Race and Ethnicity*; 2017. https://www.cdc.gov/cancer/hpv/statistics/cervical.htm.

9. Viens LJ, Henley SJ, Watson M, et al. Human papillomavirus–associated cancers in the United States, 2008–2012. *MMWR Morb Mortal Wkly Rep.* 2016;65(26):661–666.

10. Saslow D, Solomon D, Lawson HW, et al. American Cancer Society, American Society for Colposcopy and Cervical Pathology, and American Society for Clinical Pathology screening guidelines for the prevention and early detection of cervical cancer. *J Low Genit Tract Dis.* 2012;16(3):175–204.

11. American Society for Colposcopy and Cervical Pathology. *ASCCP Management Guidelines*; 2019. https://www.asccp.org/management-guidelines.

12. Massad LS, Einstein MH, Huh WK, et al. 2012 updated consensus guidelines for the management of abnormal cervical cancer screening tests and cancer precursors. *J Low Genit Tract Dis.* 2013;17(5):S1–S27.

13. Handelzalts JE, Krissi H, Levy S, et al. Multidimensional associations of pain and anxiety before and after colposcopy. *Int J Gynaecol Obstet.* 2015;131(3):297–300.

14. The National Institutes for Health. (n.d.). What is cervical cancer. National Cancer Institute. https://www.cancer.gov/types/cervical.

15. ACOG Practice Bulletin No. 147. Lynch syndrome. *Obstet Gynecol.* 2014;124(5):1042–1054.

16. ACOG Committee Opinion No. 557: Management of acute abnormal uterine bleeding in nonpregnant reproductive aged women. *Obstet Gynecol.* 2013;121(4):891–896.

17. American Cancer Society. *Cervical Cancer*; 2017. https://www.cancer.org/cancer/cervical-cancer.html.

19. American Cancer Society. *What Is Ovarian Cancer?*; 2017. https://www.cancer.org/cancer/ovarian-cancer/about/what-is-ovarian-cancer.html.

20. American College of Obstetricians and Gynecologists. Management of vulvar intraepithelial neoplasia. *Obstet Gynecol.* 2011;118(5):1192–1194.

21. American Cancer Society. *Vaginal Cancer*; 2017. https://www.cancer.org/cancer/vaginal-cancer.html.

22. Huh WK, Ault KA, Chelmow D, et al. Use of primary high-risk human papillomavirus testing for cervical cancer screening: Interim clinical guidance. *Gynecol Oncol.* 2015;136(2):178–182.

23. U.S. Centers for Disease Control and Prevention. (n.d.). *HPV-associated cancer diagnosis by age.* HPV and Cancer. https://www.cdc.gov/cancer/hpv/statistics/age.htm.

21

Breast Health

Rachel Fidino

OBJECTIVES

- Understand the basic anatomy and physiology of the breast.
- Appropriately identify and manage benign breast conditions.
- Evaluate a breast mass, including a clinical physical examination and detailed history taking including risk assessment.

- Understand breast screening recommendations and differences among organizations
- Interpret various imaging results, and provide proper management.
- Be familiar with the role primary care providers play in breast cancer prevention, diagnosis, and management.

Breast tissue is essential in reproductive function, sexuality, and feminine image. The presence of symptoms in the breast, whether the findings are benign or malignant, may cause substantial concern for a female patient. Providing adequate emotional support is just as important as risk assessment, diagnosis, and management of a breast condition. Evaluation of breast conditions requires the clinician to obtain a detailed history, perform a physical examination, properly interpret imaging results, and know when to refer the patient to a breast specialist.

BREAST ANATOMY

Ductal System

The glandular portion of the breast encompasses an independent ductal system composed of 12 to 15 ducts. Each duct drains into approximately 40 lobules. Breast lobules make up 10 to 100 milk-producing acini that drain into smaller terminal ducts. Six to eight openings are visible on the surface of the nipple. This allows for drainage of the dominant ductal systems, which consist of 80% of the breast's glandular volume. The areola has sebaceous glands called *Montgomery glands* that serve as lubrication. Montgomery glands are frequently visible as punctate projections. The breast has varying proportions of collagenous stroma and fat. The distribution

and amount of stromal components are the basis for the breast's consistency when palpated.

Lymphatic Drainage

Afferent lymphatic drainage of the breast is divided into dermal, subdermal, interlobar, and pre-pectoral systems. The drainage system can be imagined as a lattice of valveless channels that are all interconnected with every other system. These drain into one or two axillary lymph nodes. The breast drains and functions as a unit because all of these systems are interconnected. The axillary lymph nodes are responsible for receiving the majority of the lymphatic drainage and are most frequently associated with breast cancer metastases (Fig. 21.1).

BREAST DEVELOPMENT AND PHYSIOLOGY

The primordial breast ascends from the basal layer of the epidermis during development of a fetus. Before a young female reaches puberty, the breast is a rudimentary bud consisting of just a few branching ducts that are capped with alveolar buds, end buds, or small lobules. A young female typically reaches puberty between 10 and 13 years of age. Estrogen and progesterone are the dominant hormones that direct organized communication between the breast epithelial cells and mesenchymal

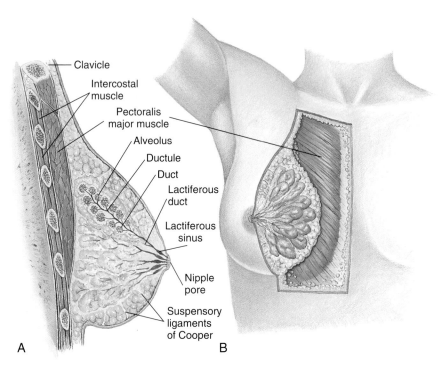

Figure 21.1 Anatomy of the breast. **A,** Internal structures. **B,** External structures and surrounding tissue. (From Ball J, Seidel HM, Dains JE, Flynn JA, Solomon BS, Stewart RW. *Seidel's Guide to Physical Examination: An Interprofessional Approach.* St. Louis: Elsevier; 2023.)

cells. This results in extensive branching of the ductal system and the proliferation of breast lobules. Progesterone and prolactin are responsible for differentiation of the breast tissue and is not completed until the first full-term pregnancy.

The terminal ducts near the acini are most sensitive to estrogen, progesterone, and prolactin. The majority of benign and malignant breast disease begins in the terminal duct-acinar structures. During the luteal phase of the menstrual cycle, breast epithelial cells proliferate. This occurs because of the natural increase in estrogen and progesterone levels. As hormone levels decrease toward the end of the luteal phase, cells undergo programmed cell death. This explains why patients often feel as if their breast tissue is full and tender the week preceding their menses.

Once an individual reaches menopausal status, ovarian estrogen production has ceased. The breast lobules undergo involution, and the collagenous stroma is now replaced with fat. After ovarian estrogen production has ceased, a postmenopausal individual will continue to produce estrogen. This occurs through the action of an enzyme called *aromatase*. Aromatase converts adrenal androgens into estrogen.

> **NOT TO BE MISSED**
>
> After ovarian estrogen production has ceased, a postmenopausal individual will continue to produce estrogen. This occurs through the action of an enzyme called *aromatase*. Aromatase converts adrenal androgens into estrogen.

BENIGN BREAST CONDITIONS

Mastalgia

Mastalgia is characterized as breast pain or mastodynia. In primary care, mastalgia is the second most common reported breast complaint.[1] Mastalgia is benign 90% of the time and accounts for 66% of provider visits for breast symptoms. Breast pain is not a risk factor for developing breast cancer. In fact, breast pain is quite common throughout life, especially during reproductive years.

Mastalgia is designated into two groups: cyclic or noncyclic. Cyclic mastalgia typically occurs in females in their twenties to thirties and composes two-thirds of all breast pain presentations.[1,2] Cyclic breast pain occurs 1 to 2 weeks before the onset of menses; thus it corresponds to the menstrual cycle and will typically improve after the onset of menses. The pain is usually related to hormonal and fibrocystic changes. This type of breast pain is often described as diffuse, bilateral, dull, and radiating to the axillae.

Noncyclic mastalgia is not related to the menstrual cycle and occurs in females in their 30s and 40s.[1,2] The etiology of most noncyclic breast pain may be inflammation or from chest wall syndromes.[1,2] Noncyclic mastalgia may be constant or intermittent, however pain-free intervals are not related to menses. The pain is often characterized as burning or sharp. Noncyclic breast pain is frequently located in the subareolar or medial portion of the breast. Common benign causes of noncyclic breast pain include cysts, fibroadenomas, mastitis, and abscess. Noncyclic breast pain is associated with oral contraceptives, hormone therapy, antidepressants, and antihypertensives.[1]

Costochondritis and Tietze syndrome are two chest wall syndromes that may exhibit breast pain.[2] Pain related to the chest wall is often localized and worsens with movement. Chest wall pain accounts for approximately 5% to 10% of mastalgia symptoms.

The provider must discern whether the breast pain is cyclic, noncyclic, or related to chest wall pain. During history taking, it is important to ask questions regarding timing, frequency, location, severity, nature, and migrating factors. A daily diary can also be used to track cyclic versus noncyclic mastalgia. The clinician should ask about associated symptoms such as nipple discharge, a palpable mass, or skin changes. It may also be helpful to ask whether the patient has had any prior breast surgeries, procedures, or biopsies. Other history-taking questions should include menstrual history, pregnancy, lactation, and current medications. Caffeine has not been definitively linked as a causal factor; however, asking about caffeine consumption can provide additional information and trends. Caffeine contains a chemical called *methylxanthine,* which causes an overstimulation of breast cells by dilating the blood vessels. This in turn can cause mastalgia.

It is important to reassure the patient that pain is generally not a common sign of breast cancer, and it does not increase the risk for developing breast cancer. A pregnancy test should be considered if indicated by the menstrual history, as mastalgia can be a sign of pregnancy. A comprehensive breast examination must be performed, including inspection and palpation of the breast tissue. Diagnostic imaging can be used for further evaluation of mastalgia. A diagnostic mammogram with ultrasonography can be performed on patients who are 30 years of age and older. A targeted ultrasound examination is recommended for patients who are younger than 30 years of age (Fig. 21.2).

Once the provider has ruled out non-breast causes of mastalgia and malignancy, the focus should be directed at reassuring the patient. Reassurance is effective in 85% of mastalgia patients. Patients can wear a supportive or well-fitted bra to provide comfort. There is limited evidence that decreasing fat or caffeine may resolve breast pain; however, neither of these dietary recommendations is likely to be harmful if attempted. Pharmacological therapies that can improve mastalgia include adjusting the dose or route of hormone therapy and/or contraceptive method depending on premenopausal or postmenopausal status. First-line treatment for mild mastalgia is topical nonsteroidal antiinflammatory drugs (NSAIDs) such as diclofenac.[1] Tamoxifen and danazol are used for moderate mastalgia symptoms. For patients with severe symptoms that are refractory to these therapies, goserelin can be used. Because of the adverse effects of tamoxifen, danazol, and goserelin, referral to a subspecialist is preferred for management of moderate to severe refractory symptoms.[1]

Evening primrose is an herbal product that is commonly recommended for mastalgia; however, the evidence is insufficient. Isoflavones and a flaxseed bread diet has also been proposed as treatment options for patients with breast pain.

> **PATIENT-CENTERED CARE:** It is important to reassure the patient that pain is generally not a common sign of breast cancer, and it does not increase the risk for developing breast cancer.

Nipple Discharge

Nipple discharge accounts for 6.8% of referrals to providers.[2] Ninety-seven percent of nipple discharge cases are caused by benign disease. Nonspontaneous discharge is

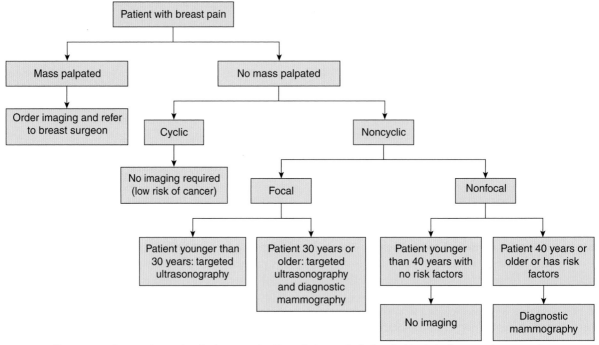

Figure 21.2 Diagnostic workup for breast pain. (From Salzman B, Collins E, Hersh L. Common breast problems. *Am Fam Physician.* 2019;99[8]:505–514.)

characterized as physiological or pathological. Physiological nipple discharge typically presents from multiple ducts, is bilateral, and is associated with nipple stimulation or breast massage.[2] During pregnancy and lactation, the patient may experience bilateral milky nipple discharge. This may persist for 1 year postpartum or following the cessation of breastfeeding.[1] Galactorrhea is a milky nipple discharge that is not associated with pregnancy or lactation. This type of discharge is multiductal and bilateral. It may occur spontaneously or during nipple manipulation. A pregnancy test should be performed in a patient experiencing galactorrhea to rule out pregnancy. Once pregnancy has been ruled out, a prolactin and thyroid-stimulating hormone (TSH) evaluation should be ordered to determine endocrinopathy. Increased prolactin levels may be physiological, pathological, or pharmaceutically induced. Physiological causes of hyperprolactinemia include sexual orgasm, nipple stimulation, exercise, sleep, and food consumption. Pathological causes include pituitary tumors, hypothalamic lesions, renal failure, hypothyroidism, chest wall trauma, and anovulatory syndromes. Certain medications can also increase prolactin levels. These include dopamine-blocking drugs

(phenothiazine and metoclopramide) and dopamine-depleting drugs (reserpine and methyldopa). Other drugs that can increase prolactin levels include certain opiates, amphetamines, and verapamil.

> **CLINICAL SURVIVAL TIP:** Medications and drugs of abuse can increase prolactin levels and cause galactorrhea. It is vital the clinician ask about the use of these drugs. A comprehensive list can be found at: https://www.uptodate.com/contents/image?imageKey=ENDO%2F75914.

Pathological nipple discharge is spontaneous and unilateral, and it may be bloody, serous, clear, or related to a breast mass. Pathological nipple discharge may arise from the nipple, areola, or breast duct.[2] Bloody nipple discharge has been associated with Paget disease. This causes erythema and ulceration of the skin surrounding the nipple. The most common finding associated with pathological nipple discharge is ductal ectasia, infection, carcinoma, or intraductal papilloma. Ductal carcinoma and ductal papilloma typically involve a single duct with serosanguineous discharge. Ductal papilloma is a benign condition that causes epithelial hyperplasia within the breast duct. Ductal carcinoma in situ is responsible for 5% to 10% of all cases of unilateral nipple discharge. If a patient presents with purulent nipple discharge, this can be a sign of infection or abscess.

NOT TO BE MISSED

Pathological nipple discharge is classified as spontaneous, unilateral, bloody, serous, clear, or related to a breast mass.

When collecting a detailed history, include age, whether the nipple discharge is unilateral or bilateral, characteristics of the discharge, current medications, duration, whether it occurs spontaneously or only with manipulation, recent pregnancy, menstrual cycle timing, menopausal status, exercise, sleep habits, and recent surgery or trauma. It is important to also inquire about symptoms of hypothyroidism (fatigue, weight gain, cold intolerance), hyperthyroidism (weight loss, nervousness, heat intolerance), pituitary tumor (visual problems, headaches), and hyperprolactinemia (infertility, irregular menses, decreased libido).

A complete clinical breast examination (CBE) is vital to determine if a palpable mass is present or if the discharge is unilateral. An inspection should also be performed to discover if there are any skin changes. The clinician should carefully palpate each quadrant of the breast to determine if the discharge is confined to a single duct.

If the patient's TSH and prolactin levels are normal and menses are normal, a diagnosis of idiopathic galactorrhea can be made. If the patient has hyperprolactinemia and menses are irregular, magnetic resonance imaging (MRI) of the brain is warranted. The posterior fossa, within the pituitary gland, should be evaluated. The most specific test in diagnostic evaluation of pathological nipple discharge is surgical duct excision. Galactography is a procedure that involves injecting a radiopaque dye into a suspicious duct. This can help determine a benign versus malignant neoplasm. Mammography should be ordered in a patient whose CBE and history are suspicious for cancer (Fig. 21.3).

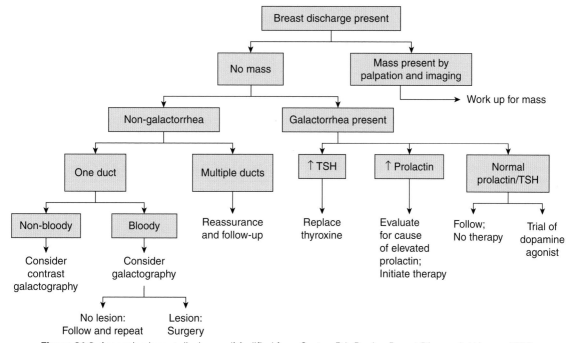

Figure 21.3 Assessing breast discharge. (Modified from Santen RJ. *Benign Breast Disease in Women;* 2018. https://www.ncbi.nlm.nih.gov/books/NBK278994/.)

Breast Infection

Breast infections are a common finding in premenopausal patients. Breast infections are typically painful, but they respond to oral antibiotics if treated early. Acute mastitis can be caused by pregnancy, lactation, and bacterial infections of unknown origin. *Staphylococcus* infections are commonly associated with acute mastitis. Treatment options for acute mastitis include oral antibiotics, warm compresses, and gentle massage. If an abscess develops or if conservative management fails, incision and drainage may be necessary. A breast abscess can be identified on physical examination or confirmed by ultrasound examination. Incision and drainage should be considered early on for breast abscess treatment.

Fibroadenoma

Fibroadenomas are a common finding throughout the reproductive years and following menopause. Fibroadenomas are typically small, discrete, smooth, round or oval, mobile, and nontender. Once a patient reaches menopause, fibroadenomas are seen as a calcified density on mammography. Fibroadenomas can change in size as a result of hormonal stimulation of combined contraceptive methods and pregnancy. The majority of fibroadenomas are confirmed by ultrasonography. An ultrasound-guided biopsy can prove a benign nature. A surgical excision may be necessary if it grows larger than 2 to 3 cm or is painful. There is no proven increased risk of developing breast cancer with a benign fibroadenoma.

Breast Cysts

Breast cysts are common throughout reproductive years and following menopause. Breast cysts are typically discrete, tender, mobile, and can fluctuate with the menstrual cycle. Simple breast cysts typically resolve without intervention. Simple cyst aspiration is required for cysts that are symptomatic and large. If a cyst is complex on ultrasound examination or associated with a solid component, a biopsy should be performed to rule out malignancy. Follow-up imaging should be performed to document a decrease in size of the cyst and complete resolution.

Breast Lipoma

Breast lipomas are an area of fatty tissue and are typically seen in later reproductive years. They are benign, generally nonpainful, discrete, soft, and may or may not be mobile. Excision is not mandatory if the CBE is consistent with a lipoma. If the clinician is concerned regarding the physical examination findings, excision or needle aspiration would be necessary.

Fat Necrosis

Fat necrosis is usually seen following trauma to the breast tissue and is often ill defined, firm, nontender, and nonmobile. Conservative management is recommended.

Phyllodes Tumor

Phyllodes tumors of the breast develop from the periductal stroma. On physical examination, these tumors are discrete, firm, round, mobile, and larger than a fibroadenoma. They are typically fast-growing masses and account for less than 1% of all breast neoplasms. Typically, phyllodes tumors are seen between 30 and 50 years of age.

Galactocele

Galactoceles are milk-filled cysts that are seen most commonly during lactation. They are round, well circumscribed, firm, and occasionally tender. They can occur up to 6 to 10 months after cessation of breastfeeding and are typically located in the central portion of the breast or directly under the nipple. Treatment typically consists of needle aspiration.

EVALUATION OF A BREAST MASS

Physical Examination

Patients who present to their primary care provider with a breast mass need a thorough physical examination and clinical history. It is impossible to distinguish whether a breast mass is benign or malignant based on clinical examination alone. However, clinical examination, in addition to imaging and pathology, contributes significantly to management decisions.

The first step in performing a CBE is by inspection (Fig. 21.4). The patient should be sitting on the edge of the table with hands placed at the hips while flexing the

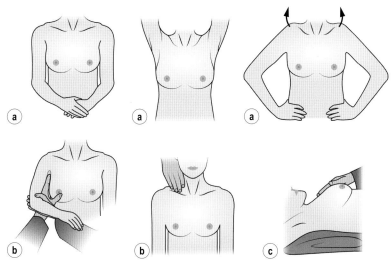

Figure 21.4 Steps of a breast examination. **A,** Visualization in three different positions. **B,** Palpation of lymph nodes. **C,** Palpation of breast tissue. (From Barber MD. Breast surgery. In: *Principles and Practice of Surgery.* Elsevier; 2023).

pectoralis muscle. This position can help identify asymmetry. The breast skin should be inspected for erythema, retraction, scaling, and edema.

After the clinician inspects the breast tissue, assessing the lymph nodes is the next step. The axillary, supraclavicular, and infraclavicular lymph nodes should be easily palpated. The lymph nodes are detected as the clinician's hand slides from high to low in the axilla and gently compresses the nodes against the lateral chest wall.

The next step during the CBE is palpation. The patient should be lying in the supine position with one hand above the head to stretch the breast tissue across the chest wall. Breast examination should include the breast tissue bounded by the clavicle, sternum, inframammary crease, and midaxillary line. The finger pads should be used in a gliding and continuous rolling movement. Palpation should be assessed both superficially and deeply. If an abnormality is noted during the CBE, the location should be described based on left or right breast, clock position, size, and distance from the margin of the areola. During the CBE, this is a great time to educate the patient on breast awareness. Patients who desire to perform a self-breast examination should be counseled regarding the benefits and limitations. One should perform a self-breast examination after the week of menses.

History

All patients who report to a clinician should be assessed for risk factors of breast cancer. The most obvious and important risk factor in assessing a patient's breast cancer risk is age. The risk of breast cancer increases with age. Family history is one of the most effective and least expensive tools in identifying a patient's risk for breast cancer, which can be categorized as sporadic, familial, or genetic causes. Approximately 10% of breast cancers can be linked with a genetic mutation from either the maternal or paternal side. A patient's risk of breast cancer is nearly doubled if there is a first-degree relative who has been diagnosed with the disease.

> **! SAFETY ALERT**
>
> All patients who report to a clinician should be assessed for risk factors of breast cancer.

Hereditary breast and ovarian cancer (HBOC) syndrome is caused by a germline mutation. The criteria in Box 21.1 should be assessed for all first-, second-, and third-degree relatives. A family cancer history should be assessed and updated on a routine basis. After collecting a detailed family history, the clinician will be more equipped to advise patients regarding risk stratification and appropriate management strategies. If the patient meets the aforementioned criteria, a genetic panel test should be performed to rule out HBOC syndrome. Even if there is no hereditary susceptibility, the patient may need

BOX 21.1   Guidelines to Evaluate Risk for Hereditary Breast and Ovarian Cancer

- Individuals with any blood relative with a known nocuous BRCA1 or BRCA2 mutation
- Individuals who have experienced any of the below conditions

Personal history of cancer
- Breast cancer with at least one of the following:
  - Diagnosed at or before 45 years of age
    - Diagnosed at or before 50 years of age with unknown family history or with less than two first- or second-degree surviving female relatives older than age 45
  - Diagnosed at age 60 or younger with triple-negative breast cancer
    - Diagnosed at any age with a first-, second-, or third-degree relative who had breast cancer at age 50 or younger or who was diagnosed with epithelial ovarian, tubal, or peritoneal cancer at any age
    - Diagnosed at any age with two or more first-, second-, or third-degree relatives with breast cancer diagnosed at any age
    - Diagnosed at any age with two or more first-, second-, or third-degree relative with pancreatic cancer or prostate cancer with a Gleason score of ≥ 7

- This cancer is a primary breast cancer and a previous primary breast cancer occurred before 50 years of age
  - Diagnosed at any age with Ashkenazi Jewish
- Epithelial ovarian, fallopian tube, or peritoneal cancer at any age
- Exocrine pancreatic cancer at any age
- Prostate cancer diagnosed at any age with metastatic, first-degree relatives of individuals diagnosed with exocrine pancreatic cancer, or high- or very-high-risk group
- Individuals who meet Li-Fraumeni syndrome (LFS) testing criteria or Cowden syndrome/PTEN hamartoma tumor syndrome testing criteria

Family history of cancer
- An unaffected individual with a first-, second-, or third-degree blood relative meeting any of the criteria listed above.
- An unaffected individual with a first-, second-, or third-degree relative with:
  - BRCA1 or BRCA2 mutation
  - Male breast cancer
  - Invasive and ductal carcinoma in situ breast cancer

Information in this box was drawn from the NCCN Clinical Practice Guidelines in Oncology, 2023 and ACOG Practice Bulletin No 182: Hereditary Breast and Ovarian Cancer Syndrome. (2017). *Obstetrics and Gynecology*, 130(3), e110-e126.

increased surveillance based on familial risk. This may include increasing breast screening at an earlier age and/or with more intensive screening than those in the general population. If the patient is found to have a genetic susceptibility, an individualized treatment plan should be developed. This includes breast surveillance, breast awareness, more sensitive screening tests, risk-reducing medications, and/or risk-reducing surgery.

NOT TO BE MISSED

Modifiable risks for breast cancer include adjusting one's lifestyle. Several important risk factors are known to be effective in reducing the risk for breast cancer. These include increasing exercise, reducing alcohol consumption, smoking cessation, and avoiding sedentary lifestyles.

The American College of Obstetricians and Gynecologists (ACOG) recommends that health care providers periodically assess a patient's breast cancer risk by collecting a detailed family history. Box 21.2 describes these risk factors.

Modifiable risks for breast cancer include adjusting one's lifestyle. Several important risk factors are known to be effective in reducing the risk for breast cancer, such as increasing exercise.[3] In postmenopausal patients, exercise and physical activity have been shown to decrease the risk for breast cancer by altering estrogen, insulin, and insulin-like growth factor 1, and it can reduce obesity and insulin resistance. A sedentary lifestyle is associated with weight gain, which in turn can increase the risk of breast cancer.

Both active and passive smokers are at an increased risk for developing breast cancer. Smoking is another risk factor that can be modifiable. Studies have shown that

BOX 21.2   Breast Cancer Risk Factors

- Family history of breast cancer or ovarian cancer
- Known deleterious gene mutation
- Personal history of breast cancer or noncancerous breast disease such as atypical hyperplasia or lobular carcinoma in situ
- Early menarche before 12 years of age
- Late menopause after 55 years of age
- First pregnancy after 30 years of age or nulliparity
- Menopausal hormone therapy with estrogen and progestin
- Not breastfeeding
- Increasing age
- Females who took diethylstilbestrol (DES) or delivered of a mother who took DES during pregnancy
- Overweight or obese after menopause
- Alcohol consumption
- Smoking
- Dense breast tissue on mammography
- Prior exposure to high-dose therapeutic chest irradiation before 30 years of age

Modified from U.S. Centers for Disease Control and Prevention. *What Are the Risk Factors for Breast Cancer?.* https://www.cdc.gov/cancer/breast/basic_info/risk_factors.htm.

females who start smoking at an early age are more susceptible to breast cancer. Those who were active smokers at the time of breast cancer diagnosis have weaker outcomes and poorer survival probability. Patients who were smokers and underwent a partial mastectomy for breast cancer are 6.7 times more likely to suffer from cancer recurrence than patients who never smoked. Smoking cessation should be recommended to all patients.

Another modifiable risk factor is alcohol consumption. Breast cancer risk increases with the amount of alcohol use. Breast cancer risk is present even with light to moderate alcohol intake. The American Cancer Society has reported an increased risk of developing breast cancer by 20% in individuals who have two to three alcoholic drinks per day compared with those who do not drink alcohol.[3]

Breastfeeding has been shown to decrease the risk of breast cancer.[3] Patients who breastfeed their infant for 12 months have a 4.3% decreased risk of developing breast cancer.

Recent studies have shown that night shift work can increase the risk of breast cancer. This is linked with increasing levels of melatonin. The data with night shift work is limited, and more research is needed to prove significance.

Socioeconomic status is associated with an increased risk of breast cancer. Females who have a higher socioeconomic status undergo more frequent visits to their medical provider. This leads to more frequent physical examinations, which leads to earlier diagnosis of breast cancer. It has been shown in some countries that females of low socioeconomic status are at a higher risk for advanced-stage breast cancer. There is inadequate screening in this population of females, which leads to poorer prognosis at the time of diagnosis.

Studies have shown that females who had their first child after 30 years of age or who have not had children are at a slightly increased risk of developing breast cancer. However, having many pregnancies and becoming pregnant at an early age reduce the risk of breast cancer.[3] The effects of pregnancy seem to be different based on the type of breast cancer. Pregnancy seems to increase the risk of developing a type of breast cancer known as *triple-negative breast cancer.*

Some birth control methods have been shown to increase the risk of breast cancer. Studies have shown that females who use oral contraceptive pills have a slightly increased risk of developing breast cancer versus females who have never used them. Once a patient stops taking oral contraceptive pills, the breast cancer risk seems to normalize over time. Some studies have linked hormone-releasing IUDs and breast cancer risk, but few studies have been conducted with the use of birth control implants, patches, or rings.[3]

Hormone replacement therapy after menopause has been studied regarding the possible increased risk of breast cancer. Females who use a combined hormone therapy after menopause have an increased risk of developing breast cancer. The use of estrogen alone after menopause does not seem to increase the risk of breast cancer.[3]

Mammography

Female patients who present with a breast mass need breast imaging. CBE findings and imaging results determine the next steps in the evaluation of a breast mass. Breast cancer screening recommendations vary based on the following organizations: American Cancer Society (ACS), U.S. Preventive Services Task Force (USPSTF), and ACOG. The American Academy of Family Physicians (AAFP) has stated that screening mammography in females before 50 years of age should be an individualized decision. The AAFP recommends biennial screening between 40 and 49 years of age for females who place a higher value on the potential benefit than the potential harm.

According to the ACS, females should begin mammography screening at 45 years of age with yearly surveillance. For females 55 and older, the ACS recommends mammography screening every 2 years until the patient's life expectancy is less than 10 years. The USPSTF requires no routine mammography in females 40 to 49 years of age. The USPSTF recommends biennial screening mammography for females between 50 and 74 years of age. The ACOG recommends screening mammography to be offered starting at 40 years of age. If the patient desires, mammography should be initiated at 40 to 49 years of age. Females should begin screening mammography by no later than 50 years of age. Mammography may be performed every 1 to 2 years after 55 years of age. The ACOG recommends females continue screening mammography until 75 years of age.

Some controversy lies in unnecessary tests and procedures by starting screening mammography at a younger age. Screening females at a younger age will allow for earlier detection and has been found to reduce the mortality rate from breast cancer. The frequency of mammography must be an individualized approach. Mammography frequency should include the patient's risk factors, benefits, limitations, and potential harm in screening.

NOT TO BE MISSED

Female patients who present with a breast mass need breast imaging. CBE findings and imaging results determine the next steps in the evaluation of a breast mass.

Mammogram interpretation is reported as a Breast Imaging Reporting and Data System (BI-RADS) score. Table 21.1 describes the result and management based on the BI-RADS classification.

Screening mammography is used as a screening tool in asymptomatic female patients with the goal of detecting breast cancer that is not yet clinically apparent. This approach focuses on identifying breast cancer at an earlier stage, obtaining a more favorable prognosis, and requiring less aggressive treatment. The potential benefits of screening are evaluated against the cost and the number of false-positive studies that prompt additional workup, biopsies, and patient anxiety.

Ultrasonography

Whole-breast ultrasonography is not the standard for routine use in breast cancer screening. Ultrasonography is the best imaging modality in differentiating between solid and cystic masses. It can be a useful tool for identifying masses in female patients who are younger than

TABLE 21.1   Breast Imaging Reporting and Data System (BI-RADS)

BI-RADS Category	Description	Examples
0	Additional views or sonography required	Focal asymmetry, microcalcifications, or a mass identified on a screening mammogram
1	No abnormalities identified	Normal fat and fibroglandular tissue
2	Not entirely normal, but definitely benign	Fat necrosis from a prior excision, stable biopsy-proven fibroadenoma, stable cyst
3	Probably benign	Circumscribed mass that has been followed for <2 years
4A	Low suspicion for malignancy, but intervention required	Probable fibroadenoma, complicated cyst
4B	Intermediate suspicion for malignancy, intervention required	Partially indistinctly marginated mass otherwise consistent with a fibroadenoma
4C	Moderate suspicion, but not classic for carcinoma	New cluster of fine pleomorphic calcifications, ill-defined irregular solid mass
5	Almost certainly malignant	Spiculated mass, fine linear and branching calcifications
6	Biopsy-proven carcinoma	Biopsy-proven carcinoma

From Hoffman BL, Schorge JO, Halvorson LM, Hamid CA, Corton MM, Schaffer JI. *Williams Gynecology*. 4th ed. McGraw-Hill Education; 2020.

30 years of age and may also be useful when a palpable mass is only partially or poorly visualized on a mammogram.

Ultrasonography can distinguish certain characteristics for breast malignancies. Certain characteristics include lesions that are taller than they are wide, irregular shape, ill-defined margins, posterior acoustic shadowing, increased vascularity, and hypoechogenicity. Ultrasonography can also diagnose a simple cyst if certain criteria are fulfilled. The criteria include round or oval shape, sharply defined margins, lack of internal echoes, and posterior acoustic enhancement.

Microcalcifications within the breast tissue are not typically seen with ultrasonography. Ultrasonography may be considered to further evaluate an area of microcalcifications seen on mammography.

Magnetic Resonance Imaging

MRI is recommended by the ACS for routine screening in certain high-risk females. The ACS recommends annual screening with MRI for any female with a 20% or greater lifetime risk for developing breast cancer based on familial risk. This includes females with a strong family history of breast or ovarian cancer and females who have received chest radiation therapy. The data is insufficient to recommend for or against routine MRI screening in females who have a personal history of breast cancer, carcinoma in situ, atypical hyperplasia, and extremely dense breast tissue noted on mammography. Annual MRI screening is recommended for female patients who have a known deleterious germline mutation or those who are a first-degree relative of a *BRCA* carrier but have not been tested.

Risk assessment is important in determining the appropriate screening tool for patients. There are multiple risk-prediction tools available including Tyrer Cuzick, Claus, and BRCAPRO models. Calculating a female patient's lifetime risk of developing breast cancer aids in the decision to incorporate MRI for breast cancer prevention.

Patients found to have a high risk using prediction models are those with a family history of breast cancer in a first-, second-, or third-degree relative; prior personal history of breast cancer; germline mutation; prior radiation therapy to the chest wall; or prior diagnosis of atypical hyperplasia or lobular carcinoma in situ. Females with a strong family history of breast cancer in a premenopausal relative should initiate screening 10 years before the youngest age of diagnosis of breast cancer in the family. Patients with a known germline mutation (e.g., BRCA) should begin breast cancer screening at 25 years of age.

Males with a known germline mutation should be managed with monthly breast self-examination, a semiannual CBE, and annual mammography. Any male patient with a personal history of breast cancer should undergo further genetic counseling and testing to rule out a hereditary cause. Table 21.2 summarizes these screening modalities.

TABLE 21.2	Screening Modalities		
Test	**Sources of Images**	**Best for Detecting**	**Limitations of Test**
Mammogram	X-rays	Calcifications, masses, and architectural distortion	Cannot show if the mass is solid or cyst; lower sensitivity in women who have dense breast tissue
Ultrasound	Sound waves	Differentiate between solid versus cystic masses	Cannot show calcifications
MRI	Magnetic fields must be enhanced with gadolinium contrast	Tissue with increased blood flow such as tumors; high sensitivity and negative predictive value	Expensive; limited to specific indications; high rate of false-positive results
Tomosynthesis	X-rays (3-D digital view); use with a standard mammogram	Architectural distortion, masses, and calcification, in dense breast tissue	Slight increase in radiation exposure versus standard mammogram

From Schuiling K, Likis FE. *Women's Gynecological Health.* 3rd ed. Burlington, MA: Jones & Bartlett; 2017.

BREAST CANCER

Primary care providers play an integral role in the prevention, diagnosis, and management of breast cancer. Primary care providers are essentially the gatekeepers to health care in the United States. Studies have shown that patients see their primary care provider more than any other specialty. These providers have a long-term relationship with their patients. Patients trust and value their family practice provider's recommendations.

Primary care providers must be familiar with the risk factors for breast cancer, how to evaluate a breast mass, imaging techniques, and when to refer to a breast surgeon for further evaluation.

Breast cancer is the most prevalent cancer diagnosed among U.S. females after skin cancer. There are more than 220,000 new invasive breast cancer cases reported annually. The risk of developing breast cancer during a female's lifetime is 1 in 8 (12%). A female's risk of developing breast cancer gradually increases with age, from 1 in 227 for females 30 to 39 years of age to 1 in 28 for those 60 to 69 years of age. Breast cancer is the second leading cause of cancer deaths among females after lung cancer deaths.

Pathophysiology

When cell growth becomes erratic and proliferation occurs, breast cancer develops. It's still unclear as to which hormones are the most critical in the development of breast cancer and why females often develop breast cancer with no identifiable risk factors.

Types of Breast Cancer

Ductal carcinoma in situ (DCIS), or intraductal carcinoma, presents in the earliest manifestation as abnormal cells that are confined to the ducts. DCIS is typically diagnosed when microcalcifications are noted on mammography. It has been referred to as a precancerous condition; however, the likelihood of DCIS progressing into invasive cancer is unknown.

Treatment options include breast-conserving surgery with or without radiation therapy and/or total mastectomy with large or high-grade tumors.

Lobular carcinoma in situ (LCIS) involves abnormal cells that are limited to the breast lobules. It is a noninvasive lesion that may present bilaterally and is often an incidental finding noted during biopsy for another lesion. Management is based on the fact that this condition is a risk factor for cancer and may not always be malignant. The following are potential treatment options: surgical excision, observation with CBE in addition to mammography, preventive therapy such as chemoprevention with tamoxifen, participation in breast cancer prevention trials, and bilateral prophylactic mastectomy for females at high risk for developing breast cancer.

The most common malignancy of the breast is invasive or infiltrating ductal carcinoma. Invasive ductal carcinoma presents as a discrete solid mass. The malignant cells are able to escape the confines of the ducts and infiltrate the breast parenchyma. The most common sites for metastasis involve the lymph nodes, bone, liver, and lungs. Invasive or infiltrating lobular carcinoma is less common and could present as a discrete mass that may be only characterized by induration or skin thickening. The margins are diffuse and often ill-defined. Invasive lobular carcinoma typically presents as bilateral involvement and causes metastatic spread to the intraabdominal region involving the uterus and ovaries, intestinal and urethral obstruction, and carcinomatous meningitis. The treatment for invasive breast cancers is multifactorial. Considerations must include the size and grade of the tumor, involvement of lymph nodes, metastases, primary versus recurrent diagnosis, and results of ER/PR/HER2 testing. Management options include surgery, chemotherapy, radiation therapy, hormone therapy, bisphosphonates, and monoclonal antibodies.

Paget disease is a rare form of breast cancer affecting only 1% of all cases. It presents with eczematous nipple changes including ulceration, itching, erythema, and nipple discharge. Approximately 50% of all female patients diagnosed with Paget disease present with a palpable mass that is typically an underlying DCIS or invasive ductal carcinoma. Paget disease must be considered in any female patient presenting with nipple symptoms. The diagnosis of Paget disease is often delayed. Treatment recommendations include breast-conserving surgery with complete excision of the nipple and areola, followed by radiation. A complete mastectomy is recommended if the margins are positive or if the disease extends beyond the central portion of the breast tissue.

> **! SAFETY ALERT**
>
> Paget disease must be considered in any female patient presenting with nipple symptoms.

Inflammatory breast cancer is a rapid and progressive type of breast cancer. Lymphovascular invasion has already occurred in one-half of all patients at the time of diagnosis. Inflammatory breast cancer presents with diffuse inflammatory changes including erythema, edema, warmth, skin thickening, and fine dimpling called *peau d'orange*. Inflammatory breast cancer can be often misdiagnosed as mastitis. Typically, there is no palpable mass noted on physical examination. If there is any suspicion that a patient has inflammatory breast cancer, immediate mammography and referral for skin biopsy is indicated. Treatment options include surgery, chemotherapy, radiation, hormone therapy, aromatase inhibitors, and monoclonal antibodies.

> **! SAFETY ALERT**
>
> If there is any suspicion that a patient has inflammatory breast cancer, immediate mammography and referral for skin biopsy are indicated.

The incidence of breast cancer diagnosed during pregnancy or within the first year postpartum has been reported as 0.2% to 3.8%. There is often a delay in diagnosis because of breast changes that occur during pregnancy and lactation. Mammography, with abdominal shielding during pregnancy, is indicated if there is a suspicion of breast cancer. Another diagnostic approach includes ultrasonography. A biopsy should be performed on any suspicious mass regardless of imaging results. The management of breast cancer during pregnancy must weigh the risks versus benefits for both the patient and fetus. Surgery can be performed during pregnancy. This may include a lumpectomy or mastectomy. Chemotherapy can be considered during the second and third trimesters but is typically discontinued at 35 weeks' gestation. However, radiation is contraindicated during pregnancy. Table 21.3 demonstrates various breast tissue sampling techniques.

> **! SAFETY ALERT**
>
> A biopsy should be performed on any suspicious mass regardless of imaging results.

Staging

Once breast cancer is diagnosed, the next step is staging to find out whether the cancer has spread within the

TABLE 21.3 Breast Tissue Sampling Procedures

Procedure	Description	Breast Target
Fine-needle aspiration biopsy	Tissue for cytology evaluation. Aspirated with a small needle. Differentiates solid versus cystic masses	Palpable mass or thickening
Stereotactic-guided core-needle biopsy	Large-bore needle used to obtain cores of tissue for histologic examination. Stereotactic mammography used for localization and targeting	Calcification seen on mammogram, masses, or other abnormalities visible only by mammography
Ultrasound-guided core-needle biopsy	Large-bore needle used to obtain cores of tissue for histologic examination. Ultrasound used for localization and targeting	Solid or indeterminate lesion
MRI-guided needle biopsy	MRI with intravenous material used for localization and targeting	Lesions visible only with MRI
Needle-localized breast biopsy	Use of a wire to localize an occult mammographic, sonographic, or MRI-detected abnormality prior to excisional biopsy	Mass or calcification seen on imaging in a location that cannot be effectively assessed with core biopsy
Excisional breast biopsy	Surgical procedure that requires a skin excision. Mass is removed with a surrounding margin of normal-appearing skin	Palpable breast mass, thickening or skin change; used for initial diagnosis only when needle biopsy is not feasible

From Schuiling K, Likis FE. *Women's Gynecological Health.* 3rd ed. Burlington, MA: Jones & Bartlett; 2017.

TABLE 21.4	**Staging Tools**
Sentinel lymph node biopsy	The removal of the sentinel lymph node during surgery. The sentinel is the first lymph node the cancer is likely to spread from the primary tumor. A radioactive substance and/or blue dye is injected near the tumor and the radioactive substance flows through the lymph ducts to the lymph nodes. The first lymph node to receive the substance or dye is removed. A pathologist will inspect the tissue under the microscope to look for cancer cells. If no cancer cells are found, removal of more lymph nodes may not be necessary.
Chest x-ray	An x-ray of the organs and bones inside the chest. An x-ray is a type of energy beam that can go through the body and onto film, making a picture of areas inside the body.
CT scan	A procedure that makes a series of detailed pictures of areas inside the body, taken from different angles. A dye may be injected into a vein or swallowed to help the organs or tissues show up more clearly.
Bone scan	This procedure checks if there are rapidly dividing cells, such as cancer cells, in the bone. A very small amount of radioactive material is injected into a vein and travels through the bloodstream. The radioactive material collects in the bones with cancer and is detected by a scanner.
PET scan	A procedure to find malignant tumor cells in the body. A small amount of radioactive glucose is injected into a vein. Malignant tumor cells show up brighter in the picture because they are more active.

From PDQ Adult Treatment Editorial Board. Breast Cancer Treatment (Adult) (PDQ®): Patient Version. In: *PDQ Cancer Information Summaries* [Internet]. Bethesda, MD: National Cancer Institute; 2022. https://www.ncbi.nlm.nih.gov/books/NBK65969/.

breast or to other parts of the body. Staging is an important component to determine the best treatment plan for the patient. Table 21.4 provides a summary of tools used in the staging process.

There are three types of breast cancer stage groups:
- The *clinical prognostic stage* is described by the TNM system, tumor grade, and biomarker status (ER, PR, HER2).
- The *pathological prognostic stage* is then used for patients who have surgery as their first treatment. This stage is based on all clinical information, biomarker status, and laboratory results from breast tissue and lymph nodes removed during surgery.
- The *anatomical stage* is based on the size and the spread of cancer as described by the TNM system. This stage is used in parts of the world where biomarker testing is not available. It is not used in the United States.

Tumor sizes are often measured in millimeters (mm) or centimeters (cm). Common items that can be used to show tumor size in millimeters include: a sharp pencil point (1 mm), a new crayon point (2 mm), a pencil-top eraser (5 mm), a pea (10 mm), a peanut (20 mm), and a lime (50 mm). Figure 21.5 presents examples of these comparisons.

CLINICAL SURVIVAL TIP: Staging for breast cancer can be quite complex. A complete explanation of TMN staging, terms used, and a description of the clinical prognostic stage can be found at: https://emedicine.medscape.com/article/2007112-overview.

Treatment
Breast-Conserving Surgery
This type surgical operation removes the cancer and some normal tissue around it, but not the breast itself. Part of the chest wall lining may also be removed if the cancer is near it. This type of surgery may also be referenced as a *lumpectomy, partial mastectomy, segmental mastectomy, quadrantectomy,* or *breast-sparing surgery* (Fig. 21.6).

Total Mastectomy. A total mastectomy is surgery to remove the whole breast that has cancer. This procedure is also called a *simple mastectomy.* Some of the lymph nodes under the arm may be removed during this procedure. This may be performed at the same time as the breast surgery or afterward (see Fig. 21.6).

Modified Radical Mastectomy. A modified radical mastectomy is surgery to remove the whole breast that

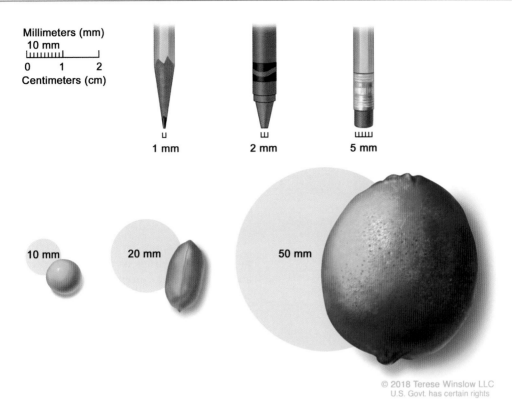

Figure 21.5 Common items representing tumor sizes. (Copyright 2010. Terese Winslow. U.S. government has certain rights.)

has cancer, many of the lymph nodes under the arm, and the lining over the chest muscles, including the chest wall muscles (see Fig. 21.6).

Radiation Therapy. Radiation therapy is a cancer treatment that uses high-energy x-rays or other types of radiation to kill cancer cells or keep them from growing. The radiation therapy given depends on the type and stage of the breast cancer being treated. External radiation therapy is used to treat breast cancer. Internal radiation therapy with strontium-89 is used to relieve bone pain caused by breast cancer that has spread to the bones.

Chemotherapy. Chemotherapy is a cancer treatment that uses certain drugs to stop the growth of cancer cells, either by killing the cells or by stopping them from dividing. When chemotherapy is taken by mouth or injected into a vein or muscle, the drugs enter the bloodstream to systemically reach the cancer cells. The amount of chemotherapy delivered depends on the type and stage of the breast cancer being treated.

Hormone Therapy. Hormone therapy is a cancer treatment that removes hormones or blocks their action and stops cancer cells from growing. Hormone therapy with tamoxifen is used in patients with early breast cancer that typically can be removed with surgery and also those with metastatic breast cancer. Hormone therapy with tamoxifen or estrogens can act on cells all over the body and may increase the chance of developing endometrial cancer. Females taking tamoxifen should undergo an annual pelvic examination to look for any signs of cancer. Any vaginal bleeding, other than menstrual bleeding, should be reported to a provider for further evaluation. Hormone therapy with an aromatase inhibitor is given to postmenopausal females who have hormone receptor–positive breast cancer. Aromatase inhibitors decrease the body's estrogen by blocking an enzyme called *aromatase* from turning circulating androgen into estrogen. The common types of aromatase inhibitors are anastrozole,

Breast-conserving Surgery

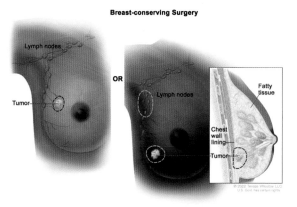

Breast-conserving surgery. Dotted lines show the area containing the tumor that is removed and some of the lymph nodes that may be removed.

Total (Simple) Mastectomy

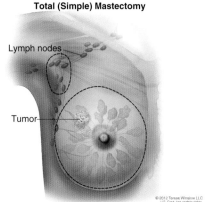

Total (simple) mastectomy. The dotted line shows where the entire breast is removed. Some lymph nodes under the arm may also be removed.

Modified Radical Mastectomy

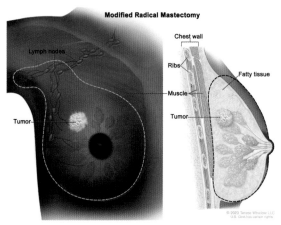

Modified radical mastectomy. The dotted line shows where the entire breast and some lymph nodes are removed. Part of the chest wall muscle may also be removed.

Figure 21.6 Breast-conserving surgery, total (simple) mastectomy, and modified radical mastectomy. (Copyright 2010. Terese Winslow. U.S. government has certain rights.)

letrozole, and exemestane. For the treatment of early localized breast cancer that can be removed with surgical intervention, certain aromatase inhibitors may be used as adjuvant therapy instead of tamoxifen or after 2 to 3 years of tamoxifen use. In females with hormone receptor–positive breast cancer, at least 5 years of adjuvant hormone therapy can reduce the risk of breast cancer recurrence.

> **! SAFETY ALERT**
>
> Any vaginal bleeding, other than menstrual bleeding, should be reported to a provider for further evaluation.

Targeted Therapy. Targeted therapy is a type of treatment that uses drugs or other substances to identify and attack specific cancer cells without harming normal cells. Targeted therapies often used in the treatment of breast cancer include monoclonal antibodies, tyrosine kinase inhibitors, cyclin-dependent kinase inhibitors, mammalian target of rapamycin (mTOR) inhibitors, and poly ADP ribose polymerase (PARP) inhibitors.

Immunotherapy. Immunotherapy uses the patient's immune system to fight cancer. This type of breast cancer treatment is also referenced as *biotherapy* or *biological therapy*. Substances made by the body or made in a laboratory are used to boost, direct, or restore the body's natural defenses against cancer.

Survivorship Program

Once patients have completed breast cancer treatment, they utilize their primary care provider for detection of cancer recurrence and management of long-term consequences. Primary care providers are essential in breast cancer follow-up because of limited secondary care facilities, a growing number of breast cancer survivors, and increasing costs. Primary care providers are essential for short-term and long-term health consequences from cancer and cancer treatment, including physical and psychological outcomes.

The National Comprehensive Cancer Network (NCCN) and the American Cancer Society/American Society of Clinical Oncology (ACS/ASCO) endorse the recommendations for breast cancer survivors found in Table 21.5.

> **PATIENT-CENTERED CARE:** Providing adequate emotional support is just as important as risk assessment, diagnosis, and management of a breast condition.

TABLE 21.5 Recommendations for Breast Cancer Survivors

	NCCN	ACS/ASCO
History and physical examination	Year 1, every 3–4 months Year 2, every 4 months Year 3–5, every 6 months Year 6+ annually	Year 1–3, every 3–6 months Year 4–5, every 6–12 months Year 6+ annually
Signs of recurrence	No recommendation	Educated and counseled about signs and symptoms
Mammography	6 months after post–breast-conserving surgery and radiation therapy Annually thereafter	Annually
MRI	No recommendation	Not recommended for routine screening unless the patient meets high-risk criteria for increased surveillance
Pelvic examination	Annually for women on tamoxifen Annual examination if uterus present	No recommendation
Routine blood tests	Not recommended	Not recommended
Imaging studies	Not recommended	Not recommended
Tumor marker testing	Not recommended	Not recommended

ACS/ASCO, American Cancer Society/American Society of Clinical Oncology; *NCCN,* National Comprehensive Cancer Network.
From Chalasani, P. (2022, Sep 20). Breast Cancer. Retrieved from https://emedicine.medscape.com/article/1947145-overview.

KEY POINTS

- Mastalgia is one of the most common reported breast complaints.
- Mastalgia is benign 90% of the time and accounts for 66% of provider visits for breast symptoms.
- Cyclic breast pain typically improves after the onset of menses. Pain is usually related to hormonal and fibrocystic changes.
- Noncyclic breast pain is associated with oral contraceptives, hormone therapy, antidepressants, and antihypertensives.
- Reassurance is effective in 85% of mastalgia patients.
- Nipple discharge accounts for 6.8% of referrals to providers; 97% of nipple discharge is caused by benign disease.
- Acute mastitis can be caused by pregnancy, lactation, and bacterial infections of unknown origin. *Staphylococcus* infections are commonly associated with acute mastitis. Treatment options for acute mastitis include oral antibiotics, warm compresses, and gentle massage.
- The most obvious and important risk factor in assessing a patient's breast cancer risk factor is age.
- Family history is one of the most effective and least expensive tools in identifying a patient's risk for breast cancer.

- Approximately 10% of breast cancers can be linked with a genetic mutation from either the maternal or paternal side.
- Breast cancer screening recommendations vary based on the following organizations: the ACS, USPSTF, and ACOG.
- Screening mammography is used as a tool in asymptomatic females with the goal of detecting breast cancer that is not yet clinically apparent.
- Ultrasonography is the best imaging modality to differentiate between solid and cystic masses.
- Patients with a strong family history of breast cancer should initiate screening 10 years before the youngest age of diagnosis of breast cancer in the family. Patients with a known germline mutation (e.g., *BRCA*) should begin breast cancer screening at 25 years of age.
- Breast cancer is the most prevalent cancer diagnosed among U.S. females after skin cancer. There are more than 220,000 new invasive breast cancer cases reported annually.
- Nurse practitioners are essential in breast cancer follow-up because of limited secondary care facilities, a growing number of breast cancer survivors, and increasing costs.

REFERENCES

1. Salzman B, Collins E, Hersh L. Common breast problems. *Am Fam Physician*. 2019;99(8):505–514.
2. Santen RJ. *Benign Breast Disease in Women*; 2018. https://www.ncbi.nlm.nih.gov/books/NBK278994/.
3. American Cancer Society. American Cancer Society Recommendations for the Early Detection of Breast Cancer. https://www.cancer.org/cancer/breast-cancer/screening-tests-and-early-detection/american-cancer-society-recommendations-for-the-early-detection-of-breast-cancer.html.
4. Hoffman BL, Schorge JO, Halvorson LM, Hamid CA, Corton MM, Schaffer JI. *Williams Gynecology*. 4th ed. McGraw-Hill Education; 2020.
5. Schuiling K, Likis FE. *Women's Gynecological Health*. 3rd ed. Burlington, MA: Jones & Bartlett; 2017.
6. PDQ Adult Treatment Editorial Board. Breast cancer Treatment (Adult) (PDQ®): Patient Version. In: *PDQ Cancer Information Summaries [Internet]*. Bethesda, MD: National Cancer Institute; 2022. https://www.ncbi.nlm.nih.gov/books/NBK65969/.
7. Chalasani P. *Breast Cancer Screening*; 2022. https://emedicine.medscape.com/article/2247407-overview.
8. National Comprehensive Cancer Network. *Genetic/Familial High-Risk Assessment: Breast, Ovarian, and Pancreatic*; 2021. https://www.nccn.org/professionals/physician_gls/pdf/genetics_bop.pdf.
9. U.S. Centers for Disease Control and Prevention. What Are the risk factors for breast cancer?. https://www.cdc.gov/cancer/breast/basic_info/risk_factors.htm.

22

Urinary Tract Problems

Kala K. Blakely and Cori Cunningham Johnson

OBJECTIVES

- Relate the anatomical and physiological components of the genitourinary (GU) system to the diagnoses and management of commonly seen GU problems.
- Identify key components of the history and physical examination necessary to diagnose common GU problems.

- Understand the diagnostic testing needed to diagnose GU problems.
- Formulate a plan of care for selected GU problems based on a focused history and physical examination as well as selected diagnostic testing.

INTRODUCTION

Many Americans are affected by urological conditions that require medical care, but the overall impact on the U.S. population is unknown. To help quantify the impact and occurrence of these conditions, the National Institutes of Health (NIH) published a report in 2012 that examined the statistics of urological conditions that required physician office visits. Of diagnoses affecting females, the most common office visit diagnoses are as follows: urinary tract infections (UTIs) (5,383,244), urinary incontinence (UI) (2,114,688), urinary tract stones (607,142), and interstitial cystitis (232,361). Of these diagnoses, the one that proved to be most costly was UTIs followed by urinary tract stones. With UTI as the most commonly diagnosed urinary condition in females, the report further specifies that White females 45 to 54 years of age who are living in the south have the highest prevalence. Females are at higher risk than males for all of the aforementioned common urinary diagnoses except for urinary tract stones. Approximately 6.5% of females are diagnosed with kidney stones in their lifetime. Bladder cancer is another frequently seen urological diagnosis; however, it is much more prevalent in males. The estimated number of new cases of bladder cancer in 2011 was approximately 70,000, but females only accounted for about 17,000 of those cases.[1] Older adult and pregnant females are considered high-risk

populations when caring for certain urinary conditions and are discussed later in this chapter.

The urinary tract serves as the body's waste management system. It is composed of the kidneys, ureters, bladder, and urethra. The kidney's role is to filter the blood, and the resulting waste product (urine) is then excreted. The kidneys filter approximately 135 quarts of blood, which results in 1 to 2 quarts of urine every 24 hours. Urine then travels through ureters and is stored in the bladder, which typically holds 250 to 500 mL of urine. When the urinary sphincter muscle relaxes, urine is eliminated from the body.[2]

FOCUSED HISTORY

Health care providers must ask focused questions about GU symptoms when eliciting a history from healthy adult patients including the following:[3]

- Onset of symptoms
- Location of symptoms
- Quality of the discomfort
- Radiation of the discomfort
- Timing (frequency, duration)
- Severity
- Aggravating and alleviating factors
- Associated symptoms
- Presence of fever

- Previous diagnosis of similar episodes
- Previous treatments
- Efficacy of previous treatments
- Sexual history and practices, including high-risk behaviors and contraception
- History of sexually transmitted infections (STIs)
- Symptoms of menopause
- Obstetrical history
- Medical history of any GU diagnoses

Information about specific symptoms should be explored, including the following:[4]

- Frequency of urination
- Amount of urine voided
- Urinary retention
- Incontinence
- Urgency
- Dysuria and its timing during voiding
- Nocturia
- Color and odor of urine
- Presence of stones or sediment in urine
- Hematuria
- Suprapubic, perineal, genital, groin, flank, or lower-back pain
- Urethral discharge
- Vaginal discharge
- Painful intercourse
- Enlarged, painful lymph nodes in the groin
- Sense of pelvic relaxation
- Lesions or persistent ulcerations to the external genitalia
- Recent antibiotic or steroid use

FOCUSED PHYSICAL ASSESSMENT

A focused female GU physical examination should be performed to determine the possible causes of urinary dysfunction. An external GU examination is necessary to identify organ prolapse, tissue atrophy, inflammation, lesions, or discharge.[5] A speculum examination can be used when symptoms are suspected to be related to STIs or pelvic organ prolapse. To assess for prolapse during a speculum examination, the clinician instructs the patient to bear down and observes for any bulging of the vaginal walls. A bimanual examination is helpful in assessing for uterine or pelvic masses that may be compromising urinary flow. An abdominal examination should be performed to assess for a palpable bladder, masses, or pain. Percussion of the costovertebral angle

for tenderness should be performed to evaluate kidney involvement.[5] Perineal sensation, rectal tone, and peripheral motor and sensory examinations should be performed to identify spinal cord or neuropathic conditions that may be contributing to urinary symptoms, such as neurogenic bladder.

FREQUENTLY USED DIAGNOSTIC TOOLS

The provider should include basic laboratory evaluation to rule out infection, malignancy, and metabolic conditions that can affect urinary function and flow (Table 22.1).

To identify bladder distention or urinary retention, a bladder scanner can be used to assess urinary volume. After voiding, the bladder should have less than 50 mL present. More than 200 mL present after voiding indicates bladder dysfunction. If a bladder scanner is not available, then a urinary catheter can be used to measure urinary volume and can relieve urinary obstruction if needed.[6]

Imaging of the urinary tract and kidneys is helpful in detecting cysts, tumors, nephrolithiasis, and obstruction. When severe flank or back pain is present, the possibility of nephrolithiasis, abscess, or obstruction causing hydronephrosis should be considered and ruled out with imaging. Renal ultrasonography or computed tomography (CT) must be used to rule out an abscess or hydronephrosis. A noncontrast helical CT scan is the best method to rule out nephrolithiasis.[7]

TABLE 22.1 Frequently Used Laboratory Tests

- Dipstick urinalysis (performed in the office, and results are obtained quickly)
- Microscopy urinalysis (collected in the office, but sent to a laboratory for testing)
- Urine culture and sensitivity
- Urethral discharge culture and sensitivity
- Pregnancy test (urine and serum human chorionic gonadotropin)
- Sexually transmitted infection screening (urine gonorrhea screening)
- Complete metabolic panel

Modified from Weber JR, Kelley JH. Assessing female genitalia and rectum. In: Richardson C, ed. *Health Assessment in Nursing.* 5th ed. Philadelphia: Lippincott Williams & Wilkins; 2014: 612–643.

Common Urinary Tract Problems

Urinary Tract Infections

Research has shown that approximately 50% of females will develop a urinary tract infection (UTI) at some point in their lifetime.[2,8] UTIs are infections caused by bacteria anywhere along the urinary tract. Lower UTIs are referred to as *cystitis*. Infection occurring in the upper urinary tract (the kidneys) is called *pyelonephritis*. There are several risk factors that place an individual at higher risk for UTIs (Table 22.2). The female urethra is in close proximity to the vagina and rectum, thus activities such as wiping from back to front and vaginal intercourse can introduce bacteria into the urethra. This may increase the risk of UTIs in some females.[8]

When a patient presents with symptoms of dysuria and/or urinary frequency, a focused history and physical examination are needed. The history can provide details of contributory factors to the symptoms and assist with ruling out diagnoses with a similar presentation, such as kidney stones or interstitial cystitis. The physical assessment should include an abdominal examination and percussion of the costovertebral angle. A pelvic examination should be performed if the patient has a normal urinalysis or if there is suspicion of vaginal infection. The pelvic examination will allow for vaginal and cervical samples to be obtained to assess for STIs.[2,8]

A dipstick urinalysis is helpful in providing quick diagnostic details at the time of the visit. Patients can leave a clean-catch urine specimen for dipstick urinalysis while in the clinic. The presence of leukocytes, red blood cells, and nitrites may indicate a UTI and a need for antibiotic treatment. Keep in mind that the urinary tract contains normal flora that can colonize, thus resulting in a urinalysis that is positive for bacteria. With this knowledge, the clinician should determine treatment based on symptom presentation, urinalysis results, and urine culture.[8]

Treatment of UTIs can include nonpharmacological and pharmacological methods. See Table 22.3 for pharmacological treatment recommendations. Pharmacological methods of prevention can be used postcoitally or continually.[8,9]

Nonpharmacological treatment and prevention of a UTI includes adequate hydration and lifestyle modifications (Table 22.4). Encourage patients to urinate when they feel the urge to void. Remind patients that holding urine in the bladder allows unwanted bacteria to stay in the bladder longer and can lead to increased bacterial

TABLE 22.2	Risk Factors and/or Associations for Urinary Tract Infections
Age	Highest incidence is in young, sexually active females 18 to 24 years of age
Sex	Community-acquired urinary tract infections occur most commonly in females[4]
Genetics	Certain HLA and Lewis blood group factors may increase the risk of urinary tract infection by altering host urinary tract defenses[4]
Other Risk Factors/Associations	
Conditions associated with reduced urine flow[4]	Prostatic hyperplasia, genitourinary malignancy, urethral stricture, outflow obstruction, or bladder calculi Neurogenic bladder Inadequate uptake of fluid
Factors that promote bacterial colonization[4]	Sexual activity Spermicide use Estrogen deficiency Antimicrobial agents that deplete indigenous flora Diaphragm contraception[8]
Factors that facilitate bacterial ascent[4]	Urinary catheterization Urinary incontinence Fecal incontinence/perineal soiling Residual urine with bladder wall ischemia
Comorbid medical conditions	Poorly controlled diabetes HIV Sickle cell disease Gout Analgesic abuse Hypokalemia Hypophosphatemia Pregnancy Spinal cord injury

Modified from *Clinical Overview. Urinary Tract Infection in Adults.* Elsevier Point of Care. Updated November 6, 2018. Copyright Elsevier BV.

growth. Voiding regularly can help decrease the risk of UTIs. Along with developing regular bathroom habits, using proper hygiene is beneficial in preventing and decreasing the risk of UTIs. Instruct females on the importance of voiding after intercourse to flush bacteria from the urethral area. Using condoms can prevent the

TABLE 22.3	Pharmacological Treatment for Urinary Tract Infections	
Cystitis	**Uncomplicated Pyelonephritis**
Nitrofurantoin; give for 7 days or for at least 3 days after urine is sterile	Oral fluoroquinolone (e.g., ciprofloxacin for 7–10 days or levofloxacin for 5 days). Give an initial one-time IV dose of a long-acting parenteral antimicrobial, such as 1 g of ceftriaxone or a consolidated 24-hour dose of an aminoglycoside if the prevalence of fluoroquinolone resistance exceeds 10%.
Trimethoprim-sulfamethoxazole for 3 days, if local resistance for *Escherichia coli* is less than 20%	Oral trimethoprim-sulfamethoxazole for 14 days if the uropathogen is known to be susceptible. If trimethoprim-sulfamethoxazole is used when susceptibility is unknown, an initial IV dose of a long-acting parenteral antimicrobial, such as 1 g of ceftriaxone or a consolidated 24-hour dose of an aminoglycoside, is recommended
Fosfomycin trometanol 3 g (1 dose)	
If Above Recommended Agents Cannot Be Used	
β-lactam agents, amoxicillin-clavulanate, cephalexin, or cefpodoxime proxetil, for 3 to 7 days	Amoxicillin-clavulanate or cefpodoxime proxetil for 10 to 14 days
Fluoroquinolones, including ofloxacin, ciprofloxacin, and levofloxacin, for 3 days; considered when no other options are available.[10] Reserve fluoroquinolones for patients who do not have other available treatment options for uncomplicated urinary tract infections; they have been associated with disabling and potentially irreversible serious adverse effects involving the central nervous system, nerves, tendons, muscles, and joints	

Modified from *Clinical Overview. Urinary Tract Infection in Adults.* Elsevier Point of Care. Updated November 6, 2018. Copyright Elsevier BV.

TABLE 22.4	Prevention of Urinary Tract Infections	
Intake and Output	**Clothing**	**Hygiene**
Drink at least 6 to 10 glasses of water daily to maintain hydration	Wear cotton underwear	Void immediately after sex
Do not hold urine	Wear loose-fitting clothes	Avoid vaginal douching
	Sleep without underwear	Wipe from front to back after voiding and bowel movements
		Use condoms for sexual intercourse
		Intercourse should be vaginal to anal, not anal to vaginal

spread of bacteria from person to person. It is also significant to instruct patients on wiping from the urethra to the rectum when cleansing after bowel movements or voiding. Wiping from front to back prevents the spread of bacteria from the rectum to the urethra and vaginal area. Intercourse should take place the same way the patient wipes (always from front to back and not from back to front).[8,9]

Avoidance of snug-fitting clothing that allows for moisture collection in the groin area can help reduce UTIs. Educate patients on wearing cotton underwear and loose-fitting clothing. Patients should avoid wearing underwear to bed. Both recommendations allow for air to freely flow in the groin area, thereby preventing bacterial growth.[8,9]

For patients experiencing more than three UTIs in 1 year, fever, or lack of symptom improvement after initial treatment, the clinician should order a urine culture to assist with determining the appropriate antibiotics. Urine culture and sensitivity will provide details on specific bacteria growing in the urine and also inform the provider of antibiotic susceptibility. The patient should be treated empirically while waiting for the urine culture results to confirm bacteria and susceptibility. If there is no improvement after treatment based on the urine culture, cystoscopy can be useful in providing an inside view of the urinary tract to rule out structural anomalies and cancer.[8,10]

Females who have undergone multiple rounds of pharmacological treatment and continue to experience UTIs should be referred to a specialist, such as a urologist or gynecologist. One specialist is not preferred over the other but is selected based on the specialist's area of expertise regarding the patient's medical needs.[9]

Cystitis

UTIs that occur in the bladder are also known as *cystitis*. Bladder infections are most often caused by bacteria found in the bowel. The bacteria spread from the rectum to the urethral area and then travel the short distance upstream to the bladder because of the shortened urethra. Common symptom presentation for cystitis includes pain with urination, pain on completion of voiding, frequent urination, and urinary urgency.[8] UTI treatment guidelines should be followed for patients with cystitis (see Table 22.3).[9,11]

Pyelonephritis

An infection located in the kidney is known as *pyelonephritis*. There are two types of pyelonephritis: uncomplicated and complicated. It is important to recognize the differences between the two to properly treat the patient (Table 22.5). Research has found that 80% of pyelonephritis cases are caused by the bacteria *Escherichia coli*. Pyelonephritis most often occurs in females 15 to 29 years of age. A universal symptom of pyelonephritis is flank pain. Additional frequently reported symptoms include fever, nausea, and vomiting. Patients who present with complaints of a possible kidney infection but no flank pain should have alternate diagnoses considered.[11]

TABLE 22.5 Types of Pyelonephritis

Uncomplicated Pyelonephritis	Complicated Pyelonephritis
Occurs in healthy individuals	Immunocompromised individuals
No anatomical abnormalities	Structural or functional abnormalities present
Causative agent has typical antimicrobial sensitivity patterns	Causative agent is multidrug-resistant
No comorbidities	Comorbidities present

Modified from Dielubanza EJ, Matulewicz RS, Schaeffer AJ. Pyelonephritis and abscesses of the kidney. In: Cohen J, Powderly WG, Opal SM, eds. *Infectious Diseases*. 4th ed. Elsevier; 2017: 547–554.e1.

The clinician should take a focused history, inquiring about urinary frequency, urgency, dysuria, and pyuria. Along with flank pain, ask if the patient has experienced any gastrointestinal symptoms such as nausea, vomiting, or abdominal pain. Also inquire about fever, chills, and malaise. Common physical examination findings for a patient with pyelonephritis can include fever greater than 100.4°F, tachycardia, hypotension, and/or costovertebral angle tenderness. Patients may also have abdominal and/or suprapubic tenderness on palpation.[11]

Diagnostic tests for patients suspected of having pyelonephritis should include a dipstick or microscopic urinalysis, urine culture, and susceptibility. The urinalysis should be performed on a clean-catch urine specimen. The clinician should look for the presence of leukocytes and microscopic hematuria, which along with physical findings will confirm acute pyelonephritis. Urinalysis resulting with gross hematuria is seen more in acute uncomplicated cystitis. Urine culture and susceptibility should be ordered to assist the clinician with any antibiotic adjustments needed based on antibiotic resistance and lack of symptom improvement.[11,12]

Initial treatment should be started based on symptom presentation, physical findings, and urinalysis results. According to the Infectious Diseases Society of America, non-pregnant patients in an outpatient setting should be treated with an oral fluoroquinolone (ciprofloxacin 500 mg orally every 12 hours for 7 days or levofloxacin 750 mg orally once daily for 5 days). In areas of known susceptibility, oral trimethoprim-sulfamethoxazole

160/800 mg twice daily for 14 days is an alternative treatment choice.[11,12]

With proper treatment and patient compliance in taking the antibiotic as prescribed, symptom improvement should occur within 48 to 72 hours of initial treatment. Changes should be made to the antibiotic regimen based on the urine culture and susceptibility results. Patients with comorbid conditions, pregnancy, hemodynamic instability, renal dysfunction or acidosis, severe flank or abdominal pain, toxic appearance, or inability to keep fluids down should be hospitalized for inpatient treatment.[11]

Interstitial Cystitis

Interstitial cystitis is a chronic condition that causes bladder pressure, bladder pain, urinary urgency, and sometimes pelvic pain lasting greater than 6 weeks. The pain ranges from mild discomfort to severe pain. With interstitial cystitis, patients also feel the urge to urinate more often and with smaller volumes of urine than most patients.[13] Although signs and symptoms of interstitial cystitis may resemble those of a chronic UTI, there is no infection.[14] The exact cause of interstitial cystitis is not known, and there is no cure, but medications and other therapies can offer relief.

Diagnosis is challenging because there is a lack of evidence in the literature for consistent findings. In diagnosing interstitial cystitis, the clinician should begin with a detailed history, physical examination, and laboratory testing to rule out other diagnoses that might be confused with interstitial cystitis. One hallmark sign is pain that worsens with specific foods or drinks or as the bladder fills and then is relieved with urination. According to evidence-based practice guidelines from the American Urological Association (AUA), the potassium sensitivity test is not a useful diagnostic test and if performed could cause symptoms to worsen. Urodynamic tests are also not helpful, as results in interstitial cystitis patients vary. Cystoscopy and/or urodynamics should be considered in complex presentations only as an aid to diagnosis to rule out other causes such as stones, malignancy, or urethral diverticula.[15] Referral to a urologist or a urogynecologist may be required for diagnosis.

No simple treatment eliminates the signs and symptoms of interstitial cystitis, and no one treatment works for everyone.[15] Trying various treatments or combinations of treatments may be required before finding an approach that relieves the patient's symptoms.[16] The

TABLE 22.6	**Interstitial Cystitis Treatment**
First-line treatments	• General relaxation/stress management • Pain management • Patient education • Self-care/behavior modification
Second-line treatments	• Appropriate manual physical therapy techniques • Oral medications; amitriptyline, cimetidine, hydroxyzine, pentosan polysulfate • Intravesical: dimethyl sulfoxide, heparin, lidocaine • Pain management
Third-line treatments	• Cystoscopy under anesthesia with hydrodistension • Pain management • Treatment of Hunner lesions if found

Modified from Hanno PM, Burks DA, Clemens JQ, et al. AUA guideline for the diagnosis and treatment of interstitial cystitis/bladder pain syndrome. *J Urol.* 2011;185(6):2162–2170.

clinician should begin with the least invasive treatment approaches and work up if symptoms do not improve. Treatment guidelines should be followed when treating patients with interstitial cystitis (Table 22.6).

Surgery is rarely used to treat interstitial cystitis because removing the bladder often does not relieve pain and can lead to other complications. Patients with severe pain that is unresponsive to therapy or those whose bladders can hold only very small volumes of urine are possible candidates for surgery.[16] This is usually only after other treatments fail and symptoms severely disturb quality of life.[15]

Nephrolithiasis

Nephrolithiasis is the presence of calculi in the kidneys, more commonly known as *kidney stones*. The AUA reports that over 8% of the U.S. population self-reported experiencing nephrolithiasis between 2007 and 2010. It is important to note that these percentage results are self-reported and therefore do not capture the percentage of individuals who did not report or who experienced asymptomatic nephrolithiasis.[17,18]

The clinical presentation is most often sudden onset of colicky pain in the flank area that radiates to the inferior and anterior areas. These patients commonly present to the emergency department because of the severity and sudden onset of pain. Patients presenting with symptoms similar to pyelonephritis with flank pain should be considered for the possibility of nephrolithiasis.[11] Physical examination findings can vary from costovertebral angle tenderness to an unremarkable abdominal examination. Patients may exhibit symptoms of pain in the groin area without visible signs or may frequently change positions because of pain. Calculi can cause pain in different regions as it moves through the urinary tract (Table 22.7).[18]

A focused history should be taken with special attention to any significant medical history that can contribute to the formation of kidney stones. Diabetes, hyperthyroidism, hyperparathyroidism, gout, and gastrointestinal malabsorption diseases can all increase the risk of developing kidney stones. It is important to assess the patient's dietary intake of calcium, sodium, fruits, vegetables, protein, and fluids. The clinician should inquire about dietary supplements that can increase the risk of kidney stones such as calcium, vitamin C, and vitamin D. The clinician should also review the medication history to determine if the patient is taking any medications that can provoke stones, such as lipase inhibitors, protease inhibitors, probenecid, triamterene, carbonic anhydrase inhibitors, or chemotherapy drugs.[17]

Diagnosis of nephrolithiasis can be made based on symptoms and physical findings. The AUA recommends dipstick urinalysis, microscopic urinalysis, and serum creatinine. The urinalysis will allow the provider to determine the presence of bacteria and the urine pH. A urine culture should be performed on patients with a UTI. A complete blood count with differential, basic metabolic panel, and 24-hour urine collection can be useful in establishing current renal function.[17-19]

TABLE 22.7 Calculi Symptom Presentation

Location of Calculus	Symptoms
Renal pelvis or calyx	Deep flank ache
Proximal or middle part of the ureter	Severe flank pain radiating to the groin
Distal end of the ureter	Flank discomfort and/or low abdominal pain
Bladder	Dysuria, frequency, urgency, retention, suprapubic discomfort

From Menckhoff, CR. Nephrolithiasis. In: Adams, JG, ed. *Emergency Medicine.* 2nd ed. Philadelphia: Elsevier; 2013.

Noncontrast CT is the diagnostic imaging tool of choice for suspected calculi. A noncontrast CT scan will provide anatomical details of the calculi that will assist the provider in developing a treatment plan. It will also rule out partial or complete obstruction caused by the calculi. Renal ultrasonography, plain abdominal radiography, renal tomography, retrograde pyelography, and nuclear renal scintigraphy also offer insight to renal anatomy and calculi location.[18]

Symptomatic care is the treatment of choice for kidney stones less than 10 mm in size. The clinician should replenish fluids and electrolytes for patients presenting with electrolyte imbalance, offer antiemetics for nausea, provide nonsteroidal antiinflammatories or corticosteroids to reduce inflammation, and address pain with non-narcotic or narcotic analgesics based on severity of pain and the patient's pain tolerance. It is recommend that patients with suspected or confirmed stones strain urine for calculi collection. Stone analysis can then be performed in the laboratory to determine composition of the calculi. More specific treatment and prevention can then be provided for the patient.[17-19]

Patients who are unable to urinate as a result of urinary tract obstruction, fever, unremitting vomiting, and/or uncontrollable pain should be directed to the emergency department for inpatient care. Approximately 80% of patients will experience spontaneous passing of calculi. Calculi that measure greater than 7 mm are not as likely as smaller calculi to pass without intervention. Intervention most often involves ureteroscopy in which a small scope is inserted into the ureter to allow for removal of the calculi. If calculi are too large to remove without further injury to the patient, lithotripsy is used. Lithotripsy is the use of a laser to break the calculi into smaller fragments for removal. Patients requiring this type treatment warrant referral to urology for further evaluation.[17,20,21]

Education is an important component of preventing nephrolithiasis. It is recommended that patients younger than 25 years of age with a history of recurrent nephrolithiasis, history of lithotripsy, or solitary kidney undergo a 24-hour urine collection for detection of hypercalciuria, hyperuricosuria, hyperoxaluria, hypocitraturia, and low urine volume. Recognition of excess or low volume can help direct which modification to make in preventing future nephrolithiasis formation. Changes can be made through diet, nutritional supplement intake, and medication.[17,20]

NOT TO BE MISSED

Patients with nephrolithiasis who are unable to urinate as a result of urinary tract obstruction, fever, unremitting vomiting, and/or uncontrollable pain should be directed to the emergency department for inpatient care.

Cystocele

A cystocele occurs when the supportive tissue that holds the bladder up and the muscle between the patient's vagina and bladder weakens and stretches, thus allowing the bladder to drop into the vagina. This is also called a *prolapsed* or *dropped* bladder.[22] A cystocele can be caused by straining the muscles that support the pelvic organs, such as straining during vaginal childbirth, heavy lifting, or with chronic constipation. This tends to be more prominent after menopause, when estrogen levels decrease.[23]

There are three grades of severity of a cystocele. Grade 1 is the mildest, and this classification is chosen when the bladder drops only a short distance into the vagina. Grade 2 is considered moderate prolapse and occurs when the bladder drops far enough to reach the opening of the vagina. Grade 3 is the most severe, and this classification occurs when the bladder protrudes out through the opening of the vagina.[22] Symptoms of a cystocele can include the sensation that something is dropping out of the vaginal opening, the sensation of pelvic fullness, urinary hesitation, feeling of incomplete urination, urinary frequency or urgency, and pain with coitus.[24] Females with a cystocele may also experience stress incontinence, urinary retention, and frequent UTIs. Many times females with a mild cystocele lack symptoms until the prolapse worsens[22] (Figs. 22.1 and 22.2).

Treatment options depend on how severe the patient's prolapse has become and the severity of the symptoms. Determining the severity of the prolapse is first established by performing a pelvic examination. The clinician should inspect for a tissue bulge into the vagina. The patient is asked to bear down as if having a bowel movement to enable the clinician determine how much this pressure intensifies the degree of prolapse. This examination can be performed with or without the use of a speculum. The clinician should also assess pelvic floor muscle strength by asking the patient to contract as if trying to stop the stream of urine. If the patient is found to have a significant prolapse, then a post-void residual test may be performed to determine how well and completely the bladder is emptying.[22] A strengthened pelvic floor provides better support for pelvic organs and relief from symptoms associated with a cystocele. Mild cases typically do not require treatment other than avoiding heavy lifting or straining with occasional visits to assess for worsening prolapse. It is important to educate patients on self-care measures to reduce the progression of the prolapse if a mild to moderate cystocele is present. Patients should be taught Kegel exercises to help strengthen the pelvic floor muscles.[25] Furthermore, teaching patients to eat high-fiber foods and maintain adequate hydration can help prevent constipation and reduce straining, which can lead to a cystocele. Avoiding heavy lifting can also prevent progression. When lifting heavy objects, it is important to educate patients on proper lifting techniques, such as lifting with the legs instead of the waist or back. Coughing can also lead to progression of a cystocele, therefore patients should be encouraged to avoid smoking and also seek treatment for a chronic cough or bronchitis.[26]

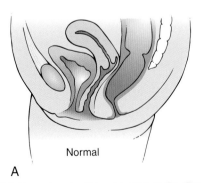
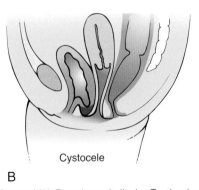

A   B

Figure 22.1 Normal vagina (A) and cystocele (B). (From Swartz MH. Female genitalia. In: *Textbook of Physical Diagnosis: History and Examination.* 8th ed. Philadelphia: Elsevier; 2021.)

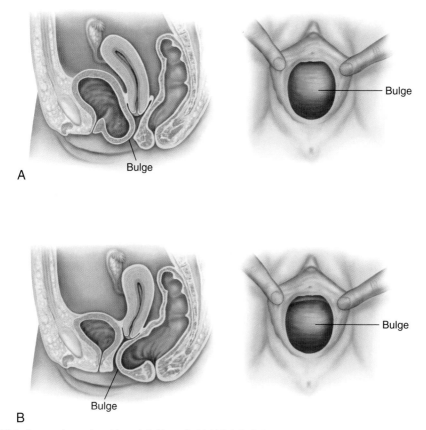

A

B

Figure 22.2 Cystocele grades. (**A and C,** From Seidel HM, Ball JW, Dains JE, Benedict GW. *Mosby's Guide to Physical Examination.* 4th ed. Mosby; 1999. **B and D,** From Symonds EM, Macpherson MBA. *Color Atlas of Obstetrics and Gynecology.* Mosby-Wolfe; 1994.)

Lastly, excess body weight can contribute to prolapse, thus the clinician should discuss avoiding weight gain and effective weight-loss strategies if the patient is overweight.[22]

Estrogen therapy is a pharmacological treatment that can be helpful, especially if the patient is postmenopausal. Estrogen helps keep pelvic muscles strong, but decreases after menopause. Vaginal estrogen therapy in a cream, tablet (oral or vaginal), or ring form is recommended.[27] See Chapter 13 for complete treatment of atrophic vaginitis and atrophic urethra. If the patient has a UTI caused by urinary retention, then antibiotics should be prescribed.

If symptoms are modest, then a pessary should be considered. A vaginal pessary is a plastic or rubber ring that is inserted into the vagina to help support the bladder. Patients should be fitted for the appropriate device and taught how to clean and reinsert it on their own. Pessaries must be removed and cleaned on a regular basis to avoid ulcers and infection.[28] Referral to a gynecologist may be needed if the primary care provider is not comfortable with fitting the patient with a pessary (Figs. 22.3 and 22.4).

When fitting a pessary, providers must rely on manufacturer guidelines, expert opinion, product availability, and clinical judgment when choosing the initial shape and style because there are no quantitative measurements to direct pessary choice and fitting. The goal of fitting a pessary is to find one that improves the target pelvic floor symptoms, is comfortable and retained during activity and toileting, and does not cause vaginal irritation or obstruction of

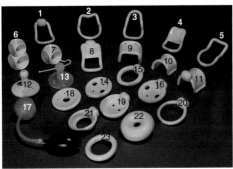

Figure 22.3 Pessary styles. (From Fowler GC. Pfenninger & Fowler's Procedures for Primary Care. Elsevier; 2020.)

voiding or defecation. A brief overview of fitting is as follows:[29]

- Before fitting, ask the patient to empty the bladder and bowels.
- Place the patient in the semi-Fowler's position.
- Apply an ample amount of water-based lubricant to the vaginal introitus.
- Digitally assess vaginal shape, size, and support.
- Select a pessary that you feel will best fit the patient, clean it with soap, and then rinse it with water.
- Apply additional water-based lubricant to the leading edge of the pessary (if needed).
- Insert the pessary by applying pressure gently toward the posterior vaginal wall and/or obliquely (at 11 o'clock and 5 o'clock positions related to the introitus) in the largest diameter, avoiding pressure on the urethra.
- Ask the patient to perform the Valsalva maneuver and cough in the lithotomy and standing positions. If fitting correctly, the pessary should be comfortable and may advance toward the introitus with pressure and recede with relaxation, but it should not come out. To assess that it is not too tight on the vaginal walls, gently rock the pessary in place.
- Ask the patient to stand, walk, and simulate normal activities to assess for any discomfort.
- Ask the patient to sit on the toilet, void, and gently perform the Valsalva maneuver to simulate defecation. The pessary should remain inside the introitus.
- If the pessary is expelled or uncomfortable, begin the fitting process again.[29]

For a mild or moderate prolapse, nonsurgical treatments are often effective. Patients should also be checked for uterine and rectal prolapse, as these can all occur simultaneously (see Chapter 19 for more details on uterine

and rectal prolapse). In more severe cases, surgery may be necessary to keep the vagina and other pelvic organs in their proper positions. If the patient has more severe symptoms, urogynecological surgery may be required, and a referral must be made for further evaluation.[22]

Urinary Incontinence

Millions of females experience UI, which is the unintentional loss of urine. The severity of UI varies as some females may lose a few droplets of urine when coughing or exercising, and others lose a large amount of urine after feeling a strong, sudden urge to urinate. Older adult females experience UI more often than younger females.[30]

There are different types of UI and therefore different ways to treat the condition. The different types of UI are *stress, urge, functional, overflow,* and *mixed* incontinence. These are defined in Table 22.8.

To determine which type of UI the patient has, the clinician should instruct the patient to keep a voiding diary that records bladder symptoms for at least 48 hours. This log should include the volume of fluid intake, timing of urination, amount of urine produced, whether the patient experienced an urge to urinate, severity, triggers, frequency of incontinence episodes, and frequency of non-incontinent voids. A urinalysis should also be performed to rule out infection as a cause or complication. A bladder stress test can be performed by asking the patient to vigorously cough as the clinician watches for a loss of urine from the urinary opening. A post-void residual can be conducted as well to help determine if there is an obstruction in the urinary tract or a problem with the bladder nerves or muscles.[6]

Once the type of incontinence, its severity, and the underlying cause are determined, a combination of treatments may be needed. The least invasive treatments are typically recommended first, and then progression to other options can be considered only if these techniques fail.[30] There are several different noninvasive behavioral techniques. Behavioral techniques are the first-line therapy and include fluid management, pelvic floor muscle training, bladder training, and bladder-control strategies.[31] For example, some patients can experience a decrease in episodes of awakening at night to urinate if they stop drinking liquids several hours before bedtime.[32] To regain bladder control, it is also important to encourage patients to minimize or avoid alcohol, caffeine, and acidic foods.[30] Losing weight can improve symptoms, as excessive weight contributes to

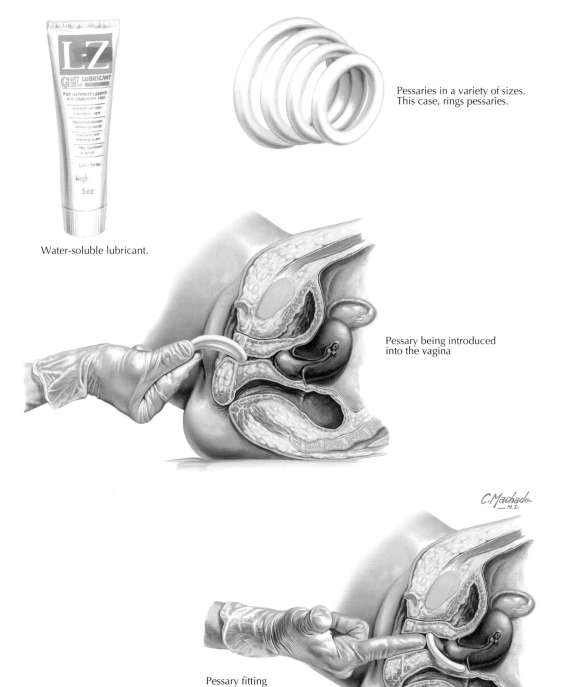

Water-soluble lubricant.

Pessaries in a variety of sizes.
This case, rings pessaries.

Pessary being introduced
into the vagina

Pessary fitting

Figure 22.4 Pessary placement. (From Roger P. Smith, *Netter's Obstetrics and Gynecology,* 3rd Edition.)

TABLE 22.8   Types of Urinary Incontinence

Type of Urinary Incontinence	Defining Factors
Stress urinary Incontinence	Complaint of involuntary urinary loss with physical exertion, sneezing/coughing, or other activities that raise intraabdominal pressure
Urgency urinary incontinence	Complaint of involuntary urinary loss associated with a sensation of urgency
Functional incontinence	Inability to toilet caused by impaired cognitive or physical function, environmental barriers, or psychological unwillingness (depression, anger, or hostility).
Overflow incontinence	The bladder is chronically distended and never empties completely. Urine may dribble out in small amounts as the bladder overflows.
Mixed incontinence	Complaint of involuntary urinary loss associated with physical exertion/increase in intraabdominal pressure *and also* with urgency

Modified from Lemack GE, Anger JT. Urinary incontinence and pelvic prolapse: epidemiology and pathophysiology. *In: Campbell-Walsh Urology.* 74: 1743-1760.e3; Gerber GS, Brendler CB. Evaluation of the urologic patient: history, physical examination, and urinalysis, In: *Campbell-Walsh Urology.* 1: 1-25.e1; Segal-Gidan, F. & Yeo, G. Geriatric Medicine. In R. Ballweg, E. Sullivan, D. Brown, & D. Vetrosky, (Eds.) *The Physician Assistant: A Guide to Clinical Practice,* 5th Ed. Philadelphia: W.B. Elsevier/Saunders. 2013

UI, although some patients may be hesitant to participate in physical activity to aid in weight reduction if they experience stress incontinence.[32] Kegel exercises are encouraged to help strengthen the pelvic floor muscles. Patients should work up to completing three sets of 10 repetitions of Kegel exercises per day.

Bladder training is a technique used to help delay urination after the patient feels the urge to urinate. Based on the patient's voiding diary, it may be helpful to suggest timed voiding, which is using the toilet at regularly timed intervals.[32] The goal is to lengthen the time between trips to the toilet until the patient is only urinating every 2 to 4 hours. Double voiding can help patients learn to empty their bladder more completely to avoid overflow incontinence.[30] For double voiding, the clinician instructs the patient to urinate, wait a few minutes on the toilet, and then try to urinate again before leaving the bathroom. Scheduled toileting or urinating every 2 to 4 hours rather than waiting for the urge to go can also be helpful.[32]

If behavioral approaches are not proven to be sufficient when treating patients, then oral medications can also be used. Medications depend on the type of incontinence. See Table 22.9 for treatment recommendations based on the type of UI.[30]

Patients who have symptoms that are not improving with behavioral and medical therapy should be referred and evaluated by a subspecialist, such as a urologist or urogynecologist, if they desire additional treatment.[31] In this case, a urethral insert or a pessary may be prescribed for stress incontinence. A urethral insert, which is a small tampon-like disposable device, can aid in prevention of activity-related stress incontinence. The device is inserted into the urethra before an activity that triggers incontinence, such as running, and acts as a plug to prevent leakage. It is then removed by the patient before urination. Once referred, other treatments, including sacral neuromodulation, peripheral tibial nerve stimulation, intradetrusor onabotulinumtoxin A (Botox) injections, and even surgical procedures, can be considered.[31]

If medical treatments are not able to eliminate the incontinence, the clinician can recommend products that help ease the discomfort or embarrassment of urine leakage. Pads and protective garments can be worn for extra protection. For patients who are incontinent because their bladder never empties completely (overflow incontinence) or because their bladder cannot empty as a result of poor muscle tone or spinal cord injury, intermittent catheterization may be recommended.[32] If catheterization is required, then the patient is at increased risk for infection.

Bladder Cancer

Bladder cancer is more common in males than in females, but it can occur in females as well. The average age at diagnosis is 73 years of age. Cigarette smoking is the leading risk factor for bladder cancer. Hematuria is the presenting symptom in the vast majority of cases. This includes gross and microscopic hematuria that may be chronic and/or intermittent. Most patients

TABLE 22.9 Treatment Recommendations for Urinary Incontinence Based on Established Cause

	ESTABLISHED CAUSE		
	Detrusor Overactivity	**Urethral Incompetence**	**Detrusor Underactivity**
First line	• Bladder training • Lifestyle modifications • Weight loss • Caffeine reduction • Timed voiding • Kegel exercises	• Lifestyle modifications • Weight loss • Caffeine reduction • Limiting fluid intake • Kegel exercises	• Double voiding • Applying suprapubic pressure
Second line	Antimuscarinic agents: • Tolterodine • Oxybutynin • Fesoterodine • Trospium chloride • Solifenacin β_3 agonist: mirabegron Onabotulinum toxin A injection into detrusor muscle	• Biofeedback • Electrical stimulation • Pessary	• Intermittent or indwelling catheter
Note	Combination of behavioral therapy and antimuscarinics have been found to be more effective than either one alone.	No medications are approved for the treatment of urethral incompetence causing stress incontinence.	In patients requiring catheterization, antibiotics should be used only for symptomatic urinary tract infection.

Modified from Qaseem A, Dallas P, Forciea MA, et al. Nonsurgical management of urinary incontinence in women: a clinical practice guideline from the American College of Physicians. *Ann Intern Med.* 2014;161(6):429–440.

do not exhibit signs of the disease. Masses, hepatomegaly, or palpable lymphadenopathy may be present in patients with advanced or metastatic disease.[33]

Urinalysis typically reveals microscopic or gross hematuria and is sometimes accompanied by pyuria. Anemia can occasionally be found as a result of chronic blood loss or bone marrow metastasis. Bladder cancer can be identified using ultrasonography, CT, or magnetic resonance imaging (MRI) to visualize a mass within the bladder. However, cancer is confirmed with cytology and biopsy.[33]

All patients with hematuria who are suspected to have bladder cancer require referral to a urologist. Hematuria many times warrants evaluation with both upper urinary tract imaging and cystoscopy, especially in high-risk patients.[33]

Population Considerations

Special consideration should be given to the older adult population when treating urinary tract symptoms because of the structural and functional changes in the urinary tract that commonly occur with age. Older adults are specifically at risk for chronic UTIs, nocturnal polyuria, and UI. The decrease in estrogen causes changes in postmenopausal females, such as loss of the protective effect of estrogen on bladder mucosa. Also, loss of tissue tone caused by the lack of estrogen may contribute to UI.[34] Female older adults are more likely to experience UI, with approximately 15% to 30% of healthy older adults experiencing urinary leakage. The prevalence increases with frailty, as approximately 50% of frail community dwellers experience UI. UI is classified as a geriatric syndrome, is often multifactorial in origin, and requires a multidimensional approach for treatment. Factors such as cognitive decline, anatomical abnormalities, and physical immobility influence continence in older adults.[6]

UI is quite common in older adult females with diabetes. More than 50% of females with diabetes experience UI. Patients with diabetes mellitus are three times more likely to experience urge incontinence and two times more likely to experience stress incontinence. Diabetes mellitus is also linked to a higher prevalence of UTI. Evidence does not yet show that tighter glycemic control improves these symptoms.[35] However, it is recommended patients with diabetes mellitus be treated with a 10- to 14-day course of antibiotics.[36]

UTIs are the most common bacterial infections among older adults. Females with UI who are older than 80 years of age and need assistance to walk have an almost 50% increased risk for developing an asymptomatic UTI.[28] Asymptomatic bacteriuria increases with advancing age and occurs in approximately 20% of females older than 80 years of age. Screening for asymptomatic bacteriuria is not regularly advised in older adults living in the community. Asymptomatic bacteriuria does not require treatment because it is not linked to adverse outcomes and can cause antibiotic resistance.[37]

Severe symptomatic UTIs in older adult female patients warrant hospitalization; however, mortality rates are low. Although classic UTI symptoms may be present, nonspecific symptoms are also common in older adult females. These symptoms include general malaise, altered mental status or delirium, or, in life-threatening cases, sepsis or septic shock. The diagnosis is based on urinalysis and urine culture, and symptomatic UTIs should always be treated.[37] Nocturnal polyuria is also prevalent in older adults, affecting an estimated 90% of adults older than 80 years of age. Nocturnal polyuria is a condition in which excessive urine is produced at night. This can cause disruption in sleep, which can then lead to daytime drowsiness, cognitive impairment, and reduced quality of life. Once infection has been ruled out as the cause, several nonpharmacological treatments can be attempted. Avoidance of diuretics and caffeine before bedtime may provide relief. Daytime use of compression stockings and elevating the lower extremities is recommended in patients with edema. In patients with chronic illnesses contributing to nocturia, such as congestive heart failure and chronic kidney disease, the primary therapy is treating the underlying disease. There are also several pharmacological treatments. First, prescribing diuretics to be taken 6 to 8 hours before bedtime may decrease a patient's overall volume status, leading to a decrease in nocturnal urine production. Specifically in females with detrusor overactivity and urge incontinence, medications such as solifenacin, propantheline, and oxybutynin can be useful.[38]

Patients who require catheterization are at increased risk for developing a UTI, therefore catheter use should be avoided in the management of incontinence when possible. Residents of long-term care facilities sometimes require chronic indwelling catheters and can be continuously bacteriuric because of biofilm formation along the catheter. When fever is present and there are no localizing findings, many times these episodes are not from a urinary source, and further evaluation is necessary. To rule out a urinary source, the catheter should be replaced if it has been present for at least 2 weeks, and the urine specimen should be collected through the new catheter. This provides a specimen of urine without biofilm contamination, and catheter replacement also improves clinical outcomes. Empirical antimicrobial therapy should be avoided when possible. It is important to avoid use of a urinary catheter whenever possible and to remove the catheter promptly when there is no longer an indication for its use.[39]

There are several STIs that mimic UTIs, therefore STIs should be differential diagnoses for sexually active females with urinary symptoms. Most females with gonorrhea do not have any symptoms, but even when a patient has symptoms, they are often mild and can be mistaken for a bladder or vaginal infection. This is because one of the main symptoms of gonorrhea is having a painful or burning sensation with urination.[40] Females with chlamydia may also present with a burning sensation when urinating,[41] and trichomoniasis can cause discomfort with urination.[42] Sexually active females, especially those who engage in risky sexual behaviors, should be tested for an STI when presenting with urinary symptoms to properly treat the correct infection. See Chapter 15 for details on STIs.

Smoking is the leading known risk factor for bladder cancer, therefore this population should be given special consideration when assessing the urinary tract. Although bladder cancer is more prevalent in males, the link to smoking occurs in both sexes. A recent study by the NIH found that approximately 50% of bladder cancer cases in females are caused by smoking, which is now equivalent to males. This study also found that past smokers were two times more likely and current smokers were four times more likely to develop bladder cancer than those who had never smoked. Smoking cessation is associated with reducing the risk of developing bladder cancer.[43]

KEY POINTS

- The urinary tract system serves as a filtration system for the body.
- A focused female GU physical examination should always be performed to determine possible causes of urinary dysfunction.

- UTIs can be prevented through adequate hydration and proper hygiene.
- Patients presenting with symptoms similar to pyelonephritis with flank pain should be considered for the possibility of nephrolithiasis.
- A cystocele, also called a *prolapsed* or *dropped* bladder, occurs when the supportive tissue that holds the bladder up weakens and stretches, thus allowing the bladder to drop into the vagina.
- Older adults are specifically at risk for chronic UTI, nocturnal polyuria, and UI.
- Sexually active females, especially those who engage in risky sexual behaviors, should be tested for STIs when presenting with urinary symptoms.

REFERENCES

1. Litwin MS, Saigal CS, eds. *Urologic Diseases in America.* U.S. Department of Health and Human Services, Public Health Service, National Institutes of Health, National Institute of Diabetes and Digestive and Kidney Diseases. NIH Publication No. 12-7865. Washington, DC: US Government Printing Office; 2012.
2. National Institute of Diabetes and Digestive and Kidney Diseases. *The Urinary Tract and How it Works.* 2013. https://www.niddk.nih.gov/health-information/urologic-diseases/urinary-tract-how-it-works.
3. Weber JR, Kelley JH. Assessing female genitalia and rectum. In: Richardson C, ed. *Health Assessment in Nursing.* 5th ed. Philadelphia: Lippincott Williams & Wilkins; 2014:612–643.
4. AMN Healthcare Education Services. *Focused Renal and Urinary Assessment*; 2004. Updated October 20, 2011 https://lms.rn.com/getpdf.php/1852.pdf?Main_Session=2a3879c7f6f1c022a18a3d32f980f0a9.
5. American Urological Association. *Female GU Exam*; Updated 2022. https://www.auanet.org/meetings-and-education/for-medical-students/female-gu-exam.
6. Gammack JK. Urinary incontinence. In: Williams BA, Chang A, Ahault C, et al., eds. *Current Diagnosis & Treatment: Geriatrics.* 2nd ed. McGraw-Hill; 2014:275–283.
7. Omar M, Abdulwahab-Ahmed A, Chaparala H, Monga M. Does stone removal help patients with recurrent urinary tract infections? *J Urol.* 2015;194(4):997–1001.
8. National Institute of Diabetes and Digestive and Kidney Diseases. *Bladder Infection (Urinary Tract Infection—UTI) in Adults*; 2017. https://www.niddk.nih.gov/health-information/urologic-diseases/bladder-infection-uti-in-adults.
9. Brusch JL, Bavaro MF, Cunha BA, Tessier JM. *Urinary Tract Infection (UTI) and Cystitis (Bladder Infection) in Females Treatment and Management*; 2017. Updated January 2, 2020 http://emedicine.medscape.com/article/233101-treatment#d8.
10. Pickard R, Bartoletti R, Bjerklund-Johansen TE, et al. *EAU Guidelines. Urological Infections*; 2021. https://uroweb.org/guideline/urological-infections/#1.
11. Colgan R, Williams M, Johnson JR. Diagnosis and treatment of acute pyelonephritis in women. *Am Fam Physician.* 2011;84(5):519–526.
12. Gupta K, Hooton T, Naber KG, et al. International clinical practice guidelines for the treatment of acute uncomplicated cystitis and pyelonephritis in women: a 2010 update by the Infectious Diseases Society of America and the European Society for Microbiology and Infectious Diseases. *Clin Infect Dis.* 2011;52(5):e103–e120.
13. Hanno PM, Erickson D, Moldwin R, Faraday MM, American Urological Association. Diagnosis and treatment of interstitial cystitis/bladder pain syndrome: AUA guideline amendment. *J Urol.* 2015;193(5):1545–1553.
14. Cody JD, Jacobs ML, Richardson K, Moehrer B, Hextall A. Oestrogen therapy for urinary incontinence in post-menopausal women. *Cochrane Database Syst Rev.* 2012;10(10):CD001405.
15. Clemens JQ, Erickson DR, Varela NP, Lai HH. Diagnosis and Treatment of Interstitial Cystitis/Bladder Pain Syndrome. *J Urol.* 2022;208(1):34-42.
16. National Institute of Diabetes and Digestive and Kidney Diseases. *Treatment for Interstitial Cystitis*; 2017. https://www.niddk.nih.gov/health-information/urologic-diseases/interstitial-cystitis-painful-bladder-syndrome/treatment.
17. Pearle MS, Goldfarb DS, Assimos DG, et al. Medical management of kidney stones: AUA guideline. *J Urol.* 2014;192(2):316–324.
18. Dave CN, Faraj K, Shetty S. *Nephrolithiasis*; 2016. Updated September 16, 2021. http://emedicine.medscape.com/article/437096-overview#a1.
19. Turk C, Neisius A, Petrik A, et al. European Association of Urology. *Urolithiasis*; 2021. https://uroweb.org/guideline/urolithiasis/.
20. Dave C, Faraj K, Shetty S. *Nephrolithiasis Treatment and Management*; 2016. http://emedicine.medscape.com/article/437096-treatment.
21. Assimos D, Krambeck A, Miller NL, et al. Surgical management of stones: American urological Association/Endourological Society guideline, Part II. *J Urol.* 2016;196(4):1153–1160.
22. National Institute of Diabetes and Digestive and Kidney Diseases. *Cystocele;* Last Reviewed August 2020. https://www.niddk.nih.gov/health-information/urologic-diseases/bladder-control-problems-women/cystocele-prolapsed-bladder.

23. Woo J. Gynecological disorders. In: Papadakis MA, McPhee SJ, eds. *Current Medical Diagnosis and Treatment.* 57th ed. McGraw-Hill; 2018:786.

24. American College of Obstetricians and Gynecologists. *Pelvic Support Problems*; October 2017. Updated November 2021. https://www.acog.org/womens-health/faqs/pelvic-support-problems.

25. Culligan PJ. Nonsurgical management of pelvic organ prolapse. *Obstet Gynecol.* 2012;119(4):852–860.

26. M. Clinic. *Anterior Vaginal Prolapse (Cystocele).* http://www.mayoclinic.org/diseases-conditions/cystocele/basics/prevention/con-20026175.

27. Nelson HD, Walker M, Zakher B, Mitchell J. Menopausal hormone therapy for the primary prevention of chronic conditions: a systematic review to update the U.S. Preventive Services Task Force recommendations. *Ann Intern Med.* 2012;157(2):104–113.

28. Doumouchtsis SK. Urogenital consequences in ageing women. *Best Pract Res Clin Obstet Gynaecol.* 2013;27(5):699–714.

29. Atnip S, O'Dell K. Vaginal support pessaries: Indications for use and fitting strategies. *Urol Nurs.* 2012;32(3):114–125.

30. Quaseem A, Dallas P, Forciea MA, et al. Nonsurgical management of urinary incontinence in women: a clinical practice guideline from the American College of Physicians. *Ann Intern Med.* 2014;161(6):429–440.

31. Lightner DJ, Gomelshy A, Souter L, Vasavada SP. Diagnosis and treatment of overactive bladder (non-neurogenic) in adults: AUA/SUFU Guideline Amendment 2019. *J Urol.* 2019;202:558–563.

32. National Institute of Diabetes and Digestive and Kidney Diseases. *Bladder Control Problems in Women (Urinary Incontinence)*; 2016. Last Reviewed June 2018. https://www.niddk.nih.gov/health-information/urologic-diseases/bladder-control-problems-women.

33. Razmaria AA. JAMA patient page. Bladder cancer. *JAMA.* 2015;314(17):1886.

34. McNamara M, Batur P, DeSapri KT. In the clinic. Perimenopause. *Ann Intern Med.* 2015;162(3):ITC1–ITC15.

35. Jackson SL, Scholes D, Boyko EJ, Abraham L, Fihn SD. Urinary incontinence and diabetes in postmenopausal women. *Diabetes Care.* 2005;28(7):1730–1738.

36. Nicolle LE, Bradley S, Colgan R, et al. Infectious Diseases Society of America guidelines for the diagnosis and treatment of asymptomatic bacteriuria in adults. *Clin Infec Dis.* 2005;40(5):643–654.

37. Nicolle LE. Urinary tract infections in the elderly. *Clin Geriatr Med.* 2009;25(3):423–436.

38. Wong MK, Campbell KH. Fluid and electrolyte abnormalities. In: Williams BA, Chang A, Ahault C, et al., eds. *Current Diagnosis and Treatment: Geriatrics.* 2nd ed. McGraw-Hill; 2014:261–268.

39. Nicolle LE. Catheter-related urinary tract infection: Practical management in the elderly. *Drugs Aging.* 2014;31(1):1–10.

40. U.S. Centers for Disease Control and Prevention. *Gonorrhea.* CDC Basic Fact Sheet; Last reviewed August 22, 2022. https://www.cdc.gov/std/gonorrhea/stdfact-gonorrhea.htm.

41. U.S. Centers for Disease Control and Prevention. *Chlamydia.* CDC Basic Fact Sheet; Last reviewed April 12, 2022. https://www.cdc.gov/std/chlamydia/stdfact-chlamydia.htm.

42. U.S. Centers for Disease Control and Prevention. *Trichomoniasis.* CDC Basic Fact Sheet; Last reviewed April 25, 2022. https://www.cdc.gov/std/trichomonas/STDFact-Trichomoniasis.htm.

43. National Institutes of Health. *Smoking and Bladder Cancer;* 2011. https://www.nih.gov/news-events/nih-research-matters/smoking-bladder-cancer.

23

Cervical Problems

Shavondra Huggins

OBJECTIVES

- Discuss current cervical cancer screening guidelines.
- Describe the rationale for the current guidelines including human papillomavirus (HPV) screening and HPV vaccination.

- Evaluate abnormal cervical screening results.
- Distinguish commonly seen cervical problems, and develop a management plan.

INTRODUCTION

The purpose of this chapter is to help the primary care provider guide the management of both cervical cancer screening and common cervical problems. Increasingly, routine gynecological care is being provided within the primary care setting. As a result, it is imperative that the primary care provider be proficient in routine gynecological health. As a result of an increased understanding of the natural history of HPV, there have been many changes in the cervical cancer screening guidelines. Not only have the guidelines changed, but the guidelines vary among the many leading professional organizations.

CERVICAL CANCER AND HUMAN PAPILLOMAVIRUS

Approximately 14,100 females in the United States will be diagnosed with invasive cervical cancer in 2022, and 4280 of these females will die.[1] Cervical cancer was one of the most common causes of cancer deaths in the United States until the past 40 years, when the cervical cancer death rate decreased by more than 50%. The main reason for this decline is the increased rate of cervical cancer screening or cervical cytology (i.e., the Pap test). The incidence of cervical cancer is highest in minority populations (Table 23.1).

Approximately one-half of cervical cancer cases diagnosed in the United States are in females who were never screened, and an additional 10% of cervical cancers occur among females who were not screened within the past 5 years.[2]

Persistent cervical infection with high-risk HPV genotypes is associated with the development of cervical cancer and its immediate precursor lesions ("precancer") cervical intraepithelial neoplasia (CIN) grade 3 (CIN3). These genotypes are referred to as high risk because of their increased risk for development of cervical cancer. Epidemiological studies suggest that nearly 100% of cervical cancer cases test positive for the high-risk HPV genotype. HPV 16 is the most carcinogenic genotype and accounts for approximately 53.5% of all cervical cancers. HPV 18 is the next most carcinogenic genotype and accounts for approximately 17.2% of cervical cancers. Approximately 10 other HPV genotypes cause the remaining 29.3% of cervical cancers.[3]

Genital HPV is acquired through sexual and genital skin-to-skin contact. In most populations, prevalence peaks within a few years after the mean age of sexual debut, which is 17 years of age in the United States. Most HPV infections (about 90%) are transient and therefore are undetectable within 1 to 2 years. Females whose infections persist are at significant risk of developing precancerous lesions. The cervical cancer precursor lesions, CIN3, has a 30% probability of becoming invasive cancer over a 30-year period, while only about 1% of treated CIN3 cases will become invasive.[4] This is

TABLE 23.1   Incidence of Cervical Cancer by Ethnicity: 2019

Race/Ethnicity	Incidence
Hispanic	9.7%
Non-Hispanic Black	8.4%
American Indian and Alaskan Native	9.0%
Non-Hispanic White	7.0%
Asian and Pacific Islander	5.7%

Modified from U.S. Centers for Disease Control and Prevention. *United States Cancer Statistics: Data Visualizations. Leading Cancers by Age, Sex, Race, and Ethnicity.* https://gis.cdc.gov/Cancer/USCS/#/Demographics/.

evidence that cervical screening is necessary in the prevention of cervical cancer.

The goal of cervical cancer screening is to prevent morbidity and mortality from cervical cancer. Ideally, screening should identify cervical cancer precursors likely to progress to invasive cancers and avoid unnecessary treatment of transient HPV infection and its associated benign lesions that are not destined to become cancerous.[5]

NOT TO BE MISSED

Screening should identify cervical cancer precursors likely to progress to invasive cancers and avoid unnecessary treatment of transient HPV infection and its associated benign lesions that are not destined to become cancerous.

As a result of the increased understanding of the association of HPV and cervical cancer risk, HPV molecular tests have been developed. These tests offer increased sensitivity (true positive results) yet lower specificity (true negative results) compared with cytology. These HPV tests may also better predict which patients will develop CIN3 over the next 5 to 15 years compared with cytology alone. The incorporation or cotesting of HPV into cervical cancer screening strategies offers the potential to allow both increased disease detection with an increase in the length of screening intervals. In terms of cervical cancer screening, HPV refers to high-risk HPV genotypes. Low-risk HPV genotypes have no clinical role in cervical cancer screening or evaluation of patients with abnormal cytology.[6]

ANATOMY AND HISTOLOGY OF THE NORMAL CERVIX

The term *cervix* is derived from the Latin word for *neck*. It is the inferior extension of the uterus and is divided into two portions. The lower portion (*portio,* or vaginal cervix) extends into the vagina and is the structure that can be visualized after speculum placement. When examined through an open speculum, the cervix appears as a raised, oval-to-circular structure. In the nulliparous (never pregnant) female, the cylindrical cervix comprises approximately 50% of the total uterine size; it is approximately 3 cm in length and approximately 2 cm in diameter. The centrally located external cervical os, or beginning of the endocervical canal, is round and measures 3 to 5 cm in diameter. During pregnancy, the cervix enlarges because of vascular congestion and proliferation of elastic fibers and smooth muscle cells. After vaginal delivery, the external os broadens into a horizontal slit with stellate lines attributable to scarring from cervical lacerations.

The majority of the cervix portio is covered by stratified squamous epithelium. This area is also known as the *ectocervix*. A single layer of tall columnar cells lines the endocervical canal and extends beyond the os in younger females and those taking oral contraceptive pills. The intersection of the stratified squamous and columnar cells is known as the *squamo-columnar junction* (SCJ). These two cell types, squamous epithelial cells and tall columnar cells, are collected for evaluation through cervical cytology.[7]

SCREENING FOR CERVICAL CANCER

The first efforts at evaluating early cytological changes as a means for detecting cervical cancer began as early as 1926. Aurel Babes from the Colthea Hospital in Romania and, 2 years later, George Papanicolaou of Cornell University in Ithaca, New York, both began using cytology as a means for screening for cervical cancer. However, Dr. Papanicolaou's *Pap smear* ultimately became the established method for cervical cancer screening. Cancer screening became more widely used after the 1943 publication of Papanicolaou and Traut's *Diagnosis of Uterine Cancer by the Vaginal Smear.*[8]

Squamous epithelial cells and columnar cells collected for cytological screening (the Pap test) can still be collected with the conventional microscope slide, yet

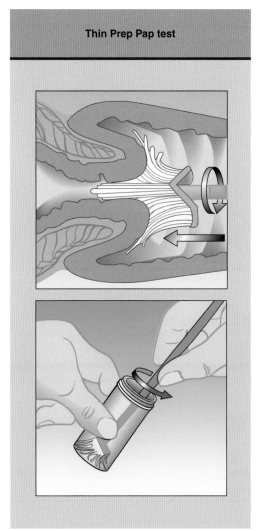

Thin Prep Pap test

Figure 23.1 Performing a Pap test. (From Bieber EJ, Horowitz IR, Sanfilippo JS. *Clinical Gynecology*. Elsevier; 2006.)

liquid-based cytology is more commonly used. The conventional Pap test consists of sampling cells from the cervix and vagina using a brush or spatula, placing the cells directly on a slide, and fixing it with a chemical fixative in the office or clinic. With conventional tests, specimens for HPV testing are collected separately. Liquid-based (Fig. 23.1) cytology consists of sampling cells in a similar manner but then suspending the cells in a liquid transport medium to be subsequently spun or filtered in the laboratory and plated as thin layers on slides. HPV testing can be performed on this specimen as well as testing for chlamydia, gonorrhea, and trichomoniasis.

Screening Interval

As the understanding of the natural history of cervical cancer and HPV has evolved, so have the recommendations regarding the timing and frequency of cervical cancer screening. At the time of publication for this text, there is still some variation in screening intervals and age of initiation (Table 23.2).

NOT TO BE MISSED

Regardless of age at first sexual encounter, cervical cancer screening should begin at 21 years of age per the recommendation of several major U.S. expert groups, with the exception of the ACS who recommends screening to begin at 25 years of age. Screening should end at 65 years of age or once a total hysterectomy is performed, whichever presents first. However, cervical cancer screenings may be necessary beyond 65 years of age or after a total hysterectomy if the patient has a history of cervical cancer, history of CIN, or no history of adequate negative testing.

Females younger than 21 years of age should not be screened regardless of age of sexual debut. Cervical cancer is rare in this age group, and the incidence of cervical cancer has not changed with the increase in screening performed over the past 40 years. Not only has the incidence remained unchanged, but there are risks associated with screening adolescents for cervical cancer. Increased screening can lead to unnecessary procedures and potential treatment of preinvasive cervical lesions that have a high probability of regressing spontaneously.[5]

Current screening guidelines extend the interval from every 3 to 5 years in females who are 30 years of age and older. Because of the high prevalence of transient, benign HPV infections and associated lesions, it is now understood that annual screening leads to very small increases in the number of prevented cancers and at a high cost of unnecessary procedures and treatments. Most of these HPV infections and associated lesions will regress within one to two years; of those that do not regress, it usually will takes many years for the lesions to progress to cancer.[5]

TESTING FOR HUMAN PAPILLOMAVIRUS

Testing for HPV along with cytological testing (the Pap test) offers the potential to increase disease detection

TABLE 23.2 Cervical Cancer Screening Intervals

Organization	Age to Initiate	Age to Discontinue	21–29 Years of Age	≥30 Years of Age
USPSTF (2018). Endorsed by ASCCP, ACOG, and SGO	21	65	Pap test every 3 years	Co-testing (Pap test and HPV) every 5 years Primary HPV testing alone every 5 years Pap test every 3 years
ACS (2020)	25	65	For females ≥25 years of age Can consider primary HPV testing every 5 years (preferred) Co-testing (Pap test and HPV) every 5 years Pap test every 3 years	
ACP (2015)	21	65	Pap test every 3 years.	Pap test every 3 years Alternative: Cotesting (Pap test and HPV testing) every 5 years

ACOG, American College of Obstetricians and Gynecologists; *ACP,* American College of Physicians; *ACS,* American Cancer Society; *ASCCP,* American Society for Colposcopy and Cervical Pathology; *SGO,* Society of Gynecologic Oncology; *USPSTF,* U.S. Preventive Services Task Force.
Modified from Crum CP, Kuh WK, Einstein MH. *Cervical Cancer Screening: The Cytology and Human Papillomavirus Report; 2022.* UpToDate. https://www.uptodate.com/contents/cervical-cancer-screening-the-cytology-and-human-papillomavirus-report#!.

TABLE 23.3 FDA-Approved Human Papillomavirus Tests for Cotesting and Reflex Testing

Test	Number of HPVs Identified	HPV Types Identified
Hybrid Capture 2 (HC2)	Pooled detection of 13 subtypes	16, 18, 31, 33, 35, 39, 45, 51, 52, 56, 58, 59, 68 (not 66)
Cervista HPV HR test Cervista HPV 16/18*	Pooled detection of 14 subtypes	16, 18, 31, 33, 35, 39, 45, 51, 52, 56, 58, 59, 66, 68
Aptima Aptima HPV 16 and 18/45†	Pooled detection of 14 subtypes	16, 18, 31, 33, 35, 39, 45, 51, 52, 56, 58, 59, 66, and 68.

*The Cervista HPV 16/18 specifically detects HPV 16 and 18.
†The Aptima HPV 16 and 18/45 specifically detects HPV 16, 18, and/or 45.
Positive pooled results indicate the detection of at least 1 HR HPV subtype. The test will not indicate which subtype or whether more than one subtype is present.
HPV, Human papillomavirus.
Modified from Crum CP, Kuh WK, Einstein MH. *Cervical Cancer Screening: The Cytology and Human Papillomavirus Report; 2022.* UpToDate. https://www.uptodate.com/contents/cervical-cancer-screening-the-cytology-and-human-papillomavirus-report#!.

and increase length of screening intervals. Testing for the presence or absence of HPV also helps triage the management of abnormal Pap results. Knowing if high-risk HPV subtypes are present or absent helps the clinician manage the follow-up of a mildly abnormal cytology result. This is discussed further in the "Management of Abnormal Results" section later in this chapter.

There are five HPV tests that are approved by the U.S. Food and Drug Administration (FDA) for use in cotesting with a Pap test (Table 23.3) and four HPV tests used in primary testing (Table 23.4). In addition to increased disease detection and increased length of screening intervals, HPV testing also allows for the triage of equivocal Pap test results (discussed in the following sections).

> **CLINICAL SURVIVAL TIP** Knowing if high-risk HPV subtypes are present or absent helps the clinician manage the follow-up of a mildly abnormal cytology result.

| TABLE 23.4 Human Papillomavirus Tests for Primary HPV Testing |||
Test	Number of HPVs Identified	HPV Types Identified
Cobas HPV*‡	12	31, 33, 35, 39, 45, 51, 52, 56, 58, 59, 66, and 68
BD Onclarity§	14	16, 18, 31, 33, 35, 39, 45, 51, 52, 56, 58, 59, 66, and 68
Cepheid Xpert HPV†‖	11	31, 33, 35, 39, 51, 52, 56, 58, 59, 66, and 68
Quiagen careHPV†	14	16, 18, 31, 33, 35, 39, 45, 51, 52, 56, 58, 59, 66, and 68

*FDA approved.
†World Health Organization prequalified.
‡Cobas HPV specifically detects HPV 16 and 18.
§BD Onclarity specifically detects 6 HR subtypes (16, 18, 31, 45, 51, and 52) and groups results for the remaining subtypes (33/58, 35/39/68, and 56/59/66).
‖Cepheid Xpert specifically detects HPV 16 and 18/45.
HPV, Human papillomavirus.
Modified from Crum CP, Kuh WK, Einstein MH. *Cervical Cancer Screening: The Cytology and Human Papillomavirus Report; 2022.* UpToDate. https://www.uptodate.com/contents/cervical-cancer-screening-the-cytology-and-human-papillomavirus-report#!.

TERMINOLOGY FOR PAP TEST RESULTS

The Bethesda system standardized cervical cytology reporting in the United States in 1988 and has been revised several times, most recently in 2014. The purpose of the standardized terminology is to decrease the variation and subjectivity of pathological interpretations of Pap tests and to decrease inconsistencies in the management of abnormal results.[9] See Table 23.5 for the current Bethesda classification.

Although management of precancerous lesions identified on the Pap test is beyond the scope of this text, interpreting Pap test results is well within the scope of the primary care nurse practitioner. According to the Bethesda system, Pap results include the following:

- A description of the specimen type and test requested: cervical or vaginal sample, conventional Pap smear, liquid-based cytology, and/or reflex HPV test
- A description of specimen adequacy
- A general categorization (optional): negative, epithelial cell abnormality, or other
- An interpretation/result: either the specimen is negative for intraepithelial lesions and malignancy (although organisms or reactive changes may be present), there is an epithelial cell abnormality as defined by the Bethesda 2014 classification, or there is another finding. The latter category may indicate some increased risk (e.g., endometrial cells in a female ≥45 years of age).
- A description of any ancillary testing or automated review that was performed (e.g., HPV, AutoPap)
- Educational notes and suggestions by the pathologist (optional)

INTERPRETATION OF CERVICAL CYTOLOGY RESULTS

Adequacy of the Sample

Pap smears are considered satisfactory for evaluation based on the number of cells in the specimen and the percentage of those cells that are obscured. Conventional Pap smears must have at least 8000 to 12,000 well-visualized squamous or squamous metaplastic cells; liquid-based preparations must have a minimum of 5000 of these cells; and post-chemotherapy, radiotherapy, postmenopausal, atrophic changes or posthysterectomy may contain <5000 cells. No more than 75% of cells may be obscured by inflammation, bacteria, blood, or lubricants to be considered satisfactory. If 50% to 75% of the cells are obscured, a disclaimer must be included with what is obscuring the cells and the percentage of cells that are obscured. If over 75% of the cells are obscured, the specimen is deemed unsatisfactory.[10]

Unsatisfactory for Evaluation

An unsatisfactory cervical cytology specimen is considered unreliable for the evaluation of epithelial abnormalities. Whether patients with an unsatisfactory cervical cytology are more likely to have intraepithelial lesions or cancer on follow-up than those with satisfactory tests is controversial. Scant cellularity may result in a false-negative HPV test.[11] Cervical cytology is reported as unsatisfactory for evaluation in approximately 1% of cases. Cervical cytology tests are designated "unsatisfactory for evaluation" for one of three reasons: scant cellularity, obscuring inflammation or blood, or unlabeled

TABLE 23.5   Bethesda 2014 Classification System for Cervical Cytology

Specimen Type

Indicate conventional smear (Pap smear), liquid-based preparation (Pap test) versus other

Specimen Adequacy

Satisfactory for evaluation (describe presence or absence of endocervical/transformation zone component and any other quality indicators, e.g., partially obscuring blood, inflammation, etc.)
Unsatisfactory for evaluation *(specify reason)*
- Specimen rejected/not processed *(specify reason)*
- Specimen processed and examined, but unsatisfactory for evaluation of epithelial abnormality because of *(specify reason)*

General categorization *(optional)*

Negative for intraepithelial lesion or malignancy
Other: see "Interpretation/results" (e.g., endometrial cells in a woman older than 45 years)
Epithelial cell abnormality: see "Interpretation/results" *(specify "squamous" or "glandular," as appropriate)*

Interpretation/results

Negative for Intraepithelial Lesion or Malignancy

(When there is no cellular evidence of neoplasia, state this in the "General categorization" above and/or in the "Interpretation/results" section of the report—whether there are organisms or other non-neoplastic findings)

Non-neoplastic Findings (Optional to Report)

Non-neoplastic cellular variations:
- Squamous metaplasia
- Keratotic changes
- Tubal metaplasia
- Atrophy
- Pregnancy-associated changes

Reactive cellular changes associated with:
- Inflammation (includes typical repair)
- Lymphocytic (follicular) cervicitis
- Radiation
- Intrauterine contraceptive device (IUD)

Glandular cells status posthysterectomy

Organisms

Trichomonas vaginalis
Fungal organisms morphologically consistent with *Candida* spp.
Shift in flora suggestive of bacterial vaginosis
Bacteria morphologically consistent with *Actinomyces* spp.
Cellular changes consistent with herpes simplex virus
Cellular changes consistent with cytomegalovirus

Other

Endometrial cells (in a woman older than 45 years)
(also specify if "negative for squamous intraepithelial lesion")

Epithelial Cell Abnormalities

Squamous cell
- Atypical squamous cells
  - Of undetermined significance (ASC-US)
  - Cannot exclude HSIL (ASC-H)

TABLE 23.5 Bethesda 2014 Classification System for Cervical Cytology—cont'd
• Low-grade squamous intraepithelial lesion (LSIL) (encompassing: HPV/mild dysplasia/CIN-1)
• High-grade squamous intraepithelial lesion (HSIL) (encompassing: moderate and severe dysplasia, CIS; CIN-2 and CIN-3)
• With features suspicious for invasion *(if invasion is suspected)*
• Squamous cell carcinoma
Glandular cell
• Atypical
• Endocervical cells (*NOS or specify in comments*)
• Endometrial cells (*NOS or specify in comments*)
• Glandular cells (*NOS or specify in comments*)
• Atypical
• Endocervical cells, favor neoplastic
• Glandular cells, favor neoplastic
• Endocervical adenocarcinoma in situ
• Adenocarcinoma
• Endocervical
• Endometrial
• Extrauterine
• Not otherwise specified (*NOS*)
Other malignant neoplasms *(specify)*
Adjunctive testing
Provide a brief description of the test method(s) and report the result so that it is easily understood by the clinician
Computer-assisted interpretation of cervical cytology
If case examined by an automated device, specify the device and result
Educational notes and comments appended to cytology reports *(optional)*
Suggestions should be concise and consistent with clinical follow-up guidelines published by professional organizations (references to relevant publications may be included)

From Nayar R, Wilbur DC. The Pap test and Bethesda 2014: "The reports of my demise have been greatly exaggerated." (after a quotation from Mark Twain). *J Low Genit Tract Dis.* 2015;19:175. Reproduced with permission from Lippincott Williams & Wilkins. Copyright 2015 American Society for Colposcopy and Cervical Pathology, The International Society for the Study of Vulvovaginal Disease, and The International Federation of Cervical Pathology and Colposcopy.

specimen or otherwise unable to be processed by the laboratory. According to the U.S. Preventive Services Task Force (USPSTF) 2018 guidelines, unsatisfactory Pap tests should be managed as follows:

• HPV testing was not done, is unknown, or is negative: Patients should repeat age-based screening (cytology, cotesting, or primary HPV test) in 2 to 4 months.
• HPV-positive without genotyping: Either repeat cytology in 2 to 4 months or colposcopy is appropriate.
• HPV positive with 16 or 18 positive: Colposcopy is recommended.

Absent Transformation Zone on Screening Cytology

Routine screening is recommended for females 21 to 29 years of age with negative screening cytology and an absent endocervical cells/transformation zone component. In females 30 years of age and older with negative screening cytology, no or unknown HPV results, and an absent endocervical cells/transformation zone component, HPV testing is preferred; however repeat cytology in 3 years is acceptable. If HPV testing is performed and negative, screening should be repeated in 5 years. If HPV testing is positive, the patient is to be managed per the most recent ASCCP management guidelines according to those results.

Squamous Cell Abnormalities

• Atypical squamous cells (ASCs) are categorized as either atypical squamous cells of undetermined significance (ASC-US) or atypical squamous cells cannot exclude a high-grade squamous intraepithelial lesion (ASC-H). The ASC-H category includes findings that are equivocal but likely consist of a mixture of true high-grade squamous intraepithelial lesions and other findings that mimic such lesions.

Approximately 5% to 10% of ASC results are designated ASC-H.

- Low-grade squamous intraepithelial lesion (LSIL). The LSIL category includes changes consistent with HPV infection and a possible histological finding of cervical intraepithelial neoplasia (CIN) 1.
- High-grade squamous intraepithelial lesion (HSIL). HSIL includes changes consistent with HPV infection, a possible histological finding of CIN 2 or 3, and HSIL involving endocervical cells; the cervical cytology report should indicate if there are features suspicious for invasive disease.
- Squamous cell carcinoma[12]

MANAGEMENT OF ABNORMAL RESULTS

In 2019, the American Society for Colposcopy and Cervical Pathology (ASCCP) guidelines shifted from utilizing results-based management algorithms to "risk-based" guidelines. These guidelines calculate an estimated risk of finding CIN 3+ lesions based on both current HPV and cytology results and all past HPV and cytology results. The current threshold for risk estimation is 4%. These newer guidelines allow for detection and treatment of CIN 3+ lesions and avoid unnecessary interventions in patients with new low-risk HPV infections. Because the estimation of risk is based on a complex calculation of past and present cytology and HPV results, a review of each possible scenario is outside the scope of this text. For an in-depth review of the guidelines, visit https://www.asccp.org/management-guidelines, and click the link for ASCCP Risk Based Management Consensus Guidelines. For use in practice, this organization has created both a mobile and Web-based application in which the clinician can input patient-specific information to determine the management of each unique patient scenario. Management of scenarios that exceed the risk threshold generally begins with a colposcopy.

> **CLINICAL SURVIVAL TIP** For use in practice, the ASCCP has created both a mobile and Web-based application in which the clinician can input patient-specific information to determine the management of each unique patient scenario.

Colposcopy is a procedure in which the cervix is examined under high magnification through a colposcope. Acetic acid is applied to the surface of the cervix to assist in visualization and subsequent biopsy of abnormally appearing and potentially cancerous or precancerous cells. Colposcopy and directed or random biopsies can be performed by physicians or advanced practice clinicians trained in the procedure.

RARE CYTOLOGY RESULTS

Nonpregnant females of any age with atypical glandular cells (AGCs) or adenocarcinoma in situ (AIS) require a colposcopy and endocervical sampling.[13] When females 35 years of age and older have any category of AGC or AIS, endometrial sampling should be performed at the same time as the colposcopy. A cytology result of atypical endometrial cells can be managed with endometrial and endocervical sampling. If no endometrial pathology is found, a colposcopy should be performed.

> **! SAFETY ALERT**
>
> When females 35 years of age and older have any category of AGC or AIS, endometrial sampling should be performed at the same time as the colposcopy.

HUMAN PAPILLOMAVIRUS VACCINES

There are three FDA-approved vaccines for HPV infection available in the United States: Gardasil, Gardasil 9, and Cervarix. Since the HPV vaccine was recommended in 2006, there has been an 88% decrease in HPV infections among adolescent females in the United States. The vaccines vary by the number of HPV subtypes they contain. Gardasil is a quadrivalent HPV vaccine and targets HPV types 6, 11, 16, and 18, whereas Gardasil 9, a 9-valent vaccine, targets the same HPV types as the quadrivalent vaccine (6, 11, 16, and 18) as well as types 31, 33, 45, 52, and 58. Cervarix protects against HPV types 16 and 18 only. Vaccination is recommended for both females and males before the age of sexual debut (11 to 12 years of age) but can be given as early as 9 years of age. The vaccine is licensed and recommended up to 26 years of age however, certain adults 27 to 45 years of age may choose to receive the HPV vaccine after speaking with their provider about their risk for new HPV infections. In addition to preventing cervical and anal cancers, the quadrivalent HPV vaccine is effective in preventing genital warts in young males and anal intraepithelial neoplasia among men who have sex with men (MSM).[14,15]

NOT TO BE MISSED

Vaccination is recommended for both females and males before the age of sexual debut: 11 to 12 years of age but can be given as early as 9 years of age.

Dosing Administration

In the United States, as of 2021, the recommended dosing schedule depends on the age of the patient. Individuals younger than 15 years of age should receive two doses of HPV vaccine between 6 and 12 months apart. Individuals 15 years of age and older should receive three doses of HPV vaccine over a minimum of 24 weeks. The minimum interval between the first two doses is 4 (Cervarix) to 6 (Gardasil) weeks, and the minimum interval between the second and third dose is 12 weeks. The quadrivalent vaccine (Gardasil) and 9-valent vaccine (Gardasil 9) are typically administered in three doses at time zero and then at 2- and 6-month follow-up.[15] Cervarix is administered at time zero and at 1 month and 6 months.

NOT TO BE MISSED

Individuals younger than 15 years of age should receive two doses of HPV vaccine between 6 and 12 months apart. Individuals 15 years of age and older should receive three doses of HPV vaccine over a minimum of 24 weeks.

Missed Doses

Patients often do not follow up for their immunizations on schedule, therefore the Advisory Committee on Immunization Practices (ACIP) recommends that if the vaccination series is interrupted for any length of time, it can be resumed without restarting the series.[16,17]

BENIGN CERVICAL FINDINGS

Ectropion

Ectropion (Fig. 23.2) occurs when columnar epithelia cells are exposed beyond the cervical os. The everted epithelium has a reddish appearance similar to granulation tissue and may be covered by a yellow turbid discharge. Ectropion is common in adolescents and in those who take combined oral contraceptives. As a female ages, the

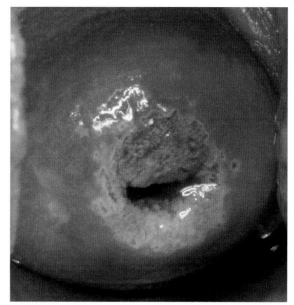

Figure 23.2 Ectropion. (From Apgar BS, Brotzman GL, Spitzer M. *Colposcopy Principles and Practice.* 2nd ed. Saunders Elsevier; 2008.)

epithelial cells dominate the surface of the cervix, and the columnar epithelium retreat into the cervical os. Ectropion is a normal finding and does not require treatment.[18]

Nabothian Cysts

Nabothian cysts (Fig. 23.3) (also called *mucinous retention cysts* or *epithelial inclusion cysts*) are discrete cystic structures that form when a cleft of columnar epithelium becomes covered with squamous cells, and the columnar cells continue to secrete mucoid material. The cysts vary from microscopic to several centimeters in size; the larger ones project above the surface of the portio. These cystic findings are benign and rarely require management.[18]

Cervical Polyps

Cervical polyps (Fig. 23.4) present as globular, friable, pedunculated lesions protruding from the external cervical os. Polyps can originate in the cervical canal or uterine endometrium, and they can be asymptomatic or present with atypical (nonmenstrual) bleeding. Polyps commonly occur during the reproductive years, especially after 40 years of age, and the etiology is unknown. Chronic inflammation of the cervical canal as well as hormonal factors may play a role. The differential diagnosis includes leiomyoma and endometrial polyps.[19]

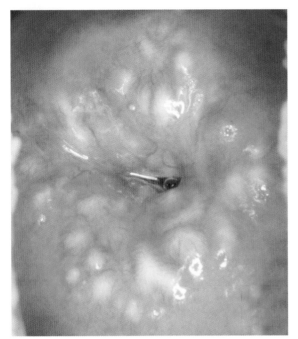

Figure 23.3 Nabothian cysts. (From Apgar BS, Brotzman GL, Spitzer M. *Colposcopy Principles and Practice.* 2nd ed. Saunders Elsevier; 2008.)

Polyps should be removed when they are symptomatic (e.g., bleeding, excessive discharge), are large (≥3 cm), or appear atypical. Polypectomy can usually be accomplished by grasping the base of the polyp with forceps and twisting it off. Caution should be taken when considering removal. Polyps can bleed after removal, so removal should be performed by a skilled practitioner. Malignancy is rarely found in a cervical polyp; however, polyps that are removed should be submitted to the laboratory for histological studies.

Cervicitis

Cervicitis (Fig. 23.5) is classified as either acute or chronic. The most common symptom, and often the only one, is purulent vaginal discharge. The appearance of the acutely inflamed cervix varies greatly, depending on the degree of involvement and the infecting organism. Mucopurulent cervical discharge, cervical friability, and cervical edema are characteristics of both gonococcal and chlamydial cervicitis; the latter is more common. Punctate hemorrhages on the vagina and cervix suggest trichomonas infection. Vesicular or ulcerative lesions suggest infection with herpes simplex virus (HSV). For further information on sexually transmitted infections, see Chapter 16.

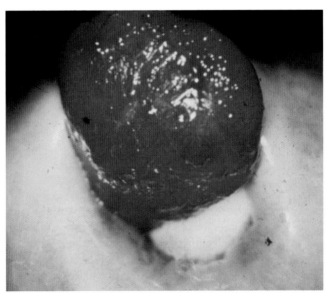

Figure 23.4 Cervical polyp. (Courtesy Dr. Henry J. Norris.)

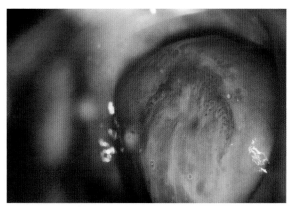

Figure 23.5 Cervicitis. (From Bennett JE, Dolin R, Blaser MJ. *Mandell, Douglas, and Bennett's Principles and Practice of Infectious Diseases.* 9th ed. Elsevier; 2020.)

KEY POINTS

- Cervical cancer screening should begin at 21 or 25 years of age and end once a total hysterectomy is performed or at 65 years of age, whichever comes first.
- Cervical cancer screening should occur, at minimum, every three to five years depending on the patient's most recent HPV result.
- Cotesting for cervical cancer screening and HPV should begin at 30 years of age.
- HPV vaccination is recommended for both females and males beginning at 11 to 12 years of age yet vaccinations may.
- Ectropion and Nabothian cysts are benign cervical findings.

REFERENCES

1. American Cancer Society. *Cancer Statistics Center.* 2022 Estimates; 2022. https://cancerstatisticscenter.cancer.org/#/cancer-site/Cervix.
2. U.S Centers for Disease Control and Prevention. *Vital Signs: Cervical Cancer Is Preventable*; 2020. https://www.cdc.gov/vitalsigns/cervical-cancer/index.html.
3. Castellsagué X. Natural history and epidemiology of HPV infection and cervical cancer. *Gynecol Oncol.* 2008;110(3 suppl 2):S4–S7.
4. Chan CK, Aimagambetova G, Ukybassova T, Kongrtay K, Azizan A. *Human Papillomavirus Infection and Cervical Cancer: Epidemiology, Screening and Vaccination—Review of Current Perspectives*; 2019. https://doi.org/10.1155/2019/3257939.
5. Saslow D, Solomon D, Lawson HW, et al. American cancer Society, American Society for colposcopy and cervical pathology, and American Society for clinical pathology screening guidelines for the prevention and early detection of cervical cancer. *J Low Genit Tract Dis.* 2012;16(3):175–204.
6. Deftereos G. Human Papillomavirus (HPV) Testing—Cervical Cancer Screening. Updated August 2022. https://arupconsult.com/content/human-papillomavirus.
7. O'Connor DM. Anatomy and histology of the normal female lower genital tract. In: Mayeaux EJ, Cox JT, eds. *Modern Colposcopy.* 3rd ed. Philadelphia: Lippincott Williams & Wilkins; 2014:14–36.
8. Cox JT. The road to cervical cancer prevention: Historical perspective. In: Mayeaux EJ, Cox JT, eds. *Modern Colposcopy.* 3rd ed. Philadelphia: Lippincott Williams & Wilkins; 2014:1–13.
9. Nayar R, Wilbur DC. The Pap test and Bethesda 2014. *Cancer Cytopathol.* 2015;123(5):271–281.
10. Crum CP, Kuh WK, Einstein MH. *Cervical Cancer Screening: The Cytology and Human Papillomavirus Report.* UpToDate; 2022. https://www.uptodate.com/contents/cervical-cancer-screening-the-cytology-and-human-papillomavirus-report#!.
11. Massad LS, Einstein MH, Huh WK, et al. 2012 updated consensus guidelines for the management of abnormal cervical cancer screening tests and cancer precursors. *J Low Genit Tract Dis.* 2013;17(5 suppl 1):S1–S27.
12. Jug R, Bean SM. *Cervix: Cytology: Bethesda System*; 2020. https://www.pathologyoutlines.com/topic/cervixcytologybethesda.html.
13. Perkins RB, Guido RS, Castle PE, et al. 2019 ASCCP risk-based management consensus guidelines for abnormal cervical cancer screening tests and cancer precursor. *J Low Genit Tract Dis.* 2020;24(2):102–131.
14. U.S. Centers for Disease Control and Prevention. *Human Papillomavirus. HPV Vaccine Schedule and Dosing.* https://www.cdc.gov/hpv/hcp/schedules-recommendations.html.
15. U.S. Centers for Disease Control and Prevention. *Vaccines and Preventable Diseases: Human Papillomavirus (HPV) Vaccination: What Everyone Should Know.* https://www.cdc.gov/vaccines/vpd/hpv/public/index.html.
16. U.S. Centers for Disease Control and Prevention. National and state vaccination coverage among adolescents aged 13–17 years—United States, 2011. *MMWR Morb Mortal Wkly Rep.* 2012;61(34):671–677.

17. Markowitz LE, Dunne EF, Saraiya M, et al. Human papillomavirus vaccination: recommendations of the Advisory Committee on immunization practices (ACIP). *MMWR Recomm Rep (Morb Mortal Wkly Rep)*. 2014;63(RR-05):1–30.

18. O'Connor DM. Anatomy and histology of the normal female lower genital tract. In: Mayeaux EJ, Cox JT, eds. *Modern Colposcopy*. 3rd ed. Philadelphia: Lippincott Williams & Wilkins; 2014:150–233.

19. O'Connor DM. Anatomy and histology of the normal female lower genital tract. In: Mayeaux EJ, Cox JT, eds. *Modern Colposcopy*. 3rd ed. Philadelphia: Lippincott Williams & Wilkins; 2014:376–398.

Exposure to Violence

Ashley L. Hodges

INTRODUCTION

The United Nations defines violence against women as "any act of gender-based violence that results in, or is likely to result in, physical, sexual, or mental harm or suffering to women, including threats of such acts, coercion or arbitrary deprivation of liberty, whether occurring in public or in private life."[1] Violence against women may manifest in a variety of ways including physical, sexual, financial, emotional, verbal, and stalking. According to the World Health Organization, intimate partner violence (IPV) and sexual violence are major public health problems and violations of women's human rights.[2] Prevalent forms of violence against women include physical violence by an intimate partner and sexual victimization by both an intimate partner and outside intimate relationships.[3]

Sexual violence and IPV of all types often occur in the reproductive years for females and can have long-term physical, reproductive, and mental health consequences. According to findings published in the National Intimate Partner and Sexual Violence Survey, 25% of females reported experiencing severe physical violence during their lifetime. Severe physical violence is defined as "hit with a fist or something hard, kicked, hurt by pulling hair, slammed against something, tried to hurt by choking or suffocating, beaten, burned on purpose, used a knife or gun.[4] IPV can occur among heterosexual or same-sex couples and is reported in every community regardless of age, economic status, race, religion, ethnicity, sexual orientation, or educational background.[5]

The etiology of violence against females is multifactorial and interactive. These elements can be based in the individual (both perpetrator and victim), family unit, the immediate community, and in the wider level of society.[2] Table 15.1 demonstrates risk factors common to both IPV and sexual violence, Box 15.1 shows elements related to IPV alone, and Box 15.2 depicts

TABLE 15.1 Risk Factors for Intimate Partner Violence and Sexual Violence	
Factor	**Perpetration or Experience**
Lower education level	Both, of sexual violence
Exposure to child maltreatment	Both
Observing family violence	Both
Antisocial personality disorder	Perpetration
Abuse of alcohol	Both
Destructive masculine behaviors such as multiple partners or condoning violence	Perpetration
Community/societal norms that put males at a higher status than females	Discriminatory laws
Low rates of females with paid employment	
Low rates of sex equality	

Modified from World Health Organization. *Violence Against Women;* 2021. https://www.who.int/news-room/fact-sheets/detail/violence-against-women.

BOX 15.1   Factors Behind Intimate Partner Violence

- Exposure to violence in the past
- Marital dissatisfaction and conflict
- Problems with interpartner communication
- Controlling behaviors of males regarding partners

Modified from World Health Organization. *Violence Against Women;* 2021. https://www.who.int/news-room/fact-sheets/detail/violence-against-women.

BOX 15.2   Factors Causing Sexual Violence

- Cultural practices and beliefs in family honor and sexual purity
- Male belief of sexual entitlement
- Weak laws against sexual violence

Modified from World Health Organization. *Violence Against Women;* 2021. https://www.who.int/news-room/fact-sheets/detail/violence-against-women.

reasons for sexual violence. Multiple sources agree that the common core cause of violence against females is sex inequality and societal norms that accept such violence.[2,6]

The health consequences of violence against females are seen as both long- and short-term physical, psychological, sexual, and reproductive problems. The worst of these are fatalities resulting from homicide or suicide. Forty-two percent of victims of IPV have reported an injury after an episode of violence. Sexual violence can result in unintended pregnancy, therapeutic abortion, gynecological issues, and sexually transmitted infections (STIs). Violence during pregnancy brings increased risk of spontaneous abortion, intrauterine fetal demise, preterm birth, and babies born small for gestational age. Depression, posttraumatic stress, anxiety, sleep disturbances, eating disorders, and suicide attempts may follow incidents of violence among females. Finally, consequences of violence can cause headaches, digestive system ailments, restricted mobility, and pain disorders of the back, abdomen, and pelvis.[2]

There are also social and economic detriments for females and society related to violence. Days lost from work resulting from injuries incur cost to both the employer and employee in the form of loss of production and lost wages. Social isolation, limited involvement in

normal activities, and limited ability to care for themselves and their children can occur as well.[2] According to Oxfam, violence traps females in poverty by restricting choices; it curbs their capacity to obtain an education, work for wages, and take part in political and public arenas.[6]

Assessing the patient's psychological status should be routine at any visit. According to the Women's Preventive Services Initiative, screening for exposure to violence is also a critical part of any history and should be completed at least annually. The U.S. Preventive Services Task Force (USPSTF) recommends that clinicians screen female patients of childbearing age for IPV and provide or refer those who screen positive to intervention services.[16]

Barriers to screening and referral include lack of provider education, time, and resources. Providers may also express discomfort in discussing the topic, or they may fear offending the patient, perceive a lack of power to change the problem, or have a misconception regarding the patient population's risk of exposure to IPV.[7] Often providers do not have the tools available or processes in place to implement efficient screening tools.

A variety of IPV screening tools are available. The USPSTF recommends potential tools with the most sensitivity and specificity. These tools are directed at patients and can be self-administered or used in a clinician interview format.

- HARK (Humiliation, Afraid, Rape, Kick), HITS (Hurt, Insult, Threaten, Scream), E-HITS (Extended-Hurt, Insult, Threaten, Scream), Partner Violence Screen (PVS), WAST (Woman Abuse Screen Tool)[7]
- OVAT (Ongoing Violence Assessment Tool), STaT (Slapped, Things, and Threaten),[7] CTQ–SF (Modified Childhood Trauma Questionnaire–Short Form)

In addition to routine screening, female patients should also be screened if they exhibit signs of depression, substance use, requests for repeat pregnancy tests when they have no desire to become pregnant, new or recurrent STIs or repeated requests to be tested, or fear about negotiating condom use with a partner.[5]

When exposure to violence is confirmed or suspected, resources should be readily available. It is critical for providers to be proactive and establish and maintain relationships with community resources. Printed take-home resource materials such as safety procedures, hotline numbers, and referral information should be kept in privately accessible areas such as restrooms and examination rooms. Most states do not mandate reporting of IPV or only mandate reporting in certain circumstances. Providers should be familiar with applicable state reporting laws.[5]

SEXUAL VIOLENCE

In the United States, 43.6% of females reported experiencing some form of sexual violence during their lifetime. Across all forms of sexual violence, most female victims reported that their perpetrators were male. The lifetime prevalence of completed or attempted rape in the United States is approximately 21.3% in females.[4] Symptoms such as anxiety and fear may manifest as physical symptoms, especially urinary and sexual complaints, even years after the abuse has occurred.[8] Regardless of the etiology or the pathophysiological or psychological basis, female patients often present to the primary care provider with urological complaints.

Females exposed to sexual violence often suffer from physical ailments long after the acute recovery phase. The long-term impact on psychological well-being is profound. From a physical standpoint, gastrointestinal symptoms are a common physical health complaint. Symptoms such as nausea, vomiting, and abdominal pain are twice as common in females who have experienced sexual violence compared with those who have not.[9] Females with a history of sexual violence are also more likely to report chronic musculoskeletal pain and somatic symptoms (headache, fatigues, insomnia).[10]

Rates of gynecological problems such as vaginal infection, pain during intercourse, sexual dysfunction, dysmenorrhea, and chronic pelvic pain are more common in females exposed to sexual violence compared with non-exposed females. Many urological dysfunctions without organic findings can be linked to a remote history or current sexual abuse. Problems such as urinary incontinence, urinary tract infection, and interstitial cystitis can occur.[11]

The exact association between bladder symptoms and psychosocial influences remains unknown. It is suggested that a combination of heritability, psychosocial factors, and environmental stress all play a part. Sanford and Rodriguez suggest that the same pathophysiological pathways involved in emotional states such as anxiety, depression, and stress are the same pathways for bladder function.[12] These pathways include activation of the hypothalamic-pituitary axis, dysregulation of the serotonergic pathways, and central sensitization. In addition, urinary syndromes, such as overactive bladder and interstitial cystitis/bladder pain syndrome involving abnormal or augmented sensory input, may also be a spectrum of the same disorder.[12]

TRAUMA-INFORMED CARE

Trauma-informed care (TIC) began in the 1970s with the return of Vietnam War veterans. The diagnosis of posttraumatic stress disorder (PTSD) was developed from the study and treatment of these patients, and the medical community became rapidly aware of the effects of trauma on the body, nervous system, and brain.[13] A landmark study in 1997 by Anda and Felitti described a compelling association between childhood trauma and abysmal health outcomes later in life.[13] We now know these childhood trauma as adverse childhood experiences (ACEs). In 1998, the Substance Abuse and Mental Health Services Administration (SAMHSA) studied various modalities for assisting females who have experienced trauma, substance abuse, and mental illness to address the lack of adequate services for females with these histories. The results of the Women, Co-occurring Disorders, and Violence Study (WCDVS) along with the ACE study helped set the stage for the development of what is now known as *TIC*.[14]

TIC is used in a variety of settings such as mental health and substance abuse treatment services, child welfare organizations, schools, and criminal justice establishments.[13] However, Varghese and Emerson report that its use in primary care is not common or well-defined.[15] In their systematic review of the literature, Varghese and Emerson identified that the employment of TIC in primary care holds much promise, and nurse practitioners can be crucial in advocating for its implementation.

REFERENCES

1. United Nations. *Declaration on the Elimination of Violence Against Women*; 1993. https://www.ohchr.org/en/instruments-mechanisms/instruments/declaration-elimination-violence-against-women.
2. World Health Organization. *Violence Against Women*; 2021. https://www.who.int/news-room/fact-sheets/detail/violence-against-women.
3. Krahé B. Violence against women. *Curr Opin Psychol.* 2018;19:6–10.

4. Smith, SG, Zhang, X, Basile, KC, et al. *The National Intimate Partner and Sexual Violence Survey 2015 Data Brief - Updated Release. State Report.* Atlanta, GA: National Center for Injury Prevention and Control, Centers for Disease Control and Prevention; 2018. https://www.cdc.gov/violenceprevention/pdf//2015data-brief508.pdf.

5. American College of Obstetricians and Gynecologists. *ACOG Committee Opinion No. 518. Intimate Partner Violence.* Reaffirmed 2022. https://www.acog.org/clinical/clinical-guidance/committee-opinion/articles/2012/02/intimate-partner-violence.

6. Oxfam International. *Violence Against Women and Girls.* Enough Is Enough; 2022. https://www.oxfam.org/en/take-action/campaigns/say-enough-violence-against-women-and-girls/violence-against-women-and-girls-enough-enough.

7. Agency for Healthcare Research and Quality. *Intimate Partner Violence Screening; Fact Sheet and Resources*; 2015. https://www.ahrq.gov/professionals/prevention-chronic-care/healthier-pregnancy/preventive/partnerviolence.html#interventions.

8. Bradley CS, Nygaard IE, Mengeling MA, et al. Urinary incontinence, depression and post-traumatic stress disorder in women veterans. *Am J Obstet Gynecol.* 2012;206(6):502.e1–502.e8.

9. Jina R, Thomas LS. Health consequences of sexual violence against women. *Best Pract Res Clin Obstet Gynaecol.* 2013;27(1):15–26.

10. Ulirsch JC, Ballina LE, Soward AC, et al. Pain and somatic symptoms are sequelae of sexual assault: results of a prospective longitudinal study. *Eur J Pain.* 2014;18(4):455–598.

11. Cichowski SB, Dunivan GC, Komesu YM, Rogers RG. Sexual abuse history and pelvic floor disorders in women. *South Med J.* 2013;106(12):675–678.

12. Sanford MT, Rodriguez LV. The role of environmental stress on lower urinary tract symptoms. *Curr Opin Urol.* 2017;27(3):268–273.

13. Curi M. *A Short History of Trauma-Informed Care.* IowaWatch; 2018. https://www.iowawatch.org/2018/06/15/a-short-history-of-trauma-informed-care/.

14. Substance Abuse and Mental Health Services Administration. Trauma-Informed Care in Behavioral Health Services. *TIP.* 2014;57. https://store.samhsa.gov/sites/default/files/d7/priv/sma14-4816.pdf.

15. Varghese L, Emerson A. Trauma-informed care in the primary care setting: An evolutionary analysis. *J Am Assoc Nurse Pract.* 2021 Oct 5. https://doi.org/10.1097/JXX.0000000000000663. Epub ahead of print. PMID: 34618717.

16. U.S. Preventive Services Task Force. (2018). *Intimate Partner Violence, Elder Abuse, and Abuse of Vulnerable Adults: Screening.* Retrieved March 9, 2023 from https://www.uspreventiveservicestaskforce.org/uspstf/recommendation/intimate-partner-violence-and-abuse-of-elderly-and-vulnerable-adults-screening.

INDEX

Note: Page numbers followed by f or t indicate figures and tables, respectively.

A

AACE. *See* American Association of Clinical Endocrinologists
Abaloparatide (Tymlos), for osteoporosis, 405t–407t
Abdominal bloating, hormonal therapy and, 271t
Abnormal uterine bleeding (AUB), 346–350, 347t, 347b
  adenomyosis, 352
  amenorrhea, 360–365, 361b–362b, 364f, 365b
  causes of, 347t
  classification system of, 347–348, 348f
  diagnostic workup for, 350–352, 350b–351b, 352t
  endometrial causes, 356
  estimating blood loss in, 349, 349f
  evaluation of, 348b, 349f
  HMB-COEIN, 353–356
  iatrogenic bleeding, 356
  leiomyomas, 353, 354f
  malignancy and hyperplasia, 353
  management of, 352, 352b
  in ovulatory dysfunction, 356
  physical examination for, 350, 350b
  polycystic ovarian syndrome, 357–360, 359f, 359b–360b, 360t–361t
  in polyps, 352, 352b
  summary evaluation of, 263, 264t
  treatment option for, 357, 357b, 358t
Abortion
  aspiration, 181, 181b
  dilation and evacuation, 181–182, 182b
  in-clinic, 179–180
  medication, 180, 180t
  options for, 179
  spontaneous, 186
Absorption, drug, in older adults, 62, 63t
ACA. *See* Affordable Care Act
Acceptance and commitment therapy, for dementia patients, 78t
Acellular pertussis, immunization for, 101b
ACEs. *See* Adverse childhood experiences
Acetabulum, 13f
Acetylcholine, for psychosis/schizophrenia, 290–291
ACIP. *See* Advisory Committee on Immunization Practices
ACOG. *See* American College of Obstetricians and Gynecologists
ACP. *See* American College of Physicians
ACS. *See* American Cancer Society
Activin, 25, 27t
Activities of daily living (ADLs), 53, 53t
Acute abnormal uterine bleeding, defined, 347

Acute pelvic pain, 388–390
  definition of, 388
  differential diagnosis of, 388–389, 390t
  history of, 389–390, 390b
  pathophysiology of, 388, 389b
Acyclovir, for herpes simplex virus, 329t, 330b
Adenocarcinoma in situ (AIS), 470
Adenomyosis, abnormal uterine bleeding, 352
Adnexa, 18–19, 20b
Adolescent women's health, 37–48
  assessment of, 38–39, 38b, 39f
  evaluation of, 37–41, 38b
  examination of, 39–41, 39b, 41b
  issues affecting, 44–45
  LGBTQ health assessment for, 246–252, 246b
    adolescent-affirming environment, 247, 247b
    role of parents and guardians, 249
    screening for personal safety, 248–249, 249b
    sexual orientation and gender identity in, 247–248, 248b
    social gender affirmation, 250–252
    support resources for, 249–250
  other reproductive health concerns to consider, 41–43
  reproductive assessment of, 37–41, 38b
  wellness and preventive health, 43–44
    primary care, 44
    vaccinations, 43–44, 43b–44b
Adolescent-affirming environment, 247, 247b
Adrenarche, 29
Adventitia, 19
Adverse childhood experiences (ACEs), violence and, 477
Advisory Committee on Immunization Practices (ACIP), 471
AFAB. *See* Assigned female at birth
Affordable Care Act (ACA), 246
AGCs. *See* Atypical glandular cells
Age, preconception care and, 115
Agender, term, 204–205, 205t
A Guide to Taking a Sexual History, 192
AIS. *See* Adenocarcinoma in situ
Alarm limit, 126
Alcohol
  abuse, 44–45, 45b
    in preconception care, 113–114
  cardiovascular disease and, 5t
  LBQ females, 208
  substance use/medication misuse of, 289
  use, screening and counseling for